Minimally Invasive Surgery

NOTICE

Medicine is an ever-changing science. As new research and clinical experience broaden our knowledge, changes in treatment and drug therapy are required. The editors and the publisher of this work have checked with sources believed to be reliable in their efforts to provide information that is complete and generally in accord with the standards accepted at the time of publication. However, in view of the possibility of human error or changes in medical sciences, neither the editors nor the publisher nor any other party who has been involved in the preparation or publication of this work warrants that the information contained herein is in every respect accurate or complete, and they are not responsible for any errors or omissions or for the results obtained from use of such information. Readers are encouraged to confirm the information contained herein with other sources. For example and in particular, readers are advised to check the product information sheet included in the package of each drug they plan to administer to be certain that the information contained in this book is accurate and that changes have not been made in the recommended dose or in the contraindications for administration. This recommendation is of particular importance in connection with new or infrequently used drugs.

Minimally Invasive Surgery

Editors

JOHN G. HUNTER, M.D., F.A.C.S.

Associate Professor of Surgery
Emory University School of Medicine
Atlanta, Georgia

JONATHAN M. SACKIER, M.B., F.R.C.S.

Associate Professor of Surgery
University of California, San Diego
School of Medicine
San Diego, California

McGRAW-HILL, INC.
Health Professions Division
New York   St. Louis   San Francisco   Auckland   Bogotá   Caracas
Lisbon   London   Madrid   Mexico   Milan   Montreal   New Delhi
Paris   San Juan   Singapore   Sydney   Tokyo   Toronto

MINIMALLY INVASIVE SURGERY

Copyright © 1993 by McGraw Hill, Inc. All rights reserved. Printed in the United States of America. Except as permitted under the United States Copyright Act of 1976, no part of this publication may be reproduced or distributed in any form or by any means, or stored in a data base or retrieval system, without the prior written permission of the publisher.

1234567890 KGP KGP 9876543

ISBN 0-07-031372-5

International Edition: ISBN 0-07-112656-2

This book was set in Berkley Old Style Medium by Kachina Typesetting, Inc.

The editors were Jane Pennington and Muza Navrozov.

The production supervisor was Clare Stanley.

The cover was designed and the project was supervised by M 'N O Production Services, Inc.

Arcata Graphics/Kinsport Press was the printer and binder.

Library of Congress Cataloging-in-Publication Data

Minimally invasive surgery / editors, John G. Hunter, Jonathan M. Sackier,
    p. cm.
   Includes index.
   ISBN 0-07-031372-5
   1. Endoscopic surgery. 2. Surgery—Technological innovations.
I. Hunter, John G. II. Sackier, Jonathan M.
   [DNLM: 1. Endoscopy—methods. 2. Surgery, Operative—methods.
WO 500 M6645 1993]
RD33.53.M56   1993
617'.05—dc20
DNLM/DLC
for Library of Congress   92-48522
                                                                                     CIP

This book is dedicated to my parents, Rhona and Ronald,
for providing me with the opportunity to further my education
at great personal sacrifice and to Susan, Natalya, and Shelley.
—Jonathan M. Sackier

This book is dedicated to my wife, Mary Ann, and daughter,
Sarah Elizabeth, who put up with much absenteeism
during the creation of this work.
—John G. Hunter

Contents

Contributors • ix
Forewords • xiii
Seymour I. Schwartz
John A. Dixon
Preface • xvii
Acknowledgments • xix

PART I NEW TECHNOLOGIES

1 Minimally Invasive High Tech Surgery: Into the 21st Century • 3
John G. Hunter / Jonathan M. Sackier

2 Fiberoptic Imaging and Measurement • 7
Daniel R. Margulies / M. Michael Shabot

3 Intraoperative, Endoscopic, and Laparoscopic Ultrasound • 15
Robert C. McIntyre, Jr. / Greg Van Stiegmann

4 Laser Physics and Tissue Interaction • 23
John G. Hunter

5 Laparoscopic Electrosurgery • 33
Roger C. Odell

6 Polymeric Biomaterials for Surgical Repair of Soft Tissue • 43
David W. Grainger

7 Technologies and Techniques for Telescopic Surgery • 57
Joseph B. Petelin

PART II OLD DISEASES

Foregut

8 Endoluminal Therapy of Esophageal Cancer • 69
Kathy Bull-Henry / David E. Fleischer

9 Perivisceral Dissection of the Esophagus • 83
Gerhard Buess / Marco Maria Lirici

10 Hiatal Hernia and Reflux Esophagitis • 87
Alfred E. Cuschieri

11 Surgical Access for Enteral Nutrition • 113
William Sangster / John G. Hunter

12 Laparoscopic Treatment of Peptic Ulcer Disease • 123
Namir Katkhouda / Jean Mouiel

Hindgut

13 Laser Therapy in Rectosigmoid Tumors • 131
J. M. Brunetaud / V. Maunoury / D. Cochelard / B. Boniface
A. Cortot / J. C. Paris

14 Laparoscopic Suturing and Tissue Approximation • 141
Zoltan Szabo

15 The Sutured Laparoscopic Gastrointestinal Anastomosis • 157
L. K. Nathanson

16 The Diagnosis and Treatment of Acute Appendicitis with Laparoscopic Methods • 171
David W. Easter

17 Laparoscopic Colon and Rectal Surgery • 179
Jonathan M. Sackier

18 Endoluminal Therapy of Rectal Tumors: Transanal Endoscopic Microsurgery • 191
Gerhard Buess / Marco Maria Lirici

Biliary Tract

19 Radiologic Procedures in the Management of Biliary Disease • 197
Franklin J. Miller

20 Endoluminal Treatment of Tumors and Stones in the Bile Ducts • 207
Jeffrey L. Ponsky

21 Laparoscopic Cholecystectomy • 213
Jonathan M. Sackier

22 Common Bile Duct Exploration • 231
Lee L. Swanstrom

Pancreas and Liver

23 Endoscopic Intervention for Pancreatic Disorders • 245
Aaron S. Fink

24 Percutaneous Approaches to Liver Neoplasms • 255
Philip D. Schneider / John P. McGahan

25 Laparoscopic Approaches to Diseases of the Liver • 265
Jonathan M. Sackier / John G. Hunter

26 Transjugular Intrahepatic Portosystemic Shunts • 269
Robert E. Barton / Josef Rösch / Frederick S. Keller / Barry Uchida

Peritoneum

27 Laparoscopic Pelvic Lymphadenectomy • 279
Ralph V. Clayman / Elspeth McDougall / Louis R. Kavoussi

28 Emergent and Urgent Laparoscopy • 291
George Berci

29 Laparoscopic Inguinal Hernia Repair • 297
Jeffrey H. Peters / Adrian E. Ortega

30 Laparoscopic Splenectomy • 309
Edward H. Phillips

Vascular System

31 Endovascular Surgery • 315
Peter F. Lawrence / Samuel S. Ahn

Thorax

32 Modern Diagnostic and Therapeutic Thoracoscopy • 329
Randolph M. Kessler

33 High Tech Surgery: Speculation on Future Directions • 339
Richard M. Satava

Index • 349

Contributors*

Samuel S. Ahn, M.D. [31]
Assistant Professor of Surgery
University of California, Los Angeles, School of Medicine
University of California, Los Angeles, Center for
 the Health Sciences
Los Angeles, California
Chief of Vascular Surgery
Olive View Medical Center
Sylmar, California

Robert E. Barton, M.D. [26]
Assistant Professor
Charles Dotter Institute of Interventional Therapy
Oregon Health Sciences University
Veterans Administration Medical Center
Portland, Oregon

George Berci, M.D., F.A.C.S., F.R.C.S. Ed. (Hon) [28]
Senior Consulting Surgeon
Cedars-Sinai Medical Center
Clinical Professor of Surgery (Emeritus)
University of California, Los Angeles
Los Angeles, California

B. Boniface, M.D. [13]
Multidisciplinary Laser Center
Clinique des Maladies de L'Appareil Digestif
Hopital C. Huriez
Laboratoire de Biomathematiques and INSERM
Lille, France

J. M. Brunetaud, M.D. [13]
Multidisciplinary Laser Center
Clinique des Maladies de L'Appareil Digestif
Hopital C. Huriez
Laboratoire de Biomathematiques and INSERM
Lille, France

*The numbers in brackets following the contributor name refer to chapter(s) authored or co-authored by the contributor.

Gerhard Buess, M.D. [9, 18]
Minimal Invasive Chirurgie
Abteilung fur Allgemeinchirurgie
Klinikum Schnarrenberg
Eberhard-Karls-Universitat
Tubingen, Germany

Kathy Bull-Henry, M.D. [8]
Instructor in Medicine
Georgetown University School of Medicine
Washington, D.C.

Ralph V. Clayman, M.D. [27]
Professor of Urologic Surgery and Radiology
Washington University School of Medicine
St. Louis, Missouri

D. Cochelard, M.D. [13]
Multidisciplinary Laser Center
Clinique des Maladies de L'Appareil Digestif
Hospital C. Huriez
Laboratoire de Biomathematiques and INSERM
Lille, France

A. Cortot, M.D. [13]
Multidisciplinary Laser Center
Clinique des Maladies de L'Appareil Digestif
Hopital C. Huriez
Laboratoire de Biomathematiques and INSERM
Lille, France

Professor Alfred E. Cuschieri, M.D., Ch.M., F.A.C.S. (Ed), F.R.C.S. (Eng), F.R.C.S. Glas. (Hon) F.I. (Biol) [10]
Professor and Head of Department of Surgery
Ninewells Hospital and Medical School
Dundee, Scotland

David W. Easter, M.D. [16]
Assistant Professor of Surgery
Division of Surgical Oncology
University of California, San Diego, School of Medicine
San Diego, California

Aaron S. Fink, M.D. [23]
Associate Professor of Surgery
Chief, Surgical Endoscopy
University of Cincinnati School of Medicine
Cincinnati, Ohio

David E. Fleischer, M.D. [8]
Professor of Medicine
Chief, Endoscopy
Division of Gastroenterology
Georgetown University
Washington, D.C.

David W. Grainger, Ph.D. [6]
Assistant Professor
Department of Chemical and Biological Sciences
Oregon Graduate Institute of Science and Technology
Beaverton, Oregon

John G. Hunter, M.D., F.A.C.S. [1, 4, 11, 25]
Associate Professor of Surgery
Emory University School of Medicine
Atlanta, Georgia

Namir Katkhouda, M.D., Ph.D. [12]
Associate Professor of Surgery
Chief, Division of Minimal Invasive Surgery
University of Nice School of Medicine
Nice, France

Louis R. Kavoussi, M.D. [27]
Assistant Professor of Urological Surgery
Harvard Medical School
Head, Section of Endourology
Brigham and Women's Hospital
Consultant in Urology
Boston Children's Hospital
Boston, Massachusetts

Frederick S. Keller, M.D. [26]
Cook Professor
Charles Dotter Institute of Interventional Therapy
Professor and Chairman
Department of Diagnostic Radiology
Oregon Health Sciences University
Veterans Administration Medical Center
Portland, Oregon

Randolph M. Kessler, M.D. [32]
Assistant Professor
Division of Thoracic and Cardiovascular Surgery
University of New Mexico School of Medicine
Albuquerque, New Mexico

Peter F. Lawrence, M.D. [31]
Professor of Surgery
University of Utah School of Medicine
Salt Lake City, Utah

Marco Maria Lirici, M.D. [9, 18]
Assistant Professor of Surgery
IV Department of General Surgery
School of Medicine
University of Rome "La Sapienza"
Rome, Italy

Daniel R. Margulies, M.D. [2]
Associate Director of Surgical Intensive Care
  and Trauma Services
Department of Surgery
Cedars-Sinai Medical Center
Los Angeles, California

V. Maunoury, M.D. [13]
Multidisciplinary Laser Center
Clinique des Maladies de L'Appareil Digestif
Hopital C. Huriez
Laboratoire de Biomathematiques and INSERM
Lille, France

Elspeth M. McDougall, M.D., F.R.C.S.(C) [27]
Instructor of Urologic Surgery
Washington University School of Medicine
St. Louis, Missouri

John P. McGahan, M.D. [24]
Head, Section of Abdominal Imaging and Ultrasound
Professor of Radiology
University of California Davis Medical Center
Sacramento, California

Robert C. McIntyre, Jr., M.D. [3]
Senior Instructor in Surgery
University of Colorado Health Science Center and Denver
  Veterans Affairs Hospital
Denver, Colorado

Franklin J. Miller, M.D. [19]
Chief, Interventional Radiology
Department of Radiology
University of Utah School of Medicine
Salt Lake City, Utah

Jean Mouiel, M.D. [12]
Professor of Surgery
Chief, Department of Surgery
University of Nice School of Medicine
Nice, France

L. K. Nathanson, M.B., Ch.B., F.R.A.C.S. [15]
Senior Lecturer in Surgery
University of Queensland
Royal Brisbane Hospital
Queensland, Australia

Roger C. Odell [5]
President, Electroscope Inc.
Boulder, Colorado

Adrian E. Ortega, M.D. [29]
Assistant Professor of Surgery
University of Southern California School of Medicine
Los Angeles, California

J. C. Paris, M.D. [13]
Multidisciplinary Laser Center
Clinique des Maladies de L'Appareil Digestif
Hopital C. Huriez
Laboratoire de Biomathematiques and INSERM
Lille, France

Joseph B. Petelin, M.D., F.A.C.S [7]
Clinical Assistant Professor of Surgery
Department of Surgery
University of Kansas School of Medicine
Shawnee Mission Medical Center
Shawnee Mission, Kansas

Jeffrey H. Peters, M.D. [29]
Assistant Professor of Surgery
University of Southern California School of Medicine
Chief, Division of General Surgery
University of Southern California University Hospital
Los Angeles, California

Edward H. Phillips, M.D., F.A.C.S. [30]
Attending Surgeon
Cedars-Sinai Medical Center
Clinical Associate Professor of Surgery
University of Southern California
Los Angeles County Hospital
Los Angeles, California

Jeffrey L. Ponsky, M.D., F.A.C.S. [20]
Director, Department of Surgery
The Mt. Sinai Medical Center
Professor of Surgery
Case Western Reserve University of Medicine
Cleveland, Ohio

Philipe Jean Quilici, M.D. [12]
Chairman, General Surgery
Saint Joseph Medical Center
Burbank, California

Josef Rösch, M.D. [26]
Professor and Director
Charles Dotter Institute of Interventional Therapy
Oregon Health Sciences University
Veterans Administration Medical Center
Portland, Oregon

Jonathan M. Sackier, M.B., F.R.C.S. [1, 17, 21, 25]
Associate Professor of Surgery
University of California, San Diego, School of Medicine
San Diego, California

William Sangster, M.D., F.A.C.S. [11]
Assistant Professor of Surgery (Clinical)
Oregon Health Sciences University
Portland, Oregon

Richard M. Satava, Colonel, M.D., F.A.C.S. [33]
Associate Professor of Surgery
Walter Reed Army Medical Center
Washington, D.C.

Philip D. Schneider, M.D., Ph.D. [24]
Associate Professor of Surgery
Division of Surgical Oncology
Department of Surgery
University of California Davis Medical Center
University of California Davis Cancer Center
Sacramento, California

M. Michael Shabot, M.D., F.A.C.S. [2]
Associate Director of Surgery
Director of Surgical Intensive Care Units
Cedars-Sinai Medical Center
Clinical Associate Professor of Surgery and Anesthesiology
University of California, Los Angeles, School of Medicine
Los Angeles, California

Greg Van Stiegmann, M.D. [3]
Associate Professor of Surgery
Chief, Surgical Endoscopy
University of Colorado Health Science Center and
   Denver Veterans Affairs Hospital
Denver, Colorado

Lee L. Swanstrom, M.D. [22]
Assistant Professor of Surgery
Oregon Health Sciences University
Director, Department of Minimally Invasive Surgery
Holladay Park Medical Center
Portland, Oregon

Zoltan Szabo, Ph.D., F.I.C.S. [14]
Director, Microsurgery and Operative Endoscopy
   Training (MOET) Institute
Associate Director, Advanced Videoscopic
   Training Center
Department of Surgery
University of California, San Francisco, School of Medicine
San Francisco, California

Barry Uchida, B.S. [26]
Assistant Professor
Charles Dotter Institute of Interventional Therapy
Oregon Health Sciences University
Portland, Oregon

Forewords

I imagine that the editors asked me to provide an introduction to their magnum opus because I have no vested interest and, as a nonparticipant, play the role of interested observer. Also I have confessed in print that I initially felt that laparoscopic cholecystectomy would not have wide applicability.

In that confession I stated, "I am certainly willing to join any Greek chorus of recantation about the applicability of laparoscopic cholecystectomy. But I hope that surgeons do not evolve into laparoscopic zealots whose efforts double when they lose sight of their goals. . . . Since the operative procedures are performed based on a two-dimensional image on a screen, binocular vision and the sensation of touch can be dispensed with. The recent generation that has devoted significant time and effort to honing skills in Nintendo computer-generated games has fortuitously been preparing itself for adeptness as technical surgeons. Lewis Carroll would have been amused to note that an amalgamation of the titles of two of his most famous works, *Adventures in Wonderland* and *Through the Looking Glass,* anticipated the future of surgery."

Although the embers had been faintly glowing for years, the catalyst for the flames of enthusiasm on the part of general surgeons was the success of laparoscopic cholecystectomy. There had arrived on the scene a technologic tool that would benefit the surgical care of hundreds of thousands of patients annually. The marketplace would permit industry's investment of research and development funds. This, in turn, resulted in the refinements in instrumentation and optics that enhanced the interest in minimally invasive surgery. As anticipated, surgeons enamored with their new tools would expand the application of these tools.

Minimally invasive surgery will remain a valuable addition to the surgical armamentarium. Although the bookshelves are rapidly being filled with monographs and more expanded works focusing on laparoscopic cholecystectomy and hernia repair, this book is unique because it provides a broad compendium of all facets of the subject.

The section on new technologies provides the surgeon with the language and appreciation necessary for a dialogue with the representatives of industry whose role is to respond to the surgeon's needs and also to seek the surgeon's endorsement and use of their product. An industrial–surgical dialogue is required; this mandates that the surgeon be informed rather than mesmerized by engineering expertise. The surgeon's appreciation of the technology will allow the surgeon to contribute to the issue of cost containment.

The section on the gastrointestinal tract, from the esophagus to the rectum, incorporates a wide variety of minimally invasive maneuvers, including endoluminal treatments, interventional radiologically controlled procedures, and laparoscopic applications. The same format pertains to hepatobiliary and other intraperitoneal disorders. The uses of endoscopic procedures for peripheral vascular diseases, laparoscopic hernia repair, and thoracoscopic operations complete the corpus. In each chapter, the minimally invasive approach is put into proper perspective in the therapeutic armamentarium, and a lucid, detailed description of the technique is provided.

The encyclopedic characteristic of the book satisfies several distinct needs. For the medical and surgical nonparticipants in the field, it provides a data base for intelligent decision making regarding the relative advantages and disadvantages of the approaches. For the practitioners of minimally invasive procedures, the book offers an in-depth presentation and critical assessment of the field and incorporates technologic information and explicit descriptions of techniques. The satisfaction of these needs certainly is praiseworthy and earns the book a position in the libraries of surgeons and other interested physicians.

Seymour I. Schwartz, M.D., F.A.C.S.
Professor and Chair
Department of Surgery
University of Rochester
School of Medicine and Dentistry
Rochester, New York

HIGH TECH SURGERY

Editors' note:
This foreword represents the last scientific writing of John A. Dixon, who died February 15, 1992. At the time of its writing, the title of this text was to have been *High Tech Surgery*. Rather than extensively revising the foreword to include a definition and discussion of *Minimally Invasive Surgery*, thereby changing the flavor of Dr. Dixon's words, the editors have chosen to leave this foreword intact. The argument for *Minimally Invasive Surgery* will be handled in Chapter 1 (vide infra).

J. H.

The editors of this volume have chosen the title *High Tech Surgery*. (See Editors' Note.) Conscientious competent surgeons try innovative methods and incorporate advances in technique in their surgical procedures. What then is unique about high tech surgery?

To conceptualize the field better, it may be well to consider two definitions from *Webster's 9th New Collegiate Dictionary* as follows:

1. *Technology:* a scientific method of achieving a practical purpose; an improvement in technical processes that increases the productivity of machines and eliminates manual operations or operations done by older machines.
2. *Surgery* (from *cheir* = hand and *ergos* = work): operative or manual procedures.

The "tech" part of the title, then, represents a scientific method of achieving a practical purpose by utilizing improvements in technical processes, which increase productivity and eliminate manual operation or operations done by older machines. From this perspective, a review of the chapters presented in this volume defines a new and vital area of surgery characterized by (1) newer, less invasive methods of visualization (e.g., fiberoptics, ultrasound, and radiologic imaging) and (2) correction of surgical lesions using innovative devices such as balloons, snares, staplers, electrodes, and lasers.

The basic science disciplines from which advanced imaging and therapeutic techniques have sprung encompass almost all of the applied sciences. Physics, electrical engineering, bioengineering, chemistry, materials science, fiberoptics, robotics, ceramics, biology, biochemistry, computer science, mechanical engineering, and pharmacology all have made significant contributions. Technologic advances have frequently been made by teams from one or more of these disciplines in cooperation with a clinician. Such cooperative ventures have generally been harmonious when directed toward "a scientific method of achieving a practical purpose."

The clinical applications side of this field (*cheir* = hand and *ergos* = work), however, has been more chaotic as newer methods of access and therapy have blurred and made irrelevant the traditional descriptions and boundaries of disciplines established nearly a century ago. Practitioners in the high tech field may have originated in either the imaging area (e.g., radiology, endoscopy, and ultrasound) or in the surgical hand-and-work area (e.g., gastrointestinal surgery, plastic surgery, and cardiovascular surgery). The researcher from the imaging field has had to learn surgical pathology, anatomy, physiology, and tissue handling from surgeons. Those primarily from the surgical area have had to learn various aspects of endoscopy and other imaging techniques from specialists in these fields.

In some cases, the interchange has been harmonious; in others, it has been fraught with great tension and hostility. It seems logical to assume that competence will ultimately prevail, regardless of the origin or background of the individual performing the procedure. It is likewise almost axiomatic that the most rapid fundamental advances will be made where integration and balance of the three supports of the field (basic science, imaging, and intervention) can be most effectively attained.

Naturally, patient interest in this field has been intense. It has been fascinating to watch laparoscopic cholecystectomy go from a unique approach of passing interest to that of becoming a procedure of choice in overwhelming demand. Traditional surgeons, who had been skeptical and resistant to nearly all types of minimally interventional techniques, were swept into performing laparoscopic cholecystectomy themselves in a brief period of less than 1 year by patients who saw the virtues of a decreased hospital stay, less pain, less time off work, and diminished cost. These objectives of high tech surgery are not new. However, the current wave of national interest in the cost of health care makes these considerations particularly pertinent now.

This very heightened visibility places special burdens on those who would work at the forefront of high tech surgery. Research must be carefully carried out, and unsubstantiated claims and unreasonably high patient expectations must be avoided. The high tech surgeon must maintain a mind that is keenly attuned to developments in the basic sciences and/or physics, fiberoptics, bioengineering, and other fields that might have application and be incorporated into new techniques of imaging and intervention. The most successful physicians in research and the practice of high tech surgery will be those that can maintain the best communication with other medical specialists using similar technology or treating similar disease processes, and continue to integrate knowledge obtained from basic research into new approaches to old diseases.

John A. Dixon, M.D., F.A.C.S.
Professor of Surgery
University of Utah
School of Medicine
Salt Lake City, Utah

Preface

Most textbooks of surgery contain warmed over summaries of standard surgical practice sprinkled with new theory, thought, and surgical technique. These texts are written by the masters of surgery and are extremely valuable to their students. Unfortunately, it is impossible to keep these tomes completely up-to-date. Close scrutiny of these texts will find little mention of any of the technologies and techniques that are described in this book. It is the aim of the authors to provide a manual of minimally invasive surgery to complement the great standard textbooks of surgery.

While we have managed to coerce some of surgery's leaders into writing chapters, we have also liberally relied upon the young surgical innovators who have carried the weight of this technological revolution on their shoulders. We are extremely proud of this volume and grateful to all our friends who authored its many chapters. We hope you will find the descriptions and illustrations helpful in your understanding and appreciation of minimally invasive surgery.

Acknowledgments

There are numerous people the editors would like to thank for their advice, guidance, and encouragement, and it is inevitable that such a list would be very long. The list of names mentioned is by no means exhaustive, and we apologize to any who have been inadvertently left off—they know who they are, and we shall be forever grateful. To our teachers and colleagues who guided us in our chosen career, we are eternally grateful: Sir Robert Shields, Pat Pattisson, Christopher Wood, Alfred Cuschieri, George Berci, and the late, sadly missed John Dixon. We thank also the members and the organization of SAGES (Society of American Gastrointestinal Endoscopic Surgeons), whose visionary approach to furthering the education of surgeons in this area and whose atmosphere of collegiality have spawned our enthusiasm. To the medical equipment companies who have helped us in our research endeavors and supported educational causes, your ethical behavior in the face of fierce financial competition is to be commended. To the secretarial staff who labored long hours and faced the challenge of interpreting our cryptic notes, we are grateful for good humor in accepting our numerous unreasonable deadlines. To our medical artist, Marilou Kundmueller, for producing such magnificent drawings and for being so diligent in ensuring their accuracy, and to Cathy Alden for supplying the style that united the syntax of authors from around the world, we acknowledge your efforts. Lastly, to Jane Pennington, PhD, for showing faith with the editors and allowing us the honor of being involved in this project—we look forward to future collaborations.

Part I

New Technologies

Chapter 1

Minimally Invasive High Tech Surgery: Into the 21st Century

John G. Hunter / Jonathan M. Sackier

MINIMALLY INVASIVE SURGERY

What's in a Name?

This volume celebrates the marriage of modern technology and surgical innovation. The offspring of the couple are many procedures that accomplish the goals of surgery (diagnosis, staging, resection, and repair) with a minimal amount of psychologic and somatic trauma. There has been much debate about the most accurate title for this new discipline. Although many of the procedures to be discussed in this volume are performed using laparoscopy, an equal number utilize an alternate route to the organ of interest. Suggested titles budding from the newly tilled surgical imagination include *less invasive surgery, video-assisted surgery, videoendoscopic surgery, telescopic surgery, endoscopic microsurgery,* and *minimal-access surgery*. A strong argument has recently been made for this latter title,[1] but it may be too late to change the nomenclature cemented in the minds of a half million practitioners of interventional therapies. The most widely recognized title for this new discipline is *minimally invasive surgery,* which first appeared in the surgical literature in 1990.[2] Despite criticism that *minimal invasion* is as much of an oxymoron as *somewhat pregnant,* the term is psychologically enticing. While acknowledging the invasiveness of surgery, it accents the reduction in trauma required to perform a conventional surgical procedure. We embrace the title, despite the paradox implied, because its ring and its resonance have pleased the ear of the surgeon and physician alike.

What Is Minimally Invasive Surgery?

If we date the "modern era" in surgery from the development of general anesthesia and aseptic technique, modern surgery is only slightly more than 100 years old. During that time, most heralded events in surgical progress, such as open heart surgery, organ transplantation, and radical cancer resections, employed maneuvers that stressed the body, often to the brink of death, to arrest a fatal disease process by heroic means. Technology was involved in these developments to the extent that life-sustaining equipment helped enact these "miracle cures." The technology that made these operations possible is well known to the surgeon and includes such things as cardiopulmonary bypass pumps, membrane oxygenators, hemodialysis machines, and positive-pressure ventilators.

Paralleling these events, an interest emerged in elucidating the subcellular mechanisms of the increased surgical stress that we were inflicting on our patients, but there was little concern by surgeons or industry in learning how to reduce that stress. The innovators who were "out there" developing minimally invasive surgical techniques were not considered to be scientists and, consequently, were rarely granted research money, selected as department chairmen, or elected to the presidency of surgical societies.

Ironically, it was the group of people we were supposed to be serving—our patients—who discovered many of the innovators in minimally invasive surgery. The public has long been looking for "seamless" surgery, operations that could be performed without an incision. Over the past decade, many readers of *Reader's Digest* and other lay journals thought that the answer was laser surgery, but it turned out that lasers did cause pain and also made nasty-looking scars. Rather than abandoning their belief in laser magic, the public, shepherded by sharp marketing managers, accepted minimally invasive surgery into the category of seamless surgery. Since the first notices of laser laparoscopic cholecystectomy hit the newspapers, patients have been coming in flocks for the new "laser gallstone surgery." But, unlike laser hemorrhoidectomy and a dozen other laser procedures, laparoscopic cholecystectomy is more substance than hype.

Incising the skin and subcutaneous tissues is a time-honored evil that is necessary to gain access to the disease process. Plastic surgery aside, the incision is rarely the goal of surgery and is the primary source of pain, infection, and psychologic stress, which often delays the performance of a needed operation. Such a delay in treatment allows the disease to advance to a point where it is either incurable or the operation is made more difficult, resulting in increased morbidity or mortality. The ability to perform conventional operations through small ("keyhole") incisions is sufficiently enticing to patients so that they are agreeable to undergo surgery earlier in the course of their disease when an operation will be easier and more effective. Although public acceptance of minimally invasive surgery may result in overuse of these procedures, the more major impact will be earlier interdiction of disease. There is evidence that this is already occurring. Literature from the 1940s and '50s suggest that choledocholithiasis was present in 10 to 20 percent of patients with cholecystolithiasis.[3,4] Although many early trials of laparoscopic cholecystectomy were selected to exclude patients with bile duct stones, newer "all-comers" data from surgeons facile with laparoscopic bile duct exploration demonstrated the incidence of common bile duct stones to be less than 10 percent in patients with gallbladder stones.[5,6] The logical conclusion is that we are operating on patients earlier in the course of cholecystitis, when bile duct stones are less likely to be found.

HIGH TECHNOLOGY

The role of technology in minimally invasive surgery has been to miniaturize our eyes and extend our hands to perform microscopic and macroscopic operations in places that could previously be reached only with large incisions. Technology has also provided new ways to look at tissue, utilizing sound waves, magnetic fields, and subatomic particles, which can be used to detect disease and guide therapy through small incisions. These same technologies, raised to a higher power or a sharper focal point, can be employed in tissue resection and destruction beyond what our hand-held instruments could ever perform.

It is vital that surgeons become familiar with the technologic principles that form the basis of this revolution so that they may reap the fruits of minimally invasive surgery and not become servants to their machines. For instance, much has been said or written about the comparative advantages of laser[7] and electrocautery[8] in laparoscopic surgery; however, it is apparent that many surgeons do not understand some of the basic concepts of energy transfer and tissue heating. Therefore, the first section of this book addresses the technologies on which our interventions are based. Although some of these chapters have been written by specialists in the field, electrical engineers, and polymer chemists, the information has been translated into the language of the general surgeon, who may have faint recollections of premedical physical science. We hope that this first section will be your reference when you are curious about "how it works."

OLD DISEASES

The second half of the book discusses the manner in which old diseases are approached after the surgeon has harnessed the new technology. This volume has been authored by a number of specialists for a couple of reasons. First, there is no single way to perform many of these operations because many of these techniques are undergoing rapid evolution. Second, the degree of subspecialization in minimally invasive surgery is so great that it is impossible for one or two surgeons to be authorities in more than one or two diseases and three or four techniques.

Broadly speaking, these new techniques fall into four categories: (1) laparoscopy, whereby a rigid endoscope is introduced through a metal sleeve into the peritoneal cavity with the aid of a carbon dioxide pneumoperitoneum; (2) thoracoscopy or mediastinoscopy, whereby a rigid endoscope is introduced either through the chest or neck to gain access to the thoracic or mediastinal contents; (3) endoluminal flexible endoscopy, whereby flexible endoscopes and other instruments are introduced into hollow organs or systems, such as the esophagus, stomach, colon, or vascular system; and (4) combined approaches, whereby visualization and treatment of the diseased organ is gained from an endoluminal and an extraluminal endoscope or other imaging device. For example, in a patient with a malignant polyp, a laparoscope may be used to visualize the exterior of the colon while a colonoscope localizes the polyp from within the lumen, thereby guiding a sleeve resection of the colon.

The old diseases effectively treated with minimally invasive techniques would fill a book many times larger than the one in your hands. To present a manageable volume of material, we have limited the scope of this volume to include only procedures that a general surgeon would be likely to perform (e.g., cholecystectomy or colectomy) or should know about (e.g., transjugular intrahepatic portosystemic shunt) to help choose the best treatment for the patients the surgeon is likely to encounter.

WHY IS MINIMALLY INVASIVE SURGERY LESS TRAUMATIC?

The easiest answer is that the wound is smaller. In most instances, it is probably true that the trauma of the surgical wound is greater than the trauma to the operative field. Similarly, the postoperative stress response is largely a response to the trauma inflicted in gaining access to the operative field. The wound is often the source of considerable morbidity, including infection, dehiscence, bleeding, and nerve entrapment. The pain suffered from the wound (bearing in mind that most of the viscera do not possess pain-sensitive fibers) leads to a longer recovery time, lethargy, and a subsequent increased incidence of deep venous thrombosis and pneumonia.

As surgeons, we have been accustomed, not only to incising the integument, but also to subjecting the patient to the additional trauma of mechanical and human retractors. It has been observed during laparoscopic cholecystectomy that stretching (retracting) the fascia to remove a thick gallbladder results in more postoperative discomfort than a short extension of the incision.[9] The same observation has been made after laparotomy or thoracotomy. Body wall retractors cause significant pain that may be greater than the pain caused by the incision alone. During laparoscopy, body wall retraction is mediated by a low-pressure pneumoperitoneum, which spreads the retraction force evenly across the entire peritoneum, minimizing trauma to any particular area.

An additional stress of open surgery is imposed by opening a body cavity to the atmosphere. Exposure injury includes dehydration and cooling of the exposed organs, with subsequent edema and interference with hemostasis and organ function. There is considerable evidence in the literature to suggest that the incidence of postsurgical adhesion formation has been reduced by the use of laparoscopy,[10] and we hope this will lead to fewer patients returning with an adhesive small bowel obstruction, intestinal ischemia, or necrosis.

Because open surgery is performed with large instruments, the amount of tissue incised with each move of the Metzenbaum scissors, for instance, is large, causing a certain amount of blood loss. When using the minimally invasive approach, however, the strokes are smaller, and the blood loss must be less to maintain adequate visualization of the operative field. The benefits of reduced blood loss extend to the operating team, who have less exposure to potentially infected blood.

DISADVANTAGES OF MINIMALLY INVASIVE SURGERY

What is the price that must be paid for less traumatic surgery? The greatest shortcomings of this burgeoning field are that we must learn to operate remote from the surgical field, using two-dimensional imaging, and that most surgeons require additional training to learn how to navigate this new landscape.

Unlike open surgery, where the interface between the doctor and patient was a small instrument held in the surgeon's hand, minimally invasive techniques usually require long instruments that are both rigid and flexible. The operation is observed through a long series of optical and electronic couples, ultimately producing a two-dimensional image on a video monitor. This leads to problems with hand–eye coordination, depth perception, and interferes with tactile sensation. These drawbacks may be addressed by future developments, such as three-dimensional television, virtual reality, and telepresence surgery (see Chap. 33).

During this phase of rapid technologic development and surgeon retraining, the shortcomings of two-dimensional imaging and remote application of energy have led to unfortunate iatrogenic injuries. Complications unreported during the era of open cholecystectomy, such as intestinal and vascular injury, are beginning to appear in laparoscopic cholecystectomy articles.[11] It appears also that bile duct injury is occurring at a greater frequency with laparoscopic than during open cholecystectomy.[12]

After performing many of these minimally invasive techniques, we are left with a large piece of tissue that has to be extracted from the body cavity. Occasionally, the extirpated tissue may be removed through a natural orifice, such as the rectum or mouth, but at other times, a novel route may be employed, such as removing a large gallbladder through the pouch of Douglas. In addition, the use of tissue morcellators, although appealing from the perspective of aesthetics, will reduce the amount of information available to the pathologist, not only hindering the ability to give the patient a full prognosis, but also interfering with the collection of patient information.

Furthermore, it is not infrequent that a minimally invasive operation is so technically challenging that the patient and surgeon are better served by conversion to an open procedure. Unfortunately, there seems to be an embarrassment or humiliation associated with this action. It is vital for surgeons to realize that conversion to an open operation is not a complication but rather reflects sound surgical judgment and is the antithesis of surgical machismo.

Although a dramatic cost savings was demonstrated with laparoscopic cholecystectomy,[13] such has not been the case with other laparoscopic procedures, especially herniorrhaphy. If minimally invasive surgery is to remain popular among medical insurers, the cost must be contained by becoming surgically efficient, reducing operating time, and limiting the use of new disposable and reusable equipment to those items that substantially add to procedure performance.

TRAINING FOR MINIMALLY INVASIVE SURGERY

Currently, there exists a knowledge deficit among surgeons in practice because many of these technologies and most of these techniques were not available when they were in medical school or residency. As a result of this deficit, some residency programs have no experienced minimally invasive surgical group at hand. With the passage of time, it is likely that every training program will offer instruction in minimally invasive techniques as they permeate general surgical practice. The second and future editions of this book will reflect these political, social, and technical changes.

Although a book such as this should provide most of the relevant information to outfit a surgeon to perform minimally invasive surgery, it is not our intention to provide a cookbook that can be set up on an easel above the operating table. Instead, training must include discussion, assistance, practice, and proctoring under the guidance of a practitioner knowledgeable about the disease in question and skilled in its treatment using minimally invasive techniques. When there are substantial risks involved, the practitioner should also be capable of performing the procedure using conventional surgical exposure.

THE WIDE IMPACT OF LOW-IMPACT SURGERY

It was stated earlier that the minimally invasive surgery revolution relied, to a great extent, on the introduction of new technologies, such as high-resolution color-accurate video cameras and specialized instrumentation, but the impact of these developments has already spread beyond minimally invasive surgery. Just as the technology of space exploration spilled over into everyday life, the technology of minimally invasive surgery is providing answers to some of the old problems familiar to all surgeons. For example, during colonic surgery, the visualization of the ureters has been a vital component of the operation but is frequently difficult. The development of an illuminated ureter probe for laparoscopic colectomy (see Chap. 17) has significantly resolved this shortcoming and will be nearly as helpful for open colectomy as for laparoscopic colectomy.

In addition, the development of laparoscopic surgical techniques, which are generally performed at laparotomy with digital dissection, may be sufficiently superior to replace the older techniques. For example, posterior esophageal dissection conventionally performed with a poke of the index finger behind the esophagus not infrequently results in esophageal perforation. It is likely that posterior esophageal dissection under direct vision, as is necessary for laparoscopic fundoplication (see Chap. 10), will reduce the incidence of such a blind error. Operations performed under direct vision are generally better operations, and minimally invasive surgery has forced us to obtain the visualization necessary to perform procedures without the use of our fingers.

CONCLUSION

Although there is no doubt that minimally invasive surgery has radically changed the practice of medicine, it has not changed the nature of disease. The basic surgical tenets still apply, including appropriate case selection, excellent exposure, adequate retraction, and performance of good operations. If a procedure makes no sense with conventional access, it makes no sense with a minimally invasive approach. In other words, because something can be done with an endoscope does not mean that it should be done with an endoscope.

It is perhaps fitting to conclude this introduction with a quotation from Sir Heneage Ogilivie (1887–1948), surgeon to Guys Hospital, London:

"There seems to be a tendency to look at change as meaning improvement, or motion as synonymous with advance. Advance means progress to something better and not progress to something new."

It is certain that minimally invasive surgery is full of something new. Time will tell if the something new is truly something better.

REFERENCES

1. Cuschieri A: "A rose by any other name . . ." Minimal access or minimally invasive surgery [editorial]. *Surg Endosc* 1992; 6:214.
2. Wickham J, Fitzpatrick JM: Minimally invasive surgery [editorial]. *Br J Surg* 1990; 77:721.
3. Bartlett MK, Waddell WR: Indications for common-duct exploration: Evaluation in 1000 cases. *N Engl J Med* 1958; 258:164–167.
4. Adams R, Stranahan A: Cholecystitis and cholelithiasis: An analytical report of 1,104 operative cases. *Surg Gynecol Obstet* 1947; 85:776.
5. Petelin JB: Laparoscopic approach to common duct pathology. *Surg Laparosc Endosc* 1991; 1:33–41.
6. Hunter JG: Laparoscopic transcystic common bile duct exploration. *Am J Surg* 1992; 163:53–58.
7. Reddick EJ, Olsen DO: Laparoscopic laser cholecystectomy. *Surg Endosc* 1989; 3:131–133.
8. Hunter JG: Laser or electrocautery for laparoscopic cholecystectomy? *Am J Surg* 1991; 161:345–349.
9. Bordelon BM, Hobday KA, Hunter JG: Incision extension is the optimal method of difficult gallbladder extraction at laparoscopic cholecystectomy. *Surg Endosc* 1992; 6:225–227.
10. Chamberlain GVP, Carron Brown JA: *Report of the Working Party of the Confidential Inquiry into Gynaecological Laparoscopy*. London, Royal College of Obstetricians and Gynaecologists, 1978.
11. Wolfe BM, Gardiner BN, Leary BF, et al: Endoscopic cholecystectomy: An analysis of complications. *Arch Surg* 1991; 126:1192–1198.
12. Southern Surgeons Club: A prospective analysis of 1518 laparoscopic cholecystectomies. *N Engl J Med* 1991; 324:1073–1078.
13. Anderson RE, Hunter JG: Laparoscopic cholecystectomy is less expensive than open cholecystectomy. *Surg Laparosc Endosc* 1991; 1:82–84.

Chapter 2

Fiberoptic Imaging and Measurement

Daniel R. Margulies / M. Michael Shabot

HISTORICAL PERSPECTIVE

Our ability to examine progressively less visible areas of the body has grown tremendously over the past two centuries. Microimaging has its roots in endoscopic imaging; this technology has improved for both diagnostic and therapeutic purposes. Endoscopy began with a candle as the initial light source, as described in 1806 by Bozzini, directed within a tin tube.[1,2] In 1870, Kussmaul demonstrated the possibility of inspecting the stomach using a rigid tube, using a professional sword swallower as his subject. Others then employed various telescopic devices that eventually led to elaborate but cumbersome flexible endoscopes. However, adequate distal illumination remained a significant problem.

The next 30 years yielded significant advances in optics and lighting.[1,2] In 1879, Nitze borrowed the idea from a dentist of using an overheated glowing platinum wire to illuminate the first cystoscope (7 mm); it had a prism on the distal end. Mikulicz used a similar system of heated (and water-cooled) platinum when he introduced the gastroscope. Although Mikulicz employed general anesthesia for his patients, others used local anesthetics (cocaine), as did Killian when he developed and successfully used the first bronchoscope in 1898. His light source was augmented with a head mirror.

These technologies were hindered still by the difficulties of negotiating anatomic curves. To overcome this problem, the first semiflexible gastroscope was designed by Wolf and Schindler in 1936 in Berlin.[1,2] This 12-mm diameter, 77-cm-long telescope contained 48 lenses. The need for progressively more flexibility with better visibility prompted the introduction of the first fiber-optic technology in medicine: a flexible Fiberglas gastroscope in 1957 developed by Basil Hirshowitz and Lawrence Curtis of the University of Michigan School of Medicine.[3] This major advance initiated the modern era of endoscopy.

OPTICAL PRINCIPLES OF ENDOSCOPY

Lens Endoscope

The purpose of the endoscope is to view the object of interest with clarity and without distortion. To understand how this is done, we first must examine the basic optics of a conventional lens endoscope (Fig. 2-1). The image, $P_1O_1Q_1$, enters the endoscope by passing through the front group of lenses, termed the *objective*, which reduces the image. The light path from point Q_1 is shown forming Q_1' after the objective lens. This inverted image then is refocused by a *relay system* to form a second image of Q_1 at Q_2'. This image then is enlarged through the *eyepiece* and focused to an appropriate distance from the *exit-pupil*, so that it can be seen by the observer's eye (E). An actual endoscope would have many relay systems between the image produced at O_1' by the objective and O_2', which is magnified by the eyepiece. For example, a typical cystoscope may have five relay stages. An odd number of relay systems is required to keep the final image at O_2' upright.[4,5]

The total amount of light that can be transmitted by this system is limited, however. Even assuming no loss from absorption by the glass lens or by reflection at the air–glass surface, the light transmitted still is reduced by the intrinsic refractive index at each interface as the light passes from one medium (air) into a different medium (glass). To help overcome this problem, a method was devised to reverse the roles of glass and air, that is, long glass spaces, curved at their ends, form essentially *air* lenses. This *Hopkins rod–lens* system more than doubles the light-transmitting capacity of the endoscope. It also has additional mechanical and manufacturing advantages.[4,5]

However, without further improvements this system would have poor overall transmission of light. Subsequent improvements allowed for dual viewing, rotation and swivel joints, and image-rotating prisms, each added in series. Each improvement added another change of medi-

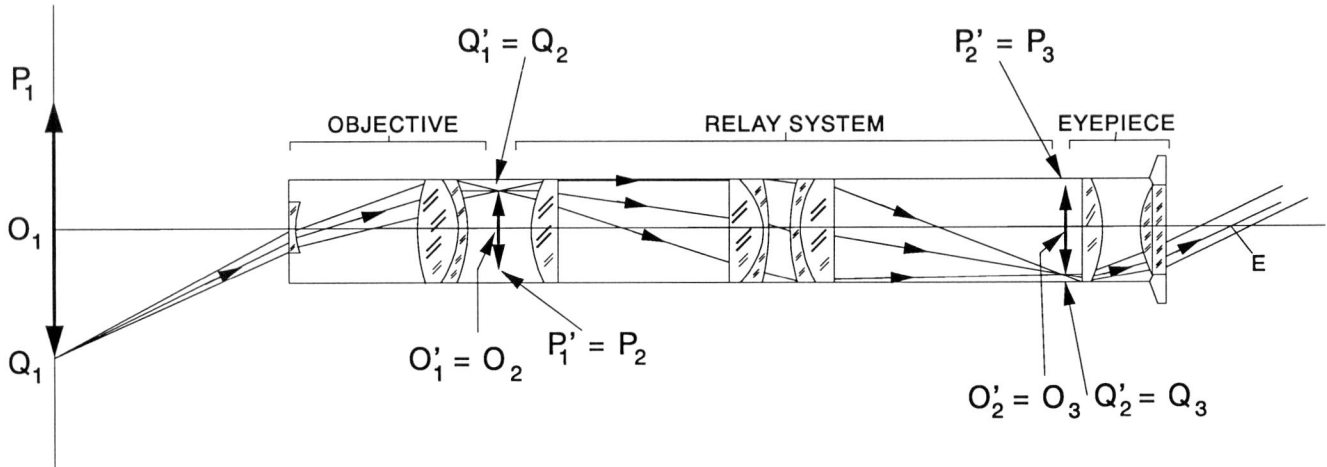

FIGURE 2-1 A conventional endoscope system. [From Berci G (ed): *Endoscopy*. New York, Appleton-Century-Crofts, 1976, p 28. Used with permission.]

um along the light path. Thus, there could be as many as 50 air–glass surfaces along one cytoscope. Because approximately 5 percent of light is reflected at each untreated air–glass interface, depending on the refractive index of the glass, as little as 20 percent of the light might be transmitted.[4,5]

The development of the antireflection coating, a thin film placed on the glass surface, substantially increased light transmission. In addition, because the rod–lens system uses more glass than a conventional endoscope, the light absorption properties of the glass are important. By selecting low-absorptive optical glass and coating the surfaces, the light transmission of a scope with 50 interfaces could be more than 80 percent. In this manner, the basic tools were developed for rigid and semiflexible endoscopes, and these principles remain useful today. However, this field expanded dramatically with the advent of fiberoptic technology.[4,5]

Fiberoptic Endoscope

Although the main advantage of an optical fiber is its ability to transmit light over large distances with extremely small losses, its flexibility and small size are also dramatic improvements. An optical fiber consists of a long core of a transparent material that can carry a beam of light. This core is covered by a coating called a cladding and another outer cover, termed a jacket or sheath. Two principles are important to understand fiberoptic light transmission: total internal reflection and numeric aperture.[5–7]

Total internal reflection is based on the physics of how light is reflected at an interface between two different mediums. Some light will be transmitted through (refracted), and some will be reflected (Fig. 2-2). Although the rigid endoscope used refracted light, the optical fiber employs reflected light. As the angle of incidence (i) increases, the refracted beam (bent to angle r) becomes more parallel to the surface of the first medium. At some critical angle (θc), the refracted ray is tangential to the surface (r = 90°) (Fig. 2-2). Any ray that is greater than this critical angle will be 100 percent reflected.

For reflected light, the angle of incidence is equal to the angle of reflection; therefore, the next angle of incidence (as the ray strikes the other side) is exactly the same as the first. Thus, the ray will again be 100 percent reflected (it remains greater than θc), and so on down the fiber. This phenomenon, *total internal reflection,* forms the basis by which optical fibers transmit light.[8]

The actual physics of this phenomenon is embodied in Snells' law of refraction, which states that $n_1 \sin(i) = n_2 \sin(r)$, where n = refractive index of the medium. Here the role of the cladding becomes apparent; it is made of a material with a lower refractive index than the fiber ($n_1 > n_2$), for example, the cladding is less dense. These materials are chosen so that the angle of incidence that propagates down the fiber is small. Therefore, only a discrete cone of light will be transmitted by one fiber.[6]

A light beam that is reflected along a 10-μm-diameter fiber over a length of 1 m may have more than 10,000 reflections; however, the phenomenon of total internal reflection makes the transmission almost loss free. Furthermore, the fiber will bend through a curve, and the light still will continue to undergo total internal reflection, emerging from the end as the same cone of rays that entered the fiber.

The numeric aperture of the fiber is determined also by the refractive index of the core material and by the critical angle. It effectively determines the cone of light admitted to the fiber and that which emerges. This becomes especially important in laser technology because it establishes the beam-divergence pattern on exiting and thus defines the

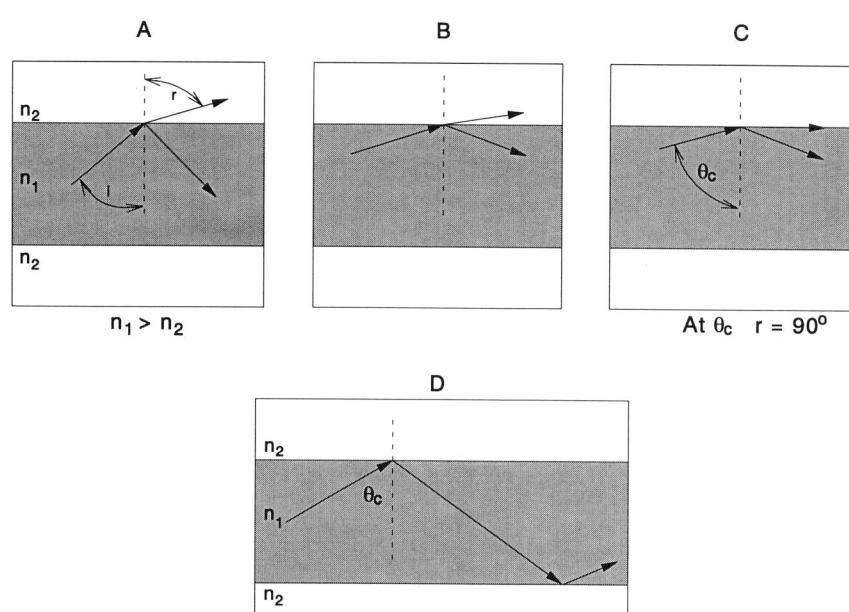

FIGURE 2-2 Any angle greater than Θ_c will result in total internal reflection.

power a laser can supply at a given distance from the fiber tip. Fiberoptic instruments that are designed with high numeric apertures are an advantage in endoscopy.[7]

The same technology is used to illuminate the object. In this situation, the optical fiber transmits a beam from a light source that itself has undergone improvements in quality. This source could be the green light of an argon laser, the ultraviolet light of an excimer laser, the near-infrared radiation of an yttrium aluminum garnet (YAG) laser, or a high-intensity visible light source, such as a xenon arc lamp. To deliver light to the distal end of an endoscope, fibers of approximately 25 μm are used, and there is no need to have any particular order in the bundle of fibers; this is termed an *incoherent* bundle. However, for an image to exit the end of the endoscope with the appearance it had when it entered the fiber bundle, the fibers must be arranged *coherently,* that is, they must maintain their alignment from one end of the bundle to the other (Fig. 2-3).[5]

An objective lens is used to focus the image onto the bundle of fibers. Each optical fiber admits only the light aligned with its axis; therefore, each fiber transmits only a small fraction of the image, a so-called picture element or pixel. Each individual fiber is only approximately 10 μm in diameter and can be as small as 6 μm. For comparison, a human hair is approximately 75 μm. Ten thousand or more fibers may be required to transmit the image properly. The ends are glued or melted together to maintain the coherence of the bundle, but the midsection may remain free to achieve flexibility. The exiting image is reconstructed by an eyepiece as in a conventional endoscope.[9]

Intrinsic loss of light transmission occurs as a result of impurities, moisture, and mechanical flaws in the otherwise transparent bundle core of the fiber. This loss is proportional to the length of the fiber and is consequently a greater problem in the field of telecommunications where fibers may extend over many kilometers. Research in this area has led to better materials; these primarily have been improved by eliminating metallic impurities (iron, nickel, and copper) and water from the silica base. Further improvements are being made using nonsilica-based fibers with particular application to lasers.[6,10]

A modern endoscope houses the illumination bundle, the image bundle, and many utility tools. These include bending wires, which, with manipulation, can bend the tip for steering. Air, water, and biopsy channels are added for suction, irrigation, and utilization of specific tools. An outer sheath integrates all components and secures the lens on each end.

NEW MEDICAL USES OF FIBEROPTICS

Currently, fiberoptics enable the transmission of light or energy back and forth across a small flexible, movable, and sterilizable system. Existing applications of this technology are in their infancy. Lasers, photodetector technology, and angioscopy all use fiberoptics and will be discussed further in subsequent chapters. A few examples of how fiberoptics currently are applied will illustrate the promise of this technology.

Fiberoptic Pressure Monitoring

Light can transmit sophisticated and encoded information in addition to simple images. Fiberoptic pressure sensors

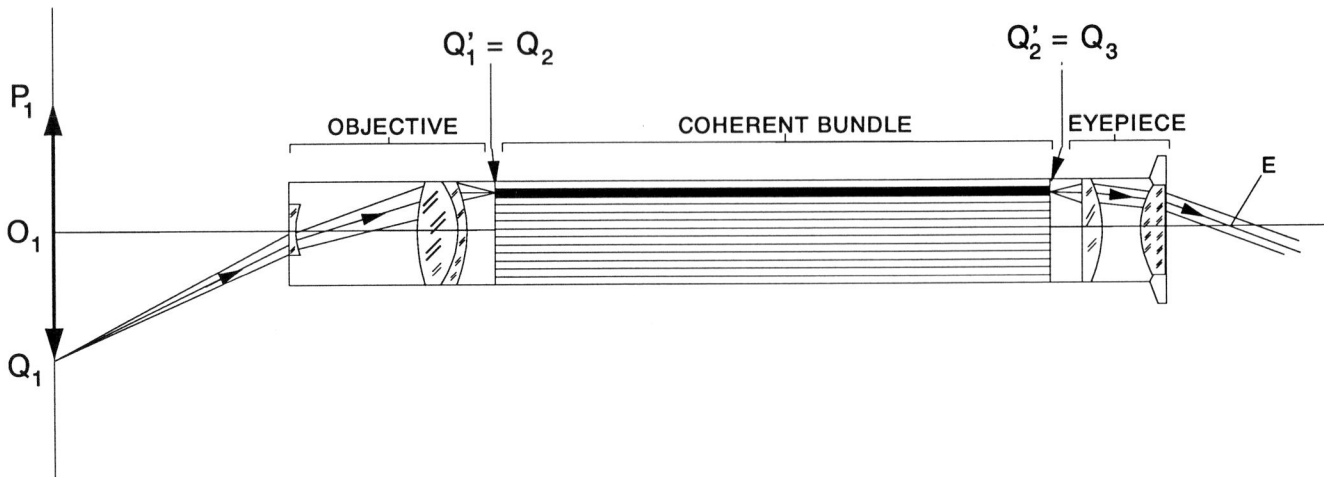

FIGURE 2-3 A fiberoptic endoscope system. [From Berci G (ed): *Endoscopy*. New York, Appleton-Century-Crofts, 1976, p 29. Used with permission.]

have been developed that detect pressure changes and transmit pressure data back to a recording instrument. Such a system has the transducer at the tip, in the actual location where pressure is to be measured. An existing example is an intracranial pressure (ICP) catheter (Camino Laboratories, San Diego, CA). This device uses a mirror–diaphragm in the tip that alters the reflection of light as the pressure changes the shape of the diaphragm (Fig. 2-4). The catheter tip can be placed in a subarachnoid bolt or an intraventricular chamber. Light is emitted from a sending fiber, reflected off the mirror–diaphragm, and received by a second receiving fiber. When the intracranial pressure changes the diaphragm's shape, the reflection of the transmitted light changes, allowing either more or less light to enter the receiving fiber. Light from the receiving fiber is analyzed by a microcomputer and displayed as a number and a continuous pressure waveform.

This system has advantages over standard ICP catheters that use a column of water to transmit pressure to a mechanical transducer. This technique primarily has been used

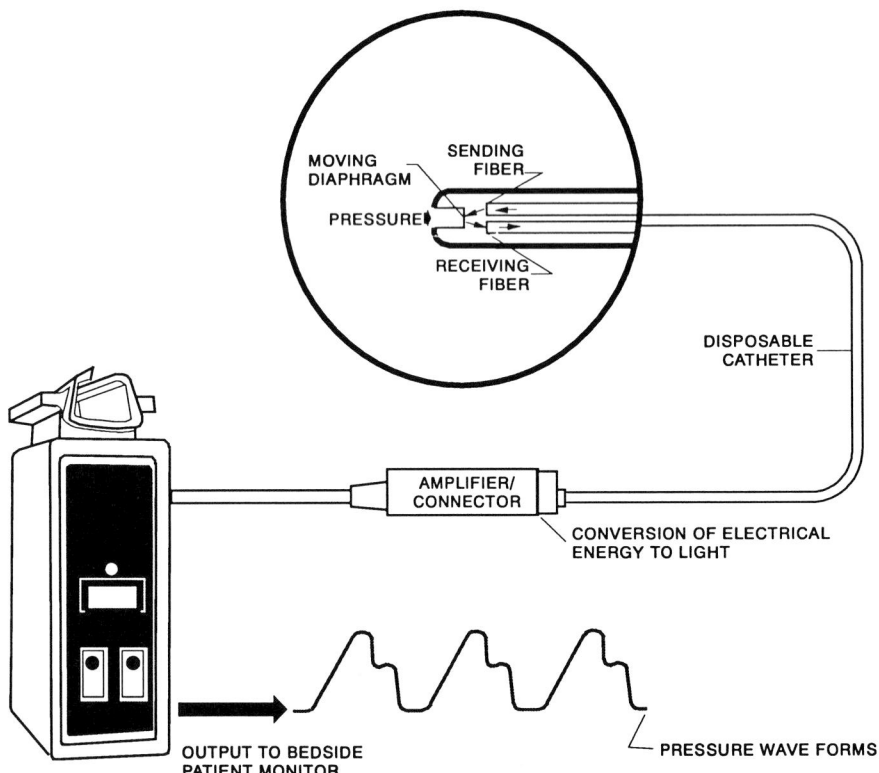

FIGURE 2-4 Fiberoptic pressure monitoring catheter system. (From Camino Laboratories, San Diego. Used with permission.)

for intracranial pressure monitoring, but it can be applied in many other areas. It has been shown to have greater accuracy with less drift, and it produces a waveform with less artifact. There is no fluid column involved, which means that the pressure waveform is not dampened by air bubbles, debris, or clots. There is no need to adjust the transducer level based on the position of the patient. Because there is no fluid involved, there may be a lower risk of infection. The catheters are completely disposable. The whole system is self-contained, and it may be transported easily with the patient, enabling continuous monitoring while the patient is away from the intensive care unit. The catheter has been shown to be safe and effective, even in children. A shortcoming of such a system is that, once it is inserted, it can not be recalibrated; should a question of accuracy arise, a new catheter must be placed.[11-16]

In Vivo Oximetry

The ratio of hemoglobin that is saturated with oxygen to total hemoglobin by volume is called the oxyhemoglobin saturation. Arterial oxygen saturation (SaO_2) is measured on the arterial side of the circulation, and mixed venous oxygen saturation (SvO_2) is measured from the venous side, preferably from a "mixed" sample that combines blood from both the superior and inferior vena cavae. Until 1965, oxygen saturation was measured only in the laboratory from blood samples drawn from arterial or venous sources. In 1965, Frommer and coworkers[17] capitalized on the principles of fiberoptic light transmission to measure oxyhemoglobin saturation continuously inside a blood vessel. In the cardiac catheterization laboratory, Frommer inserted a special pulmonary artery catheter that incorporated fiberoptic bundles connected to a light source and detector. In 1973, Cole and colleagues[18,19] at the University of Washington worked with the Physio-Control company to introduce the first commercially available in vivo oximeter.

In vivo measurement of oxyhemoglobin saturation is feasible because oxyhemoglobin and deoxygenated hemoglobin absorb light differently (Fig. 2-5). This is obvious by visual inspection; in ambient light, arterial blood is red, and venous blood is dark blue. However, inspection is not a quantitative measurement. By rapidly pulsing multiple wavelengths of light in the range of 600 to 900 nm on flowing blood using one fiber bundle and measuring the relative ratios of light reflected through a second bundle, the proportion of oxygenated hemoglobin present can be calculated (Fig. 2-6). Although early efforts were directed toward monitoring arterial saturation in adults and neonates, transcutaneous partial pressure of oxygen measurement and noninvasive pulse oximetry replaced in vivo SaO_2 monitoring. Clinicians and manufacturers then focused on the pulmonary circulation and SvO_2.

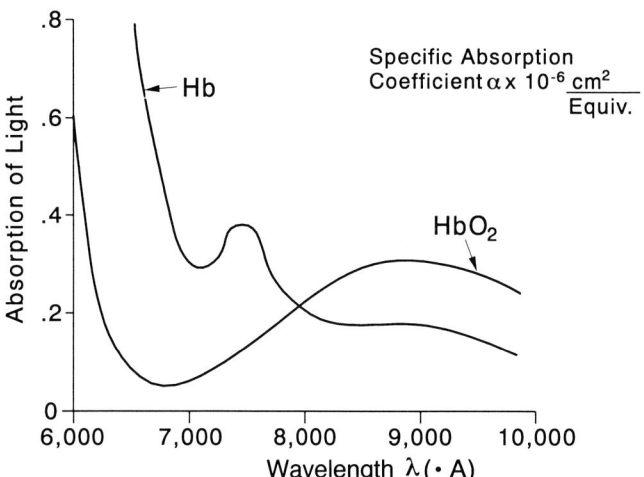

FIGURE 2-5 Relative absorption of hemoglobin and oxygenated hemoglobin. [From Schweiss JF (ed): *Continuous Measurement of Blood Oxygen Saturation in the High Risk Patient.* San Diego, Beech International, 1983, p 8. Used with permission.]

Special pulmonary artery flotation catheters (Swan-Ganz catheters, Edward Laboratories, Santa Ana, CA) were manufactured for the Physio-Control oximeter that had fiberoptic bundles running from the tip to a special optical connector. The Physio-Control oximeter used two wavelengths of light; this would seem to be adequate based on the absorption spectra of the two forms of hemoglobin. However, in practice, several factors conspired to make the two-wavelength method clinically unreliable, including Fiberglas breakage, backscatter artifact from vessel walls, catheter tip clotting, presence of carboxyhemoglobin, and hemodilution.[19] Despite these difficulties, initial studies in humans indicated that the SvO_2 could be a sensitive and early indicator of hemodynamic instability. Abnormally low SvO_2s were observed in hypotensive patients after cardiac surgery who had low cardiac output syndrome and in postoperative patients during shivering episodes.

A highly accurate three-wavelength in vivo oximeter was introduced in 1981 by the Oximetrix Company (Mountain View, CA, now part of Abbott Critical Care, Mountain View, CA). Three light-emitting diodes were packaged in an optical module that was stable over time. The third light wavelength and proprietary instrument software provided absolute calibration in the sterile package before catheter insertion, in vivo recalibration, artifact rejection, and enhanced reliability of the SvO_2 measurement. Early problems with stiff Fiberglas pulmonary artery catheters were resolved by an Oximetrix catheter, which used more compliant plastic fibers (Fig. 2-7).

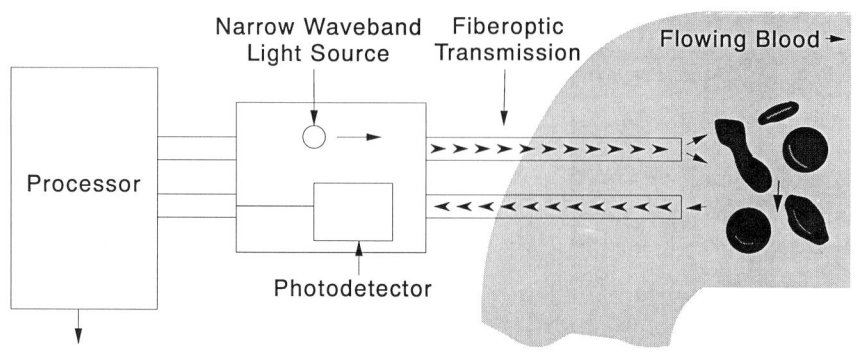

FIGURE 2-6 Principles of reflection spectrophotometry. [From Schweiss JF (ed): *Continuous Measurement of Blood Oxygen Saturation in the High Risk Patient*. San Diego, Beech International, 1983, p 9. Used with permission.]

The physiologic value of SvO_2 monitoring has remained controversial. Civetta and colleagues[20] believed that the Oximetrix instrument provided, not only additional useful data, but also was cost effective in reducing the need for cardiac output measurements and venous blood gases. Others believe that the SvO_2 is too indirect a measurement to be certain of its meaning. Mathematically, $SvO_2 = SaO_2 - (VO_2/(CO * Hgb * 13.4))$, where VO_2 is oxygen consumption, CO is cardiac output, and Hgb is the patient's hemoglobin. Thus, the SvO_2 is dependent on four other physiologic variables, making it difficult to understand, by monitoring SvO_2 alone, why the SvO_2 might rise, fall, or stay the same.[21] Some intensive care specialists routinely use continuous SvO_2 monitoring in the operating room and intensive care unit; others reserve such monitoring for specific hemodynamic or oxygenation indications. Others measure SvO_2 periodically by sending samples to the laboratory, and some do not measure it at all.

Despite the lack of consensus, in vivo oximetry is a creative and compelling example of the use of fiberoptic technology in critically ill patients. Future catheters may incorporate catheter tip dyes and other in vivo detectors, allowing for continuous fiberoptic measurement of electrolytes, glucose, blood gases, and many other parameters.

Laser Doppler

The scanning laser Doppler is a system under investigation in which laser light is transmitted onto a tissue, and reflected light is received by a sensor. In this situation, the Doppler effect is used; this is based on the finding that moving objects reflect light at a slightly different wavelength than do stationary objects. For example, laser light can be focused on a solid tissue, such as the skin. By analyzing the Doppler shift in the light reflected off the moving erythrocytes in the capillary beds or deeper arteriovenous anastomoses, a measurement of flow can be

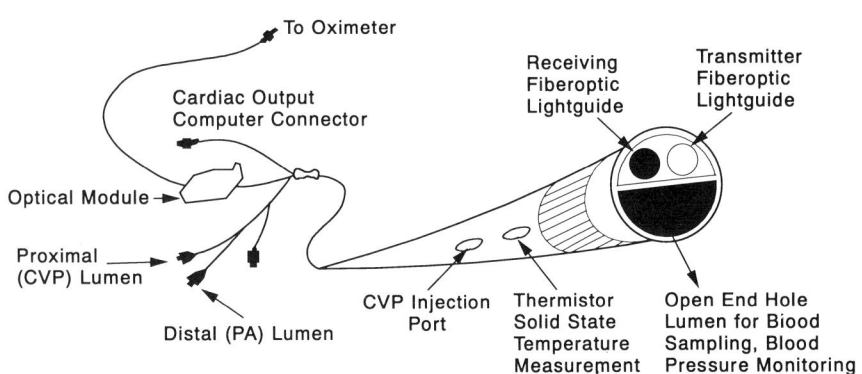

FIGURE 2-7 Fiberoptic SvO_2 monitoring catheter. [From Schweiss JF (ed): *Continuous Measurement of Blood Oxygen Saturation in the High Risk Patient*. San Diego, Beech International, 1983, p 11. Used with permission.]

obtained. This is a noninvasive method of determining tissue perfusion. Alternatively, a fiberoptic catheter can be placed in a blood vessel to determine laser Doppler blood flow, which also might elucidate specific organ perfusion. An intravascular laser Doppler probe placed in the heart offers an alternative to the thermodilution technique of measuring cardiac output.[22-28]

Videoendoscopy

When an endoscopic image is displayed on a video monitor screen, the technique is called videoendoscopy. This can be accomplished by placing the camera at the proximal end of a fiberoptic endoscope (indirect videoendoscopy) or distally at the tip (direct videoendoscopy). Instead of receiving the image in a fiber as described for the fiberoptic endoscope, light is sampled by an optoelectronic sensing device, a charge-coupled device (CCD) chip. The CCD is an array of photosensitive sensor elements that transforms each pixel into an electric charge. As the light intensity striking the sensor increases, the charge generated increases. These charges then are transformed into an image on a monitor screen. Fiberoptics are not used in a direct videoendoscopic system.

High-resolution direct videoendoscopic gastroscopes and colonoscopes have been developed that produce higher resolution images than fiberscopes. This avoids the problems of diminishing visibility by fiber damage as the fiberscope ages. Another advantage is that because the image is electronic, it could be digitalized and stored in a computer as a permanent record. However, there are still problems with these instruments that must be corrected. Reflections from particles, such as blood or food, at short focus (less than 1 cm) cause loss of resolution. this diminution of quality makes the electronic endoscope particularly poor when bleeding is brisk. It may never replace a fiberoptic endoscope in this situation. The representation of true color is another difficulty, but significant improvements have been made. Overall, electronic endoscopy offers enhancements to modern endoscopy that ultimately may replace fiberoptic technology.[2,29-32]

The same technology has been used extensively in laparoscopy and thoracoscopy. Many new microvideo cameras are available that are small, light, and easily sterilized. The resolution of the camera is measured by the number of pixels filling a chip; current cameras use chips with up to 300,000 pixels. The resolution of the monitor screen on which the picture is displayed is determined by the number of lines exhibited. A standard video screen contains 350 horizontal lines; newer monitors used in laparoscopy have approximately 700 lines of horizontal resolution. While proper digitalization of the record for permanent storage is being developed, current documentation of the operative procedure is being done by simply recording the image on standard or high-quality video tape.[33]

REFERENCES

1. Berci G: History of endoscopy, in Berci G (ed): *Endoscopy*. New York, Appleton-Century-Crofts, 1976, pp xix–xxiii.
2. Knyrim K, Seidlitz H, Vakil N, Classen M: Perspectives in "electronic endoscopy" past, present, and future of fibers and CCDs in medical endoscopes. *Endoscopy* 1990; 22(suppl 1):2–8.
3. Katzir A: Optical fibers in medicine. *Sci Am* 1989; 260(5):120–125.
4. Hopkins HH: Optical principles of the endoscope, in Berci G (ed): *Endoscopy*. New York, Appleton-Century-Crofts, 1976, chap 1, pp 3–26.
5. Hopkins HH: Physics of the fiberoptic endoscope, in Berci G (ed): *Endoscopy*. New York, Appleton-Century-Crofts, 1976, chap 2, pp 27–63.
6. Leon MB, Smith PD, Bonner RF: Laser angioplasty delivery systems: Design considerations, in White RA, Grundfest WS (eds): *Lasers in Cardiovascular Disease*. Chicago, Year Book Medical Publishers, 1987, chap 4, pp 44–63.
7. Drexhage MG, Moynihan CT: Infrared optical fibers. *Sci Am* 1988; 259(11):110–115.
8. Johnson BK: *Optics and Optical Instruments*. New York, Dover Publications, 1960; Chap V, pp 78–109; Chap VIII, pp 159–203.
9. Auth DC: Physical principles and limitations of fiberoptic angioscopy, in Moore WS, Ahn SS (eds): *Endovascular Surgery*. Philadelphia, WB Saunders, 1989, chap 4, pp 31–38.
10. Lines ME: The search for very low loss fiber-optic materials. *Science* 1984; 226:663–668.
11. Hollingsworth-Fridlund P, Vos H, Daily EK: Use of fiber-optic pressure transducer for intracranial pressure measurements: A preliminary report. *Heart Lung* 1988; 17:111–120.
12. Shellock FG: Transducer-tipped catheter. *Medical Electronics* 1985; 96:102–106.
13. Crutchfield JS, Narayan RK, Robertson CS, Michael LH: Evaluation of a fiberoptic intracranial pressure monitor. *J Neurosurg* 1990; 72:482–487.
14. Ostrup RC, Luerssen TG, Marshall LF, Zornow MH: Continuous monitoring of intracranial pressure with a miniaturized fiberoptic device. *J Neurosurg* 1987; 67:206–209.
15. Luerssen TG: Fiberoptic intraparenchymal pressure monitoring for the measurement of intracranial pressure in children. *Concepts in Pediatric Neurosurgery* 1990; 10:204–213.
16. Bolander HG: A new method for long-term lumbar pressure monitoring with a fiber optic catheter. *Acta Neurochir* 1990; 105:135–139.
17. Frommer PL, Ros J, Mason DT, et al: Clinical applications of an improved, rapidly responding fiberoptic catheter. *Am J Cardiol* 1965; 15:672–679.
18. Cole JS, Martin WE, Cheung PW, Johnson CC: Clinical studies with a solid state fiberoptic oximeter. *Am J Cardiol* 1972; 29:383–388.
19. Martin WE, Cheung PW, Johnson CC, Wong KC: Continuous monitoring of mixed venous oxygen saturation in man. *Anesth Analg* 1973; 52:784–793.
20. Civetta JM, Hudson-Civetta J: High tech = high quality at high cost: Is this the only equation? *Surgical Rounds* 1987; 10:67–82.
21. Norfleet EA, Watson CB: Continous mixed venous oxygen saturation measurement: A significant advance in hemodynamic monitoring? *J Clin Monit* 1985; 1:245–258.
22. Holloway GA, Watkins DW: Laser Doppler measurement of cutaneous blood flow. *J Invest Dermatol* 1977; 69:306–309.
23. Nilsson GE, Torsten T, Oberg PA: A new instrument for continuous measurement of tissue blood flow by light beating spectroscopy. *IEEE Trans Biomed Eng* 1980; 27:12–19.
24. Bonner R, Nossal R: Model for laser Doppler measurements of blood flow in tissue. *Applied Optics* 1981; 20:2097–2107.

25. Hirata K, Nagasaka T, Noda Y: Partial measurement of capillary and arteriovenous anastomotic blood flow in the human finger by laser Doppler flowmeter. *Eur J Appl Physiol* 1988; 57:616–621.
26. Jentink HW, de Mul RG, Hermsen RGAM, et al: Monte Carlo simulations of laser Doppler blood flow measurements in tissue. *Applied Optics* 1990; 29:2371–2381.
27. Jentink HW, deMul RG, Suichies HE, et al: Laser Doppler flowmetry: Measurements in a layered perfusion model and Monte Carlo simulations of measurements. *Applied Optics* 1991; 30:2592–2597.
28. Sriram P, Hanagud S, Craig J, Komerath NM: Scanning laser Doppler technique for velocity profile sensing on a moving surface. *Applied Optics* 1990; 29:2409–2417.
29. Classen M, Knyrim K, Seidlitz HK, Hagenmuller F: Electronic endoscopy—The latest technology. *Endoscopy* 1987; 19:118–123.
30. de Reunk M, Ramdane B, Jonas C, Nyst JF, van Gossum M, de Koster E, Deprez C, Deltenre M: A randomized, multi-observer, comparative evaluation of conventional fiberendoscopy and videoendoscopy in the upper GI tract. *Endoscopy* 1990; 22(suppl 1):9–12.
31. Schapiro M: Video endoscopy in clinical application: Colonoscopy. *Endoscopy* 1990; 22(suppl 1):13–14.
32. Knyrim K, Seidlitz HK, Hagenmuller F, Classen M: Color performance of video endoscopes: Quantitative measurement of color reproduction. *Endoscopy* 1987; 19:233–236.
33. Paz-Partlow M: The importance of permanent documentation of endoscopic findings. *Prob Gen Sur* 1991; 8(3):487–494.

Chapter 3

Intraoperative, Endoscopic, and Laparoscopic Ultrasound

Robert C. McIntyre, Jr. / Greg Van Stiegmann

Ultrasonography has many clinical applications, and it can be done with both extra- and intracorporeal techniques. Intracorporeal ultrasound, done in open operations, is useful for several applications in hepatobiliary and gastrointestinal surgery. Miniaturization of ultrasound transducers has opened the way for intracorporeal use of ultrasound with both flexible endoscopy and laparoscopy. This union of endoscopic and ultrasound technology has expanded the potential for clinical application of ultrasonography; it may grow in importance as additional endoscopic and less invasive surgical techniques develop and mature. The purpose of this overview is to acquaint the reader with basic principles of ultrasonography and detail clinical experiences relevant to modern surgical practice, which may be pertinent to future development.

BASIC PHYSICS AND INSTRUMENTATION

Ultrasound consists of mechanical waves with alternating regions of high and low pressure propagating through a medium. Medical ultrasound waves oscillate at frequencies from one to 30 Megahertz (MHz or millions of cycles per second). Dividing 40 by the frequency of an ultrasound device results in a rough guideline to the depth of tissue penetration in centimeters (e.g., 40 divided by a 10-MHz probe = approximately 4-cm tissue penetration). The velocity of ultrasound waves depends on the medium in which they propagate (Table 3-1). Ultrasound images are produced using the pulse–echo principle of sonar and radar. A transducer both transmits and receives the ultrasound waves (pulses). As an ultrasound pulse propagates through tissue, some of the pulse is attenuated by absorption and scattering; however, a part of the energy (echo) is reflected back to the transducer which measures the time since transmission and the amplitude of the received echo. The

TABLE 3-1 Velocity of ultrasound wave in various tissues

	Speed (m/s)
Air	333
Soft tissue	1450
Water	1480
Bone	3500

amount of energy attenuation depends on tissue impedance, a factor related primarily to tissue density. An interface is the boundary between two mediums with differing impedances. Ultrasound waves are either transmitted through, reflected by, or refracted by an interface.

The amplitude of the ultrasound echo received back by the transducer is represented by shades of gray on the video monitor. Two general types of echoes are recognized. Specular echoes arise from large reflectors in the body and have large amplitudes; diffuse echoes originate from small point reflectors and have low amplitudes as a result of scatter of the ultrasound pulse. Specular echoes define boundaries of large organ masses. Focal disease (stones, cysts, and surgical clips) have higher echo amplitudes (hyperechoic) or lower ones (hypoechoic) than the surrounding tissue.

The ultrasound transducer produces a planar, two-dimensional image that may be transverse, longitudinal, or oblique. The active element inside the transducer is a piezoelectric disk. Electric voltages are converted into slight changes in the disk thickness, resulting in generation of ultrasound waves. When an echo is received back at the piezoelectric disk, changes in disk conformation caused by the incoming echo produce similar electrical voltage changes, the magnitude of which is proportional to the pressure amplitude of the echo. Acoustic coupling of the transducer to the patient or area to be scanned is accomplished by using gel, liquid, or special solid acoustic interface materials. Modern ultrasound transducers can produce up to 15 to 30 frames (images) per second and can thus present anatomy in real time. Abdominal ultrasound devices typically operate at 15 frames per second.

Several transducer configurations are used for clinical real-time ultrasonography. The simplest is the mechanical sector scanner in which a single element oscillates back and forth. Alternatively, several elements can be mounted on a wheel that rotates around an axis. Such transducers produce a field that is sector (pie) shaped with a limited field of view for tissue close to the transducer and a wider field of view for more distant tissue. Multiple transducers also may be configured in longitudinal arrays of single elements. These linear-array transducers use groups of neighboring elements to produce parallel beams by firing and receiving sequentially along the array producing a rectangular image. Bending the transducer array onto a convex surface increases the field of view. Phased-array transducers consist of transducer heads constructed with a number of elements placed side by side. Slight time delays, that is, phase differences, allow for control of the direction of the resultant ultrasound beam. A small stationary transducer head may be used to view a large anatomic area. The phased-array transducer allows some anatomic acoustic obstructions to be avoided.

Small parts scanners produce images of limited depth for visualization of specific structures. Limited depth-penetration requirements allow the use of higher frequencies, which result in increased image detail. These transducers (usually of linear-array configuration) have small diameters with long focal zones at the required image depth and are used to examine the thyroid, breast, testis, and peripheral arteries. Intraoperative ultrasonography places transducers in close proximity to the area of interest. Such scanners are designed to incorporate the benefits associated with small parts scanners.

Most medical ultrasound techniques use the same method of collecting anatomic information. Variation is found only in the way the acoustic beam is directed into the body or in the presentation of the signals on a display. The simplest display technique is called A-mode. This is a one-dimensional image displaying the amplitude strength of the returning echo along the vertical axis and the distance from the transducer along the horizontal axis. This technique allows rapid identification of large interfaces in the body; however, it is not used commonly in clinical practice. Real-time, or B-mode, imaging is a method of displaying the amplitude of an echo by varying the brightness of a dot on an image to correspond to the echo strength. Real-time processing of images is possible because of the high speed of ultrasound transmission in soft tissue. More than 25 images can be generated per second. Below this rate of processing, the image will appear to flicker. The advantages of B-mode imaging include the abilities to observe motion of organs in the body and to alter the scan plane quickly to search through the body. A third ultrasound technique used in clinical imaging is M-scanning; this uses pulsed ultrasound waves to detect and record the motion of tissues. The echo signals are displayed as a line of bright spots that sweep across a display screen. This technology produces traces of the position of echoes versus time. M-scanning is used widely for noninvasive imaging of intracardiac structures.

Doppler ultrasonography measures the dependence of the observed pitch (i.e., frequency) of sound reflected to the transducer on the motion of the source of the reflection. The observed frequency of the sound reflected from flowing blood is higher if the blood is moving toward the receiver than when it is moving away. Two transducer elements are necessary for Doppler imaging. One continuously generates ultrasound waves that a second receives. The combination of Doppler ultrasound with B-mode ultrasound scanning is called duplex imaging. Regions of blood flow commonly are depicted in color-flow imaging techniques, with red representing movement of blood toward the probe and blue, movement away from the probe.

OPERATIVE ULTRASONOGRAPHY

The development of intraoperative ultrasonography paralleled that of extracorporeal sonography. Schlegel and associates[1] used the technique in 1961 to localize nephrolithiasis. Laparoscopic ultrasound was used by Hayashi and coworkers[2] in 1962 to diagnose cholelithiasis, presaging recent developments by three decades. The technique of ultrasound examination of the common bile duct at open operation was expanded to facilitate common bile duct exploration in 1965.[3] The latter group used a standard-sized probe and later developed a specialized smaller probe for introduction directly into the common bile duct. Using these techniques, they were able to detect 18 stones in the common bile duct in 46 patients; two patients had false-positive findings of duct stones, and two were diagnosed incorrectly as not having stones.

Early attempts at intraoperative ultrasonography using A-mode instruments did not spark enthusiasm. Interest was renewed when B-mode (real-time) scanning was introduced into clinical practice in 1978. The early probe design was improved, and a stainless-steel sector transducer was developed for intraoperative use. Japanese investigators later were able to improve imaging capability of this early sector scanner by designing an efficient linear scanning probe. Use of intraoperative ultrasound has expanded; however, the technique remains confined primarily to specialized centers despite its well-demonstrated utility.[4,5] Surgeons' limited experience in the use and interpretation of ultrasound images has impaired its widespread use.[6]

A fundamental clinical application of intraoperative ultrasound is imaging the bile ducts, liver, and pancreas. Operative cholangiography commonly is used to detect choledocholithiasis and define ductal anatomy, but this examination may result in a higher than necessary incidence of negative common bile duct explorations.[7] Intraoperative ultrasound assessment of the biliary tree has been compared with cholangiography in two large series of more than 400 patients each.[8,9] In both series, the accuracy of intraoperative ultrasound was found to be 98 percent versus 94 percent for cholangiography. Intraoperative ultrasound assessment of the extrahepatic biliary ductal system was quick to do (10 min or less), inexpensive, did not require isolation and cannulation of the cystic duct, and provided additional information about surrounding anatomy that cholangiography could not.

The most common contemporary use of intraoperative ultrasound is to facilitate various operations on the liver. Intraoperative ultrasound appears to be the most sensitive imaging modality to detect tumors. In a series of 152 patients with tumors less than 5 cm in size, intraoperative ultrasound was able to detect 198 of 203 tumors, a sensitivity of 98 percent. The sensitivities of preoperative ultrasound, angiography, and computed tomography were 89 percent, 84 percent, and 90 percent, respectively.[10] Systematic ultrasound examination of the liver during surgery for colorectal cancer appears to be more sensitive in the detection of metastatic disease than any preoperative imaging methods or direct palpation by the surgeon.[11] A technique was described for operative ultrasound of the liver, and its utility was emphasized for identification of the normal anatomic relationships in the liver, for recognition of anatomic anomalies, and for recognition of pathologic lesions and determination of their resectability.[12] The functional vascular anatomy of the liver described by Couinaud[13] is characterized by much variability. Direct intraoperative ultrasound examination is the only practical method to determine hepatic vascular anatomy rapidly. Intraoperative decision making regarding treatment of hepatic tumors may be influenced by its use in up to 49 percent of patients.[14,15] Tumors thought to be unresectable because of putative vascular involvement on the basis of preoperative imaging studies often are found to be technically resectable when examined using intraoperative ultrasound. The converse also is true. Tumors thought resectable on the basis of preoperative imaging studies occasionally are found to be inoperable. Intraoperative ultrasound examination may be helpful in determining the extent of resection. Ultrasound localization of a tumor to one of the eight hepatic segments may allow a segmental resection instead of lobectomy or trisegmentectomy.[16,17] This approach has been demonstrated to influence the outcome of patients undergoing operation for hepatocellular carcinoma positively in one series, particularly those with concomitant hepatic cirrhosis.[10]

The pancreas is one of the most difficult organs to assess adequately using extracorporeal imaging techniques. Intraoperative ultrasound may influence operative management in patients with pancreatic carcinoma.[18] New diagnostic information was added by intraoperative ultrasound examination of the pancreas and surrounding structures in 18 percent of patients in one report. This technique is especially well suited for the operative management of endocrine tumors of the pancreas.[19-22] Direct ultrasound examination of the pancreas is more sensitive than palpation in detection, localization, and characterization of pancreatic masses during exploration for endocrine tumors. Intraoperative ultrasound also has been used during surgery to detect complications of pancreatitis.[23] Operative ultrasound was useful in localizing dilated ducts, pseudocysts, abcesses, and previously unsuspected conditions, such as a second or multiple pseudocysts.

ENDOSCOPIC ULTRASOUND

The first application of A-mode ultrasound technology for use with conventional flexible gastrointestinal endoscopy occurred in 1976.[24] Real-time endoscopic ultrasound has emerged as a useful technique to evaluate the gastrointestinal tract wall and adjacent structures. It is ideally suited for evaluating lesions arising from the gastrointestinal tract mucosa, in the wall of the gastrointestinal tract, and in the pancreas and retroperitoneum. The ultrasound transducer can be applied directly to the target under endoscopic visualization, allowing high frequencies to be used and resulting in superior resolution and image detail.

Endoscopic ultrasound can be done in two ways. Ultrasound probes can be passed to the area of interest through the working channel of a standard endoscope. Alternatively, a dedicated ultrasound endoscope can be used. The former technique can be used at the time of diagnostic endoscopy without the need to change the endoscope. This *through-the-scope* technique is limited, however, by the need to make the probes small enough to fit through an instrumentation channel. Small high-frequency transducers (20 MHz) can provide high resolution but have a limited field of view and shallow tissue penetration. The dedicated ultrasound endoscope uses variable frequency transducers (7.5 to 12 MHz) that provide good resolution but have improved tissue penetration and a wider field of view. These instruments are more difficult to maneuver than a standard flexible endoscope because of the stiff thick tip and the oblique limited viewing optics. Luminal strictures (e.g., esophageal carcinomas) occasionally are difficult to traverse. Currently, the transducers used include linear and phased arrays and mechanical sector transducers. Acoustic coupling is achieved by the use of a water-filled balloon mounted over the transducer or by filling the gastrointestinal lumen with saline.

Endoscopic ultrasound identifies five layers in the wall of the gastrointestinal tract. These correspond to the mucosa, muscularis mucosa, submucosa, muscularis propria, and the serosa. These layers are seen as alternating layers of hyperechoic and hypoechoic bands. Structures can be localized accurately to the layer from which they arise in the wall of the gastrointestinal tract. Lymph nodes adjacent to the gastrointestinal lumen also can be seen, particularly if they are enlarged.

The largest experience with intraluminal endoscopic ultrasound is in staging of esophageal, gastric, and rectal cancer. Endoscopic ultrasound is uniquely suited to evaluate local tumor extension and determine whether adjacent lymph nodes are enlarged. Compared with resected specimens, data obtained from preoperative ultrasound examination were accurate in determining the size and extent of esophageal carcinomas.[25] The overall accuracy was 89 percent in 104 patients. Overstaging (six percent) and understaging (five percent) was related to local inflammatory or radiation-induced tissue changes. For evaluating metastasis to lymph nodes, endoscopic ultrasound was less accurate than for staging of the primary tumor.[26] Lymph nodes were visualized easily; however, enlargement was often the result of inflammatory changes instead of metastatic tumor. Small normal-sized nodes also could harbor occult metastases. Careful assessment of ultrasound images and correlation with histologic findings may improve the future accuracy of endoscopic ultrasound for detecting lymph node metastasis. One method uses the following criteria: (1) lymph nodes with a hypoechoic pattern and clearly delineated boundaries are considered suggestive of malignancy, (2) direct extension of the primary tumor into the lymph node is considered pathognomonic of malignancy, and (3) lymph nodes with a hyperechoic pattern and indistinctly demarcated boundaries are considered benign. Using these criteria, the accuracy of endoscopic ultrasound assessment in the presence of metastasis in lymph nodes was 81 percent with a sensitivity of 95 percent and a specificity of 50 percent. The positive predictive value was 82 percent and negative predictive value, 94 percent.[25] Ultrasound-guided endoscopic transmural needle cytologic examination may improve diagnostic accuracy further.

The accuracy of endoscopic ultrasound for preoperative staging of gastric carcinoma is similar to that observed in esophageal cancer.[25] Endoscopic ultrasound was compared with resected specimens in 79 patients. The overall accuracy was 83 percent with overstaging and understaging in nine percent and eight percent, respectively. Correct assessment of the presence of tumor in lymph nodes was accomplished in 73 percent of patients with a sensitivity of 87 percent and a specificity of 48 percent. Such information, obtained without an operation, may allow stratification of the risk for lymph node involvement in certain patients with esophageal and gastric carcinoma. The unusual early cancer without lymph node involvement hypothetically might be treated and cured with endoscopic resection techniques.[27,28]

Many submucosal abnormalities occur in the gastrointestinal tract. These lesions usually are visualized during standard endoscopic examinations but are often indistinguishable from an extrinsic mass. Conventional imaging methods are accurate only in determining the diagnosis if the lesions are large. However, a characteristic endoscopic ultrasound image is seen with myogenic tumors, cysts, lipomas, and varices.[29,30] Endoscopic ultrasound (EUS) may be particularly helpful in the diagnosis and treatment of gastric lymphoma.[31,32] This technique presents a characteristic image for lymphoma that may be confirmed by obtaining an endoscopic biopsy specimen. The response to chemotherapy or radiotherapy similarly can be monitored. Endoscopic ultrasound also may be useful in the long-term follow-up of patients with gastrointestinal tract cancers after operative resection. The technique appears to be sensitive for detecting anastamotic recurrence.[33]

Imaging the pancreas and the retroperitoneum is a technically challenging endeavor and requires scanning from several different positions in the duodenum and stomach. Small tumors less than 1 cm in diameter can be detected with high-frequency EUS transducers, making this modality highly competitive or superior to more conventional imaging techniques.[34] Yasuda and coworkers[35] compared the ability of EUS to detect pancreatic cancer in 50 patients with conventional ultrasound, CT scan, endoscopic cholangiopancreatography, and angiogram. EUS was able to detect the tumors in all 50 patients; the other techniques were less successful: conventional ultrasound, 72 percent; CT scan, 78 percent; endoscopic cholangiopancreatography, 88 percent; and angiogram, 75 percent. It was particularly better for imaging tumors less than 2.0 cm in diameter. The preoperative assessment of the ability to resect pancreatic and periampulary cancer, based on involvement of vascular structures, was correct in 12 of 14 and seven of nine patients, respectively.[36] Intraluminal endoscopic ultrasound may be particularly useful in detecting small periampullary (Fig. 3-1) and neuroendocrine tumors (Fig. 3-2).[37]

Colorectal ultrasound can be done using a rigid rectoscope, a flexible echoendoscope, or a blind insertion of rigid ultrasound probes. The accuracy of transrectal ultrasound examination in determining the size of colorectal neoplasms is 78 percent to 100 percent.[38,39] The data concerning the detection of metastatic involvement of the lymph nodes are less promising with an accuracy of 50 percent to 75 percent.[40,41] Compared with CT scan, transrectal ultrasound was superior in determining the size and status of lymph nodes in patients with rectal cancer.[41,42] Transrectal ultrasound staging may allow treatment of early superficial tumors by endotransrectal resection.[43] There are a few reports of the use of endoscopic intraluminal ultrasound to evaluate benign colorectal diseases.[44,45] An intact

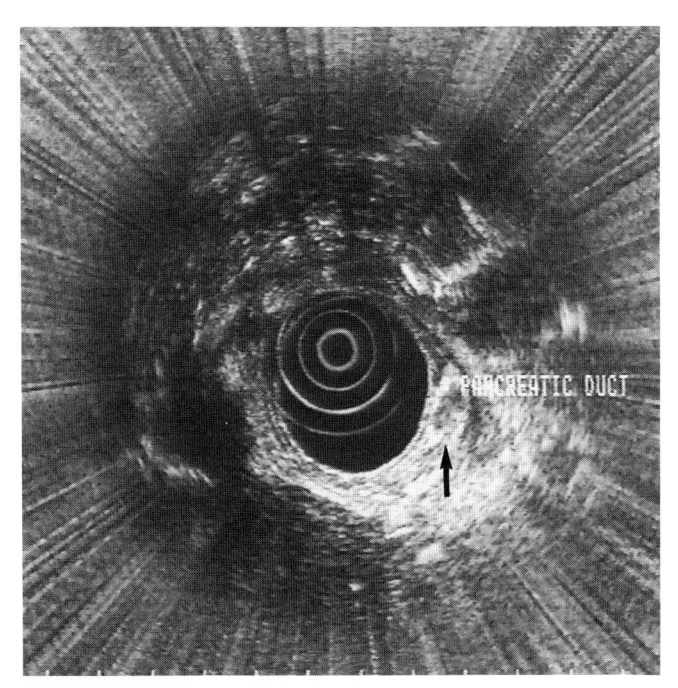

FIGURE 3-1 Endoscopic ultrasound demonstration of a small periampullary mass in a patient with epigastric pain (arrow). Extracorporeal ultrasound and CT scan showed a dilated pancreatic duct but did not reveal a mass. Attempts at endoscopic retrograde pancreatography were unsuccessful. (Photo courtesy of R. Matthew Reveille, MD.)

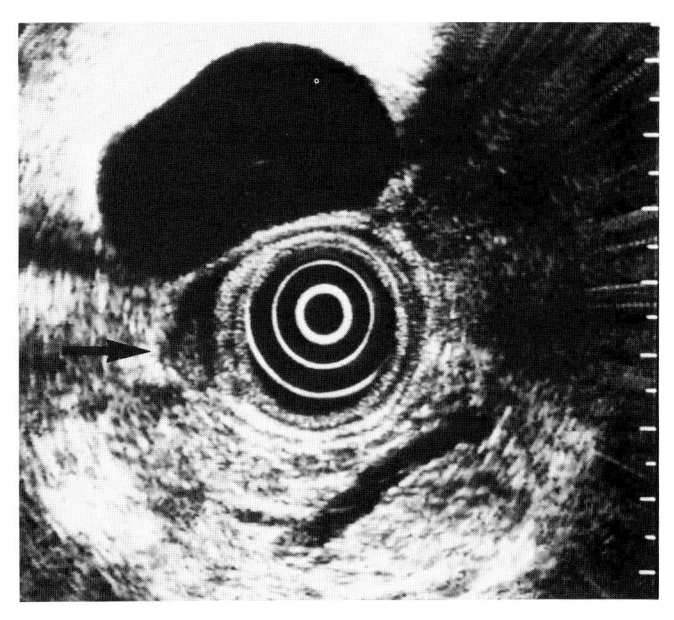

FIGURE 3-2 Endoscopic ultrasound demonstration of a mass in the wall of the duodenum in a patient with Zollinger-Ellison syndrome (arrow). The gallbladder is seen anteriorly, and the confluence of the splenic and superior mesenteric veins is visualized posterior to the duodenum. Preoperative conventional imaging modalities were unsuccessful in identifying a mass. This tumor was later confirmed to be a gastrinoma after surgical removal. (Photo courtesy of R. Matthew Reveille, MD.)

submucosa found ultrasonographically may be regarded as strong evidence in favor of benign disease. Intraluminal sonography also may be used to map anorectal abscess and fistulas accurately.[45]

The future of endoscopic intraluminal ultrasonography will be determined by both advances in technology and delineation of the clinical situation in which the ultrasound information will influence patient treatment and outcome. EUS evaluation of early esophageal, gastric, and rectal cancer may enable local endoscopic resection of tumors; however, follow-up studies are needed to determine if such therapies provide equivalent patient outcome compared with conventional operative treatment. This information also may be useful in decisions regarding preoperative or adjuvant therapy, assessment of therapeutic response, and detection of recurrent disease.

LAPAROSCOPIC INTRACORPOREAL ULTRASOUND

A logical extension of conventional intraoperative ultrasound is application of this technology to laparoscopic methods. The largest experience with laparoscopic ultrasound imaging has been in differential diagnosis of liver tumors.[46,47] Extracorporeal ultrasound and computed tomography are useful for scanning patients with mass lesions of the liver; however, both methods lack specificity. The technique of laparoscopic intracorporeal ultrasonography (LICU) uses higher frequency transducers to give more detailed images of the liver parenchyma and mass lesions. Seventy-five of 85 patients who underwent laparoscopic ultrasound examinations for suspected liver tumors had positive findings using this ultrasound technique.[48] Potential uses of this technique include directed tumor biopsy[49,50] and laparoscopic ultrasound-guided cryosurgery.[51]

LICU was useful to delineate the hepatobiliary anatomy in one animal study.[52] It was done using a 7.5-MHz linear-array 10-mm-diameter probe equipped with Doppler flow detection capability and was successful in visualizing the relationships between the cystic and common hepatic ducts and the entire common bile duct, including its entry into the duodenum. Ductal diameter measurements correlated well with those from cholangiograms and direct measurements obtained at necropsy. Portal vein and hepatic artery were identified easily using Doppler signals.

The use of LICU in humans to delineate biliary anatomy during cholecystectomy is promising.[53] This technique is done using the standard placement of trocars as in cholecystectomy. The specially designed laparoscopic ultrasound probe is introduced through the epigastric or midclavicular port (Fig. 3-3). LICU then is done by direct contact of the probe to the free edge of the hepatoduodenal ligament (Fig. 3-4). The ultrasound image and the videoscopic image from the laparoscope simultaneously is displayed on the television monitor. In one series of 22 patients, the examination was successful in 21 and required only 5 to 10 min of operating time.[53] Preliminary clinical experience from our institution confirmed the ease of this technique and the ability to determine cystic duct and common and hepatic duct relationships. A determination of the presence or absence of common duct calculi seems feasible and may obviate routine cholangiography.

COMMENTS AND CONCLUSIONS

Ultrasound is a useful, inexpensive, and safe imaging method. The accuracy and utility of intraoperative ultrasound done during conventional operations have been established in several clinical situations. Endoscopic intraluminal ultrasonography is useful both for staging gastrointestinal cancers and finding small tumors, particularly those in the peripancreatic region. New applications of intraoperative sonography during laparoscopy are being evaluated. LICU may have practical applications in the assessment of the biliary tract in patients with cholecystitis and also use in other areas.

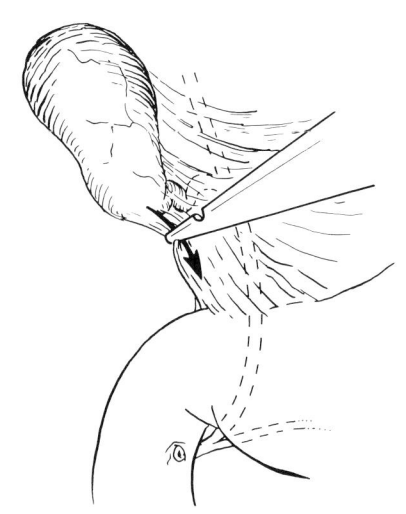

FIGURE 3-4 The probe is placed into direct contact with the free edge of the hepatoduodenal ligament. LICU is done by first visualizing the gallbladder, then tracing the cystic duct to the junction with the hepatic duct and the common bile duct to the upper border of the pancreas. Rotation of the probe clockwise allows visualization of the junction of the bile duct and duodenum.

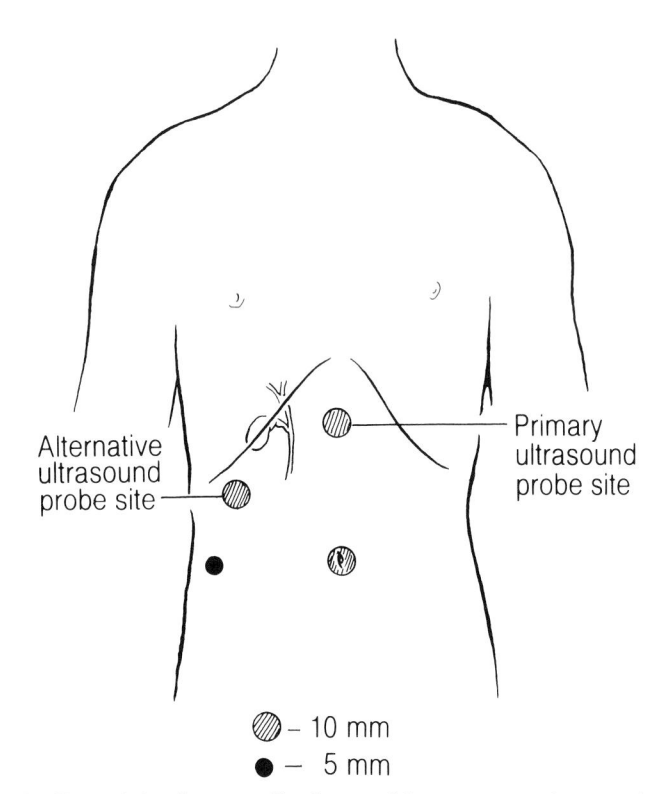

FIGURE 3-3 The specially designed laparoscopic ultrasound probe is introduced through the epigastric port, or alternatively it can be introduced through the midclavicular port.

REFERENCES

1. Schlegel JU, Diggdon P, Cuellar J: The use of ultrasound for localizing renal calculi. *J Urol* 1961; 86:367.
2. Hayashi S, Wagai T, Miyazawar R, et al: Ultrasonic diagnosis of breast tumor and cholelithiasis. *West J Surg Obstet Gynecol* Jan–Feb 1962; 70:34.
3. Eiseman B, Greenlaw RH, Gallagher JQ: Localization of common bile duct stones by ultrasound. *Arch Surg* 1965; 91:195.
4. Charboneau JW, Grant CS, James EM, et al: Diagnostic intraoperative ultrasound. *JAMA* 1985; 254:285.
5. Charnley RM, Hardcastle JD: Intraoperative abdominal ultrasound. *Gut* 1990; 31:368.
6. Sigel B: Advances in intraoperative ultrasound-introduction. *World J Surg* 1987; 11:557.
7. Doyle PJ, Ward-McQuaid JN, McEwen Smith A: The value of routine preoperative cholangiography: A report of 4000 cholecystectomies. *Br J Surg* 1982; 69:617.
8. Jakimowicz JJ, Rutten H, Jurgens PJ, Carol EJ: Comparison of operative ultrasonography and radiology in screening of the common bile duct for calculi. *World J Surg* 1987; 11:628.
9. Sigel B, Machi J, Beitler JC, et al: Comparative accuracy of operative ultrasonography and cholangiography in detecting common bile duct calculi. *Surgery* 1983; 94:715.
10. Makuuchi M, Hasegawa H, Yamazaki S, et al: The use of operative ultrasound as an aid to liver resection in patients with hepatocellular carcinoma. *World J Surg* 1987; 11:615.
11. Boldrini G, de Gaetano AM, Giovannini I, et al: The systematic use of operative ultrasound for detection of liver metastasis during colorectal surgery. *World J Surg* 1987; 11:622.
12. Castaing D, Kunstlinger F, Habib N, Bismuth H: Intraoperative ultrasonographic study of the liver-methods and anatomic results. *Am J Surg* 1985; 149:676.
13. Couinaud C: *Le foie. Etudes anatomiques et chirurgicales.* Paris, Masson, 1957.
14. Rifkin MD, Rosato FE, Branch HM, et al: Intraoperative ultrasound of the liver. An important adjunctive tool for decision making in the operating room. *Ann Surg* 1987; 205:466.

15. Parker GA, Lawrence W, Horsley S, et al: Intraoperative ultrasound of the liver affects operative decision making. *Ann Surg* 1989; 209:569.
16. Makuuchi M, Hasegawa H, Yamaziki S: Ultrasonically guided subsegmentectomy. *Surg Gynecol Obstet* 1985; 161:346.
17. Igawa S, Sakai K, Kinoshita H, Hirohashi K: Intraoperative sonography: Clinical usefulness in liver surgery. *Radiology* 1985; 156:473.
18. Plainfosse MC, Bouillot JL, Rivaton F, et al: The use of operative sonography in carcinoma of the pancreas. *World J Surg* 1987; 11:654.
19. Angelini L, Bezzi M, Tucci G, et al: The ultrasonic detection of insulinomas during surgical exploration of the pancreas. *World J Surg* 1987; 11:642.
20. Cromack DT, Norton JA, Sigel B, et al: The use of high-resolution intraoperative ultrasound to localize gastrinomas: An initial report of a prospective study. *World J Surg* 1987; 11:648.
21. Klotter HK, Ruckert K, Kummerle F, Rothmund M: The use of intraoperative sonography in endocrine tumors of the pancreas. *World J Surg* 1987; 11:635.
22. Gunther RW, Klose KJ, Ruckert K, et al: Localization of small islet cell tumors. Preoperative and intraoperative ultrasound, computed tomography, arteriography, digital subtraction angiography, and pancreatic venous sampling. *Gastrointest Radiol* 1985; 10:145.
23. Sigel B, Machi J, Kikuchi T, et al: The use of ultrasound during surgery for complications of pancreatitis. *World J Surg* 1987; 11:659.
24. Lutz H, Rosch W: Transgastroscopic ultrasonography. *Endoscopy* 1976; 8:203.
25. Tio TL, Coene PPLO, Luiken GJHN, Tytgat GNJ: Endosonography in the clinical staging of esophagogastric carcinoma. *Gastrointest Endosc* 1990; 36:S2.
26. Tio T, Tytgat GNJ: Endoscopic ultrasonography in analysing periintestinal lymph node abnormality. *Scand J Gastroenterol* 1986; 21:S158.
27. Yasuda K, Kuyota K, Nakajima M, Kawai K: Endolaser therapy (ELT) for gastrointestinal tumors: New aspects of endoscopic ultrasonography (EUS). *Endoscopy* 1987; 19:2.
28. Imacka K: Is curative endoscopic treatment of early gastric cancer possible. *Endoscopy* 1987; 19:7.
29. Yasuda K, Nakajima M, Yoshida S, et al: The diagnosis of submucosal tumors of the stomach by endoscopic ultrasonography. *Gastrointest Endosc* 1989; 35:10.
30. Yasuda K, Cho E, Nakajima M, Kawai K: Diagnosis of submucosal lesions of the upper gastrointestinal tract by endoscopic ultrasonography. *Gastrointest Endosc* 1990; 36:S17.
31. Tio T, Ad HJFC, Tytgat GNJ: Endoscopic ultrasonography of non-Hodgkin lymphoma of the stomach. *Gastroenerology* 1986; 91:401.
32. Caletti GC, Lorena Z, Bolondi L, Gruzzardi G, Brocchi E, Bulara L: Impact of endoscopic ultrasound on the diagnosis and treatment of primary gastric lymphoma. *Surgery* 1988; 103:315.
33. Lightdale CJ, Botet JF, Kelsen DP, Turnbull AD, Brennan MF: Diagnosis of recurrent upper gastrointestinal cancer at the surgical anastomosis by endoscopic ultrasound. *Gastrointest Endosc* 1989; 35:407.
34. Boyce GA, Sivack MV: Endoscopic ultrasonography in the diagnosis of pancreatic tumors. *Gastrointest Endosc* 1990; 36:528.
35. Yasuda K, Mukai H, Fujimoto S, Nakajima M, Kawai K: The diagnosis of pancreatic cancer by endoscopic ultrasound. *Gastrointest Endosc* 1988; 34:1.
36. Tio TL, Tytgat GNJ: Endoscopic ultrasound in staging local resectability of pancreatic and periampulary malignancy. *Scand J Gastroenterol* 1986; 21:S135.
37. Heyder N: Localization of an insulinoma by endoscopic ultrasound. *N Engl J Med* 1985; 312:860.
38. Tio T, Tytgat GNJ: Comparison of blind transrectal ultrasound with endoscopic transrectal ultrasonography in assessing rectal and perirectal diseases. *Scand J Gastroenterol* 1986; 21:S104.
39. Yamashita Y, Machi J, Shirouzu K: Evaluation of endorectal ultrasound for the assessment of wall invasion of rectal cancer. *Dis Colon Rectum* 1988; 31:617.
40. Saitoh N, Okui K, Sarashina H, et al: Evaluation of echographic diagnosis of rectal cancer using intrarectal ultrasonic examination. *Dis Colon Rectum* 1986; 29:234.
41. Rifkin MD, Ehrlich SM, Marks G: Staging of rectal carcinoma: Prospective comparison of endorectal US and CT. *Radiology* 1988; 170:319.
42. Beynon J, McMortensen NJ, Foy DMA, et al: Pre-operative assessment of local invasion in rectal cancer: Digital examination, endoluminal sonography, or computed tomography. *Br J Surg* 1986; 73:1015.
43. Buess G, Mentges B, Manncke K, Starlinger M, Becker HD: Technique and results of transanal endoscopic microsurgery in early rectal cancer. *Am J Surg* 1992; 163:63.
44. Doble A, Sim AJW: Endoluminal ultrasound in benign anorectal disease (abstract). *Gut* 1987; 28:A1369.
45. Tio T, Mulder CJJ, Wijers OB, et al: Endosonography of peri-anal and peri-colorectal fistula and/or abscess in Crohn's disease. *Gastrointest Endosc* 1990; 36:331.
46. Fukuda M, Mima F, Nakano Y: Studies in echolaparoscopy. *Scand J Gastroenterol* 1982; 17(suppl 78):186.
47. Fukuda M, Mima S, Tanabet S: Endoscopic sonography of the liver: Diagnostic application of the echolaparoscope to localize intrahepatic lesions. *Scand J Gastroenterol* 1984; 19(suppl 102):24.
48. Fukuda M: The role of laparoscopic ultrasonography in the differential diagnosis of liver tumors. *Clin Diagn Ultrasound* 1987; 22:151.
49. Boenhof JA, Linhart P, Bettendorf U, et al: Liver biopsy guided by laparoscopic sonography. *Endoscopy* 1984; 16:237.
50. Ido K, Kawamoto C, Ohtani M, Hitomi N, Ichiyama M, Kimura K: Tumor biopsy under the peritoneoscopic ultrasonogram guidance. *Gastrointest Endosc* 1989; 31:1528.
51. Ravikumar HS, Kane R, Cady B, et al: Hepatic cryosurgery with intraoperative ultrasound monitoring for metastatic colon carcinoma. *Arch Surg* 1987; 122:403.
52. Yamamoto M, Steigmann G, Durham J, et al: Laparoscope guided intracorporeal ultrasound accurately delineates hepatobiliary anatomy (abstract). *Surg Endosc* 1992; 6:90.
53. Jakimowicz J: Intraoperative and postoperative biliary endoscopy. Intraoperative ultrasonography and sonography during laparoscopic cholecystectomy. *Problems in General Surgery* 1991; 8:442.

Chapter 4

Laser Physics and Tissue Interaction

John G. Hunter

In the mind of the public, there is nothing that epitomizes high tech surgery more than the laser. Since the era of Buck Rogers, with his disintegrator laser beam pistol, Americans have been infatuated with the notion of destroying nasty things with silent, deadly beams of light. Although the public is able to accept that the laser is capable of instant disintegration of matter, they have not been able to make the leap to realizing that such disintegration used on their bodies might hurt. Part of the equation coupling lasers with painless surgery has been advertisements by physicians and their hospitals linking laser with minimally invasive, outpatient surgery. Thus, many patients who are seeking high technology, minimally invasive procedures will ask their physician for *laser surgery*. Once the illusion, mystery, and magic have been set aside, the laser remains a very valuable surgical tool, with a wide variety of applications, as will be discussed in subsequent chapters. In this chapter, we will introduce laser physics and discuss a variety of ways in which lasers interact with tissue.

LASER PHYSICS

Laser is an acronym for light amplification by stimulated emission of radiation. An understanding of laser physics is based on the comprehension that light acts both as a particle and a wave. The light *particle,* the photon, is responsible for initiating and amplifying a beam of light in which all light *waves* are synchronized in time and space, the *laser beam.*

The theory of laser operation was conceived by Einstein and perfected by Townes and Maiman in the late 1950s and early 1960s.[1-3] To understand how a laser works, we must start with the lasing medium (Fig. 4-1). This medium may be an elemental gas such as argon or a molecular gas such as carbon dioxide (CO_2) or argon fluoride. Another type of gas laser is the metal vapor laser; copper and gold vapor lasers are two examples of this kind of laser. The lasing medium may be a naturally occurring crystalline material, such as a ruby, or a composite crystal in which a crystalline host is mixed with other elements to form a "doped" crystal. The most common crystalline host is yttrium aluminum garnet (YAG). Doping YAG crystals has allowed the creation of several lasers that are used in medicine and industry, the neodymium (Nd) YAG, the holmium (Ho) YAG, and the erbium (Er) YAG lasers. The laser medium may be a liquid dye, such as rhodamine (red) or coumarin (green). Lastly, we are beginning to see the development of high-power diode lasers. Diodes are layers of semiconductors that will produce photons (and laser beams) when subjected to an electrical charge. The principal advantage of diode lasers are their tremendous efficiency, requiring only battery power when used in a laser pointer.

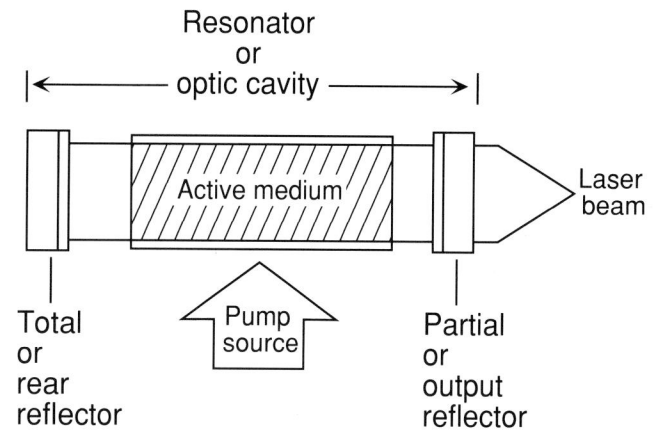

FIGURE 4-1 The basic components of a laser include the laser medium and optical cavity, with a total reflecting mirror and a partial reflecting mirror. The lasing medium is activated by an external energy source.

When a bright light or an electrical spark is discharged into a lasing medium, the light or electrical energy is transferred to the laser medium by raising electrons to unstable, high-energy states (Fig. 4-2). When one of these electrons spontaneously returns to its ground state, this transition will be heralded by the release of a photon. As this photon encounters another unstable electron, a second (stimulated) decay event occurs, resulting in two electrons with

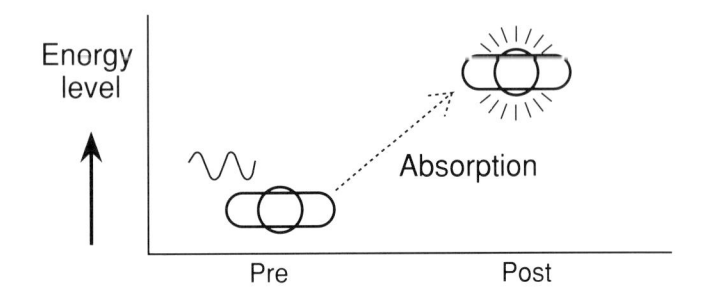

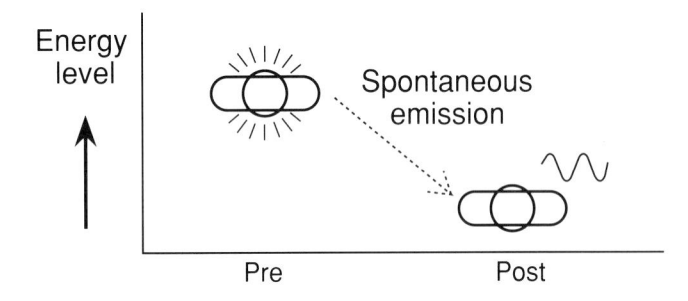

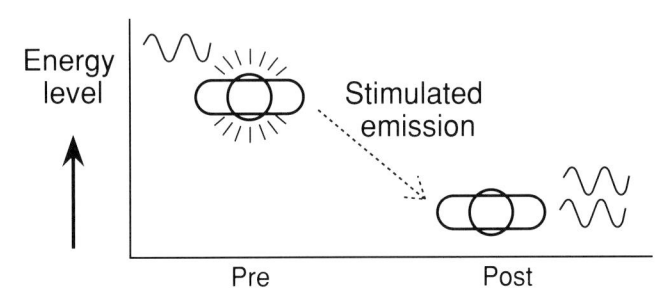

FIGURE 4-2 An electron in its ground state, orbiting the nucleus, receives energy from the pump. This energy raises the electron to an unstable energy state. When the electron spontaneously returns to its ground state, a photon of light that is characteristic of that atom is emitted. When this photon strikes a second excited electron, a stimulated decay event occurs, resulting in two photons that are in phase across time and space.

identical wave properties. They will have the same wavelength, the waves will be parallel, and the wave crests will be synchronized across time and space. As these two photons encounter two more unstable electrons, two more decay events occur, producing four photons with identical energies and wave properties. As this binomial growth occurs, a population explosion of a single "clone" of photons creates a beam of *coherent* light.

Coherent light is light of a single wavelength (monochromatic), in which all the wave fronts are in phase across time and space (Fig. 4-3). A laser beam is nothing more than a collimated beam of coherent light. The reason why a laser beam has a greater ability to heat tissue than an equivalent amount of noncoherent light is that the crests of all the light waves traveling together create a wave amplitude that is the sum of the individual wave energies. An analogous macroscopic situation is the meeting of two ocean wave crests. The size (amplitude) of the wave increases substantially at the meeting point. Imagine the size if several million 2-foot ocean waves were fused into a single wave! The power of the laser beam is determined by the number of waves (photons) that are marching in rank. This number is determined by the number of unstable electrons available for stimulated emission. The number of unstable electrons is determined by the chemical and physical properties of the laser medium and the amount of energy applied by the electrical power source.

In the lasing medium, coherent light is emitted in all directions. For lasing to occur, a laser cavity must be designed around the lasing material. Photons that align themselves along the axis of a laser cavity encounter mirrors at either end that allow the beam to resonate and amplify until a high energy level is reached. One of the mirrors is designed to allow a portion of the energy to escape, forming the laser beam. Photons emitted in directions away from the laser cavity are not amplified and are dissipated as heat. In some laser systems, greater than 99 percent of the input energy is dissipated as heat. Only one percent becomes the laser beam. Because of such tremendous inefficiency, most lasers require extensive electrical power sources and cooling systems.

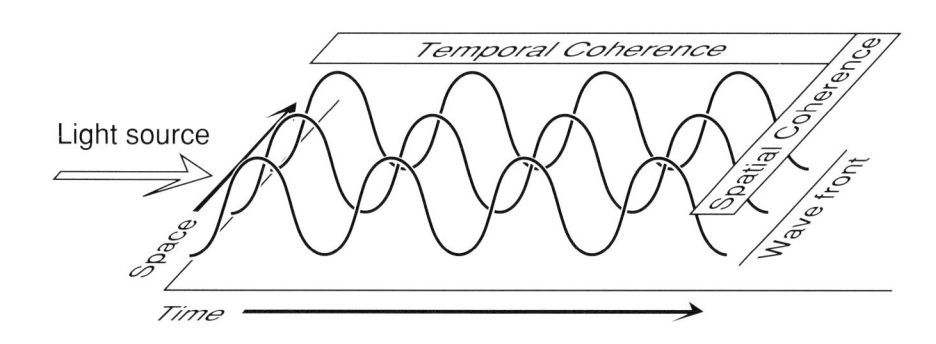

FIGURE 4-3 The unique feature of a laser beam is its coherence. Its power is derived from the fact that all wave crests are in phase across time and space.

LASER PULSING

Laser beams may be emitted as a continuous wave or a chopped wave. They may be rapidly or slowly pulsed (Fig. 4-4). Most medical lasers are continuous-wave lasers. When the surgeon puts a foot on the laser pedal, the lasing medium is stimulated to produce laser light that will last as long as the foot is on the pedal or until an internal timer shuts off the laser. Typical laser powers range from 1 to 100 W. The total energy delivered is the product of power and time (energy [in Joules]) = power [in Watts] × time [in seconds]). Chopped laser energy is produced by moving a shutter in and out of the path of the laser beam. The peak power produced by a chopped beam is no different from that of a continuous beam.

Laser pulsing occurs when the input power and, hence, the laser beam power varies as a function of time. The medical uses of pulsed lasers will be discussed later in this chapter. High-frequency pulsed lasers, such as the copper vapor laser (6000 cycles/s), produce laser light that is, for all intents and purposes, continuous, and the peak power of the pulsed laser beam is little different from a continuous wave laser.

Most low-frequency, pulsed lasers produce extremely short (10^{-6} to 10^{-12} s) pulses with extremely high peak powers (10^4 to 10^{10} W). The short pulse is created from electrical circuitry that allows rapid discharge of large amounts of electron or photon energy into the laser medium over short increments of time. Electrical capacitors discharged into a bright xenon lamp (a flash lamp) provide the energy for flash lamp-pumped dye lasers, used with a short pulse (1 μs) for gallstone and kidney stone fragmentation or with a long pulse (100 μs) for rupturing capillary networks in cutaneous port-wine stains. When these lasers are used, dosimetry is reported as the energy delivered per pulse (1 to 100 mJ) rather than the peak power of the impulse or the total amount of energy required. Typical dosimetry for gallstone fragmentation would involve 60 mJ and 1-μs pulses. The average power over the 1-μs pulse is calculated at 60 kW.

A *Q-switch* is another type of trigger, in which the rapid discharge of electrical power is used, not to stimulate the medium, but to align the mirrors in the optical cavity so that a continuously excited population of unstable electrons is able to *lase* (i.e., spontaneous decay events are able to stimulate emission and amplification of coherent light in the optical cavity). Because the unstable, high-energy electron population is allowed to build to such extremes between pulses, Q-switching is capable of generating a very high-energy laser pulse. The length of the pulse is determined by the length of time the mirrors are aligned, and this can be as little as 1 ns.[4] Q-switching has found few medical applications but has been used in industrial Nd:YAG lasers for some time. The tissue effects of high peak power pulsed lasers which are entirely different from those achieved with continuous, chopped, and high-frequency pulsed lasers will be discussed later.

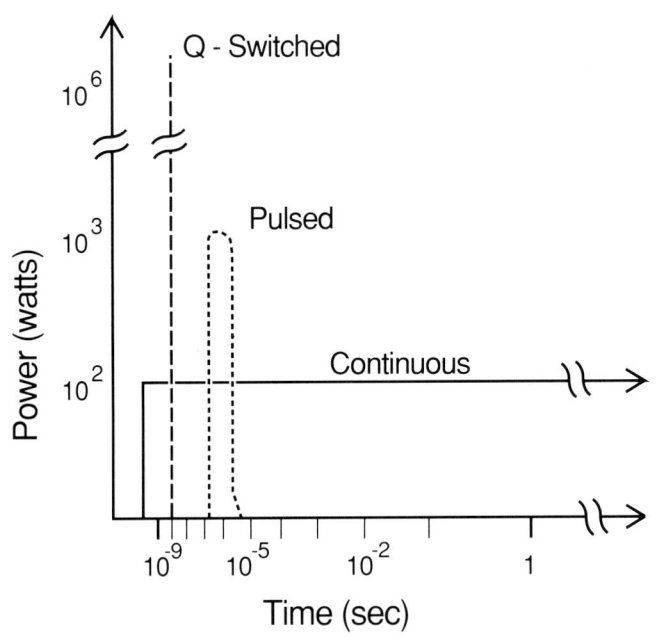

FIGURE 4-4 Laser output may be a continuous wave, in which a steady state is reached between electron excitement and stimulated emission. With a pulsed laser, a high-energy pulse is generated by dumping a large amount of energy into a lasing medium over a short period of time (microseconds). With a q-switched laser, a population of unstable electrons is allowed to build up in the tube, and then a momentary alignment of the optical cavity allows for a very high energy pulse of light to be emitted over a very short period of time (nanoseconds).

LASER DELIVERY SYSTEMS

When a laser beam is emitted from a laser chamber (tube), it will disperse unless it is focused with a lens. Many lasers have such lenses, but the purpose of the lens may vary. In a laser pointer, the lens collimates the beam so that the spot size remains the same whether it is 2 ft or 200 ft from the target. In most medical CO_2 lasers, delivered through a mechanical arm full of mirrors, an initial lens will collimate the beam, and a second lens in the handpiece will focus the laser energy to a point approximately 50 μm in diameter. Such an arrangement allows for surgical flexibility. At the focal point of the laser beam, a high concentration of coherent photons causes rapid tissue heating and vaporization. If the target tissue is beyond the focal point, the laser impact zone is much larger, allowing for more gradual tissue heating and superior coagulation (Fig. 4-5). Lastly, the lens may focus the beam on the end of a long, extruded quartz crystal, a laser fiber. The laser light, captured in the fiber, is released at the end with great-

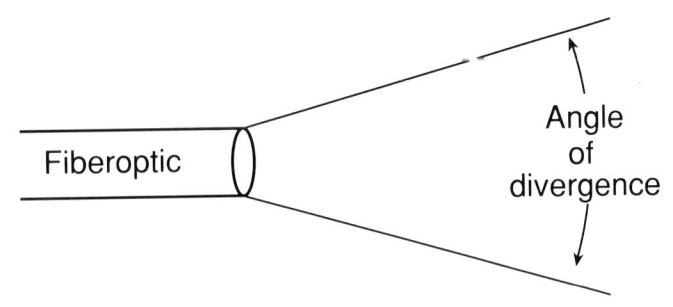

FIGURE 4-5 Energy from a quartz fiber is divergent, and the angle of divergence creates a rapidly diminishing beam intensity the further the beam is from the fiber tip. The greatest single factor in determining tissue power density is the distance of the laser fiber from the tissue.

er than 95 percent transmission efficiency. Unless a lens is placed at the end, the laser beam will diverge as it leaves the fiber, reducing the power density (in Watts/cm^2) exponentially as the distance from fiber tip to tissue increases (Fig. 4-5).

For minimally invasive surgery, fiberoptic delivery of laser energy is superior to rigid, articulating arms. The limitation of fiberoptic delivery is the optical nature of a quartz fiber. Wavelengths shorter than 250 nm and longer than 2500 nm will not transmit through quartz fibers. This limitation applies primarily to the CO_2 laser because other short- or long-wavelength lasers (e.g., excimer and Er:YAG lasers) have not been cleared or marketed for medical applications. Alternative fiber materials, such as zirconium fluoride, have been developed for infrared laser energy delivery but have not been proved to be satisfactory because of expense and fragility. Items touted to be CO_2 laser fibers have been developed for laparoscopic surgery but have really been nothing more than hollow tubes with high internal reflectance.

Another delivery system of some popularity for endoscopic application utilizes *contact tips,* in which laser light is converted to heat by absorption of the laser energy at the end of the fiber. This conversion may be effected with a piece of metal, such as that used in laser angioplasty, or a sapphire crystal that is frosted to absorb the laser light before it escapes the fiber. The simplest contact tip is a cleaved quartz fiber, which is placed in contact with the tissue until a layer of carbon (a product of tissue vaporization) builds up on the tip. The laser energy is then absorbed by the carbon and heats to the point at which the laser fiber can be used to slice through tissue like a warm knife through butter. A quartz fiber drawn down to a fine tip may be used for fine incisions, and a quartz fiber extruded into a large orb will distribute the heat over a larger area and may give better tactile feedback to keep the surgeon in the correct plane and help identify large vessels before slicing into them.

WAVELENGTHS OF MONOCHROMATIC LIGHT AVAILABLE FOR MEDICAL USE

As has been stated previously, lasers are characterized by the lasing medium from which the beam is created. Each medium emits one (occasionally several) characteristic wavelength of light, determined by the nature of the electron decay events. Lasing media have been identified that are capable of producing monochromatic, coherent light from the ultraviolet through the visible and far into the infrared portions of the electromagnetic spectrum (Fig. 4-6). Before receiving Food and Drug Administration approval for medical application, each new laser wavelength must undergo extensive testing to ensure its safety. The wavelengths currently approved or under investigation for medical use are discussed in this section.

In the ultraviolet portion of the spectrum, excimer (excited dimer) lasers produce light at 193, 266, 308, and 355 nm.[5] The dimers producing these wavelengths are argon fluoride, krypton fluoride, xenon chloride, and xenon fluoride, respectively. Visible wavelength lasers most commonly used by surgeons are the argon laser (λ = 488 and 514 nm), which produces blue-green light, and the KTP laser (Lasersonics, San Jose, CA), which produces green light (λ = 532 nm). KTP stands for potassium thionyl chloride, the components of a crystal put in the path of a standard Nd:YAG laser beam to double the frequency (or halve the wavelength) of the laser beam. The Nd:YAG laser (λ = 1064 nm) was one of the first high-power (> 100 W), continuous-wave lasers made for medical application. This laser is in the near-infrared portion of the spectrum and is invisible to the eye. (The visible spectrum ends at approximately 700 nm.) Newer YAG doped lasers, such as Ho:YAG and Er:YAG, have wavelengths in the midinfrared spectrum, 2.1 μm (or 2100 nm) and 2.9 μm, respectively.[6-8] In the far-infrared portion of the spectrum is the CO_2 laser, which produces a light wavelength of 10.6 μm.

Other medically useful lasers utilize various visible and near-infrared portions of the spectrum. Dye lasers, used with an extremely short pulse for lithotripsy or an ex-

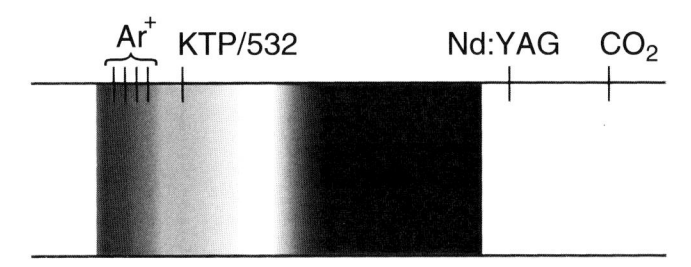

FIGURE 4-6 Lasers produce monochromatic light ranging across the entire electromagnetic spectrum from ultraviolet to infrared. Some examples of lasers to be discussed are diagrammed.

tremely long pulse for photodynamic therapy, have been filled with vital dyes ranging from violet ($\lambda = 350$ nm) through deep red ($\lambda = 650$ nm).[9] Diode lasers have characteristic wavelengths varying from 650 to 850 nm.[10-11] The copper vapor laser used by dermatologists produces yellow light ($\lambda = 566$ nm) and is used for treatment of facial telangiectasia.[12]

LASER–TISSUE INTERACTION

The medical and surgical application of new wavelengths of laser light has been driven by laser manufacturers, not by physicians. When a new wavelength of laser light is discovered, the manufacturer will turn it over to the biological scientist to "see what it can do." As physicians and other biologists better learn the nature of the interaction between light and cells, it may be possible to turn the process around and develop new lasers to fill the requirements of the biologic task.

Clearly, a single laser that could be tuned like a radio to different wavelengths across the entire magnetic spectrum, regulated like a metronome to different pulse lengths from microseconds to continuous wave, and adjusted like an amplifier from milliwatts to megawatts of power would be ideal for medical application, but no device encompassing even two of these three degrees of flexibility has been built.

The most instantly tunable laser currently in existence is the free-electron laser, which costs several million dollars to build and requires thousands of square feet of space for the hardware. The free-electron laser differs from most lasers in that the photon beam starts as an accelerated electron beam.[5] The electron beam initially has no wave characteristics but is accelerated in an axis perpendicular to its original axis by a series of electromagnets with alternating polarities, known as a *wiggler* (Fig. 4-7). If sufficiently accelerated, the electron beam, now with a sinusoidal (wave) pattern, will spontaneously emit photon energy. The emitted photon beam is, indeed, coherent, and its wavelength can be adjusted (tuned) by altering the charge on the wiggler magnets. Theoretically, the electromagnets can be adjusted to produce an electron beam with wavelengths ranging from ultraviolet to infrared; however, the tunable range of most existing free-electron lasers is only a small portion of the electromagnetic spectrum.

Given the limitations of existing technology, a surgeon in search of the ideal instrument to perform a particular task must be familiar with the range of instrument–tissue interactions available for each surgical instrument and tis-

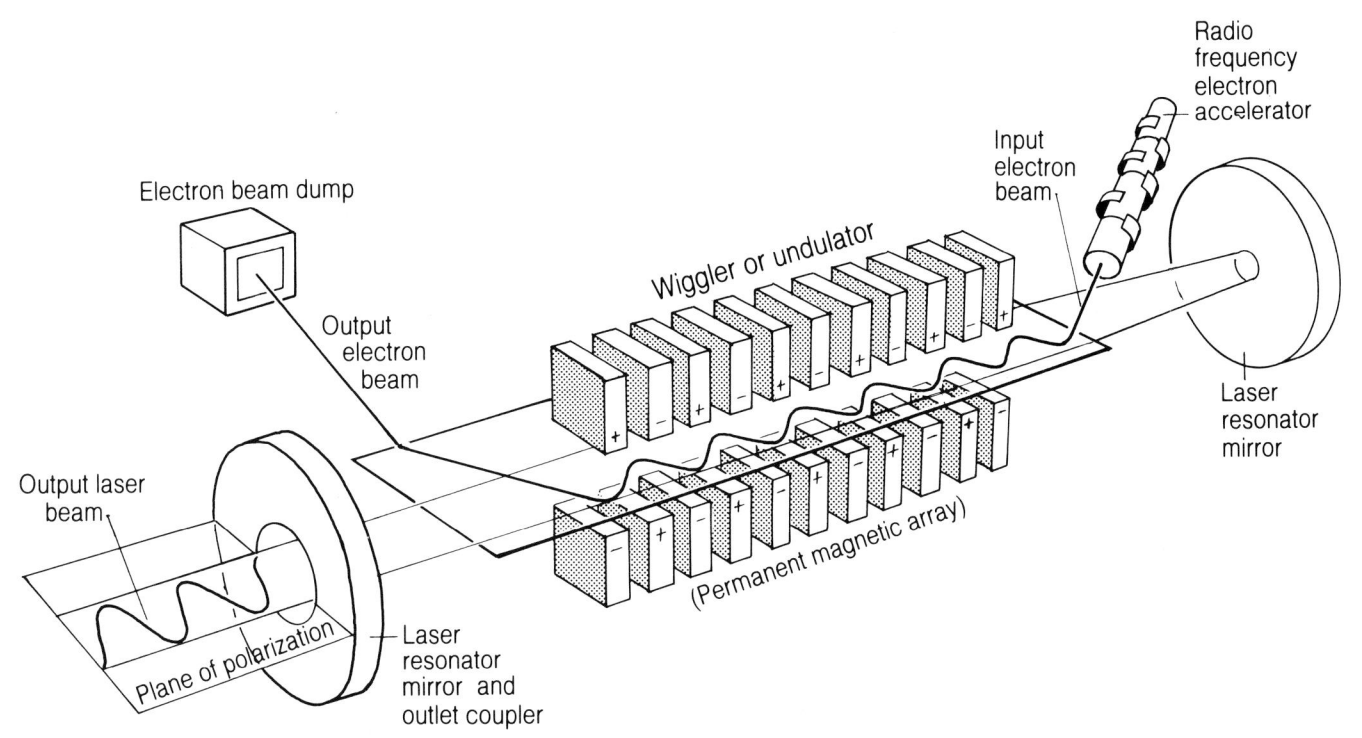

FIGURE 4-7 A free-electron laser generates a laser beam from an accelerated electron beam, which is then further accelerated between electromagnets. The excess energy generated is dissipated as a photon beam, which can be adjusted in wavelength by adjusting the charge. The beam produced is, indeed, polarized, allowing the power of the laser beam to be easily adjusted with a polarizing filter.

sue. A basic example of such a concept is the use of the scalpel. During a hepatectomy, the sharp blade of the scalpel is used to cut the dermis, and the blunt handle of the scalpel is used to separate the liver parenchyma from bile ducts and vessels bluntly. When surgeons encounter excessive bleeding, using the scalpel handle to fracture the liver, they will probably ask whether a superior technology might be available for hepatectomy. It is a goal of this book to help answer that question. In the remaining portion of this chapter, the goal is to describe the wide range of laser–tissue interactions across the electromagnetic spectrum and across pulse profiles to help the surgeon establish whether laser technology is the desired tool. We will start by discussing the nature of the interaction between light and tissue.

Absorption of Laser Light by Tissue

Tissue is composed of many chromophores, which are, as their name implies, substances that absorb light. The best understood tissue chromophores include water, hemoglobin, melanin, hematoporphyrin, and bilirubin. Each of these chromophores has a particular pattern of light absorption across the electromagnetic spectrum (Fig. 4-8). For example, water highly absorbs light in the ultraviolet and infrared portions of the spectrum. Thus, lasers designed to vaporize tissue with a high water content would utilize a wavelength in the ultraviolet or infrared portion of the spectrum. In the visible portion of the spectrum, it is "crystal clear" to anyone looking through a water glass that visible wavelengths of light are not absorbed by water. Light in the visible portion of the electromagnetic spectrum is absorbed by tissue chromophores, especially chromophores of a color complementary to the beam of light. Thus, a red lesion, such as a telangiectasia of the right colon, is well treated with a green laser, such as KTP. Dermatologists and plastic surgeons have used a yellow dye in their pulsed dye lasers to treat burgundy port-wine stains.[12] When the laser target is black, such as a pigment gallstone, all laser wavelengths will be well absorbed.

When faced with a darkly colored tissue, where almost any laser could be used, the surgeon should look beyond the target tissue and focus on the background tissue, which should be spared injury. A laser should be chosen which will be most absorbed by the desired target and least absorbed by the background tissue. Currently, this decision may be made empirically or by comparing spectrophotometric analyses of the target and the background material.[9] The ideal laser system would incorporate a spectrophotometer to scan both target and background material, calculate the ideal wavelength where this difference was greatest, and then tune the laser beam to deliver light at that wavelength. The ideal power could be calculated from the spectrophotometric profile or determined by surgical observation of tissue effect. A laser that is commercially available for endovascular application incorporates spectroscopic analysis of the vessel lumen to distinguish atherosclerotic plaque from normal arterial wall before application of laser energy (see Chap. 31).

Scattering of Laser Light in Tissue

Choosing a laser wavelength that is complementary to the color of the lesion to be treated minimizes penetration of energy and is most protective of adjacent tissue. Sometimes, the surgeon wishes to penetrate tissue deeply and may, thus, choose a laser wavelength that is poorly absorbed by tissue chromophores. When light is not readily absorbed by tissue chromophores, it is widely scattered through collision and refraction by cellular elements. Because water and hemoglobin are the predominant chromophores in tissue, laser wavelengths with the least absorption by these molecules will promote the greatest scattering in tissue and, hence, the greatest depth and width of tissue heating. If we study the plot of absorption coefficient as a function of wavelength (see Fig. 4-8), we can see that the nadir of hemoglobin and water absorption is in the near-infrared spectrum at the wavelength of the Nd:YAG laser. Nd:YAG laser energy is deeply scattered in tissue, thereby causing slow, even heating of a large volume of tissue. Predictably, the primary endoscopic application of the Nd:YAG laser is palliative ablation of obstructing or bleeding gastrointestinal cancers, where deep penetration of laser energy helps destroy the maximum volume of tumor

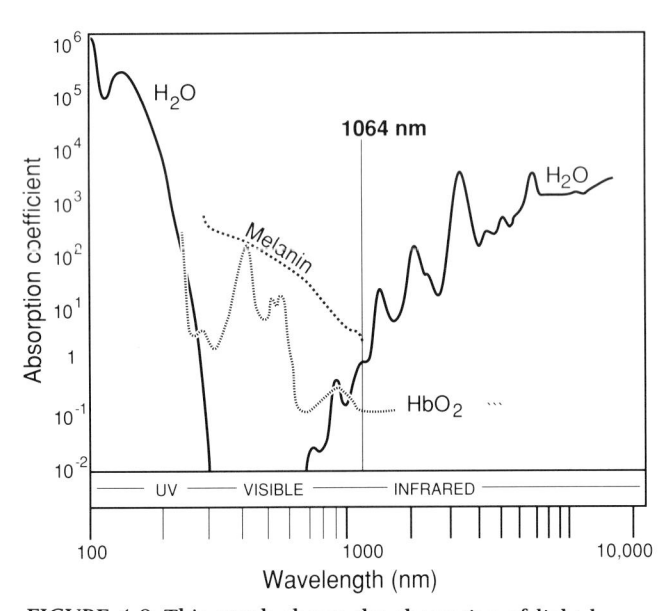

FIGURE 4-8 This graph shows the absorption of light by various tissue compounds (water, melanin, and oxyhemoglobin) as a function of the wavelength of the light. The nadir of the oxyhemoglobin and melanin curves is close to 1064, the wavelength of the Nd:YAG laser.

per treatment. In addition, uniform deep heating allows better coagulation of blood vessels than a superficially absorbed laser that may vaporize the front wall of the vessel before the column of blood is coagulated.

Tissue Effects of Laser Pulsing

After choosing a laser wavelength based on its high or low absorption by tissue chromophores, the surgeon must decide how to deliver the energy. That is, should the energy be delivered in short pulses or should it be delivered continuously? As a general rule, lasers injure tissue by heating it. The type of injury, whether coagulation or vaporization, is a direct function of the temperature achieved at any point in the tissue impinged by the laser beam (see Chap. 5, Fig. 5-1). Given a constant amount of total energy, the type and spatial confinement of injury depends on the length of the laser pulse. During a long, low-power laser pulse, the heat will spread from the point of application by radiation, diffusion, and blood flow. In a pulse lasting for 0.1 s, there will be little time for heat diffusion, radiation, and blood cooling; therefore, the injury will be confined to the spot of application. When this is taken to an extreme and pulses are shortened by several orders of magnitude (<1 ms), the tissue effects are considered to be *nonlinear*. What this means is that small amounts of energy not expected to have significant thermal effects are still capable of tissue ablation (Fig. 4-9).

In truth, with high-energy, short-pulsed lasers in the infrared portion of the spectrum, wild thermal events do occur at a molecular level. When a microsecond burst of megawatt power encounters a tissue surface molecule, immense kinetic energy is imparted to that molecule. That kinetic energy may be sufficient to break the intermolecular bonds and cause a rapid expansion of the molecule, such that it is expelled from the tissue surface in, essentially, a miniexplosion. After the surface layer is blown away, subsequent pulses may have access to deeper layers of tissue. The result is the creation of a pit in the tissue. If the laser is used on reasonably dry tissue, such as bone, the pit will be finely etched. If the tissue is vascular, blood splattering will negate any possible benefits of pulsed laser application. For this reason, high-energy pulsed lasers have little application in well-vascularized tissue. In nonvascular tissues, such as bone, cartilage, cornea, tooth, and epidermis, it may be desirable to incise tissue using a high-energy, short-pulsed laser, whose precision and strength is unmatched by a scalpel, yet causes no thermal injury which would damage healthy tissue and retard wound healing.

There are several reasons why high-energy, short-pulsed lasers cause negligible injury to the surrounding tissue. The first reason is that the amount of energy imparted per pulse (in millijoules) is insufficient to raise the temperature of 1 g of tissue by more than 0.1°C. Second, the short duration of the pulse exceeds the thermal relaxation coefficient (i.e., the rate at which heat is spread) of tissue. Finally, most of the optical energy imparted into the system is dissipated as kinetic energy during the expulsion of tissue fragments.

PHOTODYNAMIC THERAPY

When 1 J of energy is delivered as 1 W for 1 s, the tissue effect is photothermal. When 1 J of energy is delivered as 10^6 W for 10^{-6} s, the nonlinear effect is considered to be photomechanical (Fig. 4-9). When 1 J of energy is delivered as 10^{-3} W for 10^{-3} s, the effect may be a chemical reaction, catalyzed by the addition of photons but not associated with detectable temperature change (Fig. 4-10).

The most common use of lasers to initiate photochemical reactions occurs when clinicians exploit photosensitizers, which are capable, when excited, of inducing cell death. Photodynamic therapy (PDT) occurs when a physician injects a tumor-localizing agent, such as hematoporphyrin derivative (HpD), into the patient, waits for the agent to become localized in the tumor, and then initiates a photodestructive reaction in the cell using a light of appropriate wavelength.[13] This is truly "Star Wars medicine" because the effects of this low-energy (milliwatt) light on normal tissue not containing the photosensitizer are negligible. If we were able to penetrate each cancer cell with a phototoxic compound and then deliver a sufficient quantity of light to initiate cell lysis, we would have a very effective treatment for cancer.

Unfortunately, the bright hopes for PDT have not been realized. To date, a major problem limiting PDT use is in

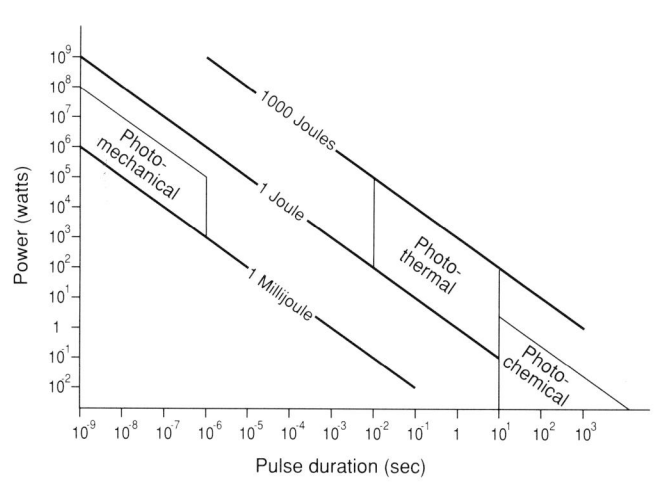

FIGURE 4-9 This graph shows the variety of tissue effects that may be obtained with a constant amount of energy by varying the pulsing parameters. Short pulses, less than 10^{-3} s, with high powers cause photomechanical or photoacoustic energy. Moderate powers (Watts) for moderate lengths of time (seconds) will cause tissue heating. Low power (milliwatts) for long durations (10^3 s) may induce photochemical reactions, especially in the presence of photosensitizing agents, such as hematoporphyrin derivative.

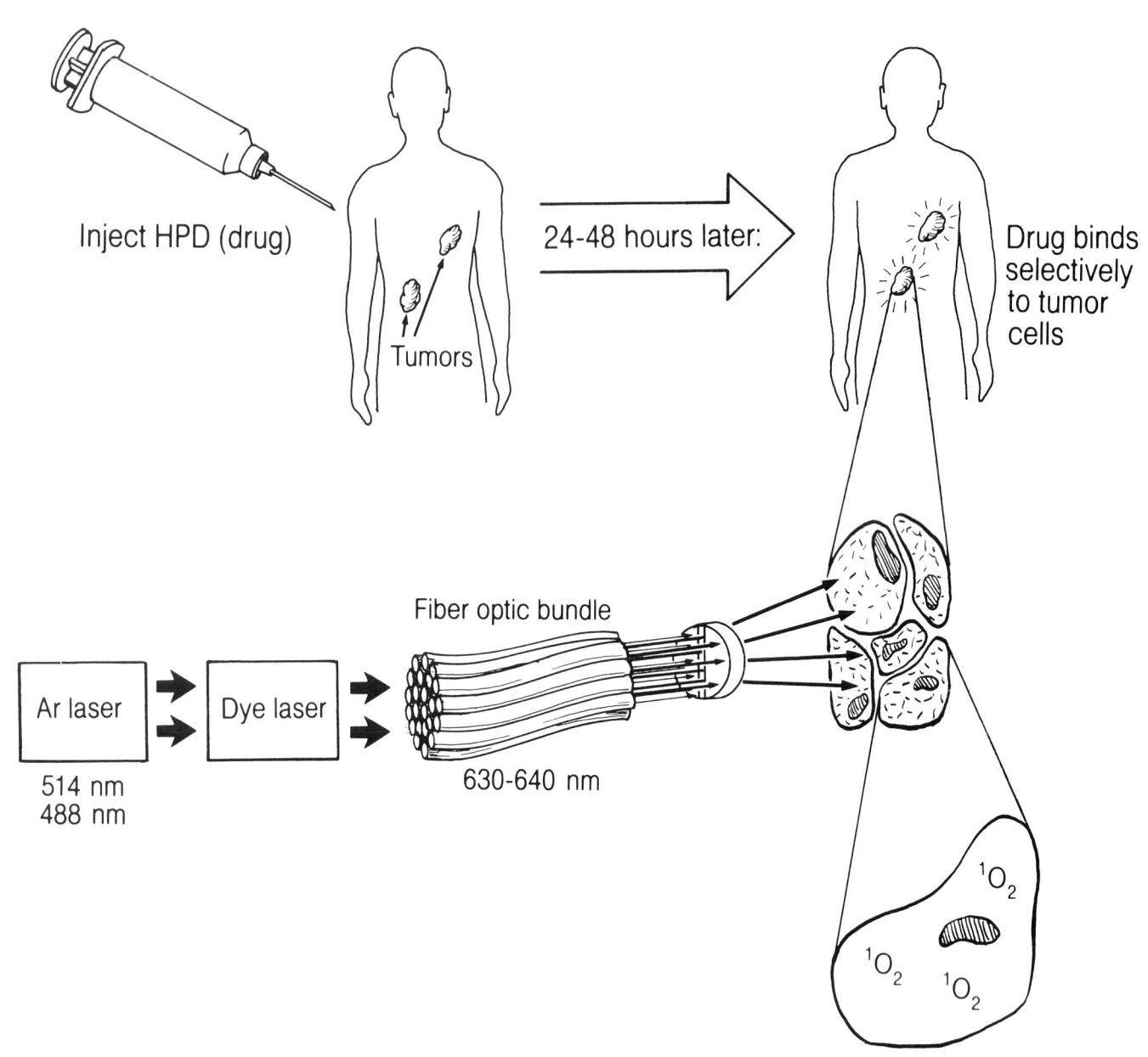

FIGURE 4-10 Photodynamic therapy is produced by injecting the photoactive drug into a peripheral vein in a tumor-bearing patient. Twenty-four to 48 hours later, the drug has concentrated in the tumor bed. A laser emitting the appropriate wavelength of light to stimulate a cytotoxic oxidative reaction is then directed at the tumor bed. The ideal photodynamic agent is one that will concentrate solely in tumor tissue; be excited at a long wavelength, where light is able to penetrate tissue deeply; and be rapidly cleared from the skin to produce a minimal amount of cutaneous photosensitivity. Some of these agents are currently under investigation. None has yet been licensed by the Food and Drug Administration.

getting the compound to every viable cancer cell, many of which are in relatively ischemic regions. A second problem is that of uniform light delivery within tissue. Although HpD is generally activated with a red laser (630 nm), because tissue penetration of red light is superior to shorter wavelengths, the depth of light penetration is still less than 6 mm, limiting the applicability of this therapy with bulky cancers. In addition, HpD is found at high levels in the skin for several weeks after treatment. Severe injury to the dermis may occur as a result of fluorescent light or sunlight, requiring PDT-treated patients to remain in dim lighting for 1 month after therapy, often one of the last months of their lives.

LASER WELDING

The contributions of laser welding to conventional anastomotic techniques are that there is no foreign body to produce an inflammatory reaction, the weld is water- or fluid-tight, and a welded anastomosis has the ability to grow, which is not the case in sutured anastomoses. A number of laser welding techniques have been developed. One technique utilizes a diode laser and a tissue solder consisting of fibrinogen and indocyanine green.[14] An automated laser tissue welding device utilizes an absorbable stent and circumferential clamping mechanism with embedded laser fibers.[15] The stent sets the edges of an end-to-end anastomosis, and a strong serosa weld is accomplished using a computer-controlled laser. Laser welding has been used to glue skin together, create vascular and gastrointestinal anastomoses, and reconstruct severed vas deferens.[16]

The mechanism of tissue welding is unknown, but there are two major competing hypotheses. The first is that welding is achieved with high temperature that induces covalent bonding of the structural proteins, such as collagen. The second is that laser-heated protein is denatured, and hydrogen or disulfide bonds are responsible for the welding bond. Regardless of the mechanism, its clinical application has been demonstrated in a series of laser welded arteriovenous fistulae. After 4½ years of follow-up, the patency rate is at least 70 percent.[17]

Here again is the theme of reconnecting a biologic cylinder, the pursuit of multiple specialties. Attempts are being made by many disciplines to connect together two ends of a cylindric structure more accurately, quickly, strongly, and efficiently with laser techniques.

REFERENCES

1. Einstein A: Zur Quantentheorie der Strahlung. *Physiol Z* 1917; 18:121–128.
2. Gordon JP, Zeigler HJ, Townes CH: The MASER—new type of amplifier, frequency standard and spectrometer. *Physiol Rev* 1955; 99:1264–1274.
3. Maiman TH: Stimulated optical radiation in ruby. *Nature* 1960; 187:93–94.
4. Fuller TA: Fundamentals of lasers in surgery and medicine, in Dixon JA (ed): *Surgical Applications of Lasers,* ed 2. Chicago, Year Book Medical, 1987, pp 16–33.
5. Enderby CE: Laser instrumentation, in Dixon JA (ed): *Surgical Applications of Lasers,* ed 2. Chicago, Year Book Medical, 1987, pp 52–78.
6. Walsh JT, Flotte TJ, Deutsch TF: Er:YAG laser ablation of tissue: Effect of pulse duration and tissue type on thermal damage. *Lasers Surg Med* 1989; 9:314–326.
7. Bass LS, Oz MC, Trokel SL, et a;: Alternative lasers for endoscopic surgery: Comparison of pulsed thulium-holmium-chromium:YAG with continuous-wave neodymium:YAG laser for ablation of colonic mucosa. *Lasers Surg Med* 1991; 11:545–549.
8. Kopchok GE, White RA, Tabbara M, et al: Holmium:YAG laser ablation of vascular tissue. *Lasers Surg Med* 1990; 10:405–413.
9. Hunter JG, Bruhn E, Goodman G, et al: Reflectance spectroscopy predicts safer wavelengths for pulsed laser lithotripsy of gallstones (abstract). *Gastrointest Endosc* 1991; 37:273.
10. Peyman GA, Naguib KS, Gaasterland D: Transscleral application of a semiconductor diode laser. *Lasers Surg Med* 1990; 10:569–575.
11. Oz MC, Bass LS, Chuck RS, et al: Strength of laser vascular fusion: Preliminary observations on the role of thrombus. *Lasers Surg Med* 1990; 10:393–395.
12. Tan OT, Stafford TJ, Murray S, et al: Histologic comparison of the pulsed dye laser and copper vapor laser effects on pig skin. *Lasers Surg Med* 1990; 10:551–558.
13. Straight RC: Photodynamic therapy in laser surgery and medicine, in, Dixon JA (ed): *Surgical Applications of Lasers,* ed 2. Chicago, Year Book Medical, 1987, 310–349.
14. Treat MR, Oz MC, Bass LS: New technologies and future applications of surgical lasers. *Surg Clin North Am* 1992; 72:705–742.
15. Sauer JS, Hinshaw JR, McGuire KP: The first sutureless laser-welded, end-to-end bowel anastomosis. *Lasers Surg Med* 1989; 9:70–73.
16. Shanberg AM, Tansey L, Baghdassarian R, et al: Laser-assisted vasectomy reversal: Experience in 32 patients. *J Urol* 1990; 143:525–529.
17. White RA, Kopchok GE: Laser vascular tissue fusion: Development, current status and future perspectives. *J Clin Laser Med Surg* 1990; 47:54.

Laparoscopic Electrosurgery

Roger C. Odell

The current wave of enthusiasm for laparoscopic surgery has spawned a renewed interest in the biophysics and dangers of monopolar electrosurgery. Speculation about the dangers of electrosurgery in laparoscopy began during the late 1960s when gynecologists encountered a number of misadventures in the course of performing single-puncture and later multiple trocar laparoscopic procedures using monopolar electrosurgery.[1] The investigations of these incidents generated much concern about the use of monopolar electrosurgery in laparoscopy. As a consequence, laparoscopic use of monopolar electrosurgery has been discouraged for the past two decades.

The objectives of this chapter are to address the biophysics of electrosurgical energy used for tissue cutting, fulguration, and dessication and the techniques used to deliver this source of energy efficiently. Another key objective will be to review the complications of laparoscopic electrosurgery, explain the physics of how they occurred, and discuss ways of minimizing hazards and eliminating their repetition in the future.

History

The surgical use of high-frequency electrical energy dates back nearly 1 century. Electrosurgery utilizes the generation and delivery of radiofrequency current between active and dispersive electrodes to elevate tissue temperature to perform vaporization (cutting), fulguration, and desiccation. In contrast, with electrocautery, the electrical current passes through a high-resistance wire, which heats the wire to cauterize tissue. The same therapeutic effect could be attained by passing the wire over a Bunsen burner flame. The biophysics of electrosurgical currents was documented by the Germans and French in the late 1800s.[2] In 1910, general surgeon William L. Clark[3] of Philadelphia reported the removal of large growths of the skin, head, neck, and breast using electrosurgery.

Harvey W. Cushing,[4] with the assistance of William T. Bovie, recorded the principles of electrosurgery in 1927. These early documents supported the use of Dr. Bovie's electrosurgical device and the versatility of this energy source. Their work changed the course of neurosurgery and, ultimately, all other surgical disciplines.

Temperature and Tissue

Energy can be neither created nor destroyed, but it can be converted. Electrosurgical current is converted into heat for the purpose of vaporizing (cutting), and coagulating tissue. The principles are similar to the conversion of laser energy into heat within tissue.

At or above 44°C, tissue necrosis starts. Between 50 and 80°C, coagulation occurs as collagen is converted into glucose. Between 80 and 100°C, tissue becomes dehydrated, and desiccation takes place. At or above 100°C, tissue turns into a vapor. Above 200°C, carbonization begins, with a black eschar as the result of fulguration (Fig. 5-1).

How Electrical Energy Affects Tissue Temperature

The three electrical properties that cause a rise in temperature are as follows:

1. Current = I (in amperes)
2. Voltage = V (in volts)
3. Resistance (impedance) = R (in ohms)

To explain these electrical energy terms, an analogy will be made to a hydraulic energy source. The water tower shown in Figure 5-2 is a source of work, which is analogous to an electrosurgical tower, and the electrical terms *current, voltage,* and *resistance* are demonstrated. Such a model diminishes the mystique of the electrosurgical principles that follow.

By Ohm's law,

$$I = V/R$$

Temperature (°C)						
	34 - 44°	44 - 50°	50 - 80°	80 - 100°	100 - 200°	> 200°
Effect: Visible	None	None	Blanching	Shrinkage	Steam "popcorn"	Carbonization cratering
Delayed	Edema	Necrosis	Sloughing	Sloughing	Ulceration	Larger crater
Mechanism	Vasodilitation, inflammation	Disruption of cell metabolism	Collagen denaturation	Dessication	Vaporization	Combustion of tissue hydrocarbons

FIGURE 5-1 The tissue effects of heating are best categorized by the immediate visible effect (surgeon feedback mechanism), the delayed effects, and the mechanism of injury. The delayed manifestation of full-thickness intestinal injury from thermal energy is the major cause of morbidity and mortality after accidental bowel burn.

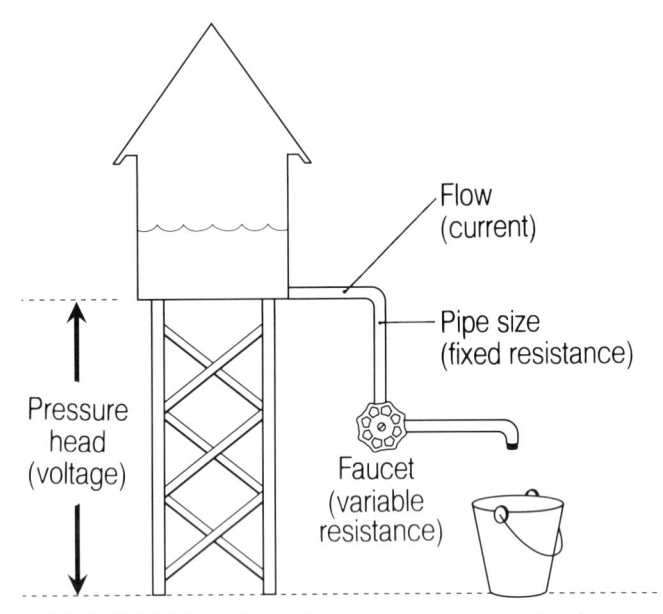

FIGURE 5-2 Voltage is analogous to the pressure head on a column of water. Current (flow) is dependent on the pressure head and resistance in the system.

the relationship between the properties of electrosurgical energy is shown.

The power formula, with energy given in Watts, is as follows.

$$W = V \times I$$

This is valuable in understanding the tissue effects of electrosurgery. Tissue heating is a function of the amount of current flowing through a given cross-sectional area of tissue, the current density.

The power density is the wattage delivered to a particular cross-sectional area of tissue and is equal to the current density (I/cm^2) times the voltage. Substituting for voltage, using Ohm's law, produces the following equation:

$$W/cm^2 = (I/cm^2)^2 \times R$$

At a fixed energy setting (wattage constant) and fixed tissue resistance (R constant), tissue heating is a function of the size of the active electrode in contact with the tissue. The larger the contact area, the less the current density and the slower the heating. In noncontact modalities, for example, cutting and fulgurating, this would be equivalent to the sparking area between the active electrode and the tissue. During cutting and fulgurating, the electrode is not in contact; therefore, the power density can only be approximated. It is only during desiccating that the exact surface area of the electrode in contact with the tissue is important in calculating power density. In general, the larger the electrode surface area is, the lower the power density that occurs, and the smaller the electrode surface area, the higher the power density.

The element of time is the primary determinant in the depth and degree of tissue necrosis at a given energy setting. Specific elements of its role will be demonstrated next.

TECHNIQUE OF LAPAROSCOPIC ELECTROSURGERY

Vaporization (cutting), fulguration, and desiccation are the three available therapeutic effects of electrosurgery. Unfortunately, the labeling on most electrosurgical units designates only two modes: called *cut* and *coag*. These terms cause confusion about the optimal use of electrosurgical energy.

Vaporization

Vaporization (cutting) requires a high-current, low-voltage (continuous) waveform, which elevates the tissue temperature rapidly, producing vaporization or division of tissue with a minimal effect on coagulation (hemostasis) of the walls of the incision (Figs. 5-3 and 5-4, cutting waveform with electrosurgical unit [ESU] set at 50 W). During optimal electrosurgical cutting, the current travels through a steam bubble between the active electrode and the tissue. Therefore, it is important to recognize that electrosurgical cutting is a noncontact means of dissection. The electrode floats through the tissue, and there is very little tactile response transmitted to the surgeon's hand.

The dynamics or velocity of the electrode dictates the depth of necrosis. Depths of necrosis under 100 μm are attainable using electrosurgical energy during dissection. The continuous waveform is analogous to the garden hose valve shown in Figure 5-2, with its even flow of water. The ratio of high current to low voltage in dissection minimizes the width and depth of necrosis to the walls of the incision. If the electrode is allowed to remain stationary or is slowed, the maximum temperature increases, augmenting the width of thermal damage to the tissue.

By interrupting the current and increasing the voltage, the waveform can be modified to promote blending and increase hemostasis during dissection (see Figs 5-3 and 5-4). In the garden-hose analogy, this would be comparable to increasing the height of the water tower to make up for a reduction in hydraulic energy resulting from the reduced time that the water was allowed to flow.

In utilizing the blended modes, again the electrode should float through the tissue. The blending waveforms require a longer period of time than the cutting waveforms to dissect the same length of incision as a result of the interrupted delivery of current at the same power setting. With this increased time comes an increase in thermal spread from the voltage component of the blending waveform, which improves coagulation of small vessels during dissection. Blend 1 yields a slight increase in hemostasis; Blend 2, a moderate increase; and Blend 3, a marked increase in hemostasis during dissection. When needed, these blending modes are a valuable option in controlling bleeding, but if they are used unnecessarily, a greater width of necrosis may promote increased postoperative infection. Additionally, laparoscopic use of high blending or coagulating modes can result in an increased amount of smoke plume.

When using the cutting or blending modes, the ESU should be activated first before the electrode touches the tissue. This allows maximum power density as the electrode approaches the tissue and facilitates initial vaporization and dissection. The touch should simulate the feathering or light stroking used in painting with a two-bristle paint brush for touching up or fine detail work. With optimum technique and control setting, the force required to dissect the tissue should, in theory, be 0 g of pressure between the electrode and the tissue.

Fulguration

Fulguration employs a high-voltage, low-current, noncontinuous waveform (highly damped), which coagulates by means of spraying long electrical sparks to the tissue (see Figs. 5-3 and 5-4, coagulation/fulguration waveform set at 50 W). By drawing the electrode away from tissue, defocusing of the power density occurs, and the power density goes down. With fulguration, a very superficial eschar is produced; the depth of necrosis is minimal. Much of the energy dissipates in heating of the air between the electrode and the tissue.

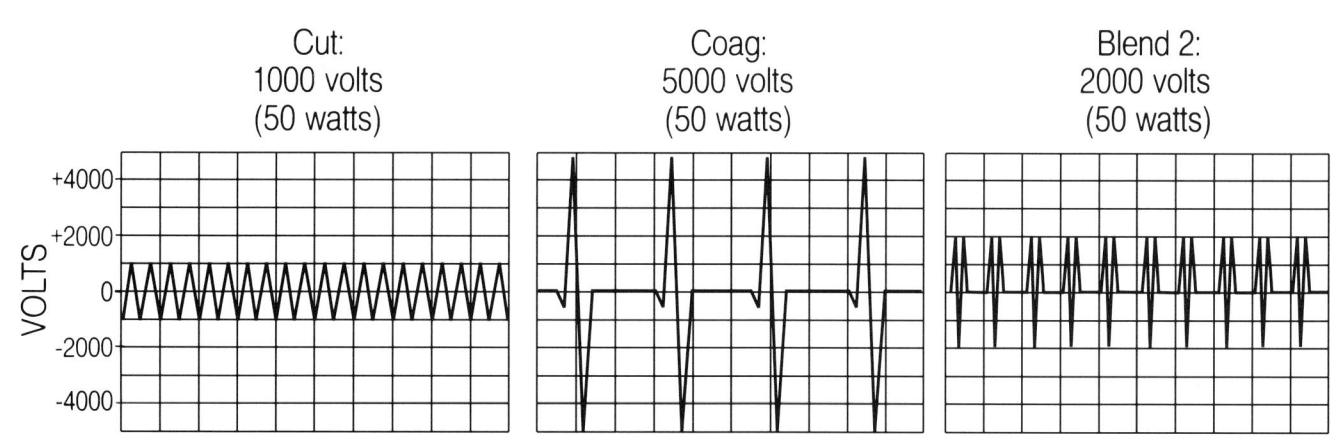

FIGURE 5-3 With the electrosurgical unit in the *cut* mode at 50 W, 1000 V of continuous current will be delivered. In the *coag* mode, 50 W will be delivered as 5000-V pulses. Blend 2 provides an interrupted chain of pulses, each 2000 V to give equivalent power. This voltage represents open circuit conditions. Loading the circuit will cause the voltage to drop to a different level depending how heavy or light the load is.

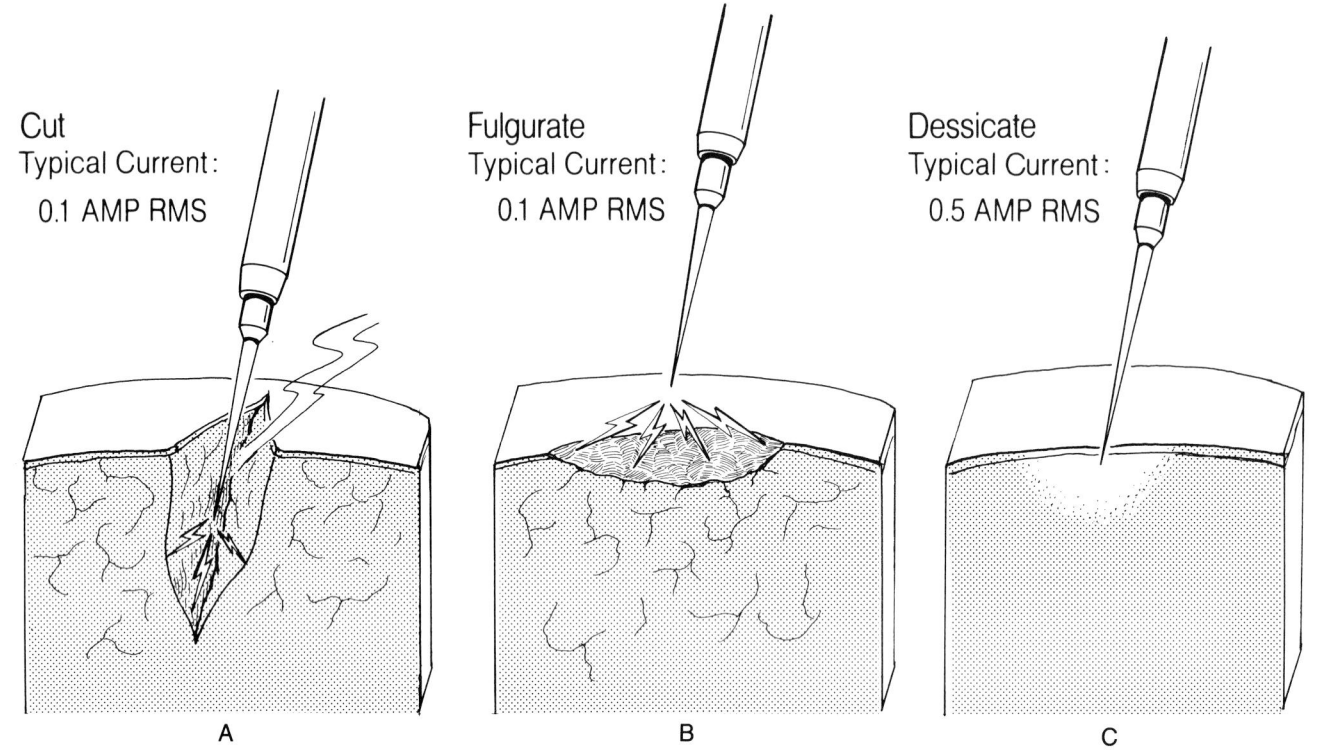

FIGURE 5-4 A. Cutting current (low voltage, high amperage) provides optimal tissue vaporization with a shallow zone of thermal injury. B. Fulguration is performed with coagulating (high voltage, low amperage) current, which discharges across the gap between electrode and tissue, arresting superficial bleeding. C. The greatest volume of tissue necrosis is produced by dessication (coag or cut waveform), in which all electrical energy is converted into thermal energy in the tissue. The volume of necrosis is dependent on the power and time settings.

The most common use of fulguration is in coagulating a large, oozing area, such as a capillary or arteriole bed, where a discrete bleeder cannot be identified. Cardiovascular, urologic, and general surgeons utilize fulguration for their most demanding oozing and capillary applications, such as surface bleeding on the heart, bleeding from a bladder tumor resection, and hepatic resections.

Fulguration and electrosurgical cutting are both noncontact modalities. Fulguration can be initiated in two ways: (1) by slowly approaching the tissue until a spark jumps to the tissue, whereby a raining effect of sparks is maintained until the electrode is withdrawn or the tissue is carbonized to the point where the sparks cease or (2) by bouncing the electrode off the tissue, resulting in a similar raining effect of sparks to the tissue, but avoiding the painstaking effort of approaching the tissue until a spark jumps without touching.

Dessication

Dessication will occur with any waveform when the electrode is placed in contact with the tissue (see Fig. 5-4). The current-to-voltage ratio is irrelevant; it is the energy wattage that is important. Desiccation is another means of coagulation. Most surgeons do not make a distinction between fulguration and desiccation but refer to both as coagulation. In desiccation, however, direct contact wih the tissue results in conversion of all of the electrosurgical energy into heat within the tissue. This contrasts with both cutting and fulgurating, where a significant amount of the electrical energy goes into heating up the atmosphere between the electrode and the tissue. Thus, coagulation and desiccation results in a deep, wide necrosis where the electrode makes surface contact.

The most common application of desiccation is treating a discrete bleeder. A hemostat is first introduced to occlude the vessel with mechanical pressure, and then electrosurgical energy is applied to the body of the hemostat. In this way, the current passes through the hemostat into the tissue grasped by the jaws of the instrument and back to the patient return electrode. The resulting coaptation of vessels has been documented as producing a collagen chain reaction, resulting in a fibrous binding of the dehydrated, denatured cells of the endothelium.[5]

In desiccation, the electrode is in contact with the tissue, and the voltage-to-current ratio is not nearly as important as in cutting and fulguration. However, in practical applications, cutting and blending waveforms are superior to fulgurating waveforms when desiccation is desired. The primary reason is that the fulgurating waveforms tend to spark through the coagulated tissue, resulting in voids in the bonding to the ends of the vessels. Additionally, when sparks occur at the electrode in contact or near contact, the metal in the electrode will heat up rapidly, causing tissue to adhere to the electrode when drawn off the target site. Bleeding will continue each time the eschar is pulled off as a result of adhesion from heat in the electrode.

In bipolar desiccation, the waveform plays a far more important role. Currently, for the most part, manufacturers have incorporated a continuous, low-voltage, high-current waveform in the bipolar output to maximize desiccation. With the older models, the surgeon could select either a continuous cutting, blending, or fulgurating waveform when bipolar desiccation was needed. A lack of understanding by physicians, in combination with ambiguous evaluations in the literature of the effects of these waveforms on bipolar desiccation, led to a number of associated problems.[6]

Therefore, at this time, the generally accepted waveform for bipolar desiccation is a continuous, low-voltage, high-current one. The author recommends that when bipolar desiccation is critical a newer-model ESU with a dedicated, continuous, bipolar waveform be utilized. If using an ESU that allows selection of both cutting and blending and fulguration and bipolar (coagulation) currents, beginning with the pure cutting (continuous) waveform will provide the best results.

When performing desiccation, patience is the key to good results. Typically, the power density is very low in desiccation; therefore, the active electrodes will be very large. The larger electrode or contact area to tissue requires longer activation times to attain the desired therapeutic effect. If higher energy is introduced to speed up the process, this most likely will be counterproductive because higher energy levels increase the temperature to the tissue adjacent to the electrodes, potentially forcing the current to spark through the necrosis and resulting in fulguration instead of desiccation. Fulgurating or sparking stops the deep heating process and causes carbonization of the surface of the tissue only. Therefore, when sparking is observed during desiccation, the surgeon should stop, reduce the power, or pulse the current by keying on and off the ESU to overcome this natural tendency of electrosurgical energy.

An ammeter (Model EM-2, Electroscope, Inc., Boulder, CO) may be used to measure the amount of current flowing through the circuit. The ammeter will show current flow only when tissue contains electrolytic fluid. When current stops flowing, complete desiccation (coagulation) has occurred, and it is safe to divide the tissue with a pair of scissors.

RESULTS

Inherent Risks

In monopolar electrosurgery, there are three areas at risk for electrosurgical burn. The first is at the site of the active electrode, where the unit is used to cut, fulgurate, or desiccate the tissue. To heat the tissue rapidly, the electrode has a high power density, which, if not kept in control at all times, can severely burn the patient. Therefore, the author strongly recommends that the active electrode, when not in use, be stored in an insulated holster or tray.

A second accidental burn that can occur involves division of the current. To avoid this problem, it is essential, when using a ground-referenced electrosurgical unit, that current division to alternate ground points from the patient's body be eliminated (explained subsequently).

A third cause of electrosurgical burn is a faulty patient return electrode, that is, with partial detachment or a manufacturing defect in the return of the current to the ESU by a high-current density. When properly applied, the patient return electrode (ground plate) has a surface area approximately 20 in^2 or larger, ensuring minimal temperature rise under normal conditions.

These latter two burn risks have been mitigated by improved ESU design during the last two decades. Safety circuits or features have been available for most units sold within the past 10 years. The two major advancements have been isolated electrosurgical outputs and contact quality monitors. These two technologic improvements have reduced the potential for patient burns during electrosurgical procedures. These features currently are incorporated on ESUs produced by major manufacturers, including Aspen, Birtcher, and Valleylab.

Isolated electrosurgical units were introduced in the early 1970s. Their primary purpose was to prevent alternate ground-site burns, resulting from current division. With the use these isolated ESUs, these burn risks have essentially been eliminated. Some hospitals utilize ground-referenced ESUs; therefore, it is wise for surgeons to determine the type of ESU that is in service at their hospitals.

Contact quality monitoring circuits were introduced in the early 1980s. Their primary purpose was to prevent burns at the patient return electrode site. The contact quality monitor incorporates a dual-section patient return electrode and circuit for the purpose of evaluating the total impedance of the patient return electrode during surgery. Therefore, if the patient return electrode were to become compromised, the contact quality circuit would inhibit the electrosurgical generator output. This feature has essentially eliminated accidental burns at the site of the patient return electrode.

Laparoscopic Issues

As stated in the previous section, electrosurgery (primarily bipolar) has been employed laparoscopically by gynecologists[1] for the past two decades. With the recent innovations in laparoscopic techniques used by general, urologic, and other surgeons, a major question has arisen. Can monopolar electrosurgical energy safely be used in laparoscopy? This section will address its potential hazards, the options available to minimize or eliminate the potential of unintended burns within the peritoneal cavity, and common misconceptions about laparoscopic electrosurgery.

There are three potential hazards in the use of electrosurgical energy during laparoscopy, resulting from three factors as follows: (1) access is obtained to the peritoneal cavity through trocars; (2) the laparoscope views less than 10 percent of the electrosurgical probe; and (3) the laparoscope is conductive (metal) and cannot be seen after it enters the trocar. Passing the electrosurgically active electrode through these access channels under such limited visualization carries these three risks of accidental burn.

The first risk stems from the fact that most laproscopic accessories are approximately 35-cm long and the laparoscopic images viewed on the monitor typically show less than 5 cm of the distal end of the device (Fig. 5-5). The active electrode used to deliver the electrosurgical energy has an insulated covering, but 90 percent or more of this insulation is out of the viewing range. If a breakdown of the insulation occurs on the shaft of the electrode, the organs touching the electrode at this site can suffer severe burns (Fig. 5-6). These burns may not be noticed during surgery but may result in severe postoperative complications. It is essential that a routine inspection of these electrodes be done periodically.

A second hazard results from capacitive coupling of energy into other metal laparoscopic instruments or trocar cannulas. The principle of capacitance in electrical physics is beyond the scope of this chapter, but 5 to 40 percent of the power that the electrosurgical unit is set to deliver can be coupled or transferred into a standard 10-cm long trocar cannula (Fig. 5-7). The energy in itself may not be dangerous, providing it is allowed to pass through a low power density pathway, such as an all metal (conductive) trocar cannula inserted into the abdominal wall, and returned to the patient return electrode.

The problem arises when this energy is allowed or made to pass through a high-power density pathway. This can happen, for example, with the partially plastic (nonconductive) and partially metal (conductive) trocar cannulas that are available. Some trocar manufacturers supply a plastic thread to the metal cannula tube to help hold the cannula in the abdominal wall while the laparoscopic electrode is

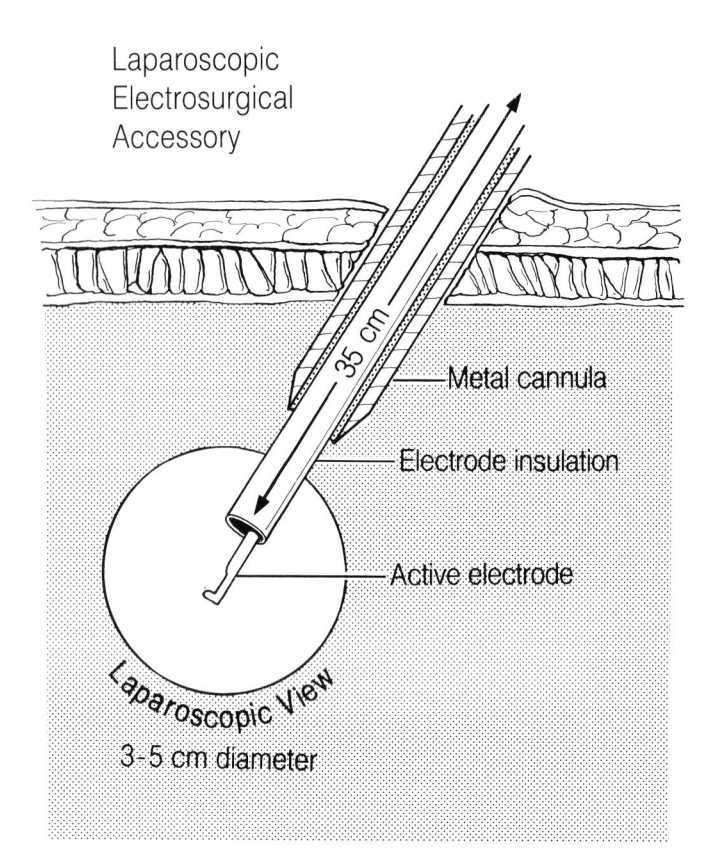

FIGURE 5-5 The limited laparoscopic field should include all uninsulated portions of electrosurgical electrodes.

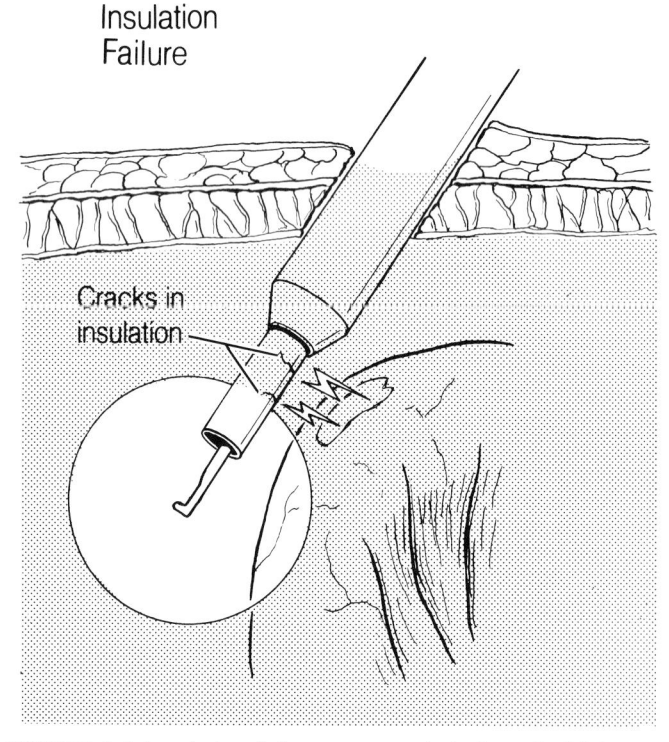

FIGURE 5-6 Insulation failure may result in intestinal injury outside the laparoscopic field of vision.

$$C = \frac{2\pi\varepsilon_0 K L}{L_N\left(\frac{b}{a}\right)}$$

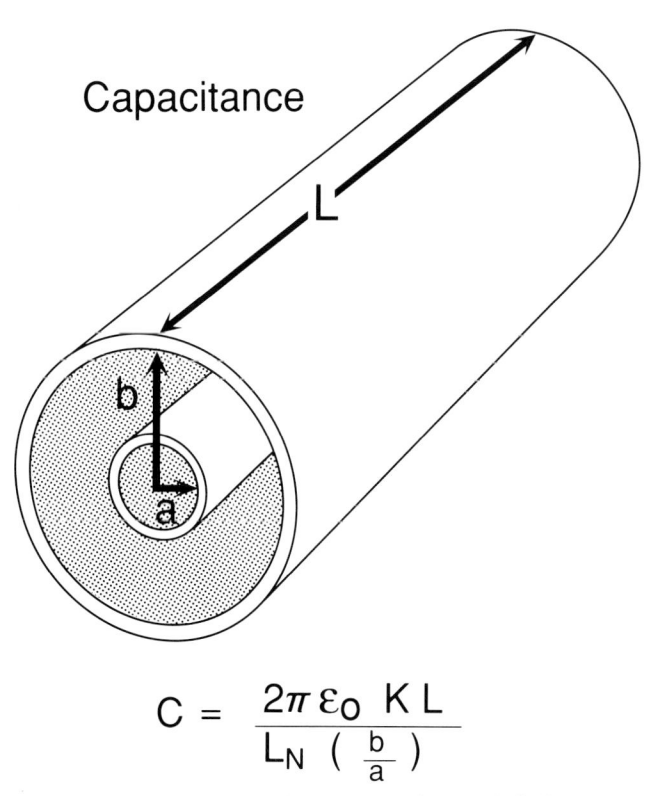

FIGURE 5-7 In a trocar, the capacitively coupled charge increases directly with the length of the metal sleeve and inversely with the fraction of trocar radius (b) to electrode radius (a). In other words, the closer the electrode and cannula (or operating telescope) are to being the same diameter and same long length, the more capacitance the system possesses.

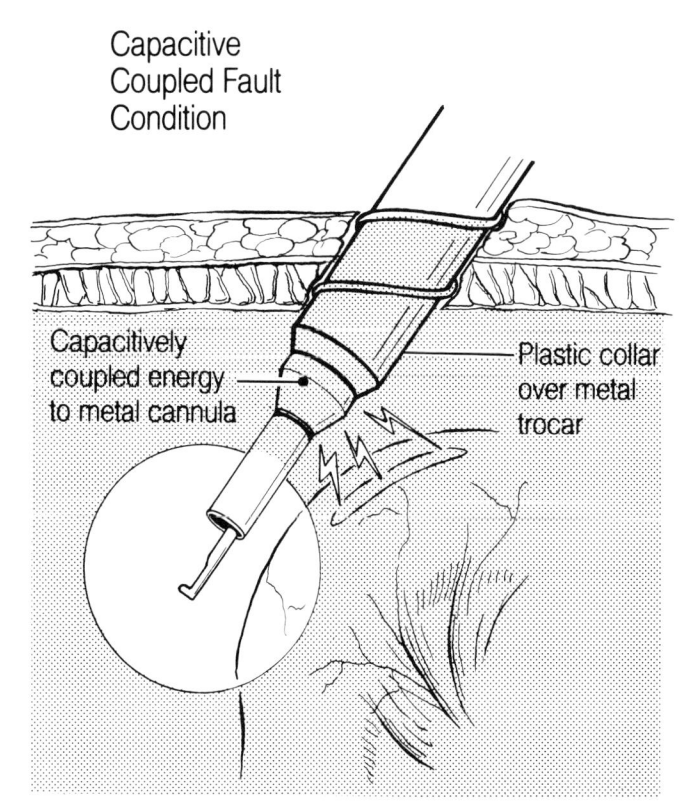

FIGURE 5-8 Capacitive coupling injury occurs when a plastic collar insulates the abdominal wall from the capacitive current. This current will be bled off the metal sleeve into adjacent bowel, outside the laparoscopic field of vision.

positioned in and out of the cannula port (Fig. 5-8). To avoid this hazard, the author strongly recommends the use of all-metal or all-plastic trocar cannulas through which to pass the electrosurgically active laparoscopic electrode.

Capacitive coupling can occur to a lesser degree in crossing another laparoscopic instrument, for example, the atraumatic grasper with the electrosurgical laparoscopic electrode within the peritoneal cavity. The energy transfer to these instruments can range from 1 to 10 percent of the power set on the ESU. Caution must be observed in these situations, especially during long activation times.

The phenomenon of capacitive coupling was first detected during single-puncture laparoscopic procedures.[7] Operating laparoscopes developed for these procedures have a 30- to 40-cm-long operating channel through which various instruments are passed. It was observed that when plastic 10- to 12-mm cannulas were used to pass the operating laparoscope, the distal end of the metal laparoscope could deliver 40 to 80 percent of the power set on the ESU, with resulting burns to adjacent tissue. Consequently, the Food and Drug Administration issued a strong recommendation in the late 1970s that only all-metal trocar cannulas be used under these circumstances to pass the laparoscope and electrosurgical electrode into the peritoneal cavity.

To prevent the occurrence of these hazards in the delivery of monopolar energy, Electroscope, Inc. (Boulder, CO), developed an Electroshield® Monitoring System. The Electroshield System features a reusable shield (Fig. 5-9) that surrounds dissecting and coagulating laparoscopic electrodes. The Electroshield Monitor EM-2 dynamically detects insulation faults and shields against capacitive coupling. If an unsafe condition exists, the Electroshield System automatically deactivates the ESU before a burn can occur. This technology shields hazardous stray energy and permits safe laparoscopic use of monopolar electrosurgical energy.[8,9]

A third potential hazard that is inherent in the use of monopolar electrosurgical energy occurs when the active electrode is accidentally touched to the laparoscope. A metal trocar cannula will allow this energy to pass safely into the abdominal wall through a low-power density pathway. However, if a plastic trocar cannula is used, the current may exit to the bowel or other organs touching the laparoscope, out of view of the monitor (Fig. 5-10). The plastic cannula may block the directly coupled energy from

40 PART I New Technologies

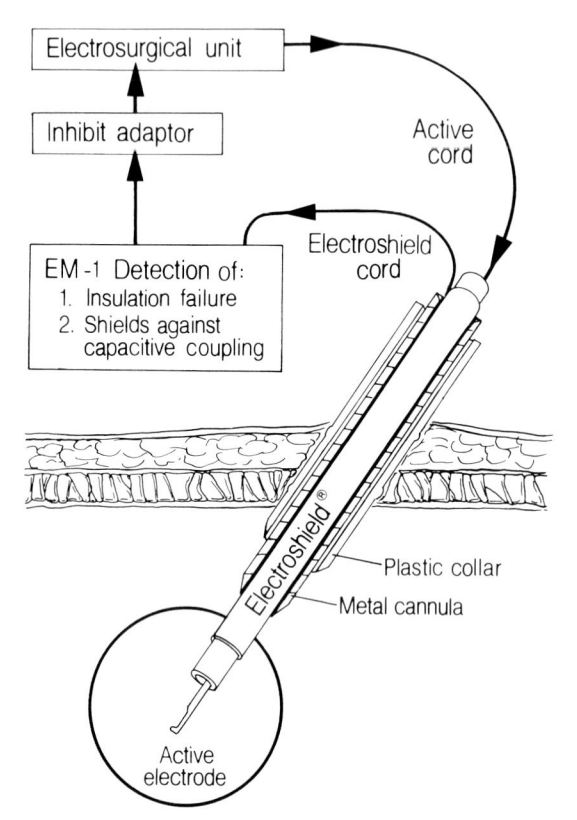

FIGURE 5-9 Current leaks and capacitive current can be detected and eliminated by the use of a shield that contains circuitry for detecting and alerting the surgeon to dangerous current division.

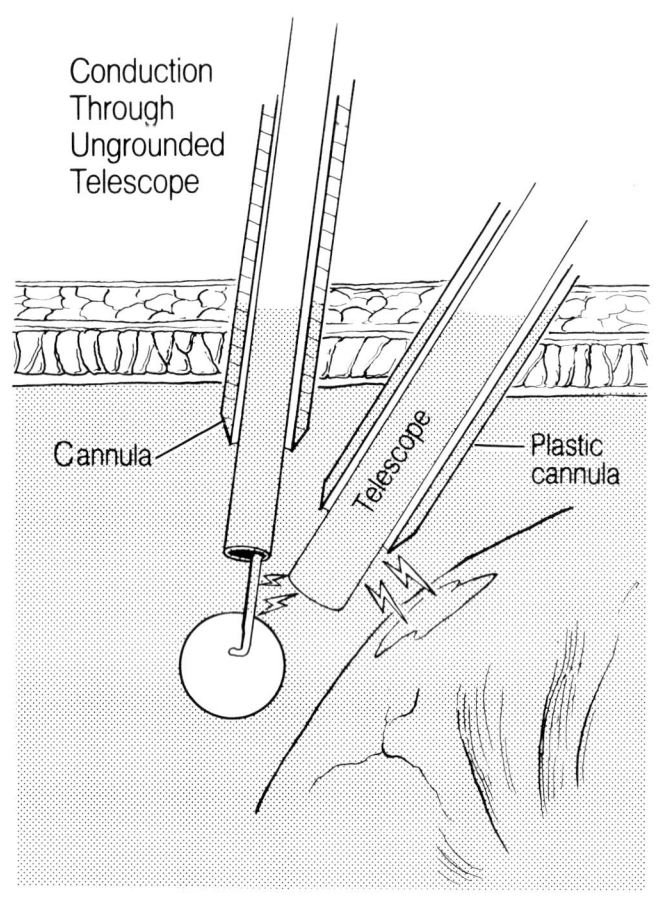

FIGURE 5-10 If the telescopic sleeve is made of a nonconductive material, electrical current may be passed to bowel through the metal laparoscope either by mechanisms depicted in Figures 5-6 or 5-8 or by direct coupling to a portion of the activated electrode just out of the field of laparoscopic vision.

being safely passed into the abdominal wall and back to the patient return electrode. Therefore, only metal cannulas are recommended for the laparoscope ports.

Misconceptions

There are two misconceptions that need to be addressed regarding the laparoscopic delivery of monopolar energy. The first misconception is that the electrosurgical current when it is delivered to the target site, for some strange reason, behaves differently in laparoscopy compared with open surgical procedures. We hear statements to the effect that, during laparoscopic procedures, the current is delivered to one organ and mysteriously exits into an adjacent organ and burns at the exit or entry points. In actuality, however, the biophysics of both open and laparoscopic electrosurgical applications are identical regarding the current paths taken to the patient return electrodes, and if this phenomenon were real, it would have occurred in classic open procedures decades ago.

Genuine complications, on the other hand, can occur in both open and laparoscopic procedures when a pedicle of tissue is created by stretching or otherwise and the current is reconcentrated through this narrow cross-section of tissue, causing a temperature rise in the tissue at that point. A case in point involved female laparoscopic sterilization.[10] Following examination of these incidents, it appears that the complications could have been avoided if the surgeons had obtained a better understanding of the biophysics of electrosurgical energy.

A second misconception is that the peak voltage that is necessary (3000 to 5000 V) at maximum control settings (120 W) results in uncontrollable sparking, rendering delivery of monopolar energy unsuitable for laparoscopic procedures. Physics textbooks, however, indicate that it takes 30,000 V to spark 1 in in air under the best conditions.[11,12] In a carbon dioxide atmosphere, approximately 30 percent more voltage is required to spark 1 in, that is, 9000 V more compared with normal air. Therefore, sparking from the active tip of the electrode can actually be better controlled in the moisture-rich laparoscopic atmosphere than in an open procedures.

CONCLUSION

Electrosurgical energy has been the "gold standard" for hemostatic tissue division for the past 50 years, offering more diverse capabilities than any other energy source. With technologic advancements in safety and performance, it has become one of the most useful tools available to the surgeon. It is the opinion of the author that electrosurgical energy will take on a similar role in laparoscopy. As with any surgical tool or energy source, education and skill are required. This introduction to the biophysical principles of electrical energy is a start to furthering our understanding and advancing the art of electrosurgery.

REFERENCES

1. Rioux JE: Laparoscopic tubal sterilization: Sparking and its control. *La Vie Medicale au Canada Français* 1973; 2:760–766.
2. d'Arsonval A: Sur les effets physiologiques comparés des divers procèdés d'électrisation; nouveaux modes d'application de l'énergie électrique, la voltaïsation sinusoïdale; les grandes fréquences et les hauts potentiels. *Bull Acad Natl Med* 1892; 27:424–433.
3. Clark WL: Oscillatory desiccation in the treatment of accessible malignant growths and minor surgical conditions: A new electrical effect. *J Adv Therap* 1911; 29:169–183.
4. Cushing H, Maton DD, German WJ: *Harvey Cushing: Selected papers on neurosurgery*. New Haven, Yale University Press, 1969.
5. Sigel B, Dunn MR: The mechanism of blood vessel closure by high frequency electrocoagulation. *Surg Gynecol Obstet* 1965; 121:823–831.
6. Soderstrom RM, Smith MR, Hayden GE: The snare method of laparoscopic sterilization: An analysis of 1,000 cases with 4 failures. *J Reprod Med* 1977; 18:246–250.
7. Corson SL: Electrosurgical hazards in laparoscopy. *JAMA* 1974; 227:1261–1262.
8. Voyles CR, et al: Education and engineering solutions for potential problems with laparoscopic monopolar electrosurgery. *Am J Surg* 1992; 164:57–62.
9. Tucker RD, et al: Capacitive coupled stray currents during laparoscopic and endoscopic electrosurgical procedures. *Biomed Instrum Technol* 1992; 26:303–311.
10. Engel T, Harris FW: The electrical dynamics of laparoscopic sterilization. *J Reprod Med* 1975; 15:33–42.
11. Gallagher TJ, et al: *High Voltage Measurements Testing and Design*. New York, John Wiley & Sons, 1983, pp 44–56.
12. Pearce JA: *Electrosurgery*. New York, John Wiley & Sons, 1986, pp 60–90.

Chapter 6

Polymeric Biomaterials for Surgical Repair of Soft Tissue

David W. Grainger

The wide range and increasing clinical applications of both synthetic and natural materials in medical devices, instruments, and implants is testimony to the significant contributions of improved materials to medical practice. Over 5 million prosthetic parts are implanted into patients in the United States and Europe each year to repair natural and traumatic injuries. This does not include transient exposure of tissues and fluids to foreign materials during surgery, including surgical sponges, wound dressings, instruments, sutures, filters, and tubing. Materials are used to replace both physical and functional aspects of body tissues. In addition, implantable pumps and polymer devices controlling the release of drugs and bioactive compounds are ever more frequently used.

No common denominator exists among successful biomaterials in terms of composition, microstructure, surface properties, or molecular construction. Past materials selection and patterns of current use are largely a haphazard result of both commercial availability and acceptable function in vivo. Optimization and de novo rational design of materials for improved surgical performance are only recent developments. However, only by characterizing and understanding the biomaterials–tissue interface will rational development of new materials with improved long-term stability and improved biological performance continue.

Chemical and plastics industries have developed and contributed many new materials with requisite properties for biomedical applications, but their use in medicine requires lengthy, costly, and complex series of evaluations to achieve regulatory approval. Less than 10 percent of the American plastics market involves the medical industry. Additionally, the majority of medical plastics are produced by traditional-materials manufacturing techniques. Higher-cost, low-volume advanced materials with nontraditional structures and properties for biomaterials applications are not yet economically viable in the medical market. The industrial sector may be unwilling to shoulder the burden for development of approved new medical materials without significant input from and interaction with multidisciplinary teams of physical and materials scientists, biomedical engineers, and surgeons. The materials industry, like any other industry, is profit motivated and requires that new biomaterials for surgery be manufactured reproducibly on a mass scale to specific standards at reasonable cost. The surgeon, on the other hand, is patient- and clinically oriented and expects materials manufacturers to accommodate the needs of a stringent, yet often poorly defined, biological scenario to satisfy very human needs. Without a facilitated exchange of technologic parameters for implantation, histologic environment, and functional requirements, new materials development on behalf of medicine will satisfy very few needs. Efforts among scientists, surgeons, and engineers must be continually emphasized and nurtured to provide the technical environment most conducive to successful implant design and performance.

Living tissues are dynamic, cellular, water-swollen, viscoelastic (having fluid deformation and recovery under strain), highly intricate, and nonuniform in ultrastructural design and provide a unique materials quality—regenerability. Materials typically applied in medicine for tissue replacement are generally acellular, dehydrated, synthetic or nonliving, isotropic (generally homogeneous), stiff, or elastic structures of relatively primitive architecture and with limited properties. Current tissue materials substitutes are, at best, crude approximations in both form and function to natural tissue. This fundamental tissue–materials incongruence often manifests itself in functional impairment and material rejection after implantation. Additionally, the limits of current state-of-the-art materials technologies define the limits of reasonable expectations of the surgeon in the near future. Until materials engineers are able to produce "intelligent materials" for medicine that self-renew and respond to external biological stimuli in predictable and controlled modes, surgeons should not expect implant materials to mimic the physiological function of living tissue. While this should continue to be a long-term demand of medical practitioners, near-term goals will focus on two dramatic improvements in current biomaterials: (1) longer-lasting, more inert, novel materials that match tissue and organ mechanical properties for increasingly durable and dynamic structural implants, and (2) synthetic, absorbable matrices and scaffolds in forms that encourage full corporeal integration, cellular ingrowth, and tissue regeneration to re-create original tissue function and configuration while the implant is gradually eliminated from the implant site.

BIOCOMPATIBILITY: DEFINITION OF TERMS

Biomaterials are natural or synthetic materials used to direct, supplement, or replace living tissue structure and function. The following definition for *biomaterials* has been recently forwarded as a modification of standing American and European definitions:[1]

> "Biomaterials are materials of synthetic or natural origin used alone or in combination with drugs as part of a device in the treatment, augmentation, or replacement of tissues or organs without causing acute or chronic harm to the host, while maintaining their intended biological and physical effectiveness during their useful service *in vivo*."

Only those materials that elicit a minimal level of deleterious biological response from the host are called biomaterials and termed *biocompatible*. It is significant to note that use of the term biocompatible as a classifying tool is inherently flawed; compatibility connotes a level of harmonious interaction. Current use of the term biocompatible often suggests an acceptable or harmonious level of interaction between tissue and material without reference to a standard. Alternatively, the use of *biological performance* has been proposed as the descriptive term to include both components of host and materials responses to implantation. Included in this definition are designated reference materials for standard testing to quantify relative levels of response. *Biocompatibility* is then defined relative to a standard material set as a suitable or acceptable level of biological performance in any specified application. Determining exactly what biological responses are elicited after implantation is yet another methodological complication with many techniques in use[2-4] but little agreement over their worth or relationships to long-term biological performance. Absence of any true bio- or blood compatibility in nearly all current medical materials is the motivation to create hybridized composite materials consisting of synthetic scaffolds and viable cells or tissue as implant biomaterials.

It is also important to consider briefly the biological environment of the host into which the implant is placed. Although conditions of homeostasis and the biochemical aspects of healthy autologous tissue with regard to pH, temperature, partial pressure of oxygen, hydrostatic and osmotic pressure, and fluid chemical content are often well characterized, the local environment around the implant is poorly understood. Because introduction of a foreign body (the implant) always elicits a host response, a wide range of local variations are induced in the environment around the implant that are difficult to predict or control. Dynamic response mechanisms of the body—coagulation, inflammation, and allergic and immune reactions—manifest themselves in the biological environment of the implant site, resulting in significant changes in many or all physiological conditions locally. Thus, the implant experiences drastic changes in environmental conditions, although systemic function of the host may be normally maintained. Moreover, the biological environment of the host responds to the chemical and physical presence of the implant. Material degradation and corrosion products, impurities and contaminants, formulating and sterilization agents, and soluble leachants will spread and diffuse into the area surrounding the implant. Defining the actual environment of the implant then becomes problematic because leaching materials diffuse over time into larger tissue areas and can, in some cases, elicit a systemic response. Lastly, mechanical effects of the host response to the biomaterial, which are separate but related to physiological or biochemical reactions, must be considered. When presented with an implant, a typical host response includes fibrous tissue encapsulation and/or ingrowth. Compromise of the functional and mechanical properties of the implant often ensues.

The long-term stability of the biomaterials–tissue interface is a critical determinant of the long-term viability and success of every implanted device and material. Historically, biomaterials have been chosen for their bulk properties, often limited to materials "borrowed" from other commercial applications. Although all materials may have the desired bulk properties required for an application (i.e., rubbery, elastomeric qualities, rigid fracture toughness, suturability, electrical conduction, or inert barrier properties), surface properties of the material are now recognized as perhaps the most important aspect of a material to minimize problems with host tissues and fluids.[5-7] A significant focus of new biomaterials research is directed at understanding what occurs at the tissue–implant interface—the chemical and mechanical responses that determine the fate of both patient and prosthesis. Currently, almost every surface property has been implicated in achieving successful implant performance.[8] Controlling behavior at this materials–tissue interface is a primary goal of much of this research. A brief description of some basic, useful surface and interfacial chemistry concepts is relevant to this approach.

BIOMATERIAL SURFACES: AN UNUSUAL ENVIRONMENT

Generally, within a material's bulk, interatomic forces act equally in all directions on atoms of the material, resulting in a homogeneous distribution of atomic- and molecular-level forces acting within a material. At a material's surface, the outermost atoms remain unsatisfied in their bonding capabilities as a result of the interface, and the molecules or atoms in this region experience a force differential across an interface caused by differences in the respective bulk environments on either side. The net result in any material at any interface is an anisotropic or asymmetric force field, causing an attraction of the surface atoms inward toward the bulk of the material. The material interface, locally depleted of a normal atomic density, is placed under tension by this net inward attraction, resulting in a localized change of energy per unit surface area, called *surface free energy*. This quantity, in terms of unit surface length, is better known as *surface tension*. Although liquids and solids have fundamental differences in how surface tension is defined, liquids aptly demonstrate the property. Water and mercury, two liquids with high surface tensions, rapidly form round drops in air as these substances attempt to respond to their interface with air by minimizing their interfacial area. The rise of blood in a glass capillary held by a phlebotomist is another example of the action of blood's surface tension pulling the liquid up the capillary tube. This phenomenon leads logically to a discussion of surface wetting, hydrophilic surfaces, and hydrophobicity. Wetting occurs when a liquid readily spreads over a solid surface (water on clean glass, for example). Hydrophilic surfaces are those that are easily wetted by water; that is, the solid surface or interfacial free energy is compatible with the high surface tension of water to allow spreading to maximize their interaction. Metals and ceramics generally have high surface energies and are, therefore, usually wetted by aqueous media. Hydrophobic surfaces such as Teflon, silicones, polyethylene, polypropylene, and polystyrene, have much smaller surface energies and do not wet as a rule, although surface modifications can easily change surface properties without affecting their bulk chemistry.

Because the structure of the outermost atomic layers of a material is structurally dissimilar to its bulk interior, the surface of solid materials has been described as a unique state of matter. Moreover, under operating room conditions, a material's surface is continually bombarded with ambient atmospheric components. Each surface atom will experience about 50 million collisions per second. Some of these colliding atoms will penetrate, adsorb, or chemically modify the surface. The combination of unique surface chemistry and structure can only be found in this outer region. The unique properties of surfaces can then be attributed to thermodynamic forces attempting to minimize an otherwise high-energy situation that produces surfaces. Surfaces compensate for their higher energy in the following ways: (1) translation and rotation of lower energy molecules in the vicinity of the interface toward the outside, (2) adsorption of contamination to or reaction of exposed surface groups (e.g., oxidation) to create a lower energy surface, and (3) diffusion or migration of low-energy components (e.g., low molecular weight additives, processing aids, and contaminants) from the bulk to the surface region. *All these processes produce a surface where the chemical and physical structure is much different than the bulk material.* The primary point is that, despite most efforts, surfaces of biomaterials are often of significantly different chemistry than their bulk.[9–11] Moreover, an exact determination of what the implant environment is, both at and around the interface, is a very difficult problem.

SURFACE INTERACTIONS AS DETERMINANTS OF IMPLANT PERFORMANCE

The instant any implant material is in contact with the biological milieu, its surface is assailed with the thousands of components present, both soluble and insoluble. Hence, the ultimate performance of any material may be determined by early events in its implantation history.[12] The adsorption process is very dynamic and interactive and, because of its complexity, remains poorly understood. It must be governed by two primary factors, both determined by interfacial chemistry: (1) a thermodynamic propensity to minimize interfacial tension (reduce surface energies), molecular organization, and structure, which cost a lot in terms of energy, and (2) a hierarchy of molecular and cell body absorption processes at the interface dependent on diffusion rates and affinities. Hence, surfaces of high interfacial energy (i.e., metals and ceramics) would show greater reactivity than lower energy surfaces (polymers); this driving force for adsorption is higher in the former case than the latter. This does not mean that low-energy surfaces are always nonadsorptive. In fact, more protein adsorption is seen on hydrophobic (lower energy surfaces) polymers than on hydrophilic polymers as a result of strong, predominant hydrophobic driving forces. These forces tend to reduce the amount of high energy structuring of water molecules at surfaces and around molecules and cells, resulting in surface adsorption on hydrophobic surfaces where water must form ordered arrays. Many properties of both surface and adsorbate interact in the implant environment during adsorption phenomena. Ultimately, these molecular events manifest themselves in clinical presentations all relevant to such biofouling: clogging of biliary stents and other shunts, thrombosis on catheters, dialysis membranes, and heart valves, pacemaker corrosion, and many other implant materials problems.

The diffusion properties of substances are generally related to the square of their size. Therefore, a simplified sequence for diffusion to and arrival at a surface from biological fluids might be the following: dissolved gases initially, followed by water, ions, small polar organic solutes, proteins, and finally cell bodies. Transport and binding are sequential components of the adsorption process and each may be rate controlling. In addition to this sequence, the surface populations of each species are constantly evolving and changing, with exchanges of loosely bound adsorbates with higher affinity adsorbing species occurring as conditions dictate. Adsorbed proteins confined to the interface undergo denaturing processes over time, exposing new residues and structures at the material surface that play a role in host response.

Many fine reviews detail the adsorption of biological compounds on medically relevant surfaces.[13–15] The importance of these adsorption responses in determining the biological performance of materials cannot be understated, nor can it be adequately addressed within the scope of this chapter. Suffice it to say that small molecules, primarily water and ions, will become structured at interfaces, creating surface potentials and ion fluxes that contribute to biological responses. Moreover, larger proteinaceous adsorbed layers are inevitable, coupled to the adsorption of smaller molecules, and form a denatured protein carpet or conditioning overlayer that governs longer-term events in biocompatibility.[16] Subsequent cell ingrowth, adhesion, thrombosis, complement activation, bacterial adhesion, foreign-body responses, and ultimately, biocompatibility, are all subsequent events determined by adsorption of solutes at the biological surface materials interface.

The nature of the material surface of the implant, therefore, is a large determinant of its compatibility. Exposing polymers, metals, and ceramics to biological fluids results in the adsorption of molecules on the surface, eventually replacing the original interface with adsorbed layers and altering the interfacial properties of the material irreversibly. Surface properties govern these responses and possibly the long-term biological response of the implant (Fig. 6-1). Currently, however, none of the many thermodynamic models proposed to account for adsorption processes from biological fluids based on interfacial properties can fully explain experimental observations. Experimental evidence suggests that adsorption of specific proteins has specific consequences. Different surfaces react to the complex mixture of host proteins in varying ways, leading to different combinations of proteins and cellular elements adhered at surfaces. Hydrophobic surfaces seem to adsorb more protein than hydrophilic surfaces. With time, fibrinogen, for example, seems to adsorb rapidly out of blood serum onto most hydrophobic surfaces, eventually being replaced by other proteins, including high molecular weight kininogen.[17,18] The timing of fibrinogen adsorption and removal by blood may be clinically relevant because human platelet adsorption is correlated with fibrinogen deposition.[19,20] Albumin adsorption, by contrast, has been shown to protect surfaces from platelet adhesion[14,21,22] and promote blood compatibility of implanted materials.[23,24] Woven polyester vascular grafts, with a bioerodible albumin precoating that eliminates the need for graft preclotting, seem to be less likely to leak, and endothelialization is improved.[23] However, given the hundreds of proteins in biological fluids, the interactions of one or even several proteins with a surface fall far short of providing a complete description of the implant environment and dynamics.

With its proteins, ions, and cellular components, blood serum responds in many ways to microenvironments at the implant surface based on both surface chemistry and physical surface topology. Surface roughness on a molecular scale influences protein adsorption, transport, and cell adhesion drastically. Thus, in the formulation of new materials for biomedical purposes, scientists must consider chemical composition, dynamic surface restructuring, mechanical requirements, and suitable surface topology for each application. Current gaps in the general understanding of adsorption-mediated biological performance are the relationships among: (1) surface properties and both ion adsorption and later protein adsorption events, (2) adsorbed protein and platelet adhesion, (3) adsorbed protein and granulocyte adhesion, and (4) adsorbed protein, complement activation, and the subsequent mobilization of white cells.

POLYMERIC BIOMATERIALS IN SURGERY

Polymeric and plastic materials have made a substantial impact as materials for implantation. A 1947 review listed only three commercially available plastics and one natural rubber as promising surgical implant materials.[25] Currently, over 50 materials are approved for application in equally as many types of prosthetic devices. Recent developments in polymer chemistry and engineering continually make new materials available with properties much more sophisticated and appropriate for surgical use than any past or current implant materials. Nevertheless, as much as ever, new polymeric materials for surgery need to satisfy the following basic criteria: (1) they must be reproducibly synthesized as a pure material at reasonable cost; (2) they must be fabricated into the desired form within the required tolerances without degradation or adverse transformations; (3) they must exhibit the required chemical, physical, and mechanical properties for their application within a suitable performance lifetime; and (4) they must not induce

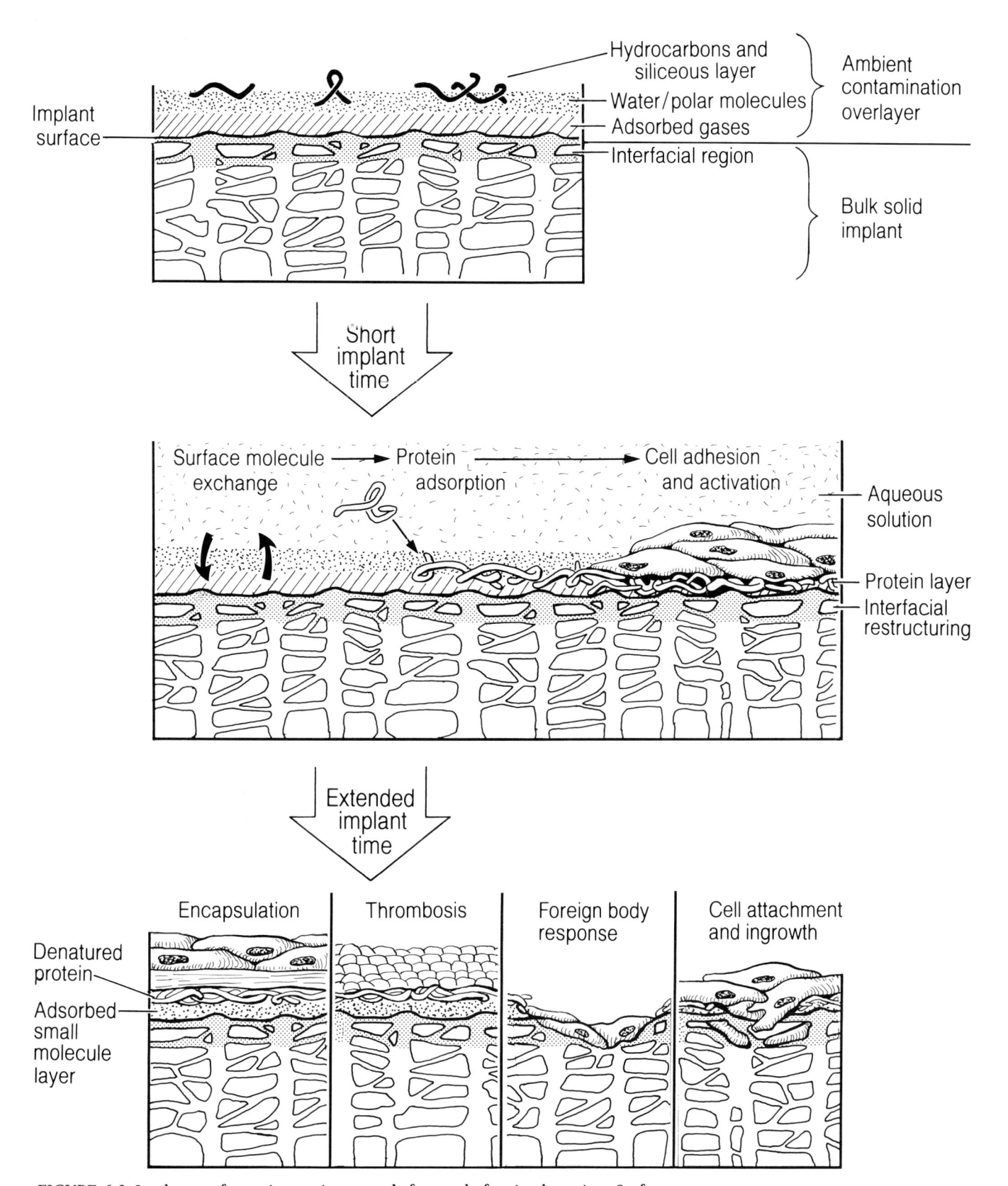

FIGURE 6-1 Implant surface microenvironment before and after implantation. Surface contamination from material fabrication, processing, sterilization procedures, and adsorption of ambient airborne molecules creates a poorly defined interfacial region. After surgical implantation, this surface reacts and is further modified by biological adsorption and exchange phenomena, contributing to a highly complex dynamic biomaterials interfacial environment.

thrombosis or activate the coagulation cascade, alter the function of any cellular function leading to host sensitivity or reaction (unless desired), induce adverse inflammatory or foreign-body responses, or be carcinogenic.

These are extremely stringent, selective materials criteria. Currently, no material implanted into a host has satisfied all of these criteria; few implants can satisfy even some of them—a source of disillusionment among many surgeons! Yet to the uninitiated investigator seeking materials as tissue substitutes, commercial sources offer a dazzling array of polymers with countless properties. Teflon, Dacron, and medical-grade silicone rubber are the most widely used soft tissue-replacement materials in surgery presently. All are adaptations of industrial polymers produced for other purposes. Because of the equally diverse list of applications of materials in surgery, this chapter cannot attempt to address each material specification and surgical need. Rather, the hope is to present an outline of materials issues in surgery and to point out directions by which the surgeon might contribute to materials development and in which materials development is heading to assist surgery.

Polyurethanes

Biomedical interest in polyurethanes is based both on their desirable range of mechanical properties and a wide number of commercially available formulations with specifically tailored properties. These materials find applications currently in vascular prostheses, blood tubing and bags, catheters, artificial hearts and assist devices, and a number of soft tissue implants.[26] Generally, polyurethanes comprise a class of highly durable, low-reactive materials. Blood–polyurethane reactivity has been shown to correlate with polyurethane surface chemistry. Polyurethane chemistries, however, are subject to biological degradation mechanisms, including hydrolysis and oxidation, calcification, and fatigue. Moreover, polyurethane surfaces often differ radically in composition from their bulk, leading to confusion over what chemistry contributes to observed tissue responses. Poly(ether urethanes) and poly(ether urethaneureas), those polyurethanes most favored in biomedical applications, are dominated in their surface regions by the soft polyether segment. The high mobility of these segments allows this polymer surface to respond to interfacial environments by moving to and from the interface, changing surface composition dynamically over time. This has implications for very dynamic material interfacial responses to protein adsorption and cell adhesion which, in turn, determine biological performance. Some aspects of polyurethane histocompatibility have been recently investigated.[27]

Silicone Rubbers

Medical-grade silicones have become one of the most extensively utilized synthetic materials in implant applications.[28] The chemistry of these materials is based on the dimethylsiloxane unit and is the basis for their accepted chemical name, poly(dimethylsiloxane). Unaltered siloxane polymers are fluids until they reach very high molecular weights. Fluid silicones are applied in surgery as defoaming agents for blood, lubricants for needles and catheters, and in plastic and reconstructive surgery applications. Medical-grade solid silicone elastomers (silicone rubbers) are produced by crosslinking high molecular weight polydimethylsiloxane polymers in mixtures with large-surface-area fumed silica particles (30-μm diameter). Compounding with varying ratios of crosslinking and particle filler contents creates siloxane materials with wide ranges of mechanical properties. It is also notable that medical-grade siloxanes are perhaps the only medical material available in highly purified form. Medical-grade polyurethanes and Dacrons all are substantially contaminated from processing aids and other low molecular weight impurities that affect their biological performance and contribute to wide variances in implant response.

Silicone elastomers are used currently in many surgical applications. Shunts for treating hydrocephalus and ascites are probably the best recognized. Surface induction of bacterial colonization in these shunts is a current research interest. In cardiovascular applications, silicones have not performed as well, with notable failures as valve, graft, and artificial heart prostheses. Part of this problem is caused by the use of silica as a filler material in this polymer. Other problems are derived from infiltration of fatty components of blood into siloxanes, cracking and fissuring, and thrombosis. Blood-contacting applications, such as gas-permeable oxygenator membranes, are more successful because of siloxane's inherently high gas permeability, although fundamental problems with blood compatibility remain unresolved. Silicone materials are used in long-term catheterization; their mechanical flexibility is better than other materials, and bacterial adherence is low. Applications of this material in the genitourinary system are prevalent, including penile, ureter, and bladder implants and urinary catheters. Despite some setbacks, general siloxane implant success as the past and current material of choice across a wide range of clinical applications is indicative of silicone's relative benign biological response and acceptable tissue interactions. Toxicity and biological performance issues have been reviewed recently.[29]

Suture Materials

Because virtually every surgical procedure requires the use of suture materials in wound closure, a large variety of materials have been developed with various chemical, physical, mechanical, and biological properties. Two broad categories are recognized: absorbable and nonabsorbable. Absorbable sutures include reconstituted collagen (from bovine tendon), collagen derived from sheep intestinal submucosa (catgut), and synthetic, hydrolyzable polymeric materials, including polyglycolic acid and its lactide copolymers, polydioxanone and poly(glycolide-trimethylene carbonate). Nonabsorbable sutures are divided into natural fibers (silk and cotton), synthetic polymer fibers (polyethylene, polypropylene, polyamide, polyester, and polytetrafluoroethylene), and stainless steel. Tissue reactivity is a function of material geometry and topology (round versus square or monofilament versus braided), tissue–suture interface movement, leukocyte reactions and degranulation, and resulting degradation products. Silk, for example, prompts a cellular invasion and degrades very slowly, leaving insoluble fragments, which may lead to granulomas; synthetic sutures break down in water to innocuous products eliminated through the kidneys. Although most natural materials (collagen) require infiltration of site-specific cellular enzymes for degradation, synthetic degradable polymers hydrolyze readily in the physiological milieu, resulting in more consistent, reliable degradation kinetics. The prediction is toward increased use of synthetic suture materials for this reason. Nevertheless, degradation properties of synthetic sutures can be tailored by changes in chemistry (anhydride versus ester), fabrication (density and crystalline properties of polymer chains), molecular weight of polymer, and degradation enhancing additives (acids, bases, and enzymes). Recent reviews of both suture–tissue responses and suture materials[30] and degradation studies on new suture materials are available.

Wound Dressings

Advances in polymer chemistry and in the understanding of wound healing physiology have prompted an explosion of new wound dressing materials. Wound dressing classification is difficult because of the complex construction of most dressing materials. A recent review[31] categorized these biomaterials based on product type: film dressings, foams, polysaccharide dressings, hydrogels, biological dressings, and hydrocolloid dressings. Film dressings are transparent, adhesive-coated polymer films (typically polyurethanes), which are readily permeable to water vapor and air but impermeable to microbes. Foams include synthetic sponge-like polymer foam sheets and reactive foam precursors, which set directly into the wound site. Polysaccharide dressings are derived from naturally occurring starches and form gel-like wound occlusion or covering materials that are often absorbable. Hydrogel dressings are water-swollen, insoluble, crosslinked polymer networks with high levels of water absorption and permeability that are easily adaptable to various dressing designs. Biological dressings are a relatively new development and consist of collagenous composite networks or liquids based on natural materials. These materials attempt to approach a synthetic skin substitute in design, and some actually incorporate live dermal cells. Hydrocolloid dressings are the latest development in wound dressings, incorporating design principles of adhesion, occlusion, and absorbency, plus an attempt to avoid damage to healing tissues. A polymer film backing is coated with a hydrocolloid mass—typically gelatin, pectin, or carboxymethylcellulose—which is in turn covered with a hydrophobic adhesive to promote an initial dry tack. At the wound site, the hydrocolloid mass absorbs wound fluids, replacing the dry tack with a wet tack and promoting liquefaction of the gel over the wound surface.

Cardiovascular Materials

A wide variety of cardiovascular repair products are currently marketed or under investigation for implant use. Types include autogenous vein grafts, pretreated heterografts, synthetic weaves, nonwoven synthetic polymer grafts, and bioresorbable vascular scaffolds. After 25 years of implantation, however, Dacron fabric (polyethylene terephthalate) remains the most widely used material for vascular prostheses[32,33] and is fabricated in a number of forms. Dacron grafts are either macro- or microporous; are constructed in woven, conventional knit, and velour types; and are available in crimped and noncrimped forms. Regardless of the type of Dacron material used, Dacron itself is a thrombogenic material. This mandates that Dacron meshes, weaves, and fabrics in contact with blood be deactivated by overcoating with synthetic polymers, such as silicones or polyurethanes, or undergo preclotting to cover the surface with a neointima consisting of coagulation products or albumin before implantation.

Surgical Mesh

In the absence of suitable autologous tissue alternatives, surgeons often require surgical mesh to reconstruct major defects that result from trauma-induced injury, congenital deficiencies, tumor resection, or tissue necrosis. Until the development of Marlex (a polyethylene mesh), Teflon mesh (polytetrafluoroethylene) was the material of choice because it was inert and routinely covered and incorporated with granulation tissue during wound healing. Additionally, wound healing with this mesh was often complete even in the presence of infection. Teflon suffered from its poor tensile strength, however, particularly when sutured under tension. Unfortunately, changing the weave to improve strength decreased tissue ingrowth into this mesh material. Marlex mesh exhibits a tensile strength much higher than nylon, Teflon, Dacron, or silk; is extremely porous and resistant to unraveling as a mesh (as opposed to the Teflon fabric); and can be sutured close to its edges, which are readily sealed by cauterization. Marlex's performance in animals and humans in functional roles has been reported and compared with Teflon fabrics. Because Marlex's low softening point requires boiling for sterilization, surgical meshes from polypropylene have supplanted the original polyethylene Marlex because they withstand repeated autoclave sterilizations and show superior performance in clinical use. Additionally, a Dacron surgical mesh, Mersilene, although not as well characterized as other synthetic meshes, is available commercially (Ethicon, Somerville, NJ) and has been evaluated in abdominal wall reconstruction.

Marlex meshes have found successful applications in both chest and abdominal wall reconstructions and as tracheal replacements. Dacron fabrics and crimped nylon and stainless-steel meshes have been reported for use in tracheal and esophageal reconstruction and dura and small bowel repair. Dacron velour and bioabsorbable polylactide or glycolide tubes and shunts have been used in genitourinary surgery, although tissue ingrowth has impaired function of porous mesh urinary prostheses. Long-term follow-up studies on the biological performance of most of these materials are not yet available, although most clinical reports affirm earlier studies showing biological inertness, resistance to infection, tissue integration, and permanent bonding. Dexon and Vicryl, both new commercial absorbable mesh materials, have also been tested. Such an absorbable mesh provides a temporary scaffold to promote ingrowth, tissue regeneration, and scarring while the supporting material is slowly degraded, reducing latent infection and foreign-body responses. New developments for biodegradable materials of this type are detailed in the next section.

Biological and Biodegradable Polymeric Materials

Biopolymer materials, including proteins or synthetic polypeptides, polysaccharides (cellulose and starches), and glycosaminoglycans (heparin and chondroitins) are being increasingly investigated as improved biocompatible and reabsorbable materials for various surgical applications.[34] Their synthesis, fabrication techniques, and implant design can have a large effect on degradation rates in vivo, and problems associated with foreign-body responses are alleviated as the implant material is removed from the site of implantation. Combinations of different biodegradable materials with synthetic nonresorbable polymers or with each other as composites or sandwich structures also affect their lifetime and biological performance. Thus, properties can be tailored over a wide range to meet specific implant specifications.

Collagens are a series of structural proteins secreted from fibroblasts and found primarily in all connective tissues. Collagens were applied as some of the first surgical biomaterials in the form of catgut sutures. Recent elucidation of collagen's molecular structures, compositions, and properties have stimulated development of new preparation, processing, and utilization of this material in surgical and implant applications.[35] Although suitable for a variety of applications, collagen's proteinaceous nature is capable of eliciting an immune response, limiting heterologous transplants as sources of material. The antigenic domains on collagen have been characterized and antigenicity appears to be related to the collagen type. Immunorecognition also appears to be altered by treatment with chemical crosslinkers (e.g., glutaraldehyde) to cover old epitopes and create new ones. Nevertheless, the host reaction to collagen implantation is different from that observed with other polymeric implant materials, primarily because collagen itself is an important component of the host's wound healing response. Cells show good adhesion to collagen implants. However, collagen is a potent activator of the coagulation cascade, triggering both platelet aggregation and Hageman factor activation. Therefore, blood contact with collagen-containing implants must be carefully considered because of its hemostatic behavior. In fact, various collagen preparations are used as hemostatic agents to control bleeding in areas such as the liver where structural support for blood clots is poor.

Collagen has been mentioned as a wound dressing type (biological) because of its abilities to clot blood, promote cell adhesion, stimulate cell migration and ingrowth, mechanically alleviate surface tissue stress and strain, and gradually degrade in the wound site. Synthetic skin replacement tissues have also been reported,[36] the most recent being a promising new composite consisting of a crosslinked collagen matrix filled with glycosaminoglycans, chondroitin-6-sulfate, and covered with an impermeable film of crosslinked siloxane polymer.[37] This matrix can also be seeded with epidermal cells and growth factors to promote regeneration of native tissue in a biodegradable structure. Other pseudodermal collagenous replacement materials, some containing live cells, have also been reported.

Collagens are also solubilized using enzymes or formulated as fibrillar suspensions for injection. Injectable collagens are used to induce an initial, stabilizing fibrotic response to stimulate tissue generation, with longer term degradation and elimination from the injection site. Applications are primarily cosmetic, and adverse responses to collagen immunogenicity or other sensitivity are reported complications.

Perhaps the most significant use of collagen biomaterials currently is as bioprosthetic heart valves derived from xenografted tissue. Typically derived from bovine pericardium or porcine aortic valve tissue sources, trileaflet valve implants closely simulating natural valve function, structure and hemodynamic properties can be readily produced. Although glutaraldehyde crosslinking stabilizes valve integrity and reduces immune and platelet-activating responses, longer-term tissue thinning, degradation, and calcification are still major problems.

Compression-molded fibrin implants constitute yet another resorbable material that has a substantial history already as a new biomaterial.[38] Absorption rates are influenced by the implant site, device geometry, and fabrication conditions. Because the breakdown products are fibrin and glycerol, the implants are relatively innocuous.

APPROACHES TO IMPROVE POLYMERS IN SOFT TISSUE SURGERY

The ultimate biomaterial must fulfill a diverse set of functional and structural criteria. Materials chemistry cannot yet create advanced materials that are able to function acceptably in many implant applications. Still, many implant environments have not been defined adequately enough to permit rational new biomaterials design. From the preceding survey of the polymeric biomaterials currently used in surgery, it is readily apparent that all synthetic implant materials present a relatively primitive, unsophisticated structure, both in bulk and surface, compared with native tissues. The next generation of biomaterials, while still a far cry from mimicking the complexity of tissue architecture and function, will attempt to integrate with the body to prevent a diverse array of adverse host reactions and mechanically match the structural aspects of tissue replacement with relatively complex synthetic designs. Figure 6-2 outlines a biomaterials development strategy incorporating both natural and synthetic materials.

Natural materials are consistently designed and built on principles of supramolecular assembly.[39] These architectural structures integrate organized groups of molecules that spontaneously self-assemble to form the functioning units necessary for life. This creates highly organized materials from a consecutive hierarchy of highly specific molecular-level assembly events, presenting higher order structures (membranes, cells, matrices, tissues, organs, and organisms) as well defined as their molecules. Unfortunately, our ability to manipulate the molecular architecture of materials to yield novel ultrastructures with sophisticated properties cannot approach Mother Nature's mastery. The materials research community has only recently begun to study the hierarchic character of natural materials with the intention of duplicating these architectural principles in new synthetic systems.[40,41] Most recent approaches attempt to improve surgical materials by coating, grafting, or modifying the surfaces of biomaterials in a wide variety of ways.[42] These strategies focus primarily on altering the interfacial character of the material without changing the bulk material properties. Molecular self- or supramolecular assembly will be an exciting future area of investigation for the biomaterials research community.

Biomembrane Surfaces

With the contention that natural membranes present an ideal passive biological interface, two groups have recently reported biomaterials surface modification strategies based on lipid membrane or membrane-like coatings on im-

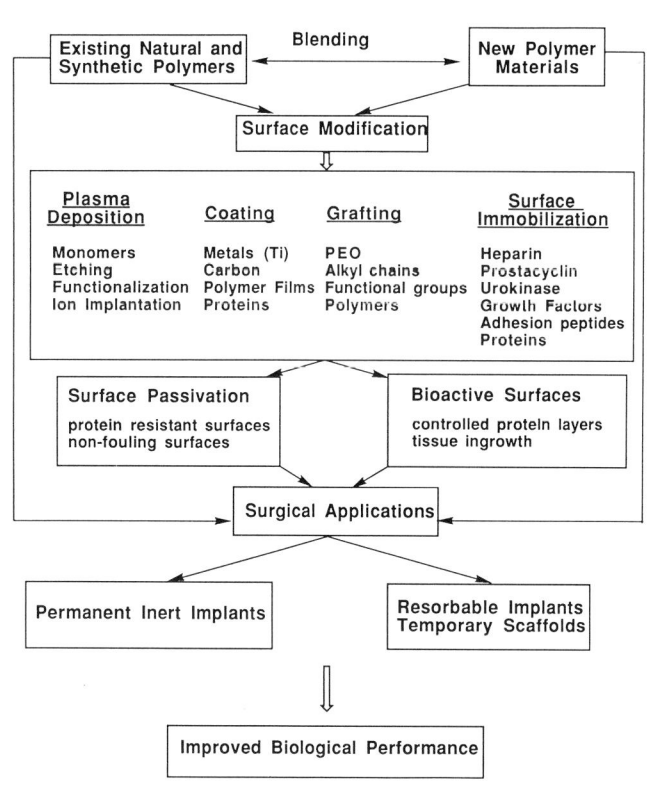

FIGURE 6-2 Strategy for the development of improved polymeric biomaterials for surgical applications. A basic design dichotomy between ingrowth promoting and nonfouling (protein- or cell-resistant) surfaces is presented for applications as resorbable or integrated materials scaffolds or nonreactive, inert permanent implants, respectively.

plants.[43,44] Reduced protein adsorption and activation of coagulation components are found on these surfaces, and there are striking improvements in blood compatibility. Polymerizable lipid membranes are thought to stabilize organized lipid arrays on implant surfaces to make a durable cell membrane-like interface inert to biodegradation (Fig. 6-3).

Cell Seeding and Adhesion

Just as no one material has found universal applicability in surgical use, no one approach will answer all demands for improved new materials for surgery in the future. Moreover, as cellular and molecular biology provide increasing understanding and insight into the molecular basis of biochemistry and physiological processes, new techniques and material aimed at controlling molecular aspects of materials compatibility will be developed. One initial attempt at this strategy is based on the recent elucidation of some cell attachment domains in cell adhesion proteins (fibronectin, vitronectin, and collagen).[45] The tetrapeptide

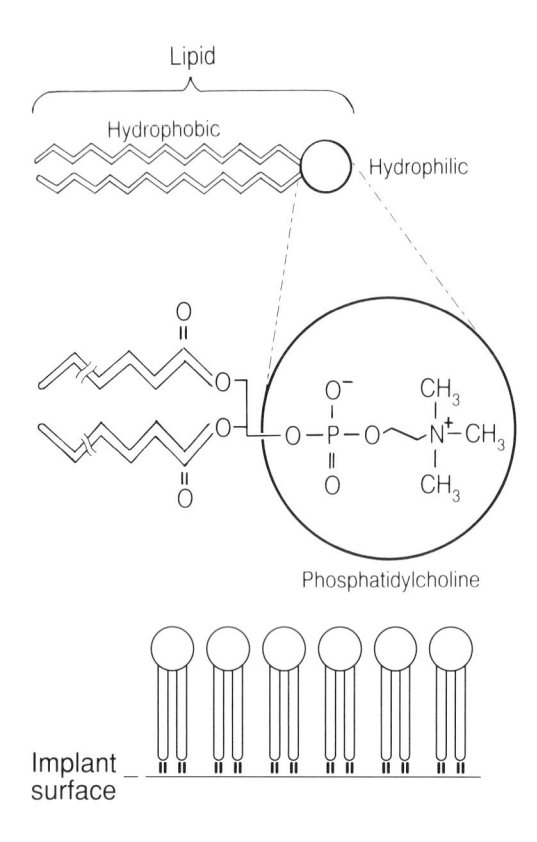

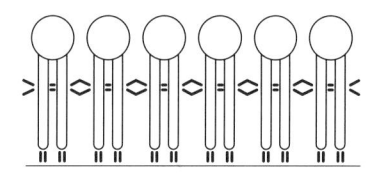

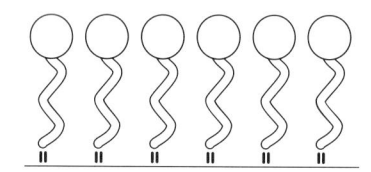

FIGURE 6-3 Biomimetic approach to optimizing biomaterials interfacial reactivity by using phospholipid chemistry *(top)* to modify implant surfaces. Each strategy would ideally present a membrane-like phospholipid surface to the biological milieu, masking the synthetic nature of the implant and reducing adverse host responses. A. Anchoring dense, organized lipid coatings to surfaces. B. Polymerization of lipid coatings on surfaces. C. Grafting of lipid-like groups to surfaces.

Arginine-Glycine-Aspartic Acid-Serine sequence has been synthesized and used as a surface modification agent on polymer surfaces to promote cell attachment and growth. Although the strategy has numerous applications, cell ingrowth into implants serves to stabilize the tissue–material interface mechanically and promotes tissue regeneration around the implant. Surfaces patterned with adhesion peptides could promote directional growth of cells, particularly for nerve guides and cell-based biosensors. A newer concept utilizes immobilized or controlled release of tissue-specific growth factors at biomaterials surfaces to promote cell growth and integration at the implant interface.

Many developments continue to improve clinical applications of vascular prostheses.[46] Nevertheless, vascular grafting could benefit greatly from surface modification strategies that promote rapid cell growth to assist in anastomotic stabilization, prevention of infection, and neointima formation. Currently, few, if any, human vascular grafts have demonstrated successful formation of complete neo- or pseudointima. Seeding of vascular graft beds with cells harvested and cultured from the host has attempted to duplicate the vascular endothelium and its ideal blood-contacting properties. Two difficulties are currently encountered as follows: (1) cultured endothelial cells appear to differentiate or, at least, modify their normal function when seeded and (2) few seeded cells remain anchored to the graft surface after implantation in flowing blood.[47]

At the beginning of this chapter, it was mentioned that select new materials in surgery should promote full integration with existing tissue and tissue regeneration. A vascular endothelial lining is capable of regeneration and renewal and is ideally blood compatible, yet vascular prostheses seem incapable of supporting such a layer in humans. Preclotting and coating with collagens or fibronectin have been used to "condition" grafts before implant for rapid cell growth. Biochemical or chemical surface modification methods may be able to promote endothelialization and cell colonization for intima generation. In this regard, newer modifications of graft surfaces involving immobilization of cell-adherent molecules, heparin, and gaseous plasma deposition methods may prove clinically viable.

Some additional new materials strategies to enhance prosthetic biological performance include thin polymeric coatings[10,11,48] over existing materials, poly(ethylene oxide)[48] and ionomer grafting methods, and new polymer developments. Bioresorbable vascular prostheses and temporary supporting scaffolds are continually evolving, incorporating new biodegradable polymers with new properties,[34,49] and attempting to eliminate many of the obstacles encountered when vascular implants are fabricated from more permanent materials.

Knit or woven Dacron large-diameter grafts are currently the synthetic design of choice for clinical application and are generally successful where flow rates are high. There are no convincing data to suggest superior performance of knitted over woven designs, nor Dacron over Teflon in large-diameter prostheses. Small-diameter vascular grafts must satisfy viscoelastic criteria; currently no acceptable synthetic prostheses are available for applications smaller than 6 mm in diameter. These materials must satisfy stringent interfacial and mechanical requirements that are not necessary for large-diameter grafts. Adaptations of large graft designs and materials have failed, and various types of polyurethanes have become candidate materials. This area, and the problem of calcification of blood-contacting materials, are two areas where new materials are critically needed.

Cell Encapsulation

Immobilization and release of cell growth factors and peptides may also assist in the development of artificial organs and tissue replacement based on transplant and/or encapsulation of live cells as implants.[50,51] The development of asymmetric polymer encapsulation membranes of controlled porosity has reduced problems associated with histocompatibility and immune recognition. Current problems with live cell transplants include posttransplant cell growth inhibition, cell differentiation, and reduced viability and response to biochemical stimuli (i.e., insulin and dopamine production) over time. Live encapsulated cell transplant technologies hold significant promise in organ replacement and repair strategies, provided that new materials and encapsulation methods support cell growth and tissue regeneration.

Bioactive Surfaces

A pharmacologic approach based on surface-immobilized bioactive molecules has been utilized to improve blood–materials compatibility.[52] Heparin, prostaglandins, heparin–prostaglandin conjugates, and albumin–heparin conjugates have all been reported to improve surface-induced thrombogenesis when immobilized at blood-contacting materials surfaces. Polymers incorporating heparin into their backbone structure[10,11] and synthetic heparin-like surfaces are also under investigation. These new materials can be coated as thin bioactive films over existing materials or used as stand-alone implant surfaces. In all cases, bioactivity of the pharmacologically active moiety is compromised by surface binding. Use of spacer chemistry, however, improves the bioactive properties of these surfaces. Additionally, such an approach provides localized anticoagulant effects, alleviating the requirement for systemic heparinization.

Polyethylene Oxide Surfaces

Polyethylene oxide (PEO)—a synthetic, nontoxic, water soluble polymer—is actively being investigated as a hydrophilic, nonfouling coating material for biomedical implant devices, including vascular grafts, contact lenses, catheters, and guide wires. These surfaces exhibit low frictional coefficients (slipperiness) and low degrees of adsorbed proteins, adhered cells, and platelets, for reasons not well understood. The PEO surfaces are readily prepared by a number of routes, including simple coating, solution adsorption, surface chemical grafting, plasma deposition, and crosslinking, facilitating their application in biomaterial interfacial applications. This surface mobility, immobilization densities, and molecular weight effects are all active areas of investigation attempting to elucidate PEO's apparent efficacy as a biomaterial. The PEO-modified surfaces appear to have a bright and versatile future in biomaterials applications.

Vapor-Deposited Carbon Coatings

Impermeable thin coatings of carbon (Biolite carbon) have demonstrated benign acute and chronic responses in contact with tissue. Carbon implants are also inert and eventually become incorporated into the host site. Moreover, carbon surfaces show promising responses in blood. As a surface modification agent over existing surgical materials, ULTI carbon deposition can be controlled in terms of density, crystallite size, and film isotropy to yield pure carbon coatings 0.1- to 1-μm thick. As a result of their dimensions, carbons can be coated over highly flexible biomaterial polymeric substrates, such as polyesters, nylons, and surgical meshes and sutures, without affecting their bulk properties. Controlled deposition can yield a pure carbon interfacial layer without affecting the porosities or physical properties of the underlying biomaterial. Although several carbon biomedical implants (e.g., heart valves) are extensively used, further applications in surgery using this material seem inevitable.[52]

Titanium Surfaces

Although the alloyed form is used primarily in orthopedic implants, pure titanium has been recently recognized as having unique interactions in the host that lend themselves to other implant applications. The outer surface of clean titanium is actually titanium dioxide, which changes and thickens as a function of implantation time. Autoclaving sterilization generally contaminates the oxide layer with quantities of carbon, nitrogen, and other components that may actually assist biomaterials performance. Titanium promotes strong interfacial osteoblast adhesion, supports other cell growth when implanted, and is the only metal that remains unencapsulated by collagen after implantation. Because titanium is one of the few materials demonstrating correlations between surface properties and biological performance, it should receive increasing attention to characterize its interfacial relationships with implant environments and in applications as ultrathin coatings to modify the surfaces of polymeric implants.

New Biodegradable and Bioresorbable Polymers

The development of new biodegradable polymers is driven by their potential applications in a diverse array of medical functions. Particular needs include improved mechanical and processing properties, controlled ranges of biodegradation kinetics that integrate well with healing dynamics, and well-metabolized biodegradation products. Recent, new biodegradable polymers with interesting new properties include polyphosphates and polyphosphonates,[45] polyphosphazenes, poly(amino acids), poly(ether–esters), polyesters derived from bacterial sources,[53] and poly(ortho esters). Some engineering properties of several of these polymer materials have been reported recently.[54]

A very significant development for new biomaterials development is the rational design of new polymers using gene-splicing techniques and production of these materials in living bioreactor-based microorganism expression systems. Mass production of biodegradable poly(hydroxybutyrates) in bacteria has recently resulted in commercially available polymer materials. Manipulation of these bacteria and other phototropic organisms is being used currently to produce poly(hydroxy alkanoate) polymers using solar energy and fatty acid feedstocks to control polymer synthesis.[55] Other genetically engineered organisms are being studied to produce nonnatural polypeptides as custom-designed materials, enzymes, and proteins. The ability to control material composition and properties on a genetic level will result in novel materials with new applications.

CONCLUSIONS

In a clinical setting, surface properties are a primary factor governing the ultimate performance of implanted polymeric biomaterials. Traditional polymeric biomaterials adapted from commercial polymers in other industries have been chosen based on bulk properties with little regard for interfacial properties. New materials development strategies will improve the surface characteristics of these widely used and accepted materials by surface modification and coating techniques. Immobilization of bioactive molecules and poly(ethylene oxide), plasma and vapor deposition methods, and polymer thin film overcoats are under active investigation. New polymeric materials are also being synthesized, both as biodegradable scaffold materials to promote tissue regeneration and as inert stable materials with improved mechanical and interfacial properties for permanent repair. Significantly, increasing research activity is focused on duplicating the complex microstructural and architectural features of natural biomaterials—the cell membrane, biopolymers, hierarchic materials, and composites found in bone, teeth, and connective tissue—to produce a new generation of improved biomaterials. These new materials will advance from the relatively primitive isotropic, homogeneous, limited materials currently available toward the dynamic, interactive, anisotropic, and responsive biomaterials to be used by the surgeon of the future.

ACKNOWLEDGMENTS

The Whitaker Foundation and the Medical Research Foundation of Oregon provided support during the preparation of this chapter.

REFERENCES

1. Bruck SD: Materials or biomaterials? *Int J Artif Organs* 1990; 13:469–471.
2. Marchant RE: The cage implant system for determining in vivo biocompatibility of medical device materials. *Fundam Appl Toxicol* 1989; 13:217–227.
3. National Heart, Lung, and Blood Institute Working Group: *Guidelines for Blood-Materials Interactions.* Bethesda, MD, U.S. Department of Health and Human Services, Public Health Service, National Institutes of Health, 1985.
4. Williams DF: A model for biocompatibility and its evaluation. *J Biomed Eng* 1989; 11:185–191.
5. Hench LL, Ethridge ED: *Biomaterials: An Interfacial Approach.* New York, Academic Press, 1982.
6. Gristina AG, Naylor P, Myrvik Q: Infections from biomaterials and implants: A race for the surface. *Med Prog Technol* 1988; 14:205–224.
7. Ratner BD, Johnson AB, Lenk TJ: Biomaterial surfaces. *J Biomed Mater Res* 1987; 21:59–89.
8. Andrade JD: Interfacial phenomena and biomaterials. *Med Instrum* 1973; 7:110–120.
9. Ratner BD (ed): *Surface Characterization of Biomaterials.* Amsterdam, Elsevier, 1988.
10. Grainger DW, Knutson K, Kim SW, et al: Polydimethyl(siloxane)-poly(ethyleneoxide)-heparin block-copolymers. II: Surface characterization and in vitro assessments. *J Biomed Mater Res* 1990; 24:403–431.
11. Grainger DW, Okano T, Kim SW, et al: Polydimethyl(siloxane)-poly(ethyleneoxide)-heparin block-copolymers. III: Surface characterization and in vitro assessments. *J Biomed Mater Res* 1990; 24:547–571.
12. Vroman L: The life of an artificial device in contact with blood: Initial events and their effect on its final state. *Bull N Y Acad Med* 1988; 64:352–357.
13. Horbett TA, Brash JL: Proteins at interfaces: Current issues and future prospects, in Horbett TA, Brash JL (eds): *Proteins at Interfaces.* Washington, DC, ACS Press, 1987, pp 1–35.
14. Andrade JD, Hlady V: Protein adsorption and materials biocompatibility: A tutorial and suggested hypothesis: *Adv Polymer Sci* 1986; 79:1–63.
15. Andrade JD, Hlady V: Plasma protein adsorption: The big twelve. *Ann N Y Acad Sci* 1987; 516:158–172.
16. Anderson JM, Bonfield TL, Ziats NP: Protein adsorption and cellular adhesion and activation on biomedical polymers. *Int J Artif Organs* 1990; 13:375–382.

17. Vroman L: Protein/surface interaction, in Horbett TA, Brash JL (eds): *Proteins at Interfaces.* Washington, DC, ACS Press, 1987, pp 80–88.
18. Vroman L, Adams A, Fischer GC, et al: Interaction of high molecular weight kininogen, factor XII, and fibrinogen in plasma at interfaces. *Blood* 1980; 55:156–159.
19. Zucker MB, Vroman L: Platelet adhesion induced by fibrinogen adsorbed onto glass. *Proc Soc Exp Biol Med* 1969; 131:318–320.
20. Kim SW, Wisniewski SM, Lee ES, et al: Role of protein and fatty acid adsorption on platelet adhesion and aggregation at the blood–polymer interface. *J Biomed Mater Res* 1977; 8:23–29.
21. Packham MA, Evans G, Glynn MF, et al: The effect of plasma proteins on the interaction of platelet with glass surfaces. *J Lab Clin Med* 1969; 73:686–697.
22. Eberhart RC, Munro MS, Williams GB, et al: Albumin adsorption and retention on C18-alkyl-derivatized polyurethane vascular grafts. *Artif Organs* 1987; 11:375–382.
23. Guidoin R, Marois Y, Rao T-J, et al: An albumin-coated polyester arterial prosthesis made ready to anastomose: In vivo evaluation in dogs. *Clin Mater* 1988; 3:119–131.
24. Kottke-Marchant K, Anderson JM, Umemura Y, et al: Effect of albumin coating on the in vitro blood compatibility of Dacron arterial prostheses. *Biomaterials* 1989; 10:147–155.
25. Ingraham FD, Alexander E Jr, Matson DD: Synthetic plastic materials in surgery. *N Engl J Med* 1947; 236:362–368.
26. Lelah MD, Cooper SL: *Polyurethanes in Medicine.* Boca Raton, FL, CRC Press, 1986.
27. Brunstedt MR, Anderson JM, Spilizewski KL, et al: In vivo leukocyte interactions on Pellethane surfaces. *Biomaterials* 1990; 11:370–378.
28. van Noort R, Black MM: Silicone rubbers for medical application, in Williams DF (ed): *Biocompatibility of Clinical Implant Materials.* Boca Raton, FL, CRC Press, 1981, vol 2, pp 79–98.
29. Arkles B, Redinger P: Silicones in biomedical applications, in Szycher M (ed): *Biocompatible Polymers, Metals and Composites.* Lancaster, PA, Technomic, 1983, pp 719–768.
30. Capperauld I: Suture materials: A review. *Clin Mater* 1989; 4:3.
31. Lydon MJ: Wound dressings materials, in Williams DF (ed): *Concise Encyclopedia of Medical and Dental Materials.* Oxford, Pergamon Press, 1990, pp 367–371.
32. Sawyer PN, Stanczewski B, Mistry FD, et al: Analysis of major arterial vessel replacement in laboratory and clinical use, in Rubin LR (ed): *Biomaterials in Reconstructive Surgery.* St. Louis, CV Mosby, 1983, pp 689–734.
33. King M, Plais P, Guidoin R, et al: Polyethylene terephthalate (Dacron) vascular prosthesis—Material and fabric construction aspects, in Williams DF (ed): *Biocompatibility of Clinical Implant Materials.* Boca Raton, FL, CRC Press, 1981, vol 2, pp 177–207.
34. Williams DF (ed): *Degradation and Biocompatibility of Synthetic Degradable Polymers.* Boca Raton, FL, CRC Press, 1991.
35. Ramshaw JAM: Collagen as a biomaterial, in Williams DF (ed): *Current Perspectives on Implantable Devices.* Greenwich, CT, JAI Press, 1990, vol 2, pp 151–220.
36. Salisbury RE: Synthetic skin and skin substitutes, in Rubin LR (ed): *Biomaterials in Reconstructive Surgery.* St. Louis, CV Mosby, 1983, pp 847–854.
37. Yannas IV, Lee E, Orgill DP, et al: Synthesis and characterization of a model extracellular matrix that induces partial regeneration of adult mammalian skin. *Proc Natl Acad Sci U S A* 1989; 86:933–937.
38. Capperauld I: Bovine fibrin implants: Tissue reaction, in Rubin LR (ed): *Biomaterials in Reconstructive Surgery.* St. Louis, CV Mosby, 1983, pp 118–130.
39. Lehn J-M: Supramolecular chemistry—Scope and perspectives: Molecules–supermolecules–molecular devices (Nobel Lecture). *J Inclus Phenom* 1988; 6:351–396.
40. Ringsdorf H, Schlarb B, Venzmer J: Molecular architecture and function of polymeric oriented systems: Models for the study of organization, surface recognition and dynamics of biomembranes. *Angewandte Chemie, International Edition in English* 1988; 27:113–158.
41. Rieke PC, Calvert PD, Alper M (eds): *Materials Synthesis Utilizing Biological Processes.* Pittsburgh, PA, Materials Research Society, 1990.
42. Engbers G, Feijen J: Current techniques to improve the blood compatibility of biomaterials surfaces. *Int J Artif Organs* 1991; 14:199–215.
43. Hall B, Bird RR, Kojima M, et al: Biomembranes as models for polymer surfaces. V: Thromboelastographic studies of polymeric lipids and polyesters. *Biomaterials* 1989; 10:219–224.
44. Ishihara K, Aragaki R, Ueda T, et al: Reduced thrombogenicity of polymers having phospholipid polar groups. *J Biomed Mater Res* 1990; 24:1069–1077.
45. Pierschbacher MD, Ruoslahti E: Cell attachment activity of fibronectin can be duplicated by small synthetic fragments of the molecule. *Nature* 1984; 309:30.
46. Greenhalgh RM, Hollier LH (eds): *The Maintenance of Arterial Reconstruction.* London, WB Saunders, 1991.
47. Callow AD: Endothelial cell seeding: Problems and expectations. *J Vasc Surg* 1987; 6:318–319.
48. Nojiri C, Okano T, Jacobs HA, et al. Blood compatibility of PEO-grafted polyurethane and HEMA/styrene block copolymer surfaces. *J Biomed Mater Res* 1990; 24:1151–1171.
49. Richards M, Dahiyat BI, Arm DM, et al: Evaluation of polyphosphates and polyphosphonates as degradable biomaterials. *J Biomed Mater Res* 1991; 25:1151–1167.
50. Sun AM, Goosen MF, O'Shea G: Microencapsulated cells as hormone delivery systems. *Crit Rev Ther Drug Carrier Syst* 1987; 4:1–12.
51. Jaeger CB, Greene LA, Tresco PA, et al: Polymer-encapsulated dopaminergic cell lines as alternative neural grafts. *Prog Brain Res* 1990; 82:41–46.
52. Kim SW: Northrombogenic treatment and strategies, in Ratner BD, Hoffman AS (eds): *Biomaterials Science.* New York, Academic Press, 1992, in press.
53. Haubold AD, Yapp RA, Bokros JC: Carbons, in Williams DF (ed): *Concise Encyclopedia of Medical and Dental Materials.* Oxford, Pergamon Press, 1990, pp 95–100.
54. Lenz RW, Gross RA: Bioresorbable polyesters from bacterial polymerization reactions, in Miglioresi E (ed): *Polymers in Medicine III.* Amsterdam, Elsevier, 1988, pp 19–26.
55. Engelberg I, Kohn J: Physico-mechanical properties of degradable polymers used in medical applications: A comparative study. *Biomaterials* 1991; 12:292–304.

Chapter 7

Technologies and Techniques for Telescopic Surgery

Joseph B. Petelin

The discipline of surgery has been categorized in the past into five activities: (1) removal of tissue or material, (2) repair or addition of tissue or material, (3) replacement or rearrangement of displaced tissue, (4) separation of tissue, and (5) reunion of that which is separated.[1] This classification is still appropriate today, but the methods of accomplishing these tasks are vastly different than they were even a few decades ago. This chapter reviews techniques and technologies available for the performance of telescopic surgery.

Telescopic surgery, which had been employed by gynecologists and orthopedic surgeons for many years, became established as a general surgical endeavor after the introduction of laparoscopic cholecystectomy by Mouret in 1987.[2] In the relatively short time since then, nearly every organ has been operated on telescopically. A revolution in patient thinking about surgical approaches and their outcomes has begun. These changes are largely the result of the tremendous success of laparoscopic cholecystectomy. This new treatment plan has been made possible primarily because of the introduction of videoendoscopy into the operating room. The video enhancement achieved with CCD (see Chap. 2) technology provides the surgical team with better visualization than ever before, easily surpassing that obtained in any open surgical theater. The enhanced view, however, is only one advantage of the new approach. The lack of damage to the body wall is the most important clinical benefit to the patient. Even when multiple puncture sites are used, postoperative pain is considerably less than that encountered after open surgery, which translates into a more rapid return to normal preoperative activity; hence, this explains the success and popularity of telescopic surgery.

EQUIPMENT FOR TELESCOPIC SURGERY

Instrumentation: Video, Insufflators, and Energy Sources

A surgeon must have the appropriate equipment to perform telescopic surgery safely and effectively. Basic requirements include standard telescopic instruments (many of which have only become available during the past few years), a high-flow insufflator, good telescope, high intensity light source, camera, high-resolution monitor(s), and additional specialized instruments necessary for more advanced laparoscopic surgery. Attempting to perform some "high-end" telescopic procedures without effective equipment in good condition is fraught with difficulty, if not hazard. One of the most important necessities, the video system, has been detailed in Chapter 2.

High-flow insufflators, a necessity for laparoscopic and pelviscopic surgery, have become commonplace in telescopic surgical suites. These units are usually capable of delivering greater than 4 L/min of gas, with some generating as much as 10 L/min, and are vital when more than three ports are used for surgical intervention and loss of the pneumoperitoneum becomes a problem. An essential feature of these insufflators is an automatic shutoff valve, which activates when a preset pressure limit is reached. Obviously, insufflation is not a problem in the thorax because the use of a double-lumen endotracheal tube for ventilation allows collapse of the ipsilateral lung to provide exposure.

Telescopic instruments are available in a variety of styles from a number of manufacturers. A basic set includes forceps for tissue grasping, scissors, straight and angled dissectors, and retractors—much like their counterparts in open surgery. Additional tools are available for special applications. Some of these will be discussed in the material that follows.

A variety of energy sources can be used to isolate tissue in place of mechanical or scissors dissection. These include monopolar and bipolar electrosurgical devices (see Chap. 5). Endothermic instruments, which produce their effect by heating tissue, are also used for some applications. Argon beam coagulation devices are preferred for some maneuvers. Lasers are available in a number of wavelengths, each with its own unique tissue effect; these machines are used to cut, coagulate, vaporize, fragment, and occasionally weld tissue. To this author's knowledge, no specific energy source is preferred in every situation. In some instances, however, a given instrument does provide significant advantages over others. Surgeons will develop preferences for the instruments and energy sources found to be most effective in completing the task at hand, with which they are most comfortable.

Operating Room Setup

The operating room arrangement necessary to perform telescopic surgery is different from that used for open surgery, but the instruments must still be arranged for convenient access without obstructing maneuverability. Similarly, energy sources are located to allow ease of access without interfering with surgical manipulations. There is no absolute design which must be followed regarding the placement of this equipment. In most cases, the layout of the operating suite will determine the necessary equipment placement.

Surgical Team

One of the most important requirements for successful telescopic surgical intervention is that the surgeon have well-trained assistant(s) in the surgical suite. Some surgeons routinely prefer to work with another surgeon, in addition to the nursing staff. In some centers, resident physicians or medical students complement the telescopic surgical team. In some practice situations, the lack of availability of assistants may demand that the surgeon develop the ability to work without a large team, often with only a scrub nurse. This situation, the single-surgeon approach, will be addressed in detail later. Whatever the case, however, the members of the operating team should be familiar with the basic tenets of telescopic surgery.

PROCEDURE NOTES

Two-Surgeon Technique

In most centers, initial telescopic surgical procedures have involved the cooperation of at least two surgeons at each operation. Because the most common first procedure is laparoscopic cholecystectomy, it will be used to illustrate the two-surgeon technique (see Chap. 21).[3] In this case, the surgeon stands on the patient's left, at or slightly cephalad to the umbilicus. The assistant surgeon stands directly opposite. The scrub nurse stands to the right of the assistant surgeon. The "camera person," that is, the individual controlling the scope and camera, stands to the left of the surgeon.

In most cases, four ports are established to perform the procedure. The camera port is most commonly located at the umbilicus. The two ports used for retraction of the gallbladder are placed in the right infracostal region at the midclavicular and anterior axillary lines, respectively. An operating port is located just right of the falciform ligament in the epigastrium.

Early in a surgeon's experience, he or she will generally use the right hand to manipulate the dissector or scissors inserted through the operating port. The left hand is placed at the base of the instrument in the portal. For many, this seems to offer stability for the operating instrument. This arrangement, however, requires the assistant to control and manipulate the other two instruments. The most lateral forceps grasps the fundus of the gallbladder and retracts it in a cephalad direction, thereby exposing the Triangle of Calot; meanwhile, the medial forceps displaces the neck of the gallbladder inferiorly and laterally. These maneuvers by assistants require considerable expertise because the view is usually being generated by a camera located approximately 180° away from their point of view. This sometimes causes confusion for the assistant, whose movements "do not seem to make sense" when viewed on the monitor. The author believes that this approach is inherently less efficient than one in which the surgeon assumes control of two instruments: the operating instrument and one forceps. This will be discussed later in more detail.

In situations where more sophisticated maneuvers are required, such as suturing and securing knots, some surgeons likewise prefer a two-surgeon approach, whereby the surgeon inserts the needle into the tissue and the assistant withdraws it. They coordinate their movements so that, when tying knots, each distracts the suture in the appropriate direction. Again, this requires a highly skilled assistant who is accustomed to working with the surgeon performing the procedure.

Single-Surgeon Technique

Single-surgeon techniques for the performance of open surgery have been common for years. It seems only natural, therefore, that similar techniques would evolve for telescopic surgery. Here the concept is not that of simply replacing the assistant surgeon with a nurse or medical student but, rather, operating with only one assistant, who is the scrub nurse. Techniques and instruments have been developed to facilitate achievement of this capability.[4]

Again let us use laparoscopic cholecystectomy as an example to describe the single-surgeon technique. The basic concepts illustrated, however, are applicable to all telescopic procedures. Here the surgeon is located on the patient's left, at or slightly cephalad to the umbilicus. The scrub nurse is located directly opposite. The same ports are established as in the two-surgeon technique. The camera is held in position by a mechanical arm attached to the operating table. It is manipulated, as necessary, by the surgeon; fortunately, this manipulation is infrequent because the tissue being dissected and/or manipulated generally can be moved into the field of view by the surgeon. In this situation, the surgeon controls both the operating port and the midclavicular port instruments, just as in open surgery.

The movements associated with the gallbladder dissection are essentially identical to those performed in the two-surgeon technique. When camera adjustment is required, the surgeon merely hands off the midclavicular instrument to the scrub nurse while adjusting the camera with the left hand. The forceps introduced through the most lateral portal are controlled by another mechanical arm, leaving the scrub nurse free most of the time to pass instruments, as required. Even in situations where more sophisticated manipulations are needed, such as in laparoscopic common duct exploration, the same single-surgeon, single-scrub nurse technique works well.[5] Although the mechanical arms currently in use are rudimentary at best, they are adequate to allow safe performance of most laparoscopic procedures. We hope future developments in this area will include mechanical arms that move on command or even intuitively (see Chap. 33).

Using Both Hands

In open surgery, a surgeon would rarely choose to operate with one hand, using the other to guide the movements of the dominant hand. Most choose to work with both hands, with one hand controlling the tissue and the other operating on it. Telescopic surgical procedures, likewise, should not preclude manipulations using both hands. In fact, in most cases, telescopic maneuvers are not unlike those encountered in open surgery. Telescopic surgeons still cut, distract, and move tissue in much the same way as they do in open surgery, although the instruments and the perspective are different.

Admittedly, the two-dimensional visual field presents less spatial information than the three-dimensional open view, but this is partially offset by the ability to magnify with the scope. Tactile sensation is not changed, however, because it is not dependent on vision, except in the sense of merely finding the object to touch. However, because it is a combination of visual and tactile feedback that provides information to guide the surgeon's movements and visual feedback is altered in the two-dimensional video world, it makes sense that to use both hands doubles the amount of tactile feedback and improves surgical maneuvering skills. The surgeon is encouraged, then, to use both hands as often as possible when performing telescopic surgery.

Methods of Dissection and Resection

DISSECTING TOOLS AND THEIR APPLICATIONS

The most common tools used for dissection are the scissors, generally used in concert with forceps and retractors. The tissues are manipulated so that traction and countertraction can be performed. Tissue planes are identified and developed in much the same manner as they are in open surgery. Both cutting and teasing of the tissues can be accomplished telescopically with excellent control. Many of the telescopic scissors are also equipped with an electrical connection that allows for monopolar cauterization during the cutting procedure. This application, however, must be used very cautiously to avoid injury to surrounding structures.

Monopolar or bipolar electrosurgical devices are available in a number of other configurations, including J-hook, L-shaped hook, spatula, and blunt-tipped electrodes. Proponents of monopolar devices stress the relative ease of dissection and speed with which these instruments can be used. Those who prefer bipolar units admit that the dissection is somewhat slower, at least with current instruments, but point out the added safety inherent in the bipolar system. Surgeons each will develop a preference for that which is accessible and performs best in their hands. Either system can be used effectively and safely if the principles of operation are understood and applied.

In some cases, tissue effects, which otherwise would be impossible or difficult to obtain with purely mechanical means, can be achieved with an electrosurgical device. This is the case in biliary tract surgery, where hemostasis is much more easily achieved in the gallbladder fossa with cautery than with pressure or suture. The same concepts of traction and countertraction, with proper exposure of the tissues, are used in electrosurgical dissection as in scissors dissection. The surgeon must take special precautions, however, to avoid electrical arcing or conduction of energy to adjacent structures. This involves either manipulation with insulated instruments or retraction of adjacent organs out of the immediate vicinity of the electrode. The surgeon must always be aware of the possibility of distant conduction of electricity along the shaft of an uninsulated instrument; this may affect organs that are out of view on the video screen (see Chap. 5).

Electrohydraulic fragmentation devices have also been useful for disintegrating common duct stones, enabling their removal without resorting to enlargement of the access sites. These machines have become so sophisticated that their energy can be delivered through tiny fibers less than 1 mm in diameter. Great care must be exercised to avoid accidental damage to adjacent structures, such as the bile duct wall.

Paralleling the interest in telescopic surgery, lasers have gained popularity among general and thoracic surgeons (see Chap. 4). In the United States, many pioneers of laparoscopic surgery have used lasers routinely for laparoscopic cholecystectomy and other general surgical procedures. The safety of these machines was repeatedly documented in the early reports of laparoscopic operations. In fact, in the early days of this revolution, there was such a concern about the safety of monopolar electrosurgery that lasers became the instruments of choice when an energy source other than mechanical force was needed to achieve a particular tissue effect.

Lasers can be used to cut, coagulate, fragment, and vaporize tissue. Each wavelength produces unique tissue effects; therefore, wavelength preferences develop based on the type of tissue likely to be encountered during surgery. The Nd:YAG, Ho:YAG, argon, KTP, CO_2, and pulsed dye lasers have been the most useful for general surgical, gynecologic, and thoracic work, although many others have been developed. In most cases, with the exception of the CO_2 laser, energy is delivered through a quartz fiber, which is placed in contact with or near the tissue. By withdrawing the fiber slightly, the beam can be defocused to achieve a broader, less intense effect. This maneuver is useful for dissecting tissue planes where dense adhesions are encountered, for example, dissection of the gallbladder from the liver.

A unique application of laser energy that has been developed for the Nd:YAG wavelength is the contact tip sapphire. This device, attached to the terminus of an optical fiber, focuses the laser energy into an area, which is determined by the shape of the sapphire. Highly accurate dissection with minimal adjacent tissue damage, less than 1 mm, is possible with this modality. Sculpted quartz fibers have also been developed to achieve similar effects. In contact laser dissection, the laser beam is merely being used to heat the glass tip; thus, the tissue effect of contact laser dissection is dependent on the shape and temperature of the tip, not on the wavelength of the laser (see Chap. 4).

When used in a noncontact mode, lasers can exert tissue effects at a distance. This capability is exploited by many surgeons who use a defocused beam to coagulate the gallbladder fossa to achieve hemostasis and by thoracic surgeons who use it similarly on the lung parenchyma. Gynecologists use the CO_2 laser to ablate endometrial implants in the pelvis, especially in locations that are inaccessible with conventional instruments.

Although no immediate electrical hazard to the patient exists with these machines, the surgeon must be very careful to ensure that unwanted exposure to other organs does not occur. This can occur when tissue is displaced into the direct or reflected beam. Retraction and good exposure are essential when using these techniques. Similarly, when pulsed dye lasers are used to fragment stones, care must be taken to avoid injury to adjacent tissue, although it is generally believed that the danger of accidental adjacent damage is much less likely with this modality than it is with electrohydraulic fragmentation devices.

The argon beam coagulator (ABC, Birtcher Medical) became available for laparoscopic application in 1990. With this instrument, monopolar electrosurgical energy is evenly delivered over a broad surface of tissue through a jet of argon gas. The control of energy is such that high-power electrofulguration may be used to coagulate rapidly and effectively the large surface area oozing that may occur during hepatic or splenic trauma.[6] The ABC should not be used on the bowel because full-thickness injuries are frequent.[7]

Ultrasonic scalpels are also under development and have been used for a multitude of telescopic procedures. These devices, which produce a thermal effect on tissue, provide a higher degree of hemostasis than can be achieved with conventional scalpels or scissors. At the same time, these instruments enable more accurate dissection than is generally possible with electrosurgical hooks or spatulas. Although they are not in widespread use, there appears to be a significant potential for the application of these high tech scalpels. Here again, however, the techniques of traction and countertraction are necessary to ensure proper use of these instruments.

Two other devices employing innovative techniques in the dissection of soft tissue planes are the irrigation pump used for aquadissection[8,9] and the CO_2 gas insufflator used for pneumatic dissection.[10] Either of these tools can be used to displace loose areolar tissues from adjacent solid structures. Reich[8] commonly uses aquadissection techniques in pelviscopic gynecologic procedures, such as hysterectomy. The gentle pressure exerted by the irrigating solution lifts the peritoneum off vital structures, such as the ureters and iliac vessels. This makes subsequent scissor, cautery, or laser dissection much safer in these areas.

Phillips[10] uses preperitoneal insufflation of CO_2 to dissect peritoneum from the inguinal region in preparation for laparoscopic inguinal hernia repair. In his technique, a Veress needle is inserted into the preperitoneal space, and gentle distention with CO_2 effects a blunt avascular dissection. Preperitoneal CO_2 dissection during laparoscopic hernia repair has also been performed under direct vision using a Hasson cannula and an "open" laparoscopic approach without entering the peritoneal cavity.

Blunt dissecting instruments are often preferred in certain areas. For example, in the Triangle of Calot, a curved instrument provides ideal maneuverability in isolating the cystic artery and cystic duct. For those surgeons who prefer to use "peanut" gauze dissectors in this area, laparoscopic models attached to long 5-mm rods have been developed. Just as in open surgery, a wide variety of blunt dissecting instruments are available. Other instruments and energy sources will be marketed in the future. Their application and usefulness in telescopic surgery will continue to depend, however, on the same basic concepts used in all dissection.

RETRACTING TOOLS, ACCESSORIES, AND THEIR APPLICATIONS

The surgeon also needs to consider the choice of instruments used to provide exposure for a given procedure. In some cases, a grasping forceps is most useful to retract tissues. In others, specialized fan-shaped retractors are best. Occasionally, a device as simple as a 5- or 10-mm rod can be used to retract tissues such as the liver, stomach, or intestine. A wide variety of tools are now available, and the array of instruments seems to be growing almost daily. Some of these special devices will be highlighted in the discussion that follows. These instruments can be controlled by an assistant or held firmly in place by mechanical means. Additionally, exposure can be achieved by tilting the table or inserting a flexible scope into the esophagus or colon.

Mechanical control of retractors can be produced using a tool as simple as a towel clip by encircling the handle of the retractor with the jaws of the clip and attaching the ensemble to the drapes. Alternatively, more complex holders can be employed when more precise command of the instrument is needed. An example of such a device is shown in Figure 7-1. Although these mechanical arms are useful in their current forms, as mentioned before, we hope further development will focus on interactive devices that respond to commands, either vocal, mechanical, or electrical. Such improvements would allow the surgeon to control the movements of the retracting instruments without manual displacement.

In some instances, even with the appropriate placement of retractors, exposure is either not adequate or not as optimal as it could be. Here a second telescopic camera system can provide invaluable assistance in displaying portions of the anatomy not visible with the primary scope. This view can be displayed on a separate monitor or incorporated onto the primary video screen using a video mixer with a picture-in-picture effect. This same video-mixing device is also used to display concurrently on the monitor a digitized, fluoroscopic cholangiographic image with the laparoscopic image. This results in increased safety and improved efficiency in cholangiographic procedures. Although not reported currently, the application of video-mixing capabilities to other procedures where concurrent endoluminal (i.e., bronchoscopic, upper gastrointestinal endoscopic, or colonoscopic) and extraluminal (i.e., laparoscopic or thoracoscopic) views are desirable seems logical.

CONDUCT OF THE DISSECTION: PORTAL PLACEMENT, EXPOSURE, CUTTING, AND SECURING

By its nature, telescopic surgical intervention poses some interesting restraints on access, maneuverability, and basic technique. The first problem the surgeon encounters after insertion of the scope and identification of the pathologic lesion is in determining the sizes and sites of the secondary portals. Whereas in open surgery the surgeon is allowed to make the incision as large as necessary to gain access, in telescopic surgery, we must accurately choose the locations of these secondary portals to allow maximum maneuverability. Early in a surgeon's experience, these sites will be chosen by rote memory of descriptions of the locations presented in published articles and texts.

However, as more expertise is acquired, the surgeon will begin to experiment with the position of these portals. (See Chap. 14 for principles of port placement for laparoscopic suturing.) Commonly, an individual will find that slight alterations in the location of a port seem to enhance the performance of a given procedure. The surgeon is advised very carefully to consider portal placement, studying the telescopic view received from the monitor connected to the camera on the scope. When a surgeon realizes that the best sites have not been chosen and if the current locations are a definite impediment to the progress of the operation, it is often wise to consider placement of additional ports in the proper locations. Port placement depends on attempts to bring instruments into the cavity at right angles to the puncture site (see Fig. 21-5). Obviously, the trocars must be positioned close enough to the site so that the instruments can reach.

After the secondary portals have been placed, the next step involves establishing exposure of the operative field. In most instances, this will be accomplished by insertion and manipulation of available standard telescopic instruments through 5- or 10-mm portals. In other situations, however, retraction can be obtained through ingenious use of sutures or other uncommon devices.[11]

For example, one may retract the colon using sutures

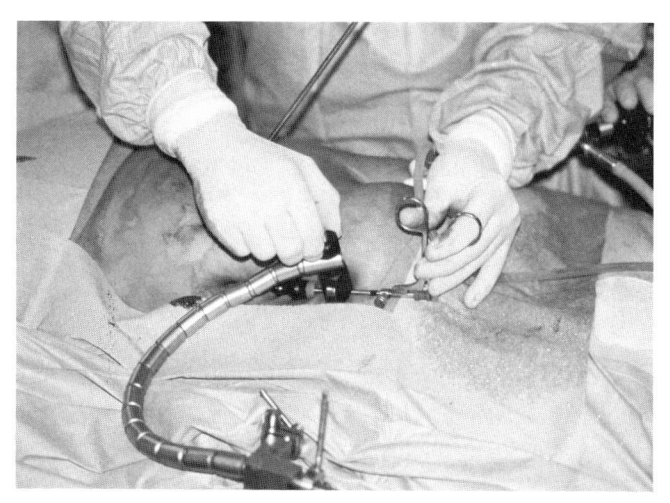

FIGURE 7-1 Wolf retractor.

of 3–0 silk placed through the abdominal wall, through the seromuscular coat, and then back out of the abdominal wall. This can be achieved either with curved needles inserted through a 10-mm portal or with straight Keith needles advanced directly through the abdominal wall. In the first instance, the suture can be brought back out of the peritoneal cavity through any of the portals available or can be fixed to the posterior aspect of the anterior abdominal wall. When the sutures are brought out through a portal, there usually is still enough room in the portal sleeve to allow easy insertion and manipulation of instruments through the same site.

After exposure is achieved, dissection of the tissue to be removed commences. As mentioned, this is most commonly performed using scissors or other mechanical devices. When tissue planes are developed and the target organ is defined, more aggressive manipulations, such as division of vascular and ductal structures, becomes necessary; this is obviously much more delicate than the displacement of loose areolar tissues with blunt techniques because highly accurate determination and assessment of the anatomy are essential. Additionally, these structures usually harbor fluids, which are considered vital to the future function of the organ and organism. Therefore, the dissection must be delicate and precise and, by its very nature, must include control of the vessels, ducts, or conduits (i.e., intestine or bronchi), which are intimately connected with the organ undergoing resection.

Conventional methods of control, such as ligating and suturing, work well here but can be time consuming, especially if the surgeon is not adept at these maneuvers under telescopic guidance. Application of ligatures can be accomplished by inserting free ligatures through any port into the cavity, placing them around the structure to be secured, and ligating either with an intracorporeal or extracorporeal method of knot tying (see Chap. 14).

Intracorporeal ligation techniques approximate the "instrument tie" of open surgery, although a number of variations have developed. When viewed on a two-dimensional monitor, such a seemingly simple task takes on a new degree of difficulty because depth of field is lost. Nevertheless, this method is quite popular among many advanced telescopic surgeons. The extracorporeal method of knot tying is preferred by other specialists. Here, a long piece of suture is advanced into the cavity through a port, placed around the structure, and brought back out of the same port, where the knot(s) are constructed under direct vision and then displaced back into the cavity through the same port with a knot pusher. This device is used to place the knot securely and accurately at the chosen location. Depending on the type of knot constructed, the surgeon may be able to place one or more knots at the given location. Pretied Roeder loop ligatures are commercially available for this purpose but require complete division of the tubular structure before their placement. Obviously, this is not always possible without adverse consequences; hence, their use is somewhat limited.

When suture ligation is necessary, it can be accomplished with almost any conventional suture material and needle configuration. Even large curved needles, ranging from 1 to 3 cm in diameter, can be inserted through most 10- or 11-mm portals and subsequently removed with minimal difficulty. Specially designed needles, such as "ski" needles, have been developed for telescopic insertion and are available with a variety of suture materials and sizes. As their name implies, the needles have the shape of a ski, allowing easier insertion through portals and easier placement into tissue than with small straight needles. In summary, telescopic suturing is not only possible but also seems to be gaining more acceptance in the surgical community as materials and techniques improve. Telescopic-guided suture placement through tissue, however, is not easily or quickly learned by the novice and requires significantly greater manual dexterity than its open counterpart. Nevertheless, most experienced advanced telescopic surgeons believe that it is a skill that should be learned by all those who seriously expect to pursue telescopic surgery.

In many instances, suture ligation can be replaced by clip application to achieve a desired result. A large array of automatic clipping devices have been adapted to this minimal-access surgical arena. These machines, when used properly, apply metal or synthetic clips in locations where a ligature or suture might otherwise have been required. The advantages afforded by these devices include time conservation, accessibility to operative sites where suturing would otherwise be almost impossible, and opportunity for less experienced telescopic surgeons to perform minimal-access surgery safely on patients who might otherwise be relegated to undergo a more painful open procedure.

After the vessels, ducts, and adjacent tissues have been controlled, detachment of the specimen from the parent organ presents the next challenge during telescopic resection. As in open surgery, where atraumatic clamps or staplers might be used for control during such a maneuver, in telescopic surgery, the same sorts of devices are employed. Many of these devices are still rudimentary but are undergoing continual improvement. The same surgical principles still apply, however. The periphery of the specimen is secured with either clamps, sutures, or staples. The development of automatic cutting and stapling devices that can be inserted through minimal access ports has allowed significant progress in the application of telescopic surgical techniques to resection of organs that would otherwise seem impossible. For example, Figure 7-2 illustrates an automatic Endo-GIA device (United States Surgical Corporation, Norwalk, CT).

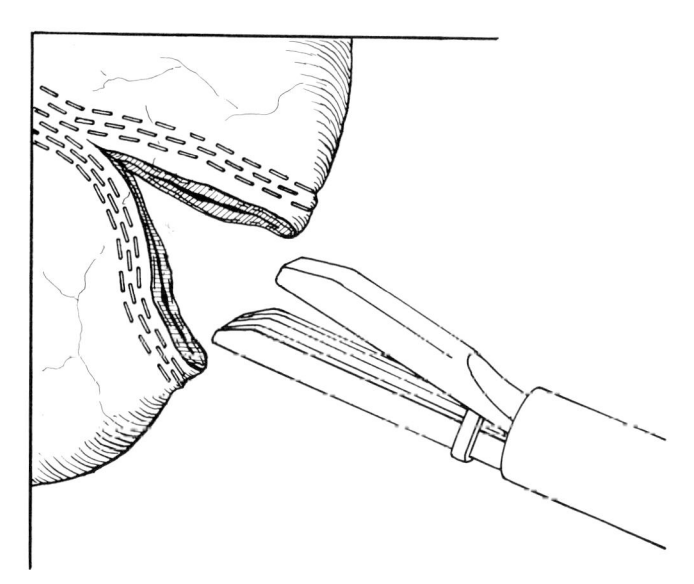

FIGURE 7-2 An endoscopic stapling device places six rows of staggered staples and cuts between the middle rows.

Methods of Removal

INCISION EXTENSION AND CONVERSION TO LARGER PORTS

In telescopic surgery, one of the most obvious potential problems after dissection and resection of an organ or part of an organ is the removal of that tissue through an orifice that appears to be smaller than the tissue specimen. This situation has engendered some of the most creative thinking in general and thoracic surgery in many years. A number of possible solutions immediately come to mind: enlarge the incision for removal; shrink, morcellate, or vaporize the tissue; crush the tissue (e.g., stones); leave the tissue in place; or remove it through another route (e.g., vagina or rectum). An array of instruments and accessories has been developed to accomplish these tasks. Their implementation is explained in the discussion of techniques that follows.

The first option, enlargement of the abdominal wall opening, is relatively straightforward. This can be accomplished by merely extending the skin and fascial incisions. As this is done, however, the loss of exposure, especially in laparoscopic cases, where CO_2 under pressure escapes through the enlarged opening, demands that the specimen be secured in a defined location so that its extraction is safe and controlled. This prevents damage to other structures, contamination, or displacement of the specimen when the pneumoperitoneum is lost. Most commonly, this extraction is performed by grasping the specimen with a forceps and withdrawing it up to the site of the puncture that is to be extended. This must be done very carefully so that the specimen is not damaged or spilled into the body cavity. The fascial opening may then be enlarged with scissors, electrocautery, laser, or scalpel. As this is done, the specimen "naturally" exudes from the wound. Another obvious drawback to extension of the incision, however, is that reduced pain, one of the advantages of telescopic surgery, can be lost in this final stage of the procedure.

An alternative to simple linear extension of the wound involves conversion of a portal to a larger size by using a blunt technique. In this situation, a blunt probe is inserted through the sheath, the sheath is removed, and then a larger-diameter sheath is threaded into position over the blunt probe. After the new sheath is in place, the blunt probe and the threaded insert are removed. This type of instrument is useful when removing an inflamed gallbladder or appendix or an enlarged fallopian tube and ovary.

CONTAINERS: BAGS, GLOVES, TUBES, AND SHUTTLES

In some cases, it is wise to place the specimen in a container while it is still in the body (infected or malignant tissue) to allow safe transport through the cavity and delivery from the wound. The author first employed this concept to remove a gangrenous gallbladder in March 1990. In this case, a simple plastic bag was constructed from a sterile camera sleeve by sectioning a 6-inch segment and ligating one end with a ligature. It was advanced into the peritoneal cavity through a 10-mm portal using an 8-mm introduction sleeve. The gallbladder was then placed in the sac which was then secured with a pre-tied Roeder loop. Figure 7-3 illustrates the use of a bag to retrieve errant gallstones.

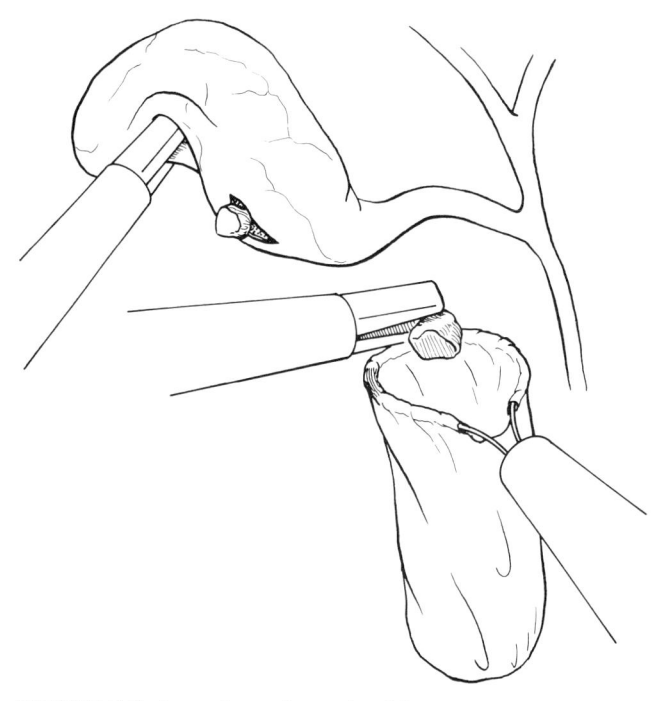

FIGURE 7-3 An endoscopic retrieval bag.

Deyo (personal communication December 1989) has advocated using a finger from a surgical glove to assist in the extraction of gallstones and other debris from the peritoneal cavity. The glove finger is used in a fashion similar to that depicted in Figure 7-3. Others have used sterile condoms to collect, store, transport, and deliver material from the peritoneal cavity. A number of commercially available bags in a variety of configurations have been developed in the past 2 years for similar purposes. One of the most useful of these is a pouch developed by Clayman and co-workers[12] to store a resected kidney. This pouch is constructed to facilitate intracorporeal morcellation of the specimen into fragments small enough to be withdrawn through a 10-mm portal.

Another interesting device, the so-called shuttle, was developed by Klaiber.[13] This 20-mm diameter instrument consists of a hollow tube, the distal end of which is capped, and the side of which contains a large distal opening to allow for placement of tissue and/or stones. The side orifice may be opened or closed, as necessary, for transport (Fig. 7-4).

MORCELLATORS

Occasionally, the tissue specimen is so large that even when it is placed in a container it cannot safely be removed from the body cavity without significantly increasing the size of the exit site or disintegrating the tissue. At least two different mechanical devices have been developed for use in this situation. The morcellator, described above for the kidney, has been used safely and effectively in a number of cases. It is pneumatically powered and reportedly cannot damage the bag containing the tissue. It is designed to remove tissue as it is morcellated. The other device, the rotary gallstone lithotrite, has been developed for gallstone fragmentation and is inserted into the gallbladder after the organ is brought to the exit site. The machine creates a vortex with its blades so that the stones in the gallbladder are delivered into the cutting edges of the rotor. Again the machine is said to be designed so as to make accidental perforation of the gallbladder nearly impossible. It is likely that other similar devices will be developed in the future because the value of preserving the integrity of the body wall has been repeatedly proved in the recent past.

CHOICE OF SITE: UMBILICUS, VAGINA, OR OTHER

The final topic to be addressed in this discussion is the choice of exit site for the tissue specimen. In the chest, the choice is relatively straightforward because any of the larger portals is adequate to allow one of the methods described. In the abdomen, the umbilicus is the most commonly chosen exit site for removal of tissue, such as the gallbladder, appendix, fallopian tube, or ovary.[14–16]

For other specimens, including the colon and uterus,

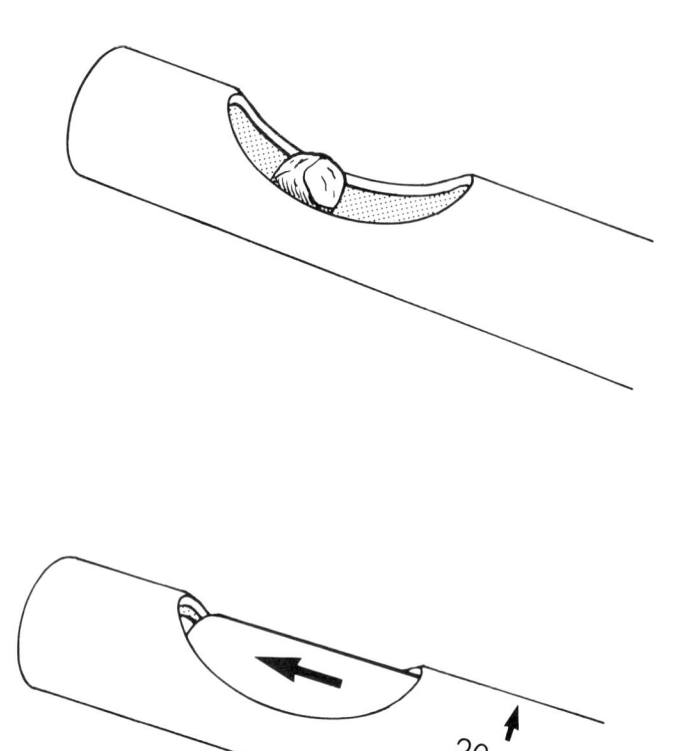

FIGURE 7-4 A 20-mm shuttle.

alternative sites may be more appropriate. In the case of sigmoid colectomy, the specimen is commonly removed from an enlarged portal site in the left lower quadrant. This allows placement of the proximal anvil of the circular stapling device into the proximal descending colon at the level of the skin after the specimen is removed.[17] The proximal remaining colon is replaced into the peritoneal cavity, the exit site is closed or occluded temporarily, and the continuity of the colon is reestablished laparoscopically. In some cases, the colonic specimen has been delivered through the remaining distal colon, rectum, and anus.[18] In the case of gynecologic surgery, large specimens, such as the uterus, can be delivered through the vagina without resorting to enlargement of any of the abdominal wall portal sites. In each instance listed, the surgeon should choose the exit site that provides the least resistance to deliverance, is least painful, and produces the best cosmetic results but does not compromise the principles of established surgical doctrine.

CONCLUSION

What was obvious to patients has become obvious to most surgeons: the degree of damage to the body wall produced in establishing access to the body cavities has a major impact on postoperative convalescence. Because the damage created by port sites in telescopic surgery is much less than that created by an open incision, a movement toward minimally invasive surgical approaches is in the best interest of patients. Numerous problems involving exposure, dissection, resection, and removal of diseased tissue have been solved, and many new devices and techniques have been developed. Much work remains to be done, however, because this new era of general surgical intervention has just begun. In some cases, the techniques that have been developed for telescopic resection and removal of tissue from body cavities appear similar to their open counterparts. In others, special problems inherent to the telescopic approach had to be overcome to accomplish the task at hand. As with other fields, necessity has often been the mother of invention.

REFERENCES

1. Dobson J: The training of a surgeon. *Ann R Coll Surg Engl* 1964; 34:1.
2. Dubois F, Icard P, Berthelot G, et al: Coelioscopic cholecystectomy: Preliminary report of 36 cases. *Ann Surg* 1990; 211:60–62.
3. Reddick EJ: *An Introductory Course in Laparoscopic Surgery*. ed 2. Chicago, EJR Enterprises, 1990, pp 6.1–6.18.
4. Petelin JB: The argument for contact laser laparoscopic cholecystectomy. *Clinical Laser Monthly* 1990; 71–74.
5. Petelin JB: Laparoscopic approach to common duct pathology. *Surg Laparosc Endosc* 1991; 1:33–41.
6. Go PMNYH, Goodman GR, Bruhn EW, et al: The argon beam coagulator provides rapid hemostasis of experimental hepatic and splenic hemorrhage in anticoagulated dogs. *J Trauma* 1991; 31: 1294–1300.
7. Go PMNYH, Bruhn EW, Garry SL, et al: Patterns of small intestinal injury with the argon beam coagulator. *Surg Gynecol Obstet* 1990; 171:341–342.
8. Reich H: Aquadissection. Presented at the Third International Meeting of the Society for Minimally Invasive Therapy, Boston, MA, Nov 10–12, 1991.
9. Popp LW: Improvement in endoscopic hernioplasty: Transcutaneous aquadissection of the musculofascial defect and preperitoneal endoscopic patch repair. *J Laparoendosc Surg* 1991, 1:83 89.
10. Phillips E: Laparoscopic hernia repair. *Laparoscopy in Focus* 1992; 1:8–11.
11. Redwine DB, Sharpe DR: Laparoscopic segmental resection of the sigmoid colon for endometriosis. *J Laparoendosc Surg* 1991; 1:217–220.
12. Clayman RV, Kavoussi LR, Soper NJ, et al: Laparoscopic nephrectomy: Initial case report. *J Urol* 1991; 146:278–282.
13. Klaiber C: The "shuttle" stone collector: A new device for collecting lost gallstones in laparoscopic cholecystectomy. *Surg Endosc* 1992; 6:84.
14. McKernan JB: Laparoscopic cholecystectomy. *Am Surg* 1991; 57:309–312.
15. Reddick EJ, Olsen DO, Daniell JF, et al: Laparoscopic laser cholecystectomy. *Laser Medicine & Surgery News & Advances* 1989; 38–40.
16. Reddick EJ, Olsen DO: Laparoscopic laser cholecystectomy: A comparison with mini-lap cholecystectomy. *Surg Endosc* 1989; 3:131–133.
17. Fowler DL, White SA: Laparoscopy-assisted sigmoid resection. *Surg Laparosc Endosc* 1991; 1:183–188.
18. Jacobs M, Verdeja JC, Goldstein HS: Minimally invasive colon resection (laparoscopic colectomy). *Surg Laparosc Endosc* 1991; 1:144–150.

Part II

Old Diseases

Chapter 8

Endoluminal Therapy of Esophageal Cancer

Kathy Bull-Henry / David E. Fleischer

Esophageal cancer has a grave prognosis. Approximately 90 percent of patients have their disease diagnosed at an advanced stage that is not amenable to curative surgical resection.[1,2] Consequently, palliative therapy becomes the goal. There are a number of modalities available as therapy for esophageal cancer, including surgery, radiotherapy, and chemotherapy. Palliative surgical resection is associated with a mortality rate of 7 to 29 percent.[3–5] External radiotherapy achieves a temporary response in 25 percent of patients with local recurrence in more than 50 percent.[2,6] Chemotherapy achieves a partial response rate of 50 percent but is associated with considerable side effects.[7,8] Combination radiotherapy, chemotherapy, and surgical resection have not significantly improved these results. These poor results have led to a continued search for better curative and palliative treatments. Because the endoscope places the physician in direct contact with the tumor, numerous palliative endoscopic therapies have become options. Endoscopic techniques are effective and have a low incidence of complications. The purpose of this chapter is to describe the various endoscopic techniques available to treat esophageal cancer.

LASER ABLATION

The word *laser* is an acronym for *l*ight *a*mplification by *s*timulated *e*mission of *r*adiation. Three types of lasers are currently being used in gastrointestinal diseases: the argon laser, the Nd:YAG, and the tuneable dye laser. These lasers have distinctive wavelengths and depths of penetration. By far, the greatest experience is with the Nd:YAG laser. Tissue destruction is caused by thermal injury. The laser–tissue interaction causes tissue molecular agitation, which leads to tissue heating. As a general rule, tissue protein coagulates at 60° and vaporizes at 100°C. The endoscopist sees tissue coagulation as blanching of the mucosa with edema, while the mucosa after vaporization is charred with smoke production (Fig. 8-1). The tissue temperature is controlled by several factors. Higher power settings (80 to 100 W), long pulse durations (1 s or longer), and short tissue–laser distances (approximately 1 cm) lead to higher tissue temperatures and vaporization. Lower power settings (40 to 50 W) cause coagulation necrosis.

Indications

There are no absolute indications for endoscopic laser therapy (ELT) in esophageal cancer versus other palliative modalities. However, there are several factors that favor a successful outcome from laser therapy (Table 8-1). The appearance and location of the tumor are important.[9]

Mucosal (exophytic) tumor lesions are more easily treated with a laser because the borders are better defined. This makes aiming of the laser beam more precise. Also, the beam of the laser will be in the axis of the lumen, making perforation less likely. Examples of these lesions include complete luminal obstruction, noncircumferential tumor involvement, polypoid masses, soft fleshy lesions, recurrence after surgical resection, and tumor overgrowth of esophageal protheses. Submucosal or extrinsic lesions, on the other hand, are not well treated. Their margins are difficult to define, making aiming more difficult. The laser beam is not parallel to the axis of the lumen, making perforation more likely. Also, we must burn through normal mucosal tissue, before reaching tumor tissue, causing pain. In addition, restenosis is more likely after treating such lesions.

Location is also important in determining the outcome of laser treatment. Straight segments of the esophagus, such as those found in the mid and distal esophagus, are easiest to treat and have the best outcomes. Lesions less than 2 cm from the upper esophageal sphincter and horizontal segments (such as those found at the gastroesophageal junc-

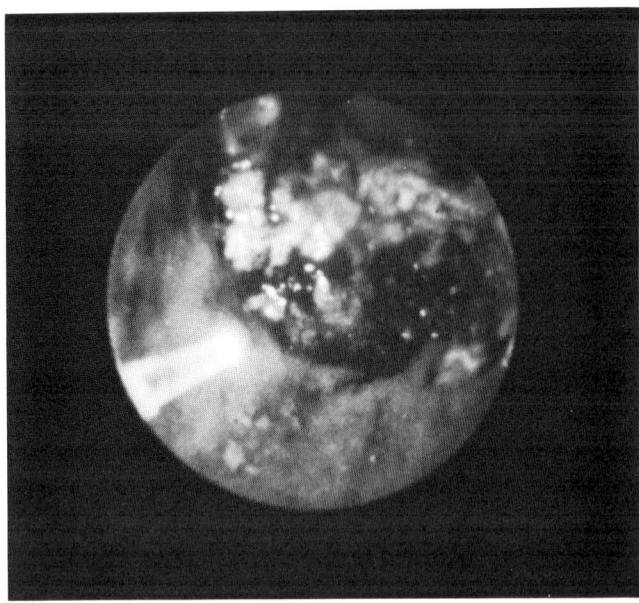

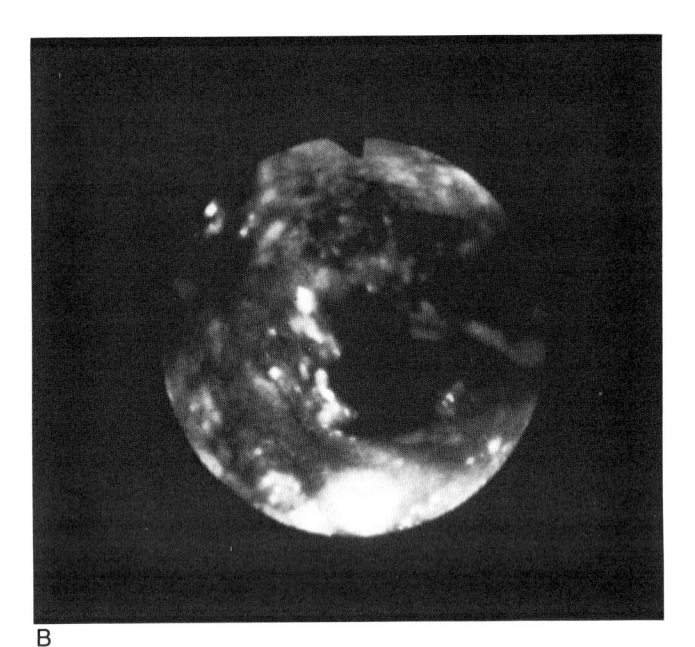

FIGURE 8-1 Endoscopic view after laser treatment. A. Coagulation produces white tissue effect and surrounding edema. B. Vaporization leads to tissue charring.

TABLE 8-1 Factors favoring successful outcome after laser treatment of esophageal cancer

1. Exophytic tumor
2. Tumor location in straight segment
3. Short length of tumor (< 5 cm)
4. Location other than cervical esophagus

tion or after surgery) are technically difficult because of the small amount of maneuvering room for the endoscope. These lesions often do not respond favorably to laser therapy. Short segments are easiest to treat and require fewer laser treatments to achieve an open lumen. In summary, the lesions most amenable to laser therapy are exophytic, short segments (< 5 cm long) in the distal and midesophagus.

An obvious contraindication to laser therapy is a fistula, unless laser therapy is required to destroy the tumor to allow for stent placement. Diffuse submucosal lesions and severely angulated lesions probably should be treated by another method of palliation.

Patient Evaluation

Patient evaluation should include a complete blood count and biochemical tests. Other tests important in the initial evaluation of patients include a barium swallow, an upper endoscopic examination, and an imaging study. The barium swallow defines the location and length of the lesion (Fig. 8-2). It is the best method to map out angulations and distortions of the lumen. The next test is the upper endoscopy, which serves to establish or confirm the diagnosis of cancer. It also allows for direct evaluation of the lesion to determine whether the lesion is exophytic, submucosal, or polypoid (Fig. 8-3). A CT scan of the chest helps to determine the extent of the disease (Fig. 8-4). For proximal esophageal lesions, views of the neck should be included. For distal esophageal lesions, views of the upper abdomen should be obtained. Although the CT scan may underestimate the extent of disease and does not accurately predict resectability, it is usually the test performed. Magnetic resonance imaging of the chest does not seem to give additional information. Endoscopic ultrasonography (EUS), if available, helps significantly in the staging process. This is a new exciting technique that uses a high-frequency transducer at the end of an endoscope to view the esophageal wall in five sonographic layers. Tio and colleagues[10] has shown that EUS is significantly more accurate than CT scan in predicting the depth of invasion (T stage) and in assessing regional node involvement (N stage) in esophageal cancer. Similar data has been reported by Lightdale and coworkers[11] in patients with esophageal cancer. Therefore, EUS permits more accurate staging of the depth of invasion of the primary tumor and local lymph node involvement (Fig. 8-5). Distant metastases (M stage) are better delineated by CT scan.

After these assessments have been completed, we determine if the patient is a candidate for ELT. If there is a possibility of resectability and the patient does not have any medical contraindications for surgery, then exploratory surgery should be performed. If resectability is not possible and ELT is being considered, then the goals of therapy need to be clear to the patient and the physician. Relief of

Chapter 8 Endoluminal Therapy of Esophageal Cancer **71**

dysphagia is a reasonable goal, but the patient must understand that ELT is only palliative and that the relief is temporary. If other therapies are planned in conjunction with ELT, then the goal may be to open the lumen just enough to relieve dysphagia.

Technique

Initial laser treatments are often performed as an inpatient procedure. After the primary laser course is complete, follow-up treatments can be performed on an outpatient basis. Conscious sedation, using intravenous meperidine and midazolam, is usually sufficient to complete the procedure. The standard left lateral decubitus position is used. Two assistants are needed for the procedure, one to monitor the patient and one to assist with the equipment and to circulate. The procedure starts with a surveillance esophagogastroduodenoscopy (EGD), and the gross appearance of the tumor is evaluated. We need to determine the location of the lesion, whether it is partially or totally obstructing, exophytic or submucosal, involves a long segment or short segment, or is sharply angulated or straight.

After this initial assessment is completed, the method of laser treatment is chosen. There are several variations of the technique as follows: (1) antegrade versus retrograde, (2) high power versus low power, and (3) contact versus noncontact. In the retrograde method,[12] an endoscope is passed beyond the malignant stricture. Laser treatment is begun at the distal tumor margin proceeding in a cephalad manner until the most proximal margin is treated. If the lumen is severely narrowed, dilation may be required before the endoscope can be advanced through the tumor. This can be accomplished in the following manner. A small-diameter endoscope is passed through the stricture and advanced to

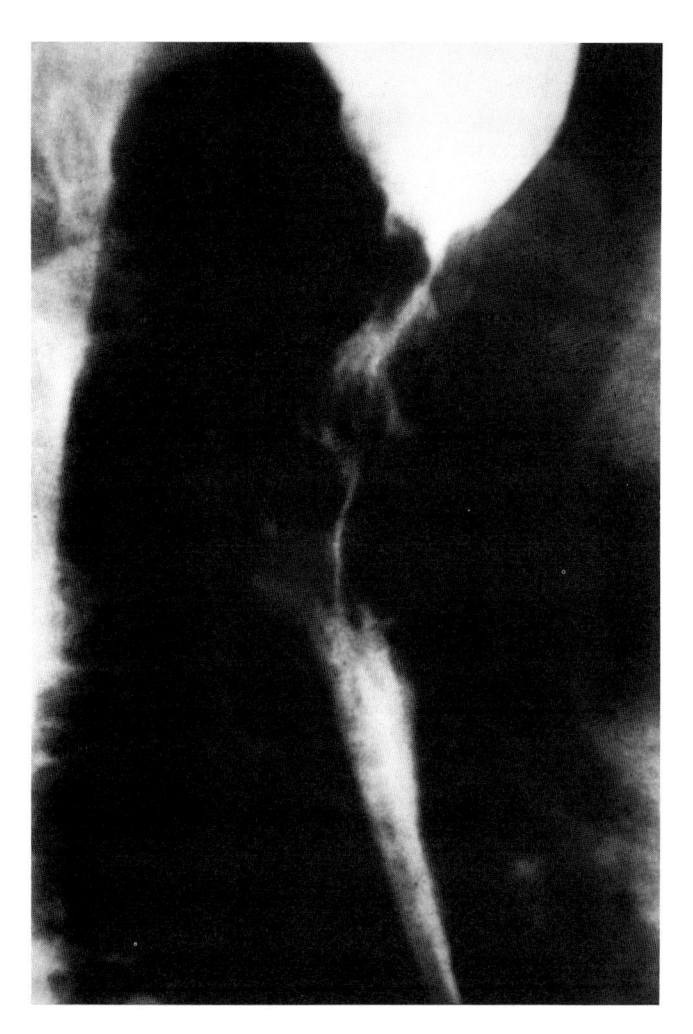

FIGURE 8-2 Barium esophagram defines location and contour of squamous cell carcinoma. A 7-cm stricture narrows the lumen and causes angulation.

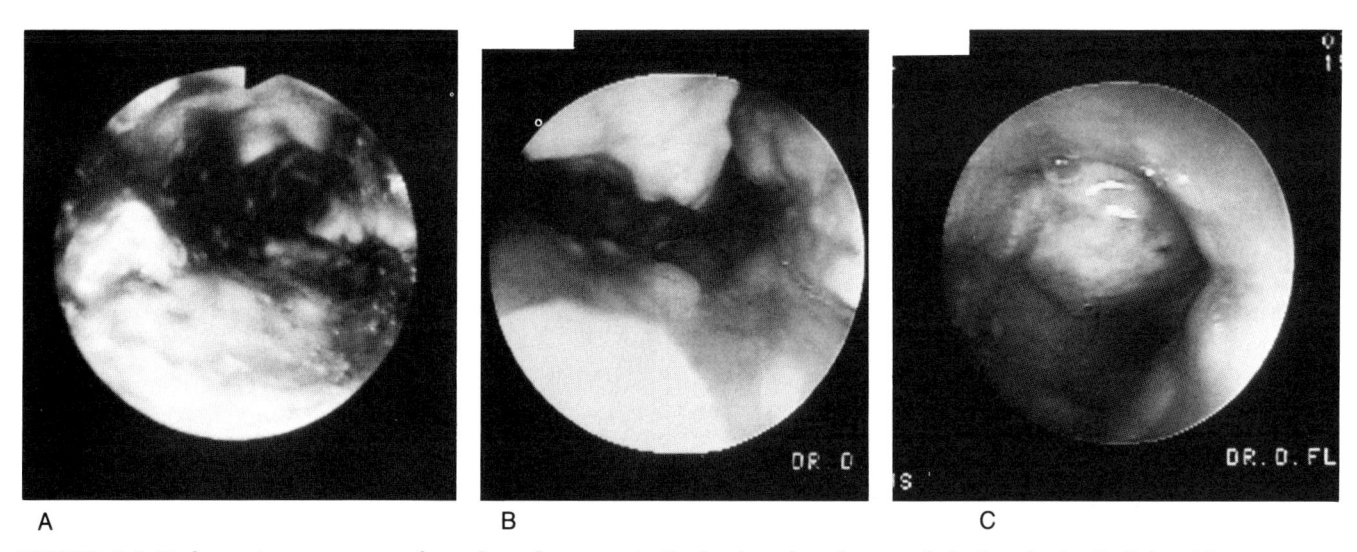

FIGURE 8-3 Endoscopic appearance of esophageal cancer. A. Predominantly submucosal. B. Exophytic. C. Polypoid.

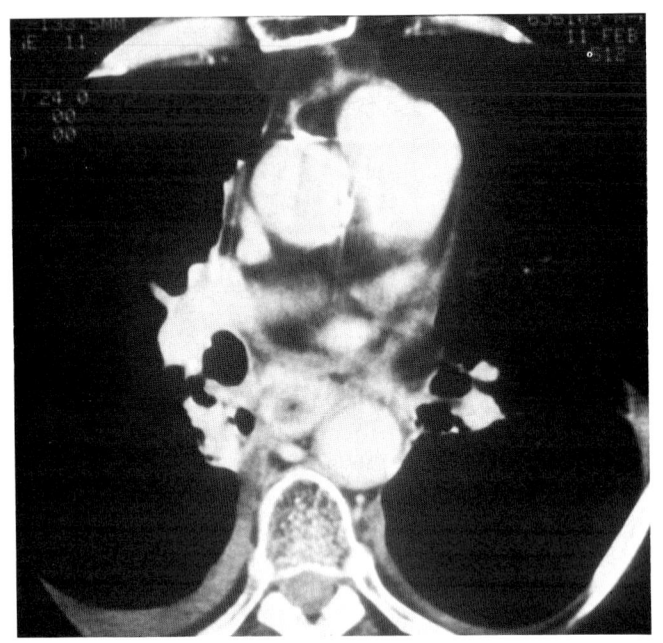

FIGURE 8-4 CT scan of patient with esophageal cancer. Depth of penetration of tumor and wall thickness assessed. Extent of metastasis is evaluated.

the antrum. A guide wire with scored markings is then passed through the biopsy channel into the antrum. The guide wire is left in place in the antrum while the endoscope is withdrawn. This is done by advancing the guide wire 10 cm and then withdrawing the endoscope by 10 cm until the endoscope is totally withdrawn. Usually, with the tip of the guide wire in the antrum, three markings, indicating 60 cm, will be seen at the incisors. Over the guide wire, progressively larger polyvinyl tapered dilators are passed so that treatment can be started at the distal tumor margin. The advantage of the retrograde method is that the entire tumor length can be treated in a single session. Disadvantages are that the endoscope has scant maneuvering room because of the narrowed lumen. This makes the procedure technically difficult and necessitates tangential treatment of tumor tissue, increasing the risk of perforation. Also, increased smoke and carbon debris accumulate because the endoscope blocks the exit pathway for the smoke. This leads to impaired vision requiring frequent removal of the endoscope for cleaning with prolongation of the procedure as a result. Bleeding, which invariably accompanies dilation, may obscure the treatment site and overdistention, as a result of the endoscope clogging the lumen, is more frequent.

In the antegrade method,[13] the laser beam is focused at the proximal margin of the tumor en face and from above (Fig. 8-6). The burn is delivered in a circumferential pattern, beginning at the center of the lumen. The laser is used to "drill" through the obstruction. The advantages are that smoke can be easily evacuated, the beam is focused perpendicular to the tumor and parallel to the lumen, and a large-diameter, two-channel endoscope can be used. The disadvantages are that edema at the proximal margin (caused by thermal injury) impedes passage of the endoscope distally so that more distal areas of the tumor cannot be treated in one session. Most experienced endoscopists use a combination of both methods.

What power setting to use must also be determined. High power settings (80 to 100 W) with 1 s or greater pulse duration at a 1-cm distance vaporizes tissue; low settings (40 to 50 W) coagulate the tissue. Coagulation of tissue may be safer and causes less smoke production, but it takes longer to destroy an equivalent amount of tumor.

Another variable to consider is whether to use the contact or non-contact method. In this method, the fiber tip does not touch tissue. The closer the tip is to the target, the smaller the target spot size is and the larger the energy density. In the contact method, sapphire or ceramic tips of varying shapes have been designed to make tissue contact. When these tips are screwed onto the quartz laser fiber and make contact with tissue, the energy density is increased;

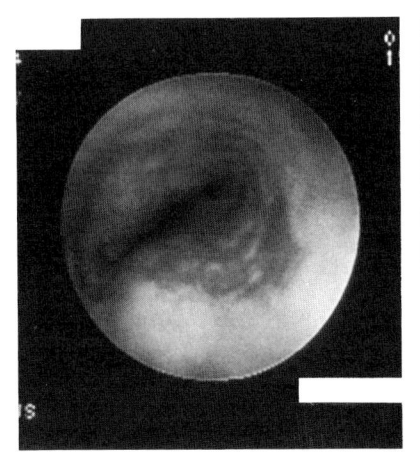

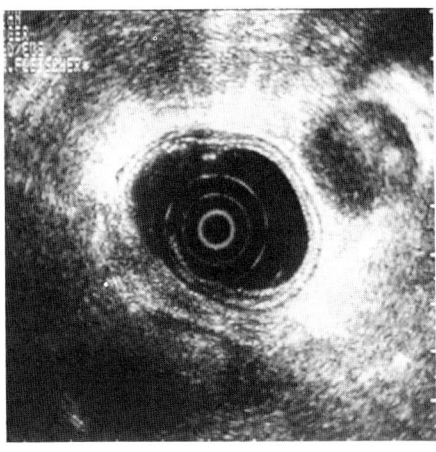

FIGURE 8-5 EUS in patient with esophageal cancer. The depth of penetration and local lymphadenopathy is best assessed with this technique. This patient has adenocarcinoma in Barrett's tissue.

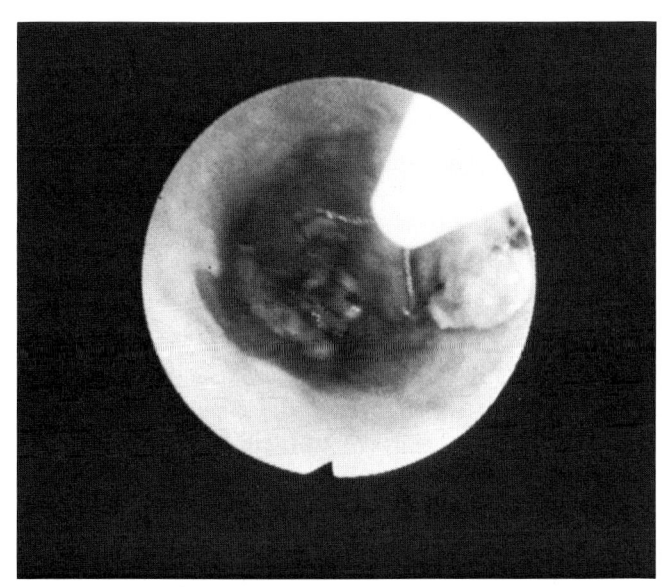

FIGURE 8-6 Antegrade method of treatment. Laser fiber is seen emitting from tip of endoscope and aiming at proximal margin of tumor.

lower power settings may be used to achieve the same effect. Contact laser treatments may be carried out with power settings from 10 to 40 W with a pulse duration from 1 to 5 s. A variation of this method is the interstitial method, in which the quartz fiber (without a specialized tip) makes contact with tissue. The advantage of the contact technique is that it is more precise, more selective, and lower power settings can be used. The disadvantage is that the treatment spot is smaller; therefore, treatment takes longer, and there is less flexibility in aiming the laser beam.

Post Procedure

After the procedure, the patient should have nothing by mouth except ice chips for 4 h. Vital signs should be checked every hour at first and then every 4 h thereafter. Chest and abdominal radiography should be performed if there is a question about perforation. If the patient remains stable, clear liquids may be started that evening and oral intake advanced as tolerated between treatments. Odynophagia may occur and can be treated with antacids or analgesics after perforation has been ruled out. Low-grade fever and mild leukocytosis may be present 12 to 36 h after laser treatment.

Subsequent Sessions

These should be scheduled at 48-h intervals. This allows time for maximum tissue necrosis and gives the patient a "day off." The subsequent sessions begin with a surveillance EGD. Laser-treated areas appear whitish-yellowish and necrotic. The area should be debrided of this necrotic tissue and then examined. The equipment used for debridement includes the endoscope, biopsy forceps, sphincterotomy baskets, polyp graspers, endoscope brushes, water jets, large-caliber suction tubes, and polyvinyl dilators. Dilators are usually used for debridement because the area can be dilated while removing the necrotic tissue at the same time. The endoscope is therefore advanced past the tumor and dilation performed. After dilation, the need for further laser treatment is determined. The end point varies from patient to patient, depending on what ancillary treatment is planned and the clinical situation, but a luminal diameter of 13 mm will generally relieve symptoms of dysphagia. On average, three laser sessions are required to achieve luminal opening. After the last laser session, a contrast swallow is ordered to document effects of therapy and to rule out perforation. Dietary recommendations depend on final luminal diameter but should include liquid nutritional supplements (e.g., milkshakes), avoidance of stringy foods, and advice to chew foods well and to drink large amounts of liquid after eating solid food. Repeat EGD should be done in 3 to 4 weeks unless earlier examination is clinically indicated.

Results

There is a consensus that laser therapy provides benefit for patients with esophageal cancer. Laser ablation relieves the obstruction in 97 percent of cases; relief of dysphagia occurs in 70 to 85 percent.[14] Residual dysphagia, despite technical opening of the lumen, may be attributed to motility disorders caused by neuromuscular damage from tumor invasion or fibrosis from prior radiotherapy or laser therapy. Sixty to 70 percent of patients have a dysphagia-free period of 3 to 6 weeks; only 20 to 25 percent have greater than 3 months without symptoms. Complications are acceptable given the type of patient usually treated. Ell and colleague[15] reported on the results of a survey of 1359 patients receiving laser treatment for malignant upper gastrointestinal stenoses. There was an overall complication rate of 4.1 percent, a perforation rate of 2.1 percent, and a procedure-related mortality of 1 percent. The incidence of fistula and hemorrhage was 1 percent and of sepsis, 0.5 to 1 percent. The perforation rate reportedly has a mean of 4 to 5 percent in other studies.[16]

Comparative studies of ELT and other endoscopic palliative modalities are scant. Buset and associates[17] compared ELT with stent placement. The success rate was similar for both modalities (100 percent versus 95 percent, respectively), but the morbidity was much higher for stent placement (13.8 percent versus 3.6 percent) as was the mortality (4.3 percent versus 0 percent). Barr and associates[18] prospectively studied laser therapy followed by endoscopic intubation with laser therapy alone. It was found that both laser therapy and intubation were equally effective in relieving dysphagia. The laser–stent group, however, had more recurrent dysphagia (45 percent versus 25 percent) and more frequent complications (40 percent versus 20 percent) compared with the laser-only group. Because these complications were considered minor and easily treated, these authors concluded that both treatments were effective in maintaining the patient's quality of life. Jensen and coworkers[19] compared low-power ELT with the bipolar electrocoagulation tumor probe (BICAP) and found the two therapies equally efficacious and safe when used for circumferential lesions. Esophageal recanalization using ELT can be achieved in a high percentage of patients compared with other nonendoscopic palliative methods with a relatively low morbidity compared with palliative surgery.

PHOTODYNAMIC THERAPY (PDT)

The unique property of lasers to generate monochromatic light makes them a promising modality to be used in selective destruction of malignant tissue. In PDT, a sensitizing agent, hematoporphyrin derivative (HpD) or photofrin II, is selectively concentrated in malignant and dysplastic cells. This drug is then activated by visible light of a specific wavelength in the drug's absorption spectrum and generates oxygen free radicals. The singlet oxygen molecules induce tissue damage. The tissue damage is from oxidative toxicity rather than thermal injury because the laser beam in PDT causes only minor elevations in tissue temperature (2 to 4°C). The efficacy of PDT depends on three factors. First, the concentration of a photosensitizing agent in the tumor cells is important. Sensitizers presently being used for PDT include a mixture known as HpD, a partly purified form (Photofrin), porphyrin, phthalocyanine derivatives, and 5-amino levulinic acid (ALA). Selective uptake and retention of porphyrins by tumors compared with normal surrounding tissue was first noted in 1924 by Policard and later confirmed in 1942 by Auler and Banzer. More recent experimental studies have shown that maximum accumulation of HpD into tumor masses occurs in 2 to 3 days.[20,21] Therefore, the optimal time for laser irradiation is 48 to 72 h after HpD injection. Photosensitizers are not only retained in tumors, however. The best concentration ratio of the sensitizer between the tumor and normal tissue is 2:1 to 3:1.[22] In this study, the difference in uptake was between the vascular stroma of the normal and tumor tissue and not between individual malignant and normal cells. Second, the depth of invasion of the tumor is important. Complete irradiation and destruction of the tumor is possible when the tumor is confined to the mucosal and submucosal layers of the digestive wall. Deeper penetration into the muscular layer reduces the possibility for tumor eradication. Therefore, patients with superficial lesions are the best candidates for PDT, and preoperative staging with endoscopic ultrasonography to determine the depth of tumor infiltration and CT scan of the chest to evaluate the extent of disease are recommended. Third, the geometry of the irradiation is critical. The position and angulation of the laser beam is very important. Activation of HPD requires an energy of 100 to 200 J/cm^2 and a power density of at least 100 mW/cm^2. Lesions in the esophagus are usually easily treated; lesions on the lesser curve and the fundus of the stomach are difficult.

Technique

An HpD, such as photofrin II, is given intravenously in a dose of 2 to 2.5 mg/kg. The tumor is then irradiated with visible light from a laser with a wavelength of 630 nm after 48 to 72 h. The laser source is a dye laser circulating rhodamine B or kitton red pumped by an argon laser or a gold vapor laser.

Results

Although use of light as a therapeutic agent dates back centuries, human studies evaluating PDT did not begin until the 1960s. In 1978, Dougherty and colleagues[23] reported complete or partial responses in cutaneous and subcutaneous malignant lesions in 25 patients. In 1984, McCaughan and associates[24] reported improvement in seven patients with obstructing esophageal cancer treated with PDT. Lambert evaluated 84 patients treated with PDT for tumors of the digestive tract (personal communication, April 1988). He found that complete tumor destruction was possible in most patients with superficial lesions confined to the mucosa or submucosa. Eighty-six percent of patients with superficial cancer had negative biopsy results at the tumor site 1 to 5 months after treatment, and 75 percent had similar findings after 2 to 40 months. The survival rate after 16 months was 50%. There were recurrences in 12 percent of patients 9 to 24 months after treatment; these were treated with repeated PDT. All patients with advanced disease had incomplete tumor destruction and poor symptomatic relief of dysphagia. Cutaneous dermatitis occurred if direct sun exposure was not avoided. He concluded that PDT could be curative in superficial esophageal cancer.

Development of more selective sensitizers to avoid skin photosensitivity will make PDT a more attractive palliative alternative. Present sensitizers are retained in the skin for 4 to 6 weeks, necessitating that the patient avoid direct sunlight. The use of ALA may solve this problem. Heme synthesizing cells convert ALA to protoporphyrin IX, which is a photosensitizer in the natural heme synthetic chain and is metabolized within 24 h. Thus, there is no delayed photosensitivity. Also, development of more efficient light delivery systems and of sensitizers activated at wavelengths greater than 630 nm to achieve greater tissue penetration may make curing more advanced cancers after PDT possible.

IRIDIUM-192 RADIOTHERAPY

Recently, interest in intraluminal radiotherapy has been growing. External-beam radiation therapy of esophageal cancer is limited because of local recurrence and distant metastasis.[25,26] The location of the esophagus prevents irradiation with sufficient doses to cause tumor obliteration without adversely effecting neighboring organs. It is not surprising, therefore, that studies have shown that more than 50 percent of patients receiving external-beam radiation therapy have local recurrence of their disease.[27] Intracavitary irradiation permits high-dose tumor irradiation and spares neighboring organs. The radioactive source used is cesium or iridium. It has been tested alone,[28] combined with external-beam radiation,[29] or combined with laser ablation therapy.[30]

Technique

An afterloading technique is employed, whereby a tube is advanced over an endoscopically placed guide wire, and its position is confirmed fluoroscopically. The tube is then fixed in place. The patient is transferred to a treatment room where the iridium or cesium source is inserted or afterloaded by remote control into the applicator tube. It is then withdrawn incrementally until the entire length of the tumor is irradiated. The dwell time of the source at any stop depends on the activity of the source and the length of the tumor. The dose given ranges from 7 to 15 Gy at 1 cm from the radiation source per treatment.

Results

Intracavitary irradiation has been found to relieve dysphagia in 60 to 70 percent of patients.[29] Some have reported permanent relief of dysphagia in treating early cancer (limited to the submucosa with no metastasis) when combined with external-beam irradiation;[30] this, however, has not been confirmed. Sander and coworkers[30] found that laser therapy combined with iridium afterloading did not shorten the length of hospital stay, prolong the survival or dysphagia-free period, or improve the quality of life of patients. In fact, the treatment significantly increased the number of endoscopic procedures performed. They concluded that endoluminal iridium irradiation could not be recommended as the sole adjunctive palliative treatment in esophageal cancer. In an ongoing study, Tytgat[31] has treated 70 patients with intracavitary radiation before and after external-beam irradiation and reported significant decreases in tumor masses. Successful treatment may depend on the depth of tumor invasion, and therefore, endoscopic ultrasonography is helpful in selecting patients and in monitoring postirradiation effects. Complications include esophagitis (found in most patients), strictures, and fistula formation.

BICAP TUMOR PROBE

The BICAP tumor probe technique was first described by Johnston and associates.[32] It is a thermal device, similar to an Eder-Puestow dilator in design, that permits circumferential destruction of large tumor masses (Fig. 8-7). It is best suited for circumferential, exophytic lesions because it may cause damage to normal tissue otherwise.

Technique

There are five tumor probe sizes. Four 360° probes with diameters of 6, 9, 12, and 15 mm. The bipolar electrical

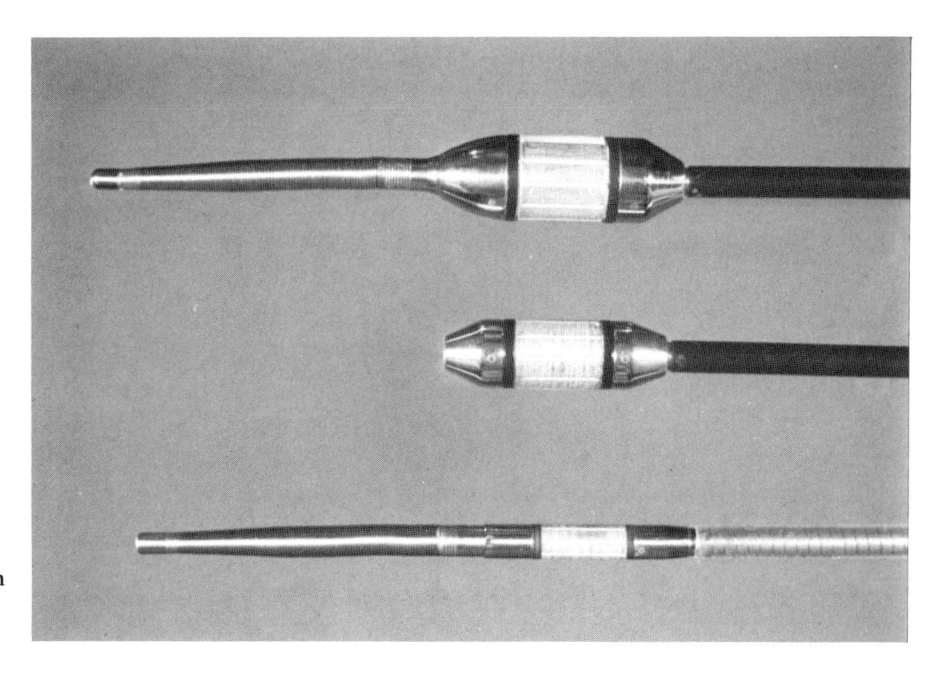

FIGURE 8-7 BICAP tumor probe. From top to bottom, probes of 15-, 12-, and 9-mm diameter are seen.

unit delivers energy circumferentially to 360° to these probes. Also, there is a 180° probe with a 15 mm diameter in which the energy is only delivered to 180°. The probes consists of a distal 6-cm flexible tip that attaches to a metal olive ball. This olive contains the electrically active segment of the probe. The olive is attached to a 60-cm semirigid shaft with markings at 1-cm intervals.

There is no consensus about which power settings should be used. The results and occurrence of complications do not differ with varying power settings or pulse durations. Power settings of 50 W with a pulse duration of 18 s for 12- and 15-mm probes, 50 W for 10 s with 9-mm probe, and 50 W for 6 s with a 6-mm probe have been used. Which size tumor probe to use is also debatable. Animal studies have shown that the 12- and 15-mm probes create similar depths of injury (approximately 1 to 2 mm).[33] Generally, the 15-mm probe is used, but if the stricture is extremely tight and resistant to dilation, then the 6- or 9-mm probe can be used. Theoretically, the 180° probe should be useful in noncircumferential lesions. The active portion of the olive is difficult to position correctly in the tumor, however, and so it is rarely effective.

Preprocedure evaluation, as in laser-treated patients, include barium swallow, CT scan of the chest, and endoscopy to better delineate the extent of disease. Also EUS is helpful in determining the depth of invasion. An esophageal wall thickness of 5 mm in all directions gives a safety margin against perforation.

The procedure should be performed with fluoroscopic support. Conscious intravenous sedation is used. A small-caliber endoscope is passed to mark the upper and lower margins of the tumor precisely. Markers are placed on the patient's skin, with the patient in the left lateral decubitus position, that correspond to the exact margins of the tumor. A guide wire is passed into the antrum and left in place as the endoscope is withdrawn as previously described. If the 15-cm tumor probe will not pass through the stricture, then the area should be dilated with polyvinyl dilators to 15 mm. Sometimes, however, the tumor probe will pass without dilation. The tumor probe is passed over the guide wire with the neck extended to allow passage of the olive through the upper esophageal sphincter. The probe is passed beyond the distal margin of the tumor and then is withdrawn. The feel of resistance, the measurements on the tumor probe shaft, and the radiopaque markers on the patient's skin assist the endoscopist in properly locating the probe in the tumor. Treatment proceeds in a cephalad direction. Using fluoroscopic guidance, the probe is pulled through the length of the tumor at 1-cm increments until the entire tumor length is treated.

Treatment of the proximal margin is observed endoscopically with a small-caliber endoscope that has been passed alongside the probe. This ensures that normal tissue is not being treated inadvertently. The tumor probe and guide wire are withdrawn and the effects of thermal injury are observed endoscopically. After treatment, the mucosa usually has an overlying circumferential white exudate, but may have a black eschar or be friable and hemorrhagic.

Postprocedure

The patient should not take anything by mouth after the procedure. Vital signs should be checked frequently. Chest and abdominal radiography should be obtained after 4 h. Clear liquids may be started that evening if the patient is clinically stable and the radiographs have excluded perforation. Chest pain frequently occurs during the first 24 h, and analgesics may be needed. Also, patients may have a low-grade fever or mild leukocytosis. Similar to laser therapy, dysphagia may temporarily worsen secondary to edema.

Follow-Up Examinations

Maximum tumor necrosis generally occurs by 48 h, and therefore, repeat endoscopy is performed at this time. The previously treated area is surveyed and then debrided by pushing necrotic tissue into the stomach with the endoscope. If an 11-cm endoscope will not pass through the stricture, then repeat BICAP treatment should be performed. At the completion of therapy, a water-soluble contrast swallow followed by a barium swallow (after perforation is excluded) is performed to document luminal patency. Monthly endoscopy follow-ups are then planned to evaluate luminal patency and determine the need for further therapy. Dietary recommendations should be given and include avoiding stringy foods, chewing food well, and following solid food ingestion with large amounts of liquid.

Results

Fleischer[34] compared endoscopic laser therapy with BICAP tumor probe therapy. He reported similar efficacy and complications with both treatments. Luminal opening was seen in 95 percent of laser-treated patients and in 80 to 90 percent of patients treated with the BICAP tumor probe. Relief of dysphagia was seen in 75 percent of laser-treated patients and 70 percent of BICAP-treated patients. Perforations were reported in both groups to be approximately 5 percent. Stricture formation after BICAP tumor probe treatment was reportedly 5 percent. Jensen and colleagues[19] compared BICAP tumor probe treatment with low-power YAG laser treatment and found them to be equally effective and safe in circumferential lesions. The BICAP tumor probe is safe, effective, inexpensive, and easy to use in circumferential tumor lesions. It is a modality that should be considered complementary to laser therapy.

ESOPHAGEAL PROSTHESIS

Indications

The first reports of esophageal stent placements were made in the 1880s.[35] Since that time, varying designs of stents have been developed with varying degrees of enthusiasm. In the early 1900s, surgically placed tubes were used. Recently, endoscopically placed stents have gained favor. There is consensus that esophageal stents are the treatment of choice in malignant esophagorespiratory fistulas. There is little consensus, however, on the role of esophageal stents in the palliation of esophageal cancer not complicated by a fistula. General indications for prosthetic insertion include strictures that are resistant to frequent dilations or are very long (> 10 cm). Contraindications include severely angulated strictures that cannot be safely dilated, lesions less than 2 cm from the upper esophageal sphincter, tumors without a proximal shelf to prevent migration, lesions with a high risk of airway compression by the stent, luminal obstruction that cannot be dilated, and horizontal orientation of a stricture at the gastroesophageal junction that would not allow good flow through a stent.

Technique

There are numerous commercially available stents of varying lengths and diameters (Fig. 8-8). They are composed of some form of plastic (latex, silicone rubber, or polyvinyl chloride) and many are reinforced with a metallic core to resist kinking. There are many ways to insert esophageal stents endoscopically. They are all variations of a single theme and involve widening the lumen using dilation or a thermal device and then forcing a stent into position. The method of a prosthesis guided over a Savary-type dilator is described next.

The procedure is performed with fluoroscopic monitoring and with intravenous conscious sedation. The proximal and distal margins of the tumor are precisely measured to determine the length of the tumor and the distance of the margins from the incisors. The distance from the proximal tumor margin to the upper esophageal sphincter is also measured since most stents have a 3- to 4-cm-long proximal flange. These are important factors in selecting the appropriate stent. The tumor is then dilated. Most stents have an outside diameter of 14 to 16 mm, and therefore, the lumen is dilated over a guide wire to a diameter of approximately 16 mm. The dilations generally should be performed over several days to lessen the risk of perforation.

A stent is chosen that has a shaft 3 cm longer than the tumor length. The proximal flange will add an additional 3 cm to the length. Therefore, a 7-cm tumor would have a 13-cm-long stent. The stent should be positioned to extend 3 cm above the proximal tumor margin and 3 cm below the distal tumor margin. The stent is readied for placement in the following manner. The 3–0 silk suture (120 cm in length) is passed through the puncture sites in the proximal end of the flange. This will aid in stent removal if there is a problem with its position. The suture is fed retrograde through the inside of the pusher tube and exits through its proximal end. The stent and the pusher tube are lubricated with silicone and then put over a stabilizing introducing tube (a modified longer dilator). Markings should

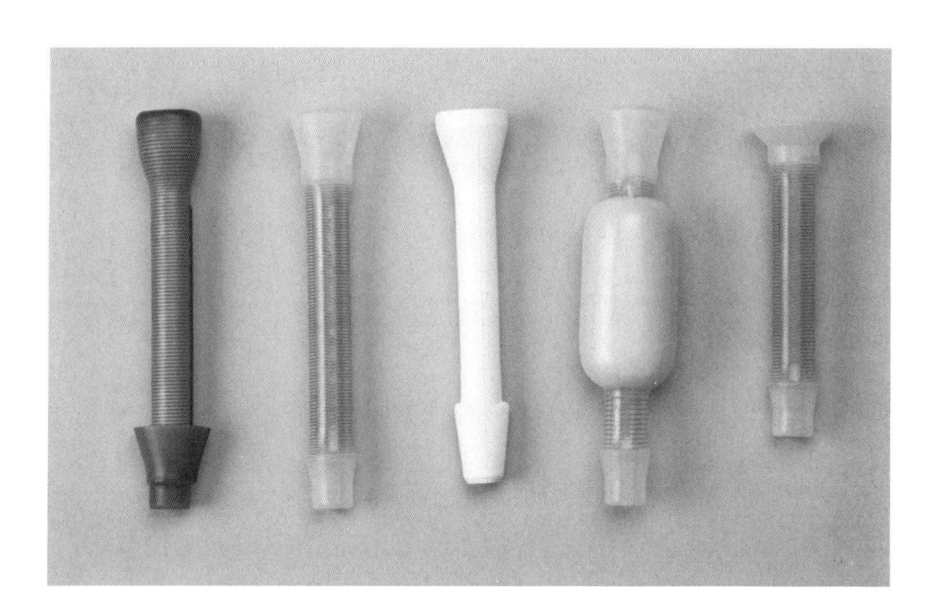

FIGURE 8-8 Commercially available prosthetic stents. Five different types of stents are pictured.

then be made on the pusher tube with an indelible marker to aid in the positioning of the stent. This is most easily performed by laying the stent-pusher tube unit on a flat surface and measuring out the distances with a ruler. The first mark on the pusher tube is the distance from the incisors to the proximal tumor margin. The second mark on the pusher tube is the distance from the incisors to the intended distal stent tip (i.e., 3 cm beyond the distal tumor margin).

The stabilizing introducing tube is passed over the guide wire, through the tumor and into the stomach. The neck is then hyperextended, and the stent-pusher tube unit is passed over the introducer tube through the pharynx. When the first mark is reached the proximal end of the tumor is reached and firm pressure is needed to overcome the resistance. When the second mark is reached, the stent is properly seated. The guide wire and stabilizing tube are carefully removed with a gentle twisting motion under fluoroscopic guidance to minimize proximal displacement of the stent. Next, the pusher tube is removed again with a gentle twisting motion and fluoroscopic monitoring to separate the stent from the pusher tube without dislodging the stent. Good lubrication of the stabilizing introducer tube and at the junction between the stent and the pusher tube helps prevent stent dislodgement during these maneuvers. If a problem develops, the stent may be removed by pulling on both ends of the 3–0 silk suture attached to the stent. If all goes well, the suture may be cut and pulled on one end to remove it.

A small-caliber endoscope is then passed to confirm the stent's proper position and to assess luminal patency. Chest radiography should be performed to look for evidence of perforation and as a reference film to evaluate for possible stent migration at a later date.

Postprocedure

The patient receives nothing by mouth except ice chips. If the patient remains clinically stable for 12 h, clear liquids may be started. Cough should be suppressed. Codeine 30 mg every 4 to 6 h for 48 h is usually successful. A water-soluble contrast study is performed within 24 h to exclude leaks. If no leak is found, free flow through the stent is checked with a barium swallow. After 24 to 36 h, the diet may be advanced. With an internal diameter of 12 to 13 mm, the patient may be able to eat a normal diet if the food is chewed well and large amounts of gassy beverages are taken after meals.

Complications

Successful intubation and relief of dysphagia after stent placement occurs in 90 to 95 percent of patients in most series.[32] Occlusion of fistula is also achieved in the majority of patients. Complications are frequent but are low in comparison to surgical alternatives. In a review by Girardet and associates,[36] the mortality for patients undergoing surgically placed Celestin tubes was 21.2 percent versus 5.6 percent for endoscopically placed tubes. The most common complications after stent placement are perforation, tube migration, tumor overgrowth, stricturing caused by reflux esophagitis, pressure necrosis, food bolus obstruction, hemorrhage, and aspiration pneumonia. A large survey by Tytgat[37] of approximately 1850 patients found that stents were successfully placed in 97 percent of patients. Complications reported were: perforation in 8.4 percent, migration in 9.7 percent (acute migration in 15 percent and late migration in 8 percent), stent obstruction in 5 percent, pressure necrosis caused by the funnel edge of the stent in 0.9 percent, hemorrhage in 1.2 percent, and procedure-related mortality in 4.5 percent. In another survey of 820 stent placements, Bennett[38] found a migration rate of 10 percent, perforation rate of 9 percent, and prosthesis obstruction rate of 8 percent.

The insertion of esophageal prostheses in patients with recurrent or progressive malignant strictures relieves dysphagia in a high percentage of patients and allows them to remain at home in the terminal stages of their disease. They are, however, associated with a high rate of complications.

New self-expanding metal stents are being designed which may overcome some of these problems (Fig. 8-9). These stents are compressed at delivery, allowing insertion into tight strictures before expanding to their final diameter after deployment. Delivery into strictures is easy and because of the small initial diameter the risk of perforation

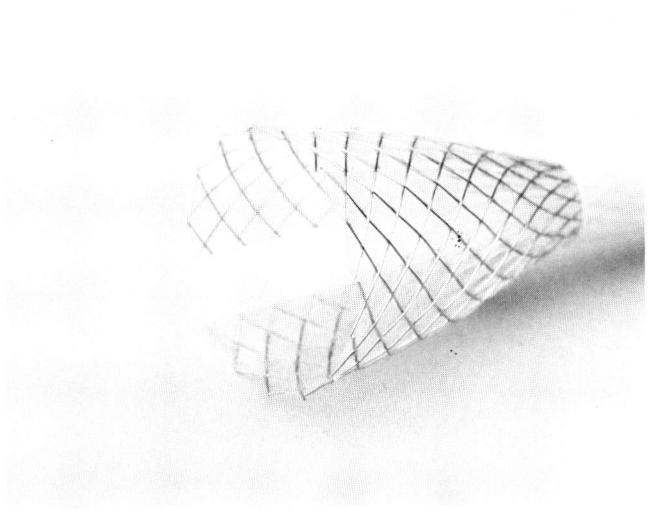

FIGURE 8-9 Self-expanding metal stents. As stent emerges from delivery catheter, it opens to fully expanded diameter.

may be less. Until self-expanding esophageal stents are approved in the United States, conventional plastic stents provide good palliation of obstructive symptoms and allow patients a good quality of life.

DILATION

Per oral esophageal dilation is simple, safe, and inexpensive. This method is frequently used when the primary therapeutic modality (e.g., radiotherapy or chemotherapy) has failed to relieve dysphagia. Numerous types of instruments are available to perform dilations, including mercury-filled Maloney bougies; tapered, over-the-guide wire Savary dilators, and balloon dilators (Fig. 8-10).

After the decision is made to dilate a malignant stricture, the anatomy of the entire stricture should be examined. If an endoscope will not pass the area, a barium swallow can be used to evaluate the anatomy. Gradual dilation should be performed, and if two successively larger dilators meet resistance, further dilation should be delayed to a subsequent session.

Any of the available dilators may be used. However, tapered dilators are more commonly used because the narrowed tip allows easier passage through strictures. Mercury-filled dilators are so flexible that they frequently pass through a stricture without successfully dilating it. This same problem may also occur with balloon dilators. There is, however, a theoretic advantage that radial dilation with balloons may lessen the risk of perforation.

When guide wires are used with dilators, fluoroscopy is generally advised to maintain their position during dilation. The risk of perforation is related more to the guide wire rather than the dilators in these cases.

Dilation is a simple palliative method in esophageal cancer. Cassidy and colleagues[39] reported a 2 percent complication rate and an 85 percent success rate. Dobbs and associates[40] reported a lower morbidity and mortality for per oral dilation compared with esophageal stent placement. They concluded that stent placement should be reserved for strictures refractory to dilation and tracheoesophageal fistulas. Aste and coworkers[41] reported an excellent response in 26 percent, a partial response in 42 percent, and no response in 31 percent of patients treated with per oral dilation. The duration of benefit ranged from 3 to 45 days (mean 11.5 days). Esophageal dilation is a simple, safe, and inexpensive procedure that temporarily relieves dysphagia in many patients. The effects are very brief, and therefore, this palliative procedure should be used in conjunction with other modalities.

INJECTION THERAPY

Injection of chemical agents into the tumor mass to cause tumor necrolysis is an option for palliative treatment. Several agents, including alcohol, polidocanol, and etha-

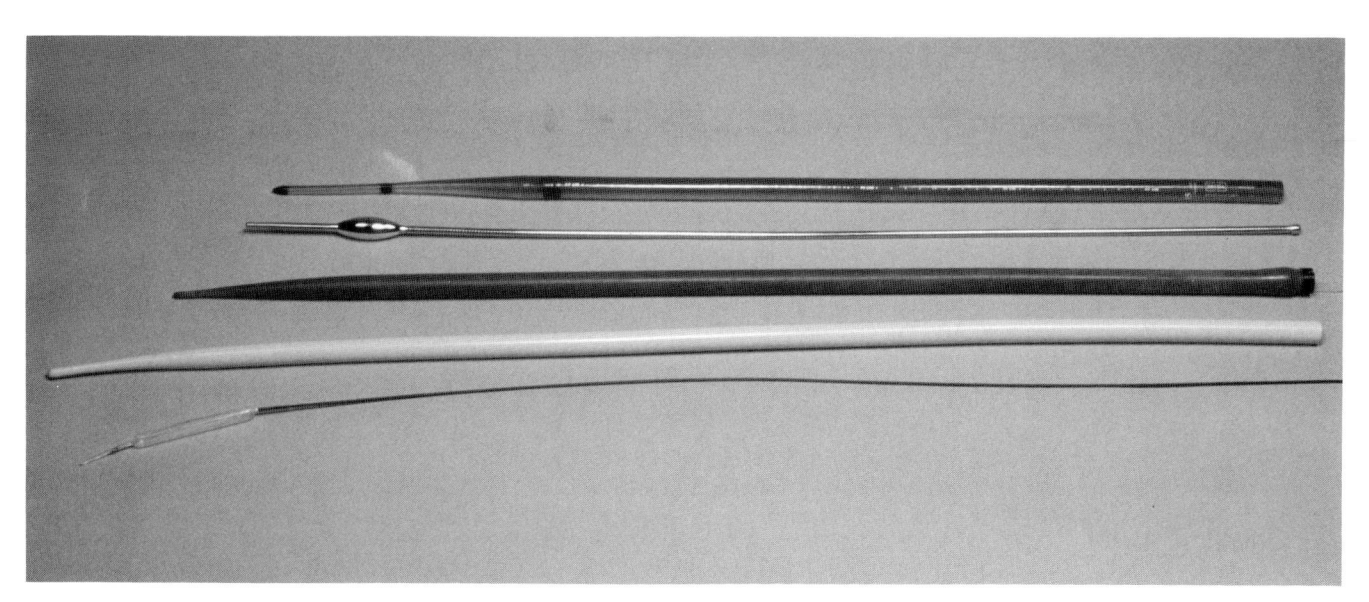

FIGURE 8-10 A variety of esophageal dilators are available.

nolamine, may be used for this therapy. In a recent study in Italy, polidocanol 3% was injected into the tumor in 1- to 2-mL boluses, using a sclerotherapy needle with an injection length of 10 to 12 mm.[42] Multiple injections were made beginning at the distal margin of the tumor and proceeding in a cephalad direction at 5-mm intervals until the entire tumor segment was treated. The area was dilated before treatment if a small endoscope could not reach the distal margin initially. Injections were made parallel to the lumen, and the sessions were scheduled at 1-week intervals. Injection therapy was equivalent to laser therapy in many aspects, including relief of dysphagia (81.2 percent versus 88.8 percent, respectively), number of sessions (3.2 versus 3.3), and the possibility of outpatient therapy. Only one complication (mediastinal fistula from too deep an injection) was reported. The fact that injection therapy is inexpensive, technically easy, and widely available may make this endoscopic palliative procedure of choice if larger studies confirm these results. Currently, the results are too preliminary to draw firm conclusions.

REFERENCES

1. Kasai M, Mori S, Watanabe T: Follow-up results after resection of thoracic oesophageal carcinoma. *World J Surg* 1978; 2:543–551.
2. Koch NG, Lewin E, Pettersson S: Carcinoma of thoracic oesophagus: A review of 146 cases. *Acta Chir Scand* 1967; 133:375–380.
3. Fein R, Kelson D, Geller N, et al: Adenocarcinoma of the esophagus and gastroesophageal junction: Prognostic factors and results of therapy. *Cancer* 1985; 56:2512–2518.
4. Belsey RHR: Palliative management of esophageal carcinoma. *Am J Surg* 1980; 139:789–794.
5. Conlan AA, Nicolaou N, Hammond CA, et al: Retrosternal gastric bypass for inoperable esophageal cancer: A report of 71 patients. *Ann Thorac Surg* 1983; 36:396–401.
6. Parker EF, Gregorie HB: Carcinoma of the esophagus: Long-term results. *JAMA* 1976; 235:1018–1020.
7. Moertel C, Reitmeier R: Mitomycin-C therapy in advanced gastrointestinal cancer. *JAMA* 1968; 204:1045–1048.
8. Kelsen DP: Chemotherapy for local regional and advanced esophageal cancer, in DeVita VT, Hellman S, Rosenberg S. *Cancer: Principles & Practices of Oncology Updates*. Philadelphia, JB Lippincott, 1988, vol 2, pp 1–12.
9. Fleischer D, Sivak MV Jr: Endoscopic Nd:YAG laser therapy as palliation for esophagogastric cancer: Parameters affecting initial outcome. *Gastroenterology* 1985; 89:827–831.
10. Tio TL, Cohen PP, Udding J, et al: Endosonography and computed tomography of esophageal carcinoma. Preoperative classification compared to the new (1987) TNM system. *Gastroenterology* 1989; 96:1478–1486.
11. Lightdale C, Botet J, Zauber A, et al: Endoscopic ultrasound compared to CT scanning for preoperative staging of esophageal cancer. *Gastrointest Endosc* 1990; 36:A191.
12. Pietrafitta JJ, Dwyer RM: Endoscopic Nd:YAG laser therapy for malignant esophageal obstruction. *Arch Surg* 1986; 121:395–400.
13. Fleischer D, Kessler F, Haye O: Endoscopic Nd:YAG laser therapy for carcinoma of the esophagus: A new palliative approach. *Am J Surg* 1982; 143:280–283.
14. Mellow MH, Pinkas H: Endoscopic therapy for esophageal cancer with Nd:YAG laser: Prospective evaluation of efficacy, complications and survival. *Gastrointest Endosc* 1984; 30:334.
15. Ell C, Demling L: Laser therapy of tumor stenoses in the upper gastrointestinal tract: An international inquiry. *Lasers Surg Med* 1987; 7:491–494.
16. Fleischer D: The Washington Symposium on Endoscopic Laser Therapy, April 1985. *Gastrointest Endosc* 1985; 31:397–400.
17. Buset M, Baise M, Bourgeois N, et al: Palliative endoscopic management of obstructive esophagogastric cancer: Laser of prothesis? *Gastrointest Endosc* 1987; 33:357–361.
18. Barr H, Krasner N, Raouf A, et al: Prospective randomized trial of laser therapy only and laser therapy followed by endoscopic intubation for the palliation of malignant dysphagia. *Gut* 1990; 31:252–258.
19. Jensen DM, Machicado G, Randall G, et al: Comparison of low-power YAG laser and BICAP tumor probe for palliation of esophageal cancer strictures. *Gastroenterology* 1988; 94:1263–1270.
20. Daniell MD, Hill JS: A history of photodynamic therapy. *Aust N Z J Surg* 1991; 61:340–348.
21. Brown SG: Phototherapy of tumours. *World J Surg* 1983; 7:700.
22. Agrev MV, Wharen RE, Anderson RE, et al: Hematoporphyrin derivative: Quantitative uptake in dimethylhydrazine induced murine colorectal carcinoma. *J Surg Oncol* 1983; 24:173–176.
23. Dougherty TJ, Kaufman JE, Goldfarb A: Photoradiation therapy for the treatment of malignant tumours. *Cancer Res* 1978; 38:2628–2635.
24. McCaughan JS, Hicks W, Laufman L, et al: Palliation of esophageal malignancy with photoradiation therapy. *Cancer* 1984; 54:2905–2910.
25. Pearson JG: The present status and future potential of radiotherapy in the management of esophageal cancer. *Cancer* 1977; 39:882–890.
26. Earlam R, Cunha-Melo JR: Oesophageal squamous cell carcinoma: II. A critical review of radiotherapy. *Br J Surg* 1980; 67:451–461.
27. Beatty JD, DeBoer G, Rider WD: Carcinoma of the esophagus: Pretreatment assessment, correlation of radiation treatment parameters with survival, and identification and management of radiation failure. *Cancer* 1979; 43:2254–2267.
28. Rowland CG, Pagliero KM: Intracavitary irradiation in palliation of carcinoma of oesophagus and cardia. *Lancet* 1985; 2:981–983.
29. Hishikawa Y, Tanaka S, Miura T: Early esophageal carcinoma treated with intracavitary irradiation. *Radiology* 1985; 156:519–522.
30. Sander R, Hagenmueller F, Sander C, et al: Laser versus laser plus afterloading with iridium-192 in the palliation of malignant stenosis of the esophagus: A prospective, randomized, and controlled study. *Gastrointest Endosc* 1991; 37:433–440.
31. Tytgat G: Endoscopic therapy of esophageal cancer: Possibilities and limitations. *Endoscopy* 1990; 22:263–267.
32. Johnston J, Quint R, Petruzzi C, et al: Development and experimental testing of a large BICAP probe for the treatment of obstructing esophageal and rectal malignancy. *Gastrointest Endosc* 1985; 31:156.
33. Fleischer D, Ranard R, Kamath R, et al: Structure formation following BICAP tumor probe therapy for esophageal cancer. Clinical observations and experimental studies. *Gastrointest Endosc* 1987; 33:183.
34. Fleischer D: A comparison of endoscopic laser therapy and BICAP tumor probe therapy for esophageal cancer. *Am J Gastroenterol* 1987; 82:608–612.
35. Earlam R, Cunha-Melo JR: Malignant oesophageal strictures: A review of techniques for palliative intubation. *Br J Surg* 1982; 69:61–68.
36. Girardet RE, Ransdell HT, Wheat MW: Palliative intubation in the

management of esophageal carcinoma. *Ann Thorac Surg* 1974; 18:417.
37. Tytgat GN: Endoscopic methods of treatment of gastrointestinal and biliary stenoses. *Endoscopy* 1980; 12(suppl):57–68.
38. Bennett JR: Intubation of gastroesophageal malignancies: A survey of current practice in Britain, 1980. *Gut* 1981; 22:336–338.
39. Cassidy DE, Juergen NH, Worth B: Management of malignant strictures. Role of esophageal dilation and per oral prothesis. *Am J Gastroenterol* 1981; 76:173A.
40. Dobbs SM, Graham DY, Zubler MA, et al: Is there a role for endoscopic placement of esophageal prosthesic devices in esophageal carcinoma? *Gastrointest Endosc* 1981; 27:134A.
41. Aste H, Munizzi F, Martines H, et al: Esophageal dilation in malignant dysphagia. *Cancer* 1985; 56:2713–2715.
42. Angelini G, Pasini AF, Ederle A, et al: Nd:YAG laser versus polidocanol injection for palliation of esophageal malignancy: A prospective, randomized study. *Gastrointest Endosc* 1991; 37:607–610.

Chapter 9

Periviseral Dissection of the Esophagus

Gerhard Buess / Marco Maria Lirici

The thoracoabdominal approach to esophageal resection for cancer carries high peri- and postoperative risks. Furthermore, most patients undergoing this procedure have pulmonary, cardiac, and/or hepatic insufficiencies at the time of surgery that increase the incidence of postoperative complications. Radical surgery in such patients is controversial because the anatomy of the mediastinum does not allow a complete node dissection and the benefit of such extensive surgery is not proved. As a consequence, blunt dissection of the esophagus has been utilized to minimize operative trauma during surgery for esophageal cancer.

The transhiatal esophagectomy is one of the only procedures in general surgery carried out without the benefit of direct visualization. Therefore, blind preparation of the esophagus results in a high rate of intra- and postoperative problems related to uncontrolled bleeding and injury of the trachea or left recurrent laryngeal nerve. A new, minimally invasive procedure called endoscopic microsurgical dissection of the esophagus (EMDE), allowing careful dissection under controlled visualization, was developed by Buess and coworkers.[1–4] In 1989, the clinical use of EMDE was initiated at the University Hospital of Tuebingen, Germany.[5]

TECHNIQUE OF PERIVISCERAL DISSECTION OF THE ESOPHAGUS

Equipment

The operating mediastinoscope (Richard Wolf, Rosemont, IL) and related instruments were developed by Buess and associates.[6] The telescope, with its obliquely offset eyepiece, can be connected to a conventional camera, enabling the surgeon to view the entire mediastinoscopic procedure on a video screen. The telescope fits inside an outer sheath in a suction–irrigation integrated system that includes a working channel for surgical instruments (Fig. 9-1). The

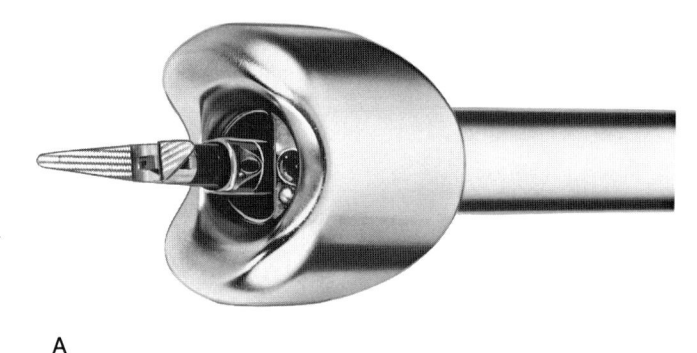

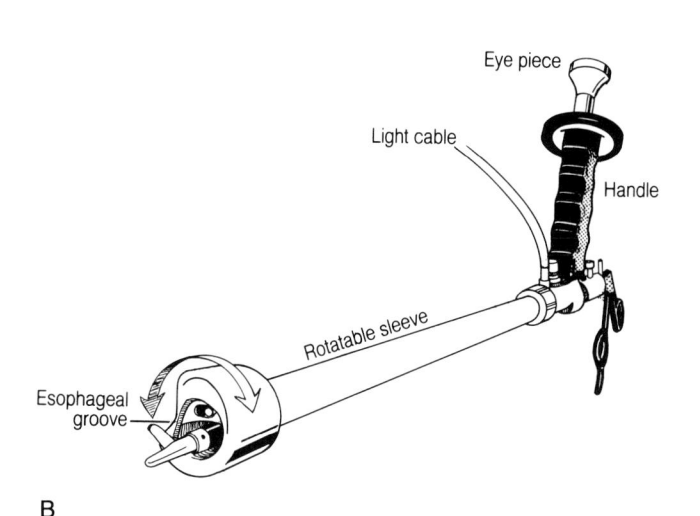

FIGURE 9-1 A. Picture of the mediastinoscope. B. Frontal view showing the retatable sleeve with esophageal groove.

tip of the outer sheath is olive shaped. Its cross-section has a groove on one side, allowing the creation of a peri-esophageal space by mechanical distraction of tissues and, at the same time, maintaining the esophagus in a central position. The olive itself turns around during dissection of the posterior, lateral, and anterior aspects of the esophagus.

Various instruments can be introduced through the working channel. Because it is impossible to insert more than one at a time, a special suction–coagulation probe with a central passage for specially designed surgical instruments has been developed. Forceps for monopolar and bipolar coagulation and straight scissors are instruments that can be introduced through the suction device. When suction or coagulation by the probe is required, the inserted instrument is just slightly retracted. This new operative concept permits continuous visualization during control of bleeding points.

Procedure Notes

PREOPERATIVE ASSESSMENT AND INDICATIONS

The diagnostic workup consists of the following.

1. Blood analysis with biochemical assessment of liver function.
2. Anteroposterior and lateral chest radiography.
3. Pulmonary function tests.
4. Electrocardiogram and cardiac evaluation.
5. Barium swallow.
6. Esophagoscopy with biopsies.
7. Chest and upper abdomen computed tomographic (CT) scans.

Because evaluation of the location, extent, and infiltration of tumor is necessary for proper decision making and because CT scanning is unreliable in detecting periesophageal structure and organ infiltration, endoluminal (endoscopic) ultrasonography should be included in the preoperative assessment. Information concerning the depth of infiltration in tumors of the middle third of the esophagus is especially important to minimize the possibility of intraoperative conversion to thoracoabdominal esophagectomy. Indications for EMDE include all T1 to T3 esophageal cancers, except for tumors of the middle third, infiltrating the trachea or extensively involving other surrounding structures.

PREOPERATIVE MANAGEMENT AND ANESTHESIA

Intensive physiotherapeutic and medical treatment is mandatory for patients with obstructive airway disease. All patients must give signed informed consent for EMDE and possible conversion to thoracotomy. An extended shave from the pubis to the chin is performed.

The operation is carried out under general endotracheal anesthesia, often combined with continuous thoracic epidural anesthesia. Endobronchial anesthesia is not necessary. Venous cannulas, a central venous catheter (right jugular) and arterial cannula, are provided. Bladder catheterization, monitoring of temperature, pulse oximetry, and end-expiratory CO_2 measurements are performed. A 30-French orogastric tube is inserted.

PATIENT, TEAM, AND THEATER SETTING

Skin disinfection and draping with a sterile, adhesive drape is performed starting from the pubis and reaching upward to the chin and laterally to the posterior axillary line. The patient is supine with the right hemithorax elevated with a 5-cm roll. The patient's head is rotated to the right. The position of the patient allows intraoperative conversion to an anterolateral thoracotomy.

The intervention is performed by two different teams that operate simultaneously (Fig. 9-2). The abdominal team consists of a surgeon on the right side and an assistant on the left. A second assistant stands at the side of the surgeon, and the scrub nurse stands to the left of the primary assistant. The mediastinal team consists of a surgeon sitting on the left side of the thorax, with the assistant sitting on the surgeon's left. The scrub nurse stands behind the surgeon. The video equipment is placed on the left and behind the mediastinal surgeon, with the light source. The suction–irrigation device is controlled with a foot pedal by the assistant. Because of the positioning and draping of the patient, access to the operating table by the anesthesiologist is generally difficult.

OPERATIVE PROCEDURE

The abdominal team performs an extensive mobilization of the stomach before constructing the gastric tube to pull it

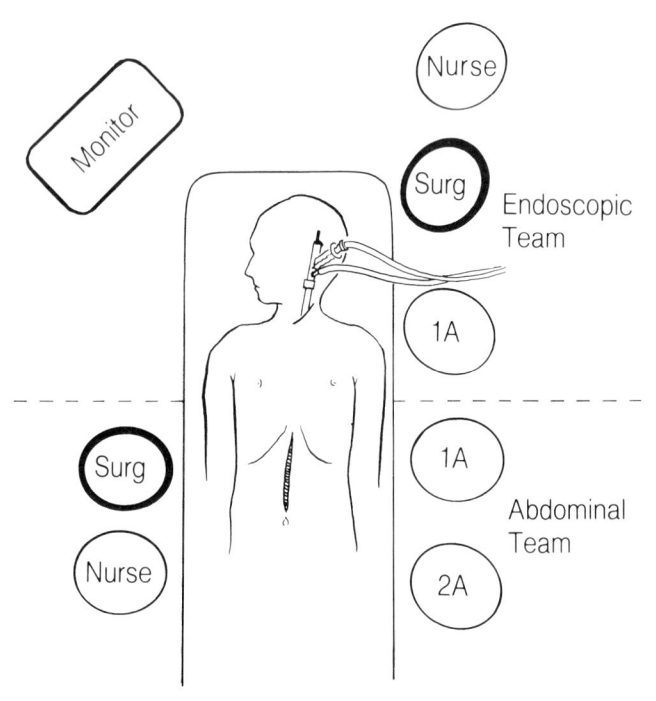

FIGURE 9-2 Positioning of the two operating teams.

up to the neck without tension. The mediastinal surgeon begins with a cervical incision along the anterior border of the sternocleidomastoid muscle. Taking care not to injure the external jugular vein and the laryngeal or left vagus nerves, the inferior thyroid artery is identified. The cervical esophagus is then identified and encircled with a rubber tape. Below the crossing of the inferior thyroid artery and the recurrent nerve, blunt dissection of the esophagus begins from the posterior aspect of the trachea. The dissection is continued 2 to 3 cm below the suprasternal notch, creating room for the introduction of the mediastinoscope.

The endoscopic perivisceral dissection begins posteriorly, and then the left side, anterior aspect, and right side are bluntly dissected, always starting from the neck. The aim is to create a tunnel alongside the esophagus down into the abdominal cavity (Fig. 9-3A). By carefully pushing the suction–irrigation device, the areolar tissue between the esophagus and surrounding structures is separated. Coagulation must be performed as soon as blood vessels contained in the perivisceral attachments are encountered and before their division. Larger vessels must be coagulated with forceps before attempting their division.

The plane of dissection is immediately adjacent to esophageal muscle fibers. Landmarks on the left side are the aortic arch and the descending aorta; landmarks during anterior dissection are the posterior aspect of the trachea and the ridges of its cartilaginous rings. On the right side, the azygos vein usually is not exposed. The parietal pleura is visible below the tracheal bifurcation and can be breached during dissection.

Dissection in the area of the tumor cannot be performed along the plane of the muscle fibers. For tumors in the upper and middle esophageal thirds, the dissection is carried out by the endoscopic surgeon. Dissection of tumors in the lower third can be done by the abdominal surgeon from below or by the endoscopic surgeon. The choice is made on the basis of the best access to the right plane of dissection. If the abdominal surgeon is to perform a digital dissection around the tumor, it is done under mediastinoscopic guidance, thus enhancing the safety of the surgical maneuvers.

When the abdominal cavity has been reached, a catheter is grasped by forceps through the mediastinoscope and pulled up into the neck incision. After withdrawal of the nasogastric tube, the cervical esophagus is transsected with a linear stapler 3 cm below the inferior thyroid artery. The mediastinal esophagus is then sutured securely to the catheter. The catheter is gently pulled by the abdominal surgeon, thus folding the esophagus on itself (Fig. 9-3B). The remaining perivisceral attachments are identified, coagulated, and divided under mediastinoscopic control, and the esophagus is removed through the diaphragmatic hiatus. Careful control of bleeding points in the esophageal bed is accomplished, and the stomach, sutured to a silicone tube, is pulled up to the neck using the mediastinoscope (Fig. 9-3C). A tension free, two-layer, end-to-end, hand-sewn anastomosis is performed, the gastric tube is once again introduced, and a Penrose drain is left in the perianastomotic area.

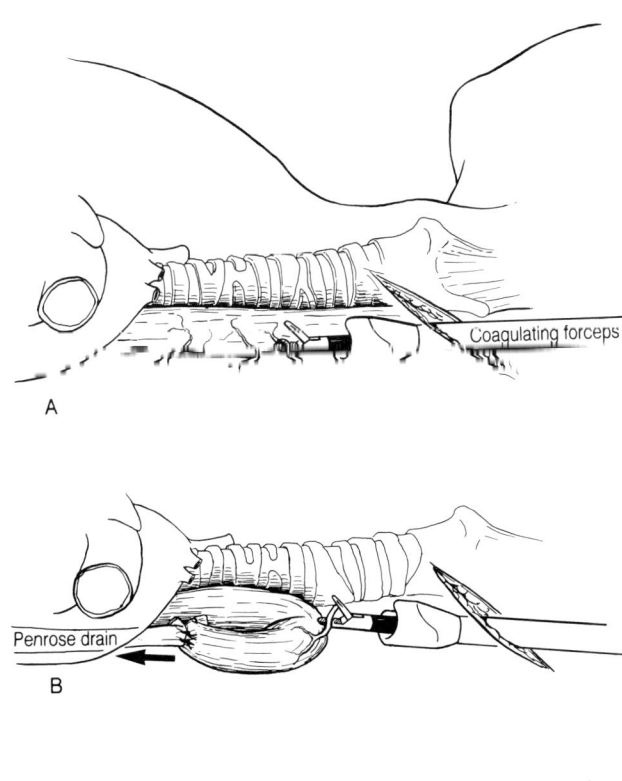

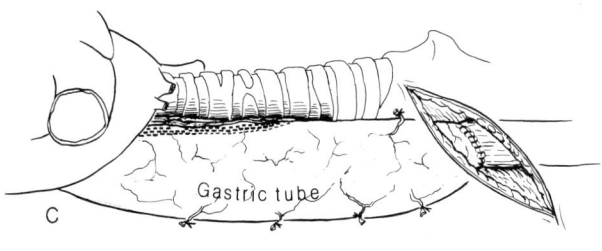

FIGURE 9-3 A. The operative mediastinoscope is inserted into the cervical incision alongside the esophagus. Blood vessels are coagulated and cut with scissors. B. The esophagus is folded on itself by gently pulling back on the Penrose drain. Mediastinoscopic dissection of the last perivisceral attachments can be performed during this operative step. C. The gastric tube is pulled up to the neck under mediastinoscopic control, and a hand-sewn or stapled anastomosis is performed.

POSTOPERATIVE MANAGEMENT

A 24-hour intensive care period providing complete monitoring and overnight assisted ventilation follows postoperatively. Chest radiography and ultrasound examination are performed to detect pleural effusions, which require drainage when greater than 300 mL. On the seventh postoperative day, a Gastrografin (diatrizoate meglumine) swallow is carried out to ensure patency of the anastomosis before oral intake begins.

RESULTS

From September 1989 to January 1992, 32 patients suffering from esophageal cancer underwent EMDE at the University Hospital of Tuebingen. Twenty-four of these patients were fully evaluated. The average age was 59.2 years, and the mean duration of symptoms was 3.9 months.

A tumor was found in the cervical third of the esophagus in 2 patients (8.3 percent); the middle third, in 14 (58.3 percent); and the distal third, in 8 (33.4 percent). Histologically, 19 patients had squamous cell carcinoma, 4 had adenocarcinoma, and 1 had malignant T-cell lymphoma. Complete TNM staging was impossible in most cases because lymph node clearance was not attempted. Using the histologic microinvasion scale of Hermanek and coworker,[7] we found pathologic Stage T1 neoplasms in eight patients, pT2 lesions in seven, pT3 in seven, and pT4 in two. In nine patients, the histologist found pN1 neoplasms.

The resection rate in these 24 cases was 100 percent; no conversion to a thoracotomy was necessary. The mean operating time was 3 hours and 20 minutes, with the mediastinoscopic procedure requiring 1 hour and 5 minutes. The average blood loss was 1300 mL, 100 mL of which was lost during the endoscopic portion of the operation.

The following intraoperative problems related to the operative mediastinoscopy were recorded: tumor infiltration of the right main bronchus in one patient, esophageal perforation in one, thoracic duct injury in one, and opening of the right pleura in 80 percent. No tracheal injury occurred during EMDE.

The postoperative mortality rate was 12.5 percent: one patient died of intravenous line sepsis and two, of necrosis of the gastric tube. Blood supply problems were unrelated to EMDE. Postoperative complications were: bleeding in two patients, one related to abdominal problems; necrosis of the gastric tube in three; pleural effusion in nine; fistulae in six; pneumonia in three; and recurrent laryngeal nerve palsy in four.

During the postoperative course, thoracic wall movement was not impaired, and most patients had a low analgesic requirement. Because of the limited follow-up period, the long-term survival rate has not been evaluated.

CONCLUSION

Minimally invasive EMDE allows careful esophageal dissection under continuous visualization, minimizing the incidence of intra- and postoperative bleeding and injury. With the application of this new technology, blunt dissection of the esophagus can reduce the operative trauma during surgery for esophageal cancer.

REFERENCES

1. Kipfmueller K, Narhun M, Melzer A, et al: Endoscopic microsurgical dissection of the esophagus: Results in an animal model. *Surg Endosc* 1989; 3:63–69.
2. Buess G: Mikroskopische endoskopische Tumorchirurgie: Was ist moeglich? *Langenbecks Arch Chir* 1989; (suppl II):553–559.
3. Buess G, Kipfmueller K, Naruhn M, et al: Endoskopisch-mikrochirurgische Dissektion des Oesophagus, in Buess GF (ed): *Endoskopie. Von der Diagnostik bis zur neuen Chirurgie*. Cologne, Deutscher Aerztverlag, 1990, pp 355–375.
4. Kipfmueller K, Buess G, Naruhn M, et al: Die endoskopisch-mikrochirurgische Dissektion der Speiseroehre: I. Eine tierexperimentelle Studie. *Chirugie* 1990; 61:187.
5. Buess G, Becker HD: Minimal Invasive Chirurgie bei Tumoren der Speiseroehre. *Langenbecks Arch Chir* 1990; (suppl II): 1355–1360.
6. Buess G, Becker HD: Perivisceral endoscopic oesophagectomy, in Cuschieri A, Buess G, Perissat J (eds): *Operation Manual of Endoscopic Surgery*. New York, Springer Verlag, 1992, pp 149–165.
7. Hermanek P, Gall FP: Early (microinvasive) colorectal carcinoma. *Int J Colorect Dis* 1986; 1:79–84.

Chapter 10

Hiatal Hernia and Reflux Esophagitis

Alfred E. Cuschieri

Indigestion and heartburn are common complaints experienced by many individuals and accepted as the temporary consequence of food and alcohol abuse. Against this background, certain individuals suffer from gastroesophageal reflux disease (GERD), which gives rise to severe and persistent symptoms. These vary in severity as does the propensity to the development of complications. It is not always possible to identify those patients at risk of complications because there is no firm relationship between the development of complicated esophagitis and the severity of reflux symptoms. The disease GERD is often considered synonymous with hiatal hernia, but this is incorrect. Although symptoms of reflux are the most commonly presenting evidence of hiatal hernia, GERD can occur in the absence of herniation, and hiatal hernias are often symptom-free.

PATHOLOGY AND CLINICAL FEATURES OF HIATAL HERNIA

The gastroesophageal junction and fundus of the stomach herniate through the esophageal hiatus of the right crus of the diaphragm into the posterior mediastinum, taking with it a peritoneal sac anteriorly. Most commonly, the gastroesophageal junction slides upward with obliteration of the gastroesophageal angle, and the proximal stomach passes, tent-like, into the chest. This is the *axial, sliding, or Type 1 hernia*. In the *paraesophageal, rolling, or Type 2 hernia*, the fundus of the stomach rotates as it herniates into the chest, passing anteriorly and to the right of the esophagus into the peritoneal sac. The gastroesophageal junction remains within the abdomen, and reflux rarely occurs. A third type of hernia is described, the *mixed type* because it has features of both. In appearance, it simulates the paraesophageal type, but the gastroesophageal junction lies above the diaphragm. This should be viewed as a large axial hernia.[1] Esophagitis occurs in patients with sliding or mixed hiatal hernias,[2] whereas the main complication of paraesophageal hernias is acute strangulation. Because the risk of this complication is high, all paraesophageal hernias require surgical treatment if the patient is fit.

The muscular sling of the right crus forming the diaphragmatic hiatus is stretched but not disrupted by the hernia. The phrenoesophageal membrane and peritoneal lining are also stretched and form the hernial sac that surrounds the anterior half of the esophagogastric junction in the posterior mediastinum. Posteriorly, the gastroesophageal junction retains continuity of attachment with the retroperitoneal tissues in which lie the branches of the left gastric vessels, the esophageal branches of the inferior phrenic vessels, and the vagal nerve trunks. The short gastric vessels are also pulled up into the sac, which when large, may include the whole stomach and rarely other organs.

Paraesophageal and mixed hernias are bulky in the hiatus and may, for this reason, produce venous constriction. Vascular congestion and submucosal edema occur in the herniated fundus. The extravasated fluid and protein are reabsorbed, but the red cell loss can lead to severe anemia. In the paraesophageal type, the lower esophagus is obstructed when the fundus is distended, and the middle sector of the stomach may be occluded at the hiatus. Volvulus of a massive hernia obstructs the pylorus or first part of the duodenum.

Axial hiatal hernia is frequently asymptomatic, especially in older patients whose physical activity is limited. When symptoms do arise, they are usually caused by GERD and, to a lesser extent, by the mechanical effects of herniation. The mixed hernia is usually symptomatic, with both mechanical and reflux symptoms. By contrast, the clinical picture of paraesophageal hernias is dominated by mechanical (pressure) symptoms, which many patients tolerate for years. The herniated stomach, by stretching the right crus of the diaphragm, produces a sharp pain deep to the xiphisternum, radiating to the back at the same level. After food, gastric distention causes pain accompanied by a bloated feeling in the epigastrium and retrosternal tightness often with anxiety, palpitations, and dyspnea. The postprandial symptoms vary in intensity because the volume of gas in the fundus varies with the amount eaten or drunk, the extent of air swallowing, and the composition of the meal. Most patients learn to modify their symptoms in this respect but they are rarely free of discomfort for long. Eructation or vomiting gives relief. Because the stomach usually slides up and down with ease, symptoms vary with posture. The symptoms can simulate those of angina, especially in the presence of arrhythmias, but the relationship to meals and bending or stooping rather than exercise should alert the surgeon to the correct diagnosis. On the other hand, it is not uncommon for myocardial ischemia and hiatal hernia to coexist, and this poses diagnostic difficulties. In patients with dual pathology, the decision on management can be difficult but is influenced by the severity of the symptoms, the nature of the hernia, and the extent of myocardial disease.

Dysphagia occurs in 20 percent of patients with paraesophageal hernias. Food is slow to pass the mechanical obstruction at the overcrowded hiatus, and low retrosternal discomfort and regurgitation are experienced. Endoscopy shows no esophagitis in these patients; its findings are distinct from the severe inflammation and stricture formation seen in patients with dysphagia associated with a sliding hernia. Obstruction to the stomach, either in the body or further distally, causes attacks of vomiting with coffee-ground vomiting or frank blood. This might be intermittent over several years, and the diagnosis is often missed even on contrast radiologic studies.

Complications of hiatal hernias present as emergencies, often without a prior diagnosis, but a detailed history usually reveals that the majority of patients have had symptoms. Previous regurgitation and nocturnal aspiration is found in 40 percent, heartburn and reflux symptoms in 86 percent, and nausea and vomiting in 40 percent of patients with massive hernias presenting acutely.[3] Some 30 percent of these patients are anemic, and overt gastrointestinal hemorrhage occurs in just under 50 percent. These patients often present diagnostic problems in the emergency setting. Retrosternal pain, hypotension, and sweating may suggest acute myocardial infarction. The electrocardiographic changes of ischemia can be produced by reflux and incarceration, adding to the confusion. In these patients, the detection of a gastric gas shadow overlying the cardiac outline on the posteroanterior chest film may be life saving. Dramatic collapse with septicemia follows perforation when basal pulmonary collapse, mediastinal emphysema, and hydropneumothorax develop rapidly. The condition is associated with a high mortality despite surgical intervention.

GERD

This is one of the commonest gastroenterologic disorders, the exact pathophysiology of which is still incompletely understood, despite intensive studies with modern sophisticated ambulatory techniques that monitor esophageal pH, transit, and motor activity. What seems certain is that a number of factors are involved in the development of the chemically induced inflammation of the esophageal mucosa. The disorder GERD may occur in association with hiatal hernia, but it is more commonly encountered in the absence of this abnormality.

Etiology

The various factors involved in the competence of the cardioesophageal junction may be grouped as mechanical or motor. The latter affect the lower high-pressure zone (sphincter) and are largely dependent on vagal reflexes. In addition to mechanical and motor abnormalities, three other factors influence the development and severity of reflux-induced damage to the esophageal squamous epithelial lining: the nature and composition of the refluxate, the esophageal mucosal resistance, and the lower esophageal clearance mechanism. To a large extent, all these variables are interrelated and often operate in concert. Controversy exists, however, with regard to the relative importance of each factor.

MECHANICAL FACTORS

In 1674, Willis[4] described the inverted horseshoe arrangement of the *oblique gastric muscle fibers,* which are arranged as a sling around the esophagogastric junction. Two functions were ascribed to this structure: angulation of entry of the lower esophagus into the gastric fundus (flap valve)[5] and sphincteric action. It is currently believed that the flap valve arrangement is not necessary for normal competence, although it is an essential component of antireflux surgical procedures. The cardiac sling fibers are the closest representation of an anatomic sphincter in humans but, despite this, they do not contribute to the manometric high-pressure zone. The cardiac sling may fulfill an auxiliary role in closing the intraabdominal segment of the esophagus.[6]

In 1813, Magendie[7] described the closure of the cardia by mucosal folds. Contraction of the muscularis mucosa was alleged to bunch the mucosal folds into a rosette-like plug.[8] Although the mucosal opposition is actually responsible for the closure of the lumen, this is a passive effect that is secondary to muscular activity. It is possible, although, that after the mucosal rosette is closed, surface tension is a factor that resists opening forces.

Chevalier Jackson[9] revived interest in the pinchcock action of the diaphragm originally described by Bohnius.[10] In 66 percent of individuals, the esophageal hiatus is formed exclusively by the right crus; in 32 percent, there is some contribution from the left crus; and in 2 percent, the hiatus arises mainly from the left.[11] The right limb of the right crus is innervated by the right phrenic nerve, whereas the left limb and the left crus are innervated by the left nerve.[12] The gastroesophageal junctional high-pressure zone persists if the left phrenic nerve is avulsed, but the normally prominent respiratory deflections disappear,[13] indicating that the hiatus contributes significantly to the manometric recording, including its radial asymmetry.

The phrenoesophageal membrane[14] comprises the fused and condensed endothoracic and endoabdominal fascia, which passes from the edge of the diaphragm into the walls of the esophagus, the fibers diverging to attach to the lower 2 to 3 cm of the esophagus. In normal subjects, the lower leaf is thin and diffuse. The upper leaf of the membrane is thicker and is inserted at a variable height above the esophagogastric junction. The insertion is high (3.5 cm) in cadavers without esophagitis and low (1 cm) in cadavers with esophagitis, whether or not hiatal hernia is present.[15] These observations are in agreement with clinical manometric studies from which the abdominal segment of the esophagus is calculated as the length of the high-pressure zone below the respiratory inversion point.[16] Manometrically, the respiratory inversion point marks the level below which the esophageal wall is exposed to the abdominal pressure. This point coincides with the attachment of the upper leaf of the phrenoesophageal membrane.[17] Although the membrane is composed predominantly of elastic fibers, it has no function in actively closing the lower esophagus. It does, however, determine the length of the lower esophagus exposed to the intraabdominal pressure. Longitudinal traction by the membrane on the esophagus results in a tendency to separation of the esophageal walls. This constitutes an important part of the mechanism, which opens the cardia for swallowing, vomiting, reflux, and regurgitation.[18] The distraction effect is less if the attachment of the membrane is above the intrinsic sphincter and greater if the pull is exerted on the walls of the high-pressure zone, which may occur with a low insertion of the membrane. Repeated traction on the phrenoesophageal membrane by retching and vomiting has been proposed as one mechanism for the development of hiatal hernia.

Passive compression of the lower esophagus by positive abdominal pressure against a posterior buttress formed by the oblique hiatus, spine, and crural tunnel is important.[19] The flutter-valve theory of lower esophageal competence is based on the observation that the intraluminal esophageal pressure is lower than the abdominal pressure, and at rest, closure of the abdominal segment is maintained by external compression. During swallowing, the bolus is propelled through the collapsed segment in the same manner as air is blown through the inlet flutter valve of a spirometer. Lower esophageal resistance is reduced by traction on the phrenoesophageal membrane. The segment is closed behind the bolus by strong contraction of the lower esophageal sphincter as the peristaltic wave passes. According to this theory, the sphincter needs to maintain closure until the full intraabdominal length of the esophagus is restored as the longitudinal muscle relaxes. Thereafter, closure is maintained hydrostatically. The flutter-valve theory implies that the sphincter primes the abdominal segment for predominantly closing forces.[18] The flutter valve theory of competence entails the presence of a sufficiently long segment of intraabdominal esophagus, which is exposed to the intraabdominal pressure. The combined importance of pressure and length is denoted by their product, which approximates the closing force. The intraabdominal length of the esophagus is an important factor in the control of reflux and in successful antireflux surgery.[20] In the maintenance of competence during abdominal compression, there is an inverse relationship between length and pressure. Shorter abdominal segments remain competent if their pressure is high, and lower-pressure zones resist reflux if they are long. The probability of reflux is very high (90 percent) if the pressure is less than 5 mmHg or the intraabdominal length is less than 1.0 cm, regardless of the corresponding length or pressure. Pressures in excess of 20 mmHg and length over 2.0 cm are associated with little chance of reflux.

SPHINCTERIC AND MOTOR FACTORS

It is currently recognized that, although there is no anatomic lower esophageal sphincter in humans, a physiologic sphincter mechanism undoubtedly exists and extends over the terminal 1 to 4 cm of the esophagus.[21–24] The circular smooth muscle of this zone is functionally different from that of the adjacent stomach and esophagus, having a lower transmembrane potential, different length–tension relationship,[25,26] and increased sensitivity to gastrin and cholinergic agents.[27,28] Manometrically, this specialized segment is demonstrated as a zone of high pressure. Many refer to it as the lower esophageal sphincter but the term *lower high-pressure zone* (HPZ) is more accurate because an anatomic sphincter is not present and competence is dependent on both sphincteric and mechanical factors, which also contribute to the manometric recording.

In part, sphincteric tone appears to be autoregulatory and independent of neural control because the length–tension response and sphincter pressure[29] are maintained in the presence of the nerve toxin, tetrodotoxin. Tone is believed to be maintained by a state of partial depolarization of the sphincteric smooth muscle cell membranes,[30] which have a lower membrane potential (–40 mV) than smooth muscles cells of the esophageal body or stomach (–50 to –60 mV). Calcium ion leakage into the cells may explain the low potential because the calcium-channel blockers, verapamil and nifedipine,[31] reduce sphincter pressure.

Many hormonal and neural control mechanisms have been postulated for the HPZ. A decrease in the HPZ pressure occurs after the administration of atropine; glucagon; secretin; cholecystokinin; vasoactive intestinal peptide, gastric inhibitory peptide, progesterone; serotonin (N-receptors); histamine (H$_2$ receptors); prostaglandins E$_1$, E$_2$, and A$_2$; enkephalins; alcohol; caffeine; antihistamines; ganglion-blocking agents; tricyclic antidepressants; or fatty foods, including chocolate.

As a group, patients with reflux are characterized by low-pressure and poor HPZ responses to stretch,[32] abdominal compression,[33] and other stimuli. However, the overlap in the pressure recorded between patients and controls is so great that an individual's reflux status cannot be predicted from the HPZ pressure alone.[34] In addition, large spontaneous variations in pressure occur normally between observations in the same individual.[35] Free reflux occurs if the HPZ pressure is absent, and this is usually found in patients with severe degrees of esophagitis.[36] Reflux can also be produced in some patients by sudden increases in the intraabdominal pressure. This is currently considered to be the result of a defective vagal reflex, which is normally responsible for the adaptive increase in the HPZ pressure in this situation.[37]

Pressure in the HPZ falls in advance of the primary esophageal peristaltic wave, and this is termed *receptive relaxation* because it is thought to be part of the coordinated neuromuscular process of swallowing. Pressure rises again as the wave passes. The HPZ pressure also falls if the esophageal body is stimulated by dilating a balloon within its lumen or if the vagus nerve is stimulated. Several studies have confirmed the original findings of Dent and associates[38] that the majority of episodes of GERD occur during periods of transient lower esophageal sphincter relaxation (TLESR), regardless of the basal HPZ pressure in both normals and patients with symptomatic reflux.[38–40] Although there is no firm evidence that the number of TLESRs is increased in patients with GERD compared with those in normal individuals, more of the TLESRs are accompanied by acid reflux episodes in patients than controls.[41] Although the exact mechanism responsible for TLESRs remains debatable, these are often preceded by pharyngeal or esophageal contractions, which are not conducted to the distal esophagus. Mittal and McCallum[43] have proposed that the contractions in the pharyngoesophageal region and the relaxations of the sphincter are mediated by a long-train subthreshold vagal stimulus.[42] An increased number of TLESRs occurs in relation to belching[43] and gaseous gastric distention. A similar increase in TLSERs is obtained if the stomach is distended by a balloon, indicating that gastric distention probably mediates the increase in TLESRs after meals.[44] Evidence that TLESRs are neurally mediated includes their abolition by vagal cooling in an experimental dog model[45] and their absence in patients suffering from achalasia.[46]

Defective vagal reflex seems, therefore, to be important in the etiology of GERD. Surgical vagotomy is commonly blamed for producing GERD. However, a significant number of patients have undiagnosed reflux preoperatively. The incidence of symptomatic reflux esophagitis is actually reduced by vagotomy.[47] Reports of the effect of vagotomy frequently confuse the issue by basing conclusions on manometric data without reflux tests. None of the standard vagotomy procedures reduces the resting sphincter pressure,[48–54] although there is evidence for impairment of sphincter function. Truncal vagotomy reduces the sphincter response to raised intraabdominal pressure, according to some studies,[55–57] but this is refuted by other reports. Parietal cell vagotomy either has no effect on the response to compression or the effect is variable.[58] In one report, reflux testing by esophageal pH monitoring showed no increase in reflux after parietal cell vagotomy.[53] In another study, the score of the standard acid reflux test increased significantly after both truncal and parietal cell vagotomy. During abdominal compression, 29 percent of patients refluxed before truncal vagotomy and 43 percent afterward. The corresponding rates for the parietal cell vagotomy group were 37 percent and 42 percent. Acid clearance was unchanged in both groups.[59]

Vagal fibers enter the esophagus at a higher level than the region of dissection and truncal division. Thus, it is likely that the afferent limb of the reflex responsible for the response to compression is interrupted by vagotomy. Because parietal cell vagotomy does not disturb the reflex, the afferents must arise outside the lower esophagus of the gastric fundus. The response is impaired even when the vagi are sectioned in the thorax or neck. When the vagi are divided in the neck, electrical stimulation of the cephalic cut ends causes sphincter contraction,[60] indicating that the motor limb of the reflex arc is not in the vagus. In dogs, vagal section in the neck produces esophageal atony, aperistalsis, lower esophageal sphincter hypotension, and delayed esophageal emptying. Similar changes are encountered in humans after cervical esophagectomy and pharyngectomy.

Autonomic nerves are either inhibitory or excitatory to the sphincter region. Our current understanding is that inhibitory preganglionic fibers are vagal, with cholinergic ganglionic transmission, but the postganglionic transmitter is unknown. Dopaminergic receptors are believed to be inhibitory to the sphincter; the administration of drugs that inhibit these receptors (domperidone and metoclopramide) cause an increase in the HPZ pressure.

ESOPHAGEAL MUCOSAL RESISTANCE

This is dependent on preepithelial, epithelial, and postepithelial defenses.[61] The first consists of a mucous layer overlying the esophageal mucosa. The deeper unstirred layer is probably derived from swallowed saliva and the secretions of the submucosal esophageal glands. Immediately overlying the cells of the stratum corneum is a hydrophobic phospholipid layer, the glycocalyx, which normally resists attack by acid. The epithelial defense mechanisms are chiefly located in the functional and prickle cell layers. The cells of the functional layer contain membrane-coated granules filled with lipid, neutral mucin, and lysosomal enzymes, including an acid phosphatase. These granules are released into the intercellular spaces in the presence of acid. This appears to be the primary epithelial defense mechanism.[62,63] The Na+/K+ ATPase located in the basolateral membranes of the cells of the prickle cell layer is also important in maintaining cellular integrity in the presence of excess acid.[64] The postepithelial defense is composed of the esophageal blood flow, which increases when the luminal acid content is elevated.[65] The exact cytoprotective mechanisms secondary to the increased blood flow remain poorly understood but are likely to be multiple, for example, increased availability of nutrients and buffers and enhanced clearance of acid.

ESOPHAGEAL CLEARANCE

The degree of esophageal injury caused by reflux is dependent on the composition of the refluxate and the contact time with the esophageal mucosa. In this respect, effective esophageal peristalsis, resulting in rapid clearance of the refluxate, is an important defense mechanism against esophageal injury. Esophageal clearance and transit are often delayed in severe esophagitis. This is often considered to be secondary to the esophagitis, but there is good circumstantial evidence that the lower esophageal dysmotility may be primary.[66]

GASTRIC FACTORS

Delayed gastric emptying and increased gastric secretory activity of acid and pepsin have been implicated in the pathogenesis of reflux disease, particularly in patients with duodenal ulcers and those suffering from the Zollinger-Ellison syndrome.[67–69] Although either of these factors may operate in these situations and in complicated disease, there is no firm evidence that delayed gastric emptying or increased gastric secretory activity are important etiologic factors in the pathogenesis of uncomplicated GERD.

PATHOLOGY OF REFLUX DISEASE

In the final analysis, reflux disease is caused by prolonged exposure of the esophageal epithelium to gastric juice. The extent of the damage depends on the duration of contact, the nature of the refluxate, and the susceptibility of the epithelium (mucosal defense). Early stages of inflammation are often difficult to diagnose, and microscopic evidence is needed. Clinicians depend largely on a visual assessment of the mucosa, and esophagitis is graded to define the potential risks of complications.

The duration of contact between gastric juice and the esophageal mucosa is determined by the frequency of reflux episodes and their duration. During 24-h pH monitoring, the normal range of esophageal pH is 5.0 to 6.8. By accepted usage, acid reflux is deemed to occur when the esophageal pH falls to 4.0 or below. This value is significant physiologically as the upper limit for optimal activity of pepsin (pH, 1.8 to 3.8).

In the upright position, normal individuals reflux 1.2 times per hour overall,[70] and most of these episodes, which are short lived, occur during the first or second postprandial hours.[71,72] In a study of reflux in normal subjects, lower esophageal pH dropped to 4.0 to 3.0 for 1 percent, 3.0 to 2.0 for 2 percent, and 2.0 to 1.0 for 0.4 percent of the time during the first 3 h postprandial. In comparison, the frequency of upright reflux episodes in patients with symptomatic disease rose to 3.3 times per hour. In refluxing infants, episodes of reflux are evenly distributed throughout the waking hours, irrespective of their position.

At rest, in the recumbent or supine position, there are normally 0.2 reflux episodes per hour, concentrated in periods of semisleep and semiarousal. By contrast, refluxing patients average 1.9 episodes per hour during this period. Although reflux is less common when lying down, its clearance is slow because there is no gravitational assistance. Esophageal motor activity and flow of salivary secretion down the esophagus are absent during sleep. Both factors exacerbate the prolonged clearance of nocturnal reflux and probably account for the mean fall in esophageal pH by 1.0 during the night.

Patterns of Reflux

Three patterns of reflux are recognized: predominantly upright, predominantly supine, and combined. The upright group experience postprandial reflux, aerophagia, and mild esophagitis. The incidence of esophagitis is higher in the supine group and highest in the combined refluxers who exhibited severe disease with a 15 percent incidence of stricture. Lichter[73] observed that 1 h of supine nocturnal reflux produced endoscopically evident esophagitis, and others have stressed the importance of nocturnal reflux in the development of esophageal mucosal damage.[74]

Gastric Juice and Duodenogastric Reflux

In vivo experiments have shown bile to be as traumatic to the esophageal epithelium as gastric secretions and for the mixture to be particularly injurious.[75] Hydrochloric acid (HCl) alone in the region of pH 4.0 causes little damage.[76,77] During in vitro studies using electron microscopy, HCl (0.1 mM) or conjugated bile acids individually cause little damage, but acid and pepsin or acid and bile salt mixtures are rapidly destructive.[78]

Readings higher than pH 7.0 are found in approximately 25 percent of patients and are the result of duodenogastric reflux, which is increased in patients with reflux disease compared with controls. High levels of intraesophageal bile acids are found in patients with severe disease, particularly in the presence of columnar metaplasia. Readings higher than pH 7.4 are rare, and for this reason, the term *alkaline reflux,* often used in relation to reflux disease associated with previous gastric surgery, is inappropriate. The alternative term *neutral reflux* is preferable. Neutral reflux associated with previous gastric surgery (vagotomy and drainage, vagotomy and antrectomy, and gastrectomy) usually causes severe esophagitis, particularly after total gastrectomy. There is indirect evidence that trypsin may be involved in the pathogenesis of the esophageal mucosal injury in these patients.[79]

Histopathology of Esophagitis

Whereas it is easy to recognize advanced complicated disease, lesser degrees of esophagitis are more difficult to define. Erythema fluctuates, and the esophagus may appear normal when viewed endoscopically in as many as 40 percent of patients.[80] When esophagitis has occurred, histologic changes will persist,[81] but their interpretation is not always easy.[82] Histologically, esophagitis is not characterized by inflammatory cell infiltrates, and polymorphs within the lamina propria are only found in 18 percent of biopsies. Lymphocytes and mononuclear cells are found in 50 to 70 percent of esophagitis specimens but also in 50 percent of normal samples. The total thickness of the epithelium is not altered, but there are significant changes in the depth of the basal zone and the vascular papillae.

The basal zone comprises the germinal or basal layer and adjacent immature cells (stratum Malpighii) with closely packed nuclei that stain darkly and contain no glycogen. The prickle and functional (flattened superficial) cell layers contain glycogen and stain with periodic acid-Schiff. The functional layer also contains numerous lipid droplets. The basal zone normally occupies 10 to 15 percent of the epithelial thickness, but esophagitis results in cellular proliferation, and the proportionate thickness of the layer increases to 50 percent, on average. Surface cells are lost, and the prickle cell layer becomes thinner. The surface roughening is seen well on scanning electron microscopy,[83] which also demonstrates damage to organelles, widened intercellular spaces containing inflammatory cells and cellular debris, and parakeratosis of the superficial cells. However, it is important to stress that thickening of the basal cell zone is encountered in 10 percent of biopsies from the distal 2.5 cm in normal subjects and in only 85 percent of symptomatic patients, highlighting the difficulties that often arise with histologic interpretation.

The papillae of the lamina propria project into the epithelium normally to a depth of up to one half the thickness of the epithelium. In esophagitis, the papillary projections extend two thirds or more of the way to the lumen and are more vascular. Loss of surface layers can give rise to an apparent increase in papillary depth, but there is a real increase in activity because there is no reduction in total epithelial thickness.

Histochemical studies of inflamed esophageal epithelium show an increase in alkaline phosphatase activity, resulting from the thickening of the papillae, the capillaries of which are rich in the enzyme. There is a decrease in the activity of the lysosomal enzyme acid phosphatase caused by enhanced exocystosis of membrane-coated granules (functional layer). The increase in β-glucuronidase activity is possibly related to the enhanced secretion of mucosubstance in response to injury.

Inflammatory changes and ulceration frequently spare the esophageal epithelium in the immediate vicinity of the squamocolumnar junction. Acute esophageal ulcers are superficial to the muscularis mucosae, covered by a thin layer of granulation tissue, and surrounded by an inflammatory cell infiltrate and submucosal edema. Healing is normally by squamous reepithelialization, but when there is submucosal fibrosis, a columnar or mixed squamocolumnar epithelium covers the damaged area. When inflammation becomes chronic, inflammatory cell infiltrates and interstitial fibrosis extend deeper into the esophageal muscular walls.

Complications of Reflux Disease

The complications of reflux disease are esophageal webs, strictures, ulcers, and columnar cell metaplasia (Barrett's change).

ESOPHAGEAL WEBS

A localized area of fibrosis confined to the submucosa can, by contraction, lead to the formation of an esophageal web. These are found at sites of esophagitis, the squamocolumnar junction, and sometimes at the level of the aortic arch. Intermittent bolus obstruction may occur. Webs are easily and usually permanently broken down by a single dilatation, but medical antireflux treatment should be administered afterward. Schatzki's ring is also caused by an incomplete submucosal fibrous web, situated usually at the squamocolumnar junction.

STRICTURES AND ULCERS

The incidence of stricture in patients with hiatal hernia and reflux is approximately 20 percent in adults and 35 percent in children. Strictures are commonest in the 60- to 80-year-old age group. Deep ulcers erode the thickened submucosa and muscular coats. The floor of the ulcer has a layer of granulation tissue with an overlying fibrinopurulent exudate. Local periesophageal blood vessels are narrowed by subintimal fibrosis and may be eroded, leading to severe hemorrhage. Both acute and chronic perforation can occur.

COLUMNAR LINED OR BARRETT'S ESOPHAGUS

Barrett[84] described heterotopic columnar epithelium in the lower esophagus, originally mistaking it for tubular stomach. Barrett's esophagus is sometimes referred to by the abbreviation CELO (columnar-epithelium-lined esophagus). The metaplasia can extend up from the esophagogastric junction to any level, either in tongue-like projections uniformly with or without islands of squamous epithelium, or in a patchy distribution. The incidence of columnar change in patients with reflux disease is 11 percent in adults and 12.6 percent in children.[84–86] It appears to be more common in male patients with a reported male-to-female ratio of 3:1. It is commonly confined to the lower two thirds of the esophagus, but there may be islands at a higher level. The endoscopic appearance is of slightly elevated patches or tongues, darker pink and more velvety than the adjacent esophagitis, streaming up from the esophagogastric junction. Esophagitis can obscure the margins of the columnar change and the location of the junction. Identification of the columnar change is facilitated by the application of Lugol's solution or toluidine blue, which stain the abnormal epithelium but not the adjacent inflamed squamous lining.[87] It is important to stress, however, that these dyes also stain dysplastic epithelium. Barrett's esophagus may be misdiagnosed from a biopsy of normal gastric mucosa at the esophagogastric junction. As a guide, gastric mucosa is normally found up to 3.0 cm above the highest recognizable gastric feature, which is usually the upper end of a rugal fold. Thus, biopsies for the confirmation of columnar change must be taken above this level.

There is no doubt that, in most instances, Barrett's esophagus is the result of long-standing acid reflux.[88,89] Duodenogastric bile reflux has also been implicated in the development of the metaplastic epithelium,[90] and certainly, higher levels of conjugated bile salts are observed in the esophageal lumen of patients with this complication. However, the exact role of bile salts in the pathogenesis of this condition remains unsettled. *Helicobacter pylori* is often present in patients with Barrett's change but only if the same organism is also present in the stomach.[91] There is no evidence that it is concerned with the development of the metaplastic change. The origin of the columnar epithelium remains speculative. The suggestion originally made by Trier[92] that the epithelium is derived from the esophageal mucosal glands has had recent backing from experimental studies in a dog reflux model in which the columnar epithelium appeared to develop from the cuboidal cells lining the esophageal gland ducts.[93]

There are three types of metaplastic epithelium: gastric fundic (contains pits, mucous glands, parietal cells, and chief cells), gastric junctional (mucous glands and pits only), and specialized intestinal epithelium with a villous structure possessing mucous glands, goblet cells, and Paneth cells. Three quarters of the patients exhibit one type, 17 percent have two, and 10 percent have all three types. In the latter instance, the three types of columnar epithelium exhibit a zonal pattern and, less frequently, a mosaic arrangement.[94] The relative proportions of each type are intestinal, 43 percent; junctional, 32 percent; and fundic, 25 percent.[95,96]

Barrett's epithelium possesses little absorptive capacity but secretes acid mucus, pepsin, pepsinogen, and possibly, gastrin, although secretion of the latter has not been confirmed by subsequent studies.[97] Although the activity of the enzyme β-glucuronidase in Barrett's epithelium is similar to that found in intestinal mucosa, the β-galactosidase activity is lower.[98]

Barrett's esophagus is frequently complicated by stricture formation, usually at the squamocolumnar junction, and ulcer formation. A Barrett's ulcer is usually a deep crater and is often situated posteriorly. It has a longitudinal configuration and is located proximally. It can penetrate deeply into the walls of the esophagus and may indeed perforate into the mediastinum or cause massive life-threatening hemorrhage. Rarely, the ulcer may erode into the aorta with a fatal outcome.

Recent studies have shown that, although intestinal metaplasia and sulfomucin secretion are common features of columnar-lined esophagus, they are not sufficiently discriminating to detect a subgroup of patients at special risk for malignant change. The reported increased activity of ornithine decarboxylase in Barrett's epithelium[99] and the higher levels of this enzyme in the presence of dysplasia compared with nondysplastic Barrett's epithelium[100] suggest a causal relationship with malignant change.

Unquestionably, the development of dysplasia is important, especially if this is severe (high grade) because this is currently regarded as carcinoma in situ. Furthermore, 30 percent of patients with severe dysplasia have invasive carcinoma in the resected specimen. Thus, the current recommendation is that severe dysplasia, if confirmed by a repeat biopsy, is an indication for esophageal resection. One report has demonstrated regression of mild-to-moderate dysplasia with successful antireflux surgery,[101] although this has not been confirmed by others. Currently, patients with mild-to-moderate dysplasia are managed with endoscopic surveillance and repeat biopsies.

Although the development of squamous carcinoma has been reported in association with Barrett's change,[102] the real risk is the development of adenocarcinoma. The exact risk is difficult to calculate, but the results from most of the large reported series indicate a 40+-fold increase in the incidence of adenocarcinoma over the expected.[103,104] Barrett's tumors are often associated with a hiatus hernia and contain endocrine cells that secrete serotonin in 31 percent as opposed to 3.8 percent of cardiac adenocarcinomas not associated with Barrett's change.[105]

CLINICAL FEATURES OF REFLUX DISEASE

Table 10-1 indicates the incidence and range of symptoms and complications drawn from reports of 2178 patients with GERD and hiatal hernia.[106,107] Heartburn, dysphagia, and regurgitation are the classic esophageal symptoms caused by reflux and its complications. There are no specific physical signs of reflux esophagitis, but there may be high epigastric tenderness, pharyngitis (caused by chronic nocturnal regurgitation), and overt regurgitation, bleeding, or pulmonary complications. At times, it may be difficult to differentiate esophageal, cardiac, pulmonary, and gastroduodenal symptoms, and detailed evaluation by specialized tests is necessary.

Heartburn

Heartburn or pyrosis is caused by chemical irritation of the esophageal subepithelial sensory nerve endings by the refluxate. Some foods, such as spices, onions, cucumber, and chocolate, are particularly prone to cause this symptom. Postural aggravation is almost a prerequisite for the diagnosis. Heartburn may wake the patient at night, but often patients sleep through reflux episodes, and the inflammation so generated is symptomatic the next day. Many observe that reflux is more likely when lying on the right side.

The burning pain is typically deep substernal in location and radiates upward, sometimes into the neck, jaws, or ears. Commonly, there is radiation of the pain to the interscapular region of the back. An epigastric location may suggest duodenal ulceration, but the pain of esophagitis is high, actually subxiphoid. Occasionally, patients complain of left subcostal gnawing aching pain, which radiates through to the back at T11/12 level. This pain is worse after meals and bending and is not typical of heartburn. It can be reproduced by gastric inflation during endoscopy and is relieved by eructation. It probably represents diaphragmatic hiatal stretching by the bulk of the stomach. Even the severest symptoms exhibit periods of exacerbation and periods of remission, and during each day, most patients with GERD have periods of freedom from pain. Relief from heartburn is obtained by washing the esophagus with a drink of water, milk, or antacid or by stimulating salivation and primary peristalsis by sucking a sweet. Sufferers of GERD tend to adopt an upright posture to encourage esophageal clearance.

Dysphagia

Swallowing may be painful or obstructed. Painful swallowing or odynophagia is either the result of irritation of the inflamed esophagus by the food bolus or is muscular in origin when it is secondary either to esophageal distention or spasm. Obstruction is caused by strictures, webs, edema, or spasm.

TABLE 10-1 Symptoms and complications of gastroesophageal reflux disease

Symptom/complication	%
Heartburn	85
Postural aggravation	81
Dysphagia	37
Stricture	19
High dysphagia	4
Regurgitation	23
Cough	47
Hoarseness	12
Sore throat	3
Nausea and vomiting	21
Bronchitis	35
Pneumonitis	16
Asthma and wheeze	16
Aspiration	8
Intermittent dyspnea	13
Hemoptysis	13
Bleeding	12
Bleeding-transfused	3
Angina-like pain	3
Arm, shoulder pain	8
Neck pain, otalgia	3

Painful Swallowing

In the presence of active esophagitis, pyrosis is caused by swallowing irritants, such as hot food or drink, coffee, alcohol, spices, acidic fruits, hypertonic or carbonated fluids, and incompletely chewed foods. The muscular pain is cramp-like or knife-like and shares the same distribution as heartburn, except that radiation to the arms is rare. The pain originates from acute dilatation of the esophagus or from a tertiary contraction. Transient hold-up of a bolus at an area of the esophagitis, partial stricture, web, or incoordinated motor activity can produce several possible sensations. Patients may simply be aware of the arrest of the bolus and the hold-up of food or fluid above. They then wait for the bolus to pass or take a drink to clear it. Esophageal dilatation above the arrested bolus can produce severe pain. Tertiary contraction or spasm are responsible for the most severe pain, which is sometimes described by the patient with a clenched fist pressed against the sternum. Spasmodic pain is not always triggered by swallowing but may be induced by repetitive reflux episodes. On occasion, a phantom sensation of bolus obstruction may be felt.

Obstructed Swallowing

Partial or complete bolus obstruction is not always painful. There are three clinical forms of dysphagia: for liquids, for solids, and high dysphagia. Dysphagia for solids indicates a stricture and dysphagia for liquids, a primary motility disorder. Esophagitis can produce all three types.

Infrequent, unpredictable, and sudden rejection of a liquid bolus results from incoordinated motor activity. The drink is thrust back from the esophagus into the mouth and nose in a hail of coughing and choking as the laryngopharynx is flooded. Incoordinated contractions along the esophagus generate this power. Esophageal spasm is not always so dramatic and usually only delays or temporarily arrests the bolus, affecting both solids and liquids. So-called first-bite dysphagia is another feature of incoordinated activity. The first few mouthfuls of a meal are slow and difficult to swallow; thereafter, the remaining food is swallowed more easily, although the individual is still the last to leave the table. Bread, meat, and vegetables are usually the first solids to give trouble, and patients frequently avoid these for some time before presentation. Patients' denials of dysphagia need to be pursued to ensure that they have not had to modify their diets.

Solid food sticks at strictures, webs, and where the esophagus is compressed by distended paraesophageal herniation of the stomach. Strictures are sometimes at the level of the aortic arch but, much more commonly, are at the lower end of the esophagus. The location of food impaction depends on the length of the stricture and the size of any hiatal hernia. For this reason, and the lack of discrimination in esophageal sensation, we cannot rely on the patient's impression of the level of obstruction in the body of the organ. Generally, the site of the obstruction is felt by by the patient to be higher than its anatomic position. Edema and spasm may cause significant hold-up at a stricture that is negotiable by an endoscope. As the stricture progresses, food empties more slowly into the stomach, accumulating in the esophagus during a meal until regurgitation or high dysphagia occurs. In time, a degree of megaesophagus develops, but this does not match the proportions found in long-established achalasia.

Complete obstruction is a late event and is more frequently encountered with a malignant stricture, but it happens when meat or a fruit stone becomes impacted in a benign stricture. The patient then seeks urgent medical attention and is in an anxious state with pain, drooling, and salivation.

High dysphagia results from cricopharyngeal spasm or incoordination. There is difficulty in transfer of the food bolus from the mouth to the pharynx with choking and spluttering during attempted swallowing. In common with spasm of the body of the esophagus, the intensity of the dysphagia is variable, being especially severe at times of stress. Before chronic GERD was recognized as the common cause, this condition was referred to as globus hystericus. Not infrequently, more than one member of the family is affected, typically mother and daughter. Chronic pharyngeal spasm may lead to the development of pharyngeal (Zenker's) diverticulum. However, a normotensive cricopharyngeus is often present in this disorder. High dysphagia indicates the need for a barium swallow to assess the risk of perforation of a high diverticulum during esophagoscopy.

Noncardiac Chest Pain

A significant number of patients, estimated at 20 to 25 percent[108] with recurrent vice-like retrosternal pain that is virtually indistinguishable in nature and radiation from that of ischemic heart disease have no objective evidence of coronary artery disease. A small percentage of these suffer from microvascular angina (syndrome X), which is associated with diminished coronary vasodilator reserve during atrial pacing and reduced esophageal and forearm muscle blood flow. Most are the result of reflux disease, esophageal motility disorders (nutcracker esophagus and diffuse esophageal spasm), or both.[109] The evaluation of these patients requires initial exclusion of significant coronary artery disease before detailed esophageal function tests are performed to determine the exact underlying abnormality.

Regurgitation

Gastric content refluxes into the esophagus for any distance as far as the cricopharyngeal sphincter. Regurgitation is the gushing of esophageal contents into the mouth. Vomiting describes the violent explusion of gastric contents directly to the outside via the mouth. As distinct from vomiting, which involves a complex series of involuntary and voluntary muscle reflexes, regurgitation occurs unexpectedly and relatively passively. There is no forceful propulsion of gastric contents into the mouth, except when an esophageal spasm occurs. There is no involvement of the abdominal or thoracic wall musculature, except in those rare individuals with megaesophagus who partially empty the overfilled organ by a soundless coughing maneuver, or the attention seekers who feign reflux and vomiting. The regurgitation of gastric juice or bile into the back of the mouth provides sure evidence of reflux. Gastric material has to be spat out or swallowed, leaving an acid or bitter taste in the throat and mouth, causing halitosis and impairing the sense of taste. The latter has been reported as the only symptom of reflux. Chronically irritated lips may have a burning sensation. Regurgitation follows eating and exertional or postural changes. The patient may find it impossible to work if bending, lifting, and carrying is involved. Regurgitation occurs silently at night, and gastric juice or bile is found on the pillow, or the patient may wake up coughing and choking as fluid enters the larynx. Alternatively, the patient may wake up with a sore throat, hoarseness, cough, or a vomit taste in the mouth.

Other Symptoms

Most of the complications of reflux are symptomatic. Respiratory complications: aspiration pneumonitis, asthma, stridor, bronchiectasis, and chronic bronchitis are present in approximately 20 percent of patients. It is difficult to ascertain whether the problems are initiated or simply exacerbated by the reflux. Repeated aspiration can lead to chronic basal pulmonary inflammatory changes, especially on the right, and to lung abscess and hemoptysis. A chronic cough or laryngitis may be traced to reflux, but other causes of hoarseness must be excluded. Brisk hematemesis results occasionally from esophagitis, but more commonly, it is from a penetrating ulcer, usually associated with Barrett's change. Approximately 20 to 30 percent of patients with paraesophageal hernia will suffer an episode of hematemesis. Melena rarely occurs alone. Most commonly, blood loss is occult and chronic and leads to an iron-deficiency anemia with positive fecal occult blood findings. Flatulence results from continued swallowing to clear the esophagus, and the resultant frequent eructation can be embarrassing. Simple aerophagia and anxiety neurosis produce atypical symptoms, and care is needed to avoid surgical treatment in these individuals because they do not do well after antireflux surgery.

Individual Variation

There is a wide variation in individual tolerance or symptoms, and the intensity does not always correlate with the extent of the organic disease. At one extreme, some complain bitterly of heartburn, and yet, there is little or no visible esophagitis found during endoscopy. At the other extreme, severe strictures may occur without any prior reflux symptoms. It is not known what proportion of the latter group conceal or minimize symptoms, and how many have a genuine diminished sensitivity of the esophageal mucosa to reflux injury. In some patients, esophagitis appears to progress rapidly to stricture formation; other patients have mild esophagitis on and off for years without the development of complications. Symptoms are not a reliable indicator of the severity of the disease, and to plan appropriate therapy, it is important to quantify the pathology by objective tests.

Symptom Scoring

The severity of the symptoms can be graded[110] for more precise assessment before and after treatment. A total numeric score can be generated with a maximum of 12, which indicates the highest severity possible (Table 10-2).

TABLE 10-2 DeMeester Symptom Scoring

Heartburn
0 None
1 Minimal, occasional only
2 Moderate, seeks medical advice or significant but tolerable limitation of activity
3 Severe, constant, disruption of normal life
Dysphagia
0 None
1 Mild, brief, occasional
2 Moderate, requires clearing with liquids
3 Severe, food impaction
Regurgitation
0 None
1 Mild, after straining or with lying down
2 Moderate, frequent, easily provoked
3 Severe, respiratory complications
Hemorrhage
0 None
1 Mild, positive fecal occult blood findings
2 Moderate, anemia
3 Severe, gross bleeding requiring transfusion

INVESTIGATIONS

For the general surgeon without a special interest in the study of lower esophageal physiology, contrast radiology and upper gastrointestinal endoscopy suffice to investigate the majority of patients with hiatal hernia and GERD. Of the other tests, 24-h pH monitoring is very useful, both in establishing the diagnosis and in assessing the results of treatment.

The important endoscopic features that provide hard evidence of esophagitis are erosions with fibrin deposits and junctional ulceration.[111] Less reliable soft criteria include circumscribed erythema without white film, pseudopapilloma at the Z line, cobblestone appearance, and mucosal friability. Other frequently annotated findings are irrelevant to the diagnosis: generalized diffuse erythema, visible vessels near the cardia, loss of normal vascular pattern, and mucosal edema. The best endoscopic classification of reflux esophagitis is that proposed by Savary and Miller (Table 10-3).

MEDICAL THERAPY

The majority of patients with reflux disease can be controlled by medical treatment. The patient's full cooperation and understanding is required for a successful outcome. Obesity must be corrected, alcohol avoided, and smoking stopped. There are two objectives in medical management. The first is to reduce or abolish esophageal contact with gastric juice to allow healing and prevent complications.

TABLE 10-3 Savary-Miller endoscopic classification of esophagitis

Grade 1	Single or isolated erosive lesion(s), oval or linear, but affecting only one longitudinal fold.
Grade 2	Multiple erosive lesions, noncircumferential, affecting more than one longitudinal fold, with or without confluence.
Grade 3	Circumferential erosive lesions.
Grade 4	Chronic lesions: ulcer(s), stricture(s), and or short esophagus. Alone or in association with lesions of Grades 1 to 3.
Grade 5	Columnar epithelium in continuity with the Z line, noncircular, star-shaped, or circumferential. Alone or associated with lesions of Grades 1 to 4.

The second is to relieve symptoms while healing is taking place. Effective therapy entails both the adoption of mechanical measures designed to reduce reflux and the administration of pharmacologic agents.

Postural and Dietary Advice

To avoid gastric distention, meals should be small and frequent, delaying drinks to at least 1 h after food. Supper should be taken at least 1 h before bedtime. There is no specific diet, except patients should avoid fats, chocolate, and coffee. Otherwise, they should simply avoid foods that they know precipitate symptoms. The patient must sleep with the torso 45° head-up. The main objective is to aid gravitational esophageal clearance during sleep.

Pharmacologic Treatment

Although most of the drugs singly and in combination are effective in ameliorating the symptoms, only omeprazole is effective in accelerating the healing of the esophagitis. Medical therapy does not alter the basic cardioesophageal incompetence, and therefore recurrence is common. Many patients require maintenance therapy over long periods.

The details of the medical therapy vary in accordance with the clinical picture. In addition to the postural and dietary advice, symptomatic patients with mild esophagitis are simply managed by administration of palatable antacid tablets, which they suck whenever heartburn occurs. This is supplemented by an antacid–alginate mixture after meals and especially before retiring to bed.

For more troublesome symptoms and in the presence of moderate-to-severe esophagitis, an H_2 blocker is added initially as a single bedtime ulcer-healing dose. This is increased and administered more frequently (e.g., cimetidine 400 mg four times a day or ranitidine 300 mg twice a day) if the response is poor. If symptoms are incompletely relieved by this regimen, additional agents are introduced. Prokinetic drugs are useful in those patients who continue to experience nausea, fullness, regurgitation, and belching, whereas mucosal protective agents may improve odynophagia and persistent heartburn. Medical treatment should be continued for 3 months. Thereafter, the medication is reduced gradually, but the majority of patients will require long-term maintenance therapy.

Omeprazole is reserved for failure of this regimen. This proton-pump inhibitor is certainly very effective in relieving the symptoms and in promoting healing. An 8-week course is administered. There are justifiable fears about prolonged treatment with this drug in view of the adverse long-term consequences of complete achlorhydria and the experimental evidence that it induces hyperplasia of the enterochromaffin cells. It is the author's opinion that recurrence of symptoms after a full course of omeprazole is an indication for surgical intervention, especially if the patient is fit and young.

LAPAROSCOPIC SURGICAL TREATMENT

Reflux disease presents a varying problem in the individual patient in terms of the requirements for a successful outcome after surgical treatment, and therefore, no one operation may be universally applicable to all patients suffering from this disease. This applies equally well to laparoscopic as it does to open antireflux surgery. Selection of the appropriate endoscopic procedure, based on the patient's build, technical feasibility, and assessment of the pathologic anatomy, is an important aspect of surgical treatment.

Indications for Antireflux Surgery

The currently accepted indications for surgical treatment are shown in Table 10-4. Practice, however, varies from center to center, and some gastroenterologists are reluctant to refer patients for surgery despite failure of medical therapy to control symptoms. The fitness of the patient for surgery and the presence of comorbid cardiorespiratory disease are important considerations in the selection of patients for surgical treatment.

Failure of Medical Therapy

This is the commonest indication: persistence of symptoms and esophagitis despite medical therapy. The problem concerns the definition of failure of medical treatment. The duration of medical therapy after which treatment is said to have failed is not generally agreed. Most antacids including H_2-receptor antagonists and alginates control reflux symptoms. These agents do not cure the reflux diathesis, and for this reason, symptoms recur on cessation of therapy. In practice therefore, patients are referred for surgery either because symptoms persist despite medication, symptoms

TABLE 10-4 Indications for surgical treatment of reflux disease

Failure of medical therapy
   Persistent symptoms despite medication
   Intractable esophagitis
   Noncompliance with treatment

Development of complications
   Stricture or Barrett's metaplasia

Reflux with motility disorders and/or esophageal chest pain
   Refluxed-induced motility disorders
   Motility disorders causing reflux
   Reflux after myotomy

Reflux in infants and children

Reflux after upper abdominal surgery
   Neutral/alkaline
   Acid

recur soon after withdrawal, or the patient is noncompliant with the medication.

In the short term (8-week course), omeprazole has proved more effective in healing esophagitis and in controlling chronic bleeding from this disorder. There are justifiable fears regarding the long-term consequences of this Na^+/K^+ ATPase inhibitor because of the total achlorhydria it induces. However, this consideration need not concern the aged patient whose esophagitis cannot be controlled by the routine medication.

Development of Complications of Reflux Disease

These usually arise on a background of a long-standing history of reflux symptoms but may, on occasion, constitute the presenting complaint, as exemplified by the onset of dysphagia from an esophageal peptic stricture in elderly patients. Although generally regarded as indications for surgical treatment, the management of patients with esophageal strictures and Barrett's esophagus is by no means standardized and, to a large extent, is influenced by the age and general condition of the patient.

Reflux Associated with Esophageal Motility Disorders

Gastroesophageal reflux may initiate nonspecific motility disorders of the esophagus and induce noncardiac chest pain. Certain motility disorders that lead to hypo- or aperistalsis of the esophageal musculature, for example, scleroderma, are often accompanied by an acid reflux that tends to be particularly severe because of the grossly defective esophageal clearance of the refluxate. Reflux may be precipitated by various myotomy procedures performed for certain specific motility disorders of the esophagus.

Reflux in Infancy and Childhood

Untreated or inadequately controlled reflux in children leads to esophageal shortening, which in the past, was confused with congenital short esophagus. Most are agreed, however, that conservative treatment should be continued whenever possible until 2 years of age because of the tendency to spontaneous resolution and the undoubted inferior results in infants.

CONTRAINDICATIONS, FUNCTIONAL, AND ANATOMIC CONSIDERATIONS TO LAPAROSCOPIC ANTIREFLUX SURGERY

Absolute Contraindications

In the author's experience, laparoscopic mobilization of the abdominal esophagus and esophagogastric junction is usually not possible after previous vagotomy or partial gastrectomy as a result of adhesions that render the dissection difficult and hazardous. Previous (failed) antireflux surgery is also an absolute contraindication. Laparoscopic antireflux surgery is difficult and often impossible in the morbidly obese patient, especially when the left lobe of the liver is enlarged from fatty infiltration. The grossly hypertrophied greater omentum adds to the difficulty of the hiatal dissection.

Relative Contraindications

The presence of significant esophageal shortening, such that the esophagogastric junction cannot be brought down to the abdomen, is a relative contraindication, although with experience, it is possible to perform a laparoscopic gastroplasty (Collis type) and then surround this with a total fundoplication. This procedure is, however, lengthy and was attempted once by the author. The operation took 6 h, although the outcome of the patient was good in the short-term follow-up. This procedure should only be attempted by the experienced esophageal laparoscopic surgeon.

Functional Considerations

When motility is grossly disturbed, for example, in aperistalsis, the nature of the antireflux operation should be considered carefully. Thus, a complete fundal wrap is likely to obstruct the gastroesophageal junction in this situation, and partial wraps (posterior or anterior) should be employed. Although not a significant feature of adult GERD, delayed gastric emptying is encountered in some children with reflux, particularly in the presence of neurologic deficits, but it occurs rarely in adult patients unless they have had previous gastric or antireflux surgery. When delayed gastric emptying is demonstrated by the appropriate isotope studies, a drainage procedure (pyloroplasty or anterior gastroenterostomy) has to be added to the antireflux operation.

Anatomic Considerations

Specifically these relate to the following: (1) absence or presence of a hiatal defect and hernia and (2) foreshortened gastrosplenic ligament or small fundus. In the absence of a hiatal hernia, the author's choice is for a partial (270°) crurally fixed fundoplication of the Toupet type because this gives the same reflux control but is accompanied by a lower incidence of gas bloat symptoms.[112]

A hiatal hernia must be reduced, the hiatal defect repaired, and added security achieved by a total loose fundoplication of the Hell-Rosetti type. When the gastrosplenic ligament is short or the fundus is small, the author's preference is for a round ligament cardiopexy.

INSTRUMENTATION FOR LAPAROSCOPIC ANTIREFLUX SURGERY

In addition to a good video imaging system, the essential instruments and consumables needed are shown in Table 10-5. Other instruments considerably facilitate the hiatal mobilization and are recommended (Table 10-6). A 30° forward-oblique 10-mm telescope is essential.[113] In the absence of the dipping endoretractor, the best and safest method of lifting the left lobe is by use of the black plastic 10-mm rod. The suture material must be of the atraumatic kind, ideally mounted on endoski needles and made of silk or braided polyamide. A pair of good needle drivers is essential, and preferably these should have the nonserrated gripping jaws because ordinary laparoscopic needle holders damage the suture material and, for this reason, can lead to breakage during knot tying.

TABLE 10-5 Essential instrumentation and consumables for laparoscopic antireflux surgery

30° forward oblique 10-mm telescope
Atraumatic straight grasping forceps × 2 (Babcock, Glassman)
Traumatic grasping forceps × 2
Distally configured curved grasping forceps (Storz, Jarit)
Plastic retractor rod or expanding retractor
Twin-action dissecting scissors
L-shaped electrosurgical hook knife
5-mm needle holders × 2
Endoski atraumatic sutures (black silk or polyamide), 2–0, 3–0.
Vascular silicone sling

TABLE 10-6 Additional equipment which facilitates laparoscopic antireflux surgery

Dipping endoretractor
Variable curvature superelastic dissector (vs. surgical)
Variable curvature sling passer

PATIENT POSITIONING AND PLACEMENT OF TROCARS

There is a choice of position of the patient: supine or lithotomy. In either situation, a slight head-up tilt of the operating table is desirable. The lithotomy position is more comfortable for the surgeon standing between the legs and creates more room around the operating table because the camera person is on the left side and the first assistant and scrub nurse are on the right side. It does, however, impose increased pressure on the calf veins, particularly during long operations. Irrespective of position, the sites of the trocar cannulae are the same (Fig. 10-1). The left lower 5.5 mm subcostal cannula should be flexible (metal or plastic).

HIATAL DISSECTION AND MOBILIZATION OF THE ESOPHAGUS AND ESOPHAGOGASTRIC JUNCTION

This is common to all antireflux procedures that require complete mobilization of the esophagus (vide infra). Unless the endoretractor is used, the left lobe liver is elevated by the 10-mm plastic rod (or expanding retractor) introduced through the 10.5-mm left subcostal port. Orientation of the anatomy is crucial. This is easy if hiatal hernia is present because the margins of the hiatus are easily identified by the smooth hollow caused by the hernial defect (Fig. 10-2). In patients without a hernia, the upper margin of the hiatus and the crural pillars are identified by close inspection. If

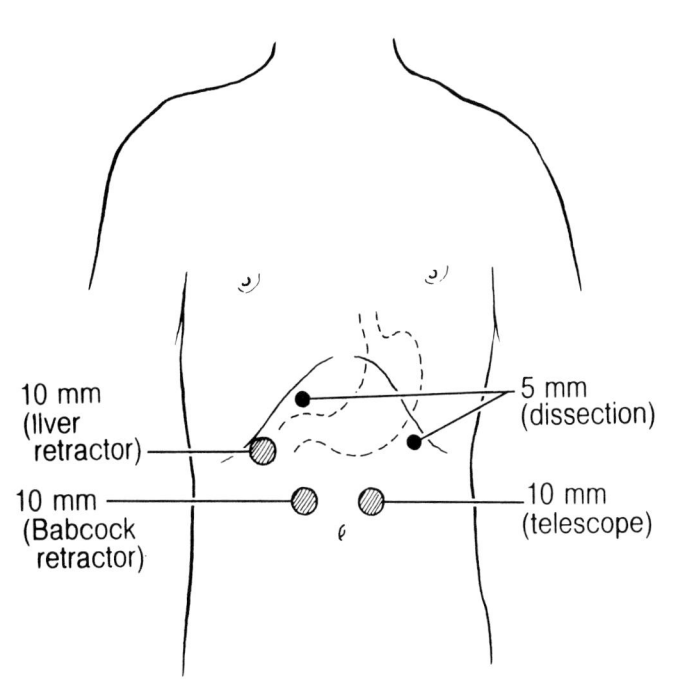

FIGURE 10-1 Five ports are placed in the supraumbilical region. All ports are approximately 15 cm from the gastroesophageal junction.

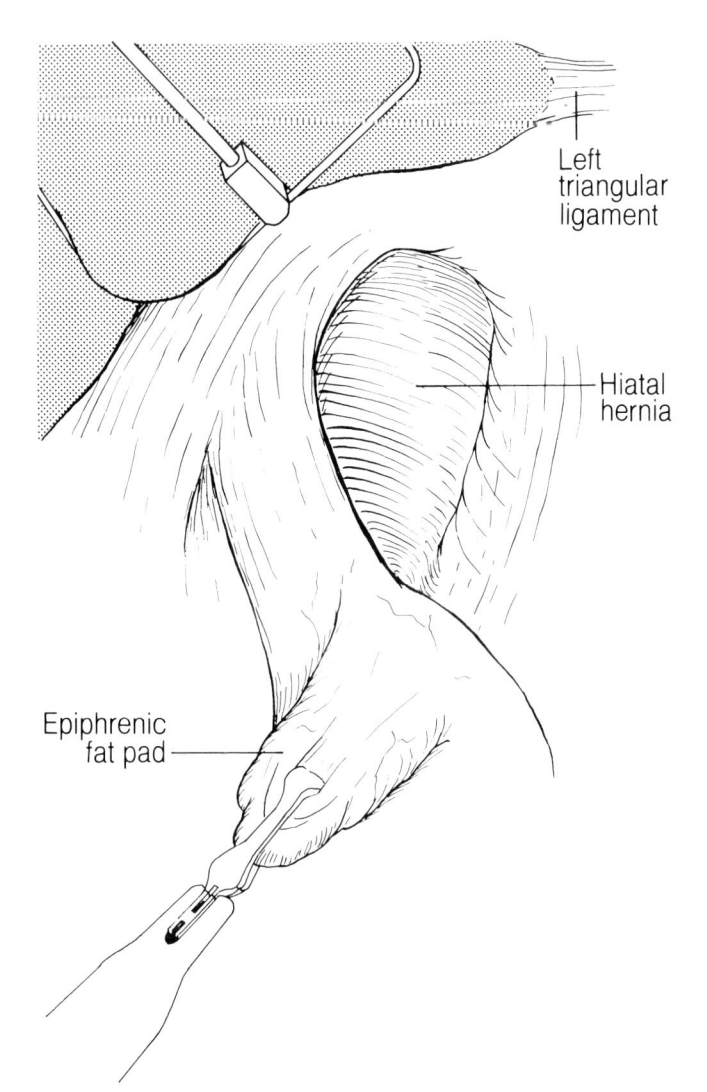

FIGURE 10-2 The initial exposure includes cephalad elevation of the left lobe of the liver with an expandable liver retractor. A grasper on the epiphrenic fat pad reduces a hiatal hernia, which is seen as a smooth hollow.

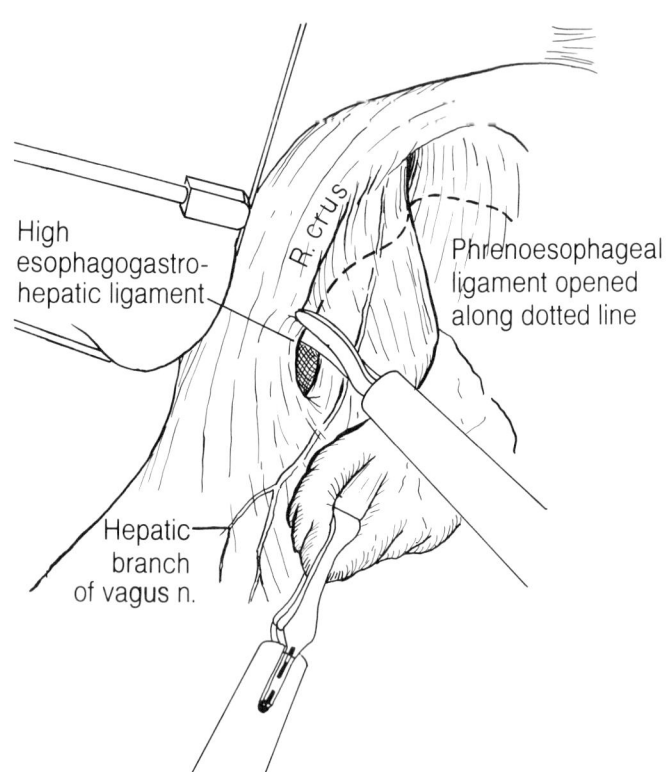

FIGURE 10-3 Dissection commences to the right of the esophagus with a monopolar electrocoagulating scissors above the hepatic branch of the vagus. After the right crus of the diaphragm has been identified, dissection is carried across the anterior wall of the esophagus.

difficulty is encountered, a 30-French orogastric tube is inserted, and after the position of the esophagus is identified, it is withdrawn into the intrathoracic esophagus because the dissection of the abdominal segment and esophagogastric junction is made more difficult with the tube in situ.

The hiatal dissection starts with high division of the peritoneum, preferably with scissors, to expose the hiatal margin and the crura (Fig. 10-3). The upper anterior wall of the stomach is then grasped by the assistant and pulled downward and to the right to expose the left margin of the hiatus. The fixation (by fibrous strands) of the esophagus and esophagogastric junction to the left crus is separated by scissors or electrosurgical hook knife. Next, the gastrophrenic peritoneum between the left crus and the superior pole of the spleen is divided by the electrosurgical hook knife (Fig. 10-4). This is the most important step in the mobilization of the fundus and, if complete, will permit a sufficient wrap of upper stomach without tension and the need for division of the upper short gastric vessels.

The stomach is then pulled downward and to the left. The peritoneum of the transparent section of the lesser omentum (pars flaccida) is divided with scissors to expose the lower part of the right crus and the loose fibroareolar tissue between it and the esophagus. Blunt dissection with pledget swab of the anterior wall of the esophagus is performed to identify the anterior vagus and the lower margin of the phrenoesophageal membrane. This is pushed proximally until the mediastinum is entered anteriorly. Several stretched strands of the phrenoesophageal membrane are divided during this stage. The dissection is then continued in the loose areolar tissue between the right margin of the esophagus and the right crus until the posterior vagus is identified (Fig. 10-5). This is separated from the esophagus, the mobilization of which is continued within the mediastinum until the aortic pulsations are encountered.

Insertion of Vascular Sling Around the Esophagus

If a variable curvature superelastic dissector (U.S. Surgical, Norwalk, CT) (Fig. 10-6A) is available, this is introduced

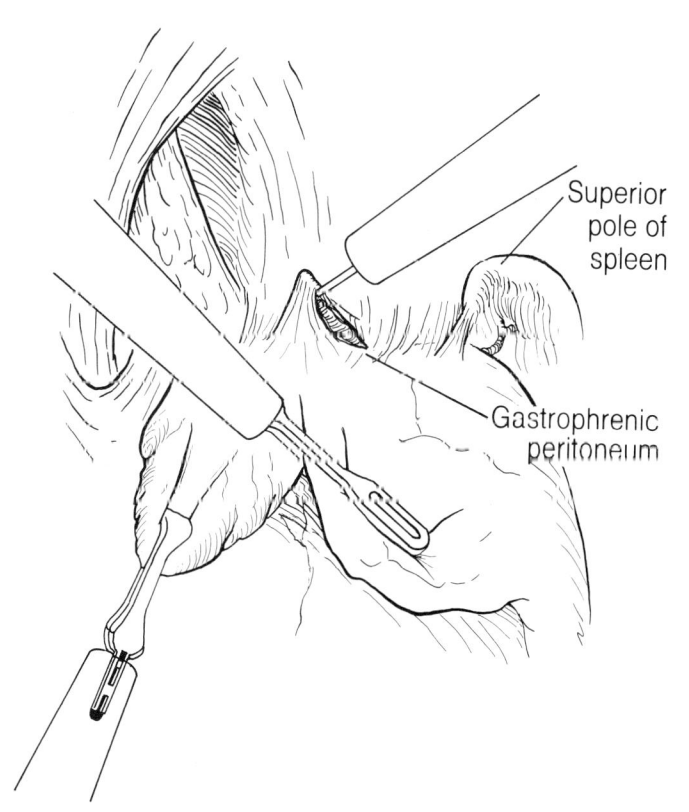

FIGURE 10-4 Division of the gastrophrenic ligament left of the esophagus is best accomplished by two-point inferior retraction of the fundus to "roll it over." The attachments are taken down with an L hook or scissors. Division of the short gastric vessels is generally not required.

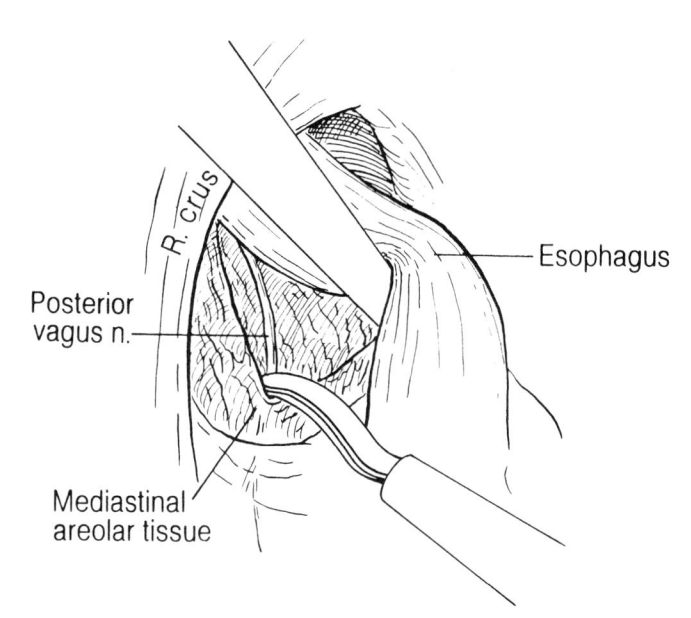

FIGURE 10-5 With a combination of blunt and sharp dissection the mediastinum is entered from the right side of the esophagus. Dissection in this plane is continued until the left crus is identified at its insertion with the right crus. The dissection is complete when the fundus or perisplenic fat can be seen through a window between the left crus of the diaphragm and the posterior esophageal wall.

through the right lower subcostal cannula, and its tip placed between the esophagus and the left crus. The tip is then extruded to the right amount until it is visualized underneath the loose stretched tissues on the right side of the esophagus, when it is extruded fully and its tip made to emerge medial to the right crus and the posterior vagus nerve. The dissector is then moved up and down to mobilize the posterior aspect of the esophagus (akin to the curved finger during open surgery). The superelastic dissector is then closed and removed. It is replaced by the distally configured curved forceps (Fig. 10-6B), which is passed behind the esophagus. The jaws are opened to grasp the silicone sling. This is introduced through the anterior abdominal wall in the immediate left midsubcostal region through a small stab wound and by means of a 3-mm needle holder. After grasping the end of the silicone sling, the curved forceps is withdrawn from behind the esophagus, and the silicone sling is transferred back to the 3-mm needle holder, which is then exteriorized. Traction on the two external ends of the sling pulls the abdominal esophagus and the esophagogastric junction forward and downward (Fig. 10-6C).

If the variable curvature superelastic dissector is not available, the esophageal mobilization is performed using a curved grasper with gentle dissection from the left side until the end of the instrument emerges on the right side of the esophagus.

Posterior Mobilization of the Crura and the Upper Stomach

A straight grasper is passed beneath the elevated esophagus and used to stretch it upward to expose the crura and the posterior surface of the stomach. Division of all fibrous attachments, especially between the stomach wall and the crura and retroperitoneal tissue, is essential, and a sufficient window must be created anterior to the left crus through which the fundus is clearly visualized (Fig. 10-7A). The fundus is then grasped and pulled through the window. A second grasper picks the fundus lower down, and more stomach is withdrawn behind the esophagus (Fig. 10-7B). The process is repeated until sufficient stomach has been herniated to permit the formation of a complete wrap without tension. At this stage, the 50-French orogastric tube is pushed down across the esophagogastric junction into the stomach.

REPAIR OF HIATUS AND TOTAL FUNDOPLICATION

The Rosetti-Hell modification was devised in an attempt to reduce the supercompetence and risk of vagal damage of the classic Nissen procedure.[114] The hiatal dissection is

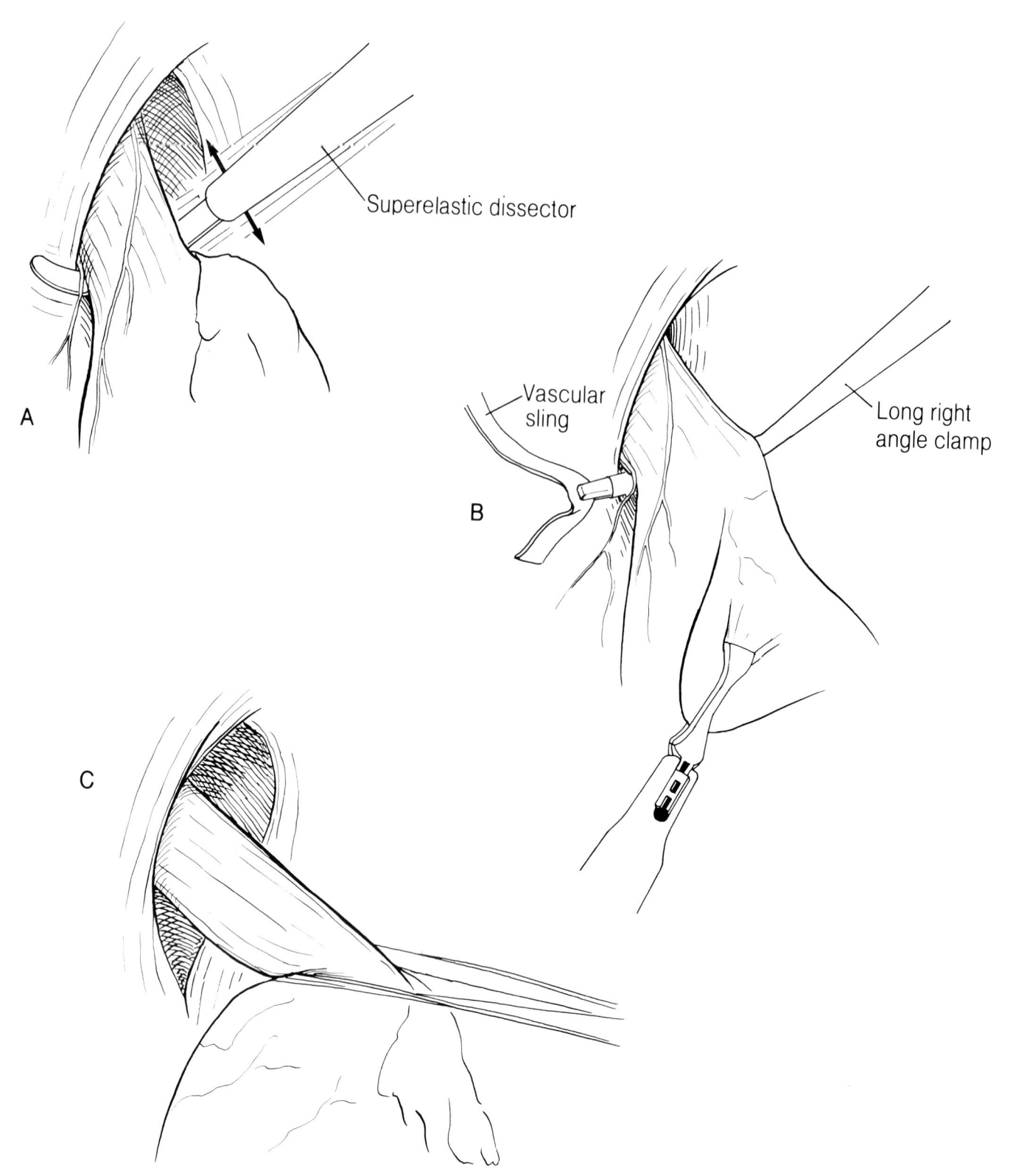

FIGURE 10-6 A. A super elastic dissector is placed behind the esophagus and gently slid up and down to increase the size of the posterior esophageal window. B. The dissector is removed and a long right-angled clamp is introduced through a flexible trocar in the left upper quadrant or introduced percutaneously after removal of the rigid trocar. After this clamp has been placed behind the esophagus, a Penrose drain or vessel loop is grasped and pulled behind the esophagus. C. The vessel loop is brought out through a small stab wound in the high epigastrium, allowing anterior retraction of the esophagus for posterior dissection.

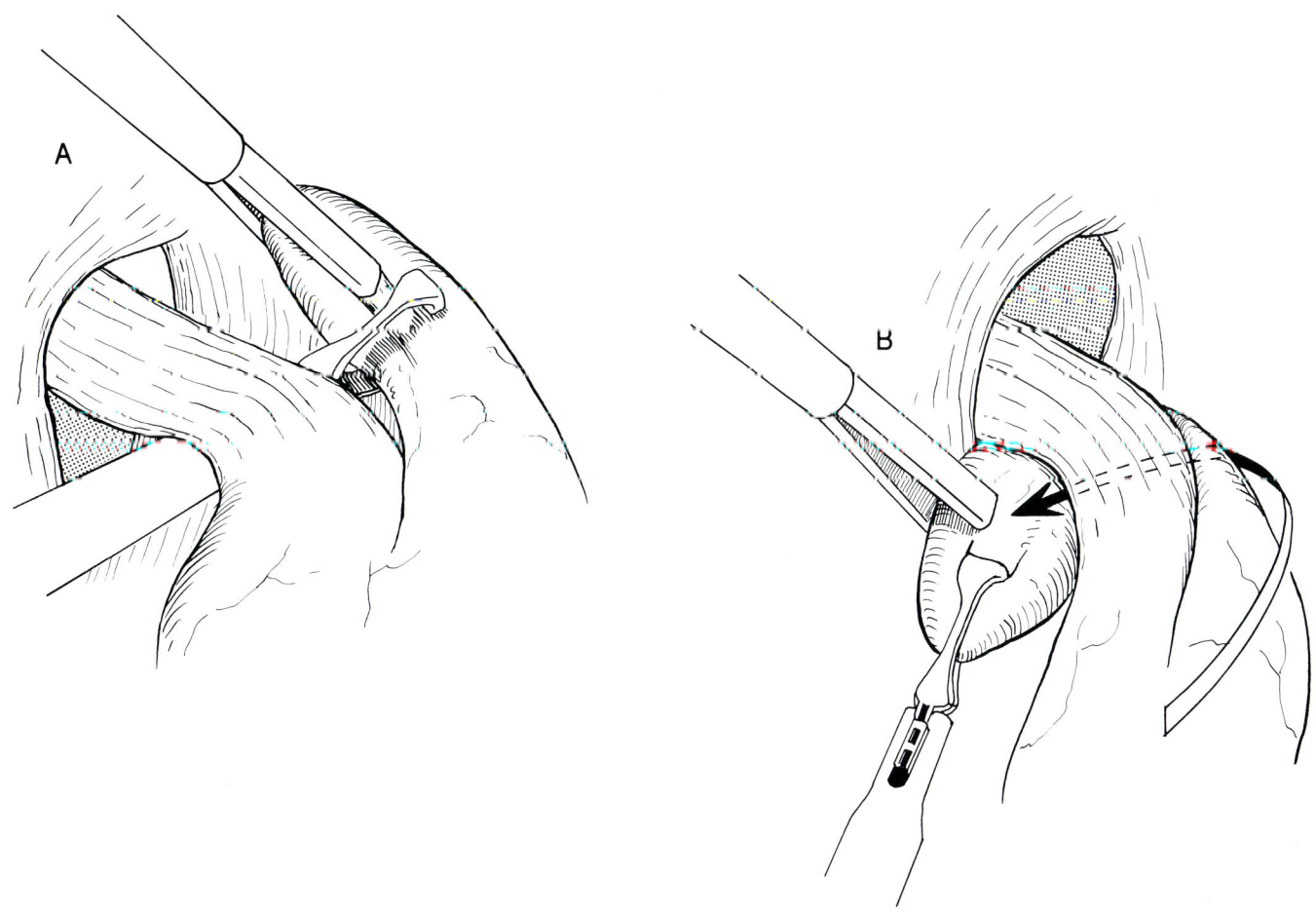

FIGURE 10-7 A. The position of the liver retractor and Babcock clamp are reversed to allow a high lateral entrance of the Babcock clamp. With the stomach elevated anteriorly, the Babcock clamp is slid behind the esophagus. With a Glassman-type clamp, the stomach is placed into the open jaws of the Babcock clamp. B. The fundus is then pulled behind the esophagus with the Babcock and "walked" forward by exchanging grasps between the Babcock and Glassman clamps to determine the portion of fundus with the greatest freedom.

limited to exposure of the crura and mobilization of the esophagus, esophagogastric junction, and posterior wall of the upper stomach, which is often adherent to the body of the pancreas by fibrous bands. These can be divided laparoscopically after elevation of the esophagus and junction by traction on the esophageal sling and insertion of a straight grasper to stretch the esophagus. Division of the short gastric vessels is unnecessary. The crural defect is repaired by one to two 2–0 black silk interrupted sutures after the insertion of a 50-French orogastric tube (Fig. 10-8). The anterior wall of the fundus is picked up by a grasping forceps and pulled behind the esophagus to emerge on its right margin, usually inside the mobilized posterior vagus. There are two techniques that can be used to produce the total loose fundoplication, which should not exceed 2.0 cm in length.

Interrupted Suturing Method

Traction on the sling is maintained to keep the esophagogastric junction down during the creation of the fundoplication using 2–0 black silk mounted on endoski needles. The most cephalad suture includes the anterior wall of the stomach (to the left of the esophagus), the anterior margin of the hiatus, the anterior esophageal wall to the right of the anterior vagus, and the apex of the wrap, in that order (Fig. 10-9A). This suture is tied using the standard microsurgical surgeon's knot or the square tumbled knot. It initiates the wrap and automatically fixes it to the esophagus and to the hiatus. The next two interrupted sutures approximate the edges of the wrap together over the esophagus, which is not included in the suture bites (Fig. 10-9B). The distal suture picks up the left edge of the wrap, esophagogastric junction, and the lower margin of the transposed fundus, in that order. When tied, it completes and fixes the fundoplication to the junction. The orogastric tube is then replaced by a size 16 nasogastric tube.

Continuous Suturing Method

This is quicker and requires the formation of the Dundee jamming loop knot at the end of a 25-cm length of suture (see Fig. 15-6).[115] The suture with terminal knot is then introduced into the peritoneal cavity. The left stomach, the anterior margin of the hiatus, the anterior esophageal wall (to the right of the anterior vagus nerve), and the apex of the wrap are traversed by the needle, and the suture is pulled, until the jamming loop impinges on the apex of the wrap (Fig. 10-10A). The right needle holder is then passed through the loop and used to pick up the long limb of the suture, which is then railroaded through the loop (Fig. 10-10B). The loop is then slipped from the tail and the knot tightened by pulling on the suture. The rest of the fundoplication is created by continuous suturing with the last bite picking up the esophagogastric junction in addition to the two edges of the wrap. The terminal knot is produced using the Aberdeen method (see Fig. 15-8).

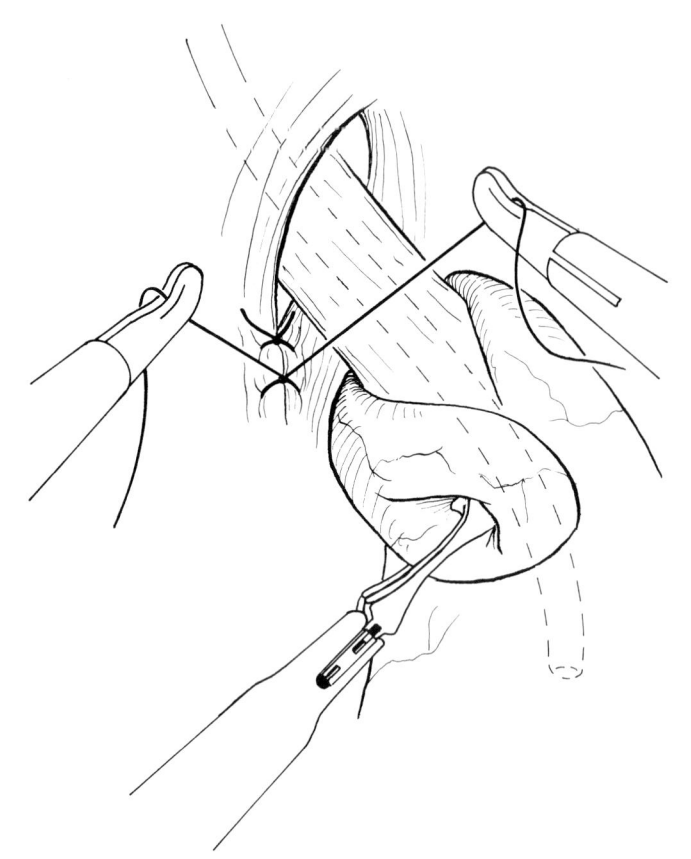

FIGURE 10-8 Posterior closure of the hiatal hernia is performed with interrupted nonabsorbable sutures.

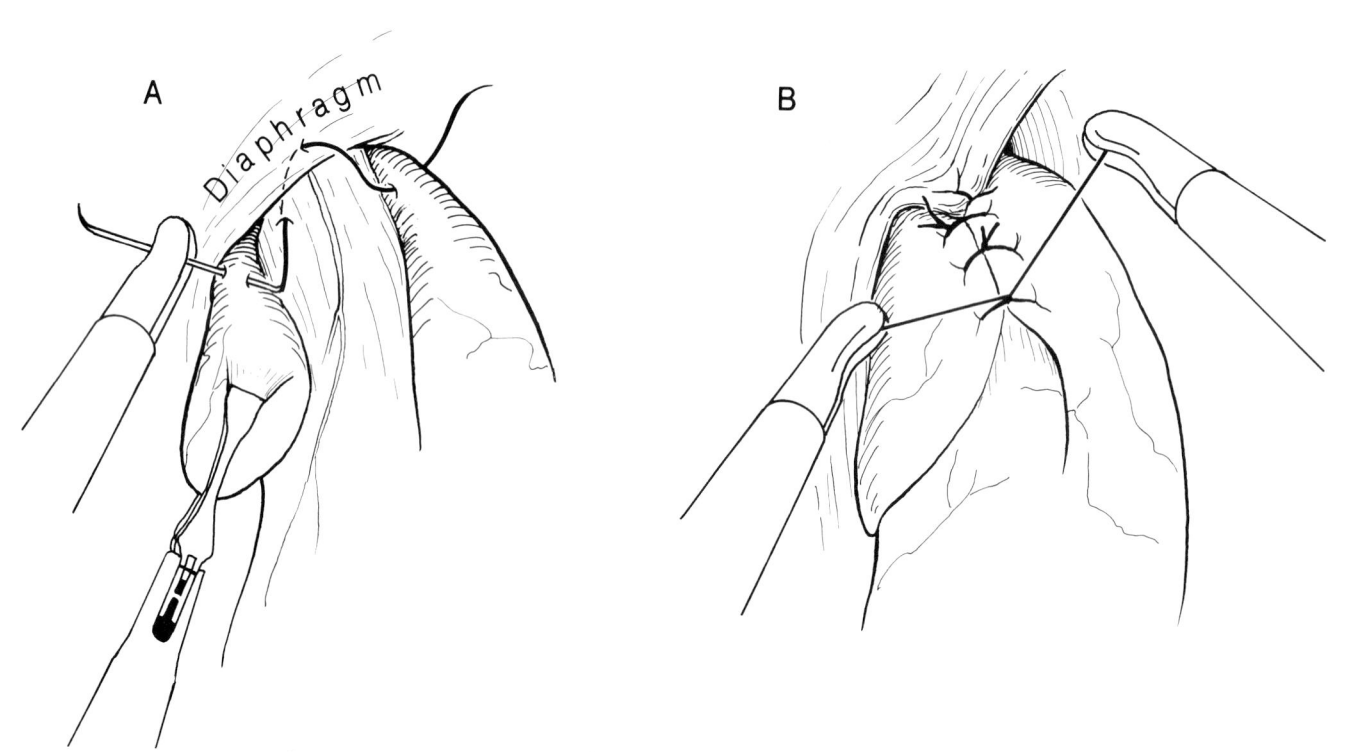

FIGURE 10-9 Interrupted suturing method. A. With a large dilator (50 to 60 French) in the esophagus the first suture incorporates the diaphragm and the anterior surface of the esophagus. B. The interrupted suture line is carried inferiorly for a distance of approximately 2 cm.

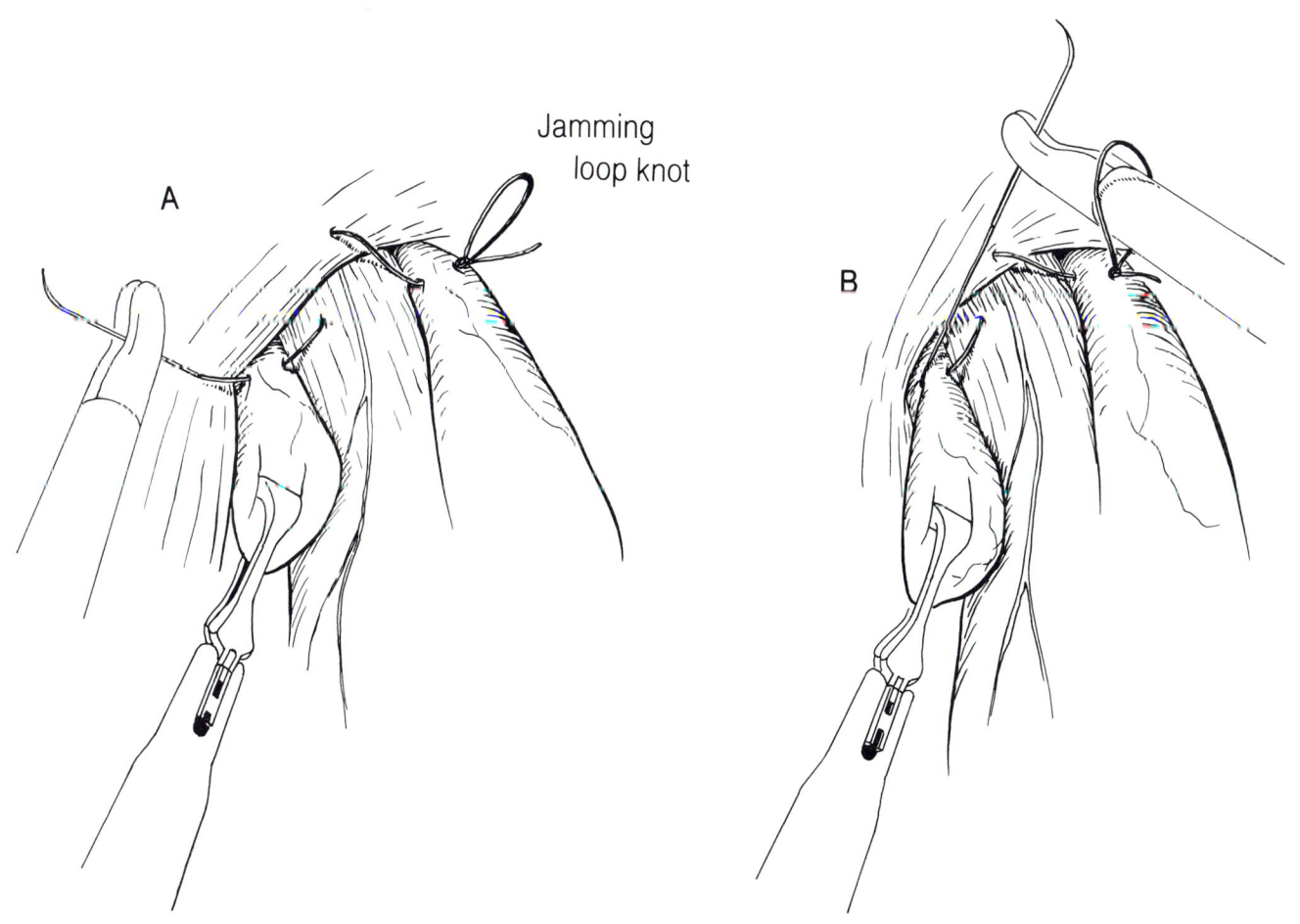

FIGURE 10-10 Continuous suturing method. A. A jamming loop knot is created extracorporeally. The first bite is identical to that performed in Figure 10-9. B. The needle is brought back through the open loop, and with firm traction on the tail, the loop is closed. After a 2-cm repair has been performed, the knot is tied off with an Aberdeen or crochet knot (see Figs. 15-6 and 15-8).

REDUCTION REPAIR AND TOTAL FUNDOPLICATION FOR LARGE HIATAL HERNIAS

These are usually encountered in elderly women. The following technique[116] has given uniformly satisfactory results in 13 such patients. The hernia is reduced by the *walking method* using two graspers. Irrespective of size, all these hernias can be reduced, although in long-standing cases associated with recurrent volvulus, adhesions to the sac need to be divided. Often the sac is adherent to the mediastinum. No attempt should be made to mobilize the sac in these cases. Its lower margin is divided to expose the crura and repair it, the sac itself is left in the mediastinum.

The best technique for repair of the large hiatal defect is continuous suturing with the Dundee preformed jamming loop knot at the end of a 30-cm length of 2–0 black silk mounted on endoski needle. The repair starts at the bottom, and deep bites are taken through the two crura until the hernial defect is reduced to a 1.0-cm gap (with a 40-French orogastric tube across the esophagogastric junction, Fig. 10-11A). The suture is then locked and the needle reversed to allow continued suturing, using more superficial bites down the approximated crura until the jamming loop is reached (Fig. 10-11B). The suture is then passed through the jamming loop, which is the closed by traction on the tail, and the knot is tightened from the long limb of the suture. The knot is reinforced by a simple hitch.

POSTERIOR CRURALLY FIXED PARTIAL FUNDOPLICATION

This repair was first described by Toupet[112] and subsequently modified by Boutelier and Jonsell.[117] The author

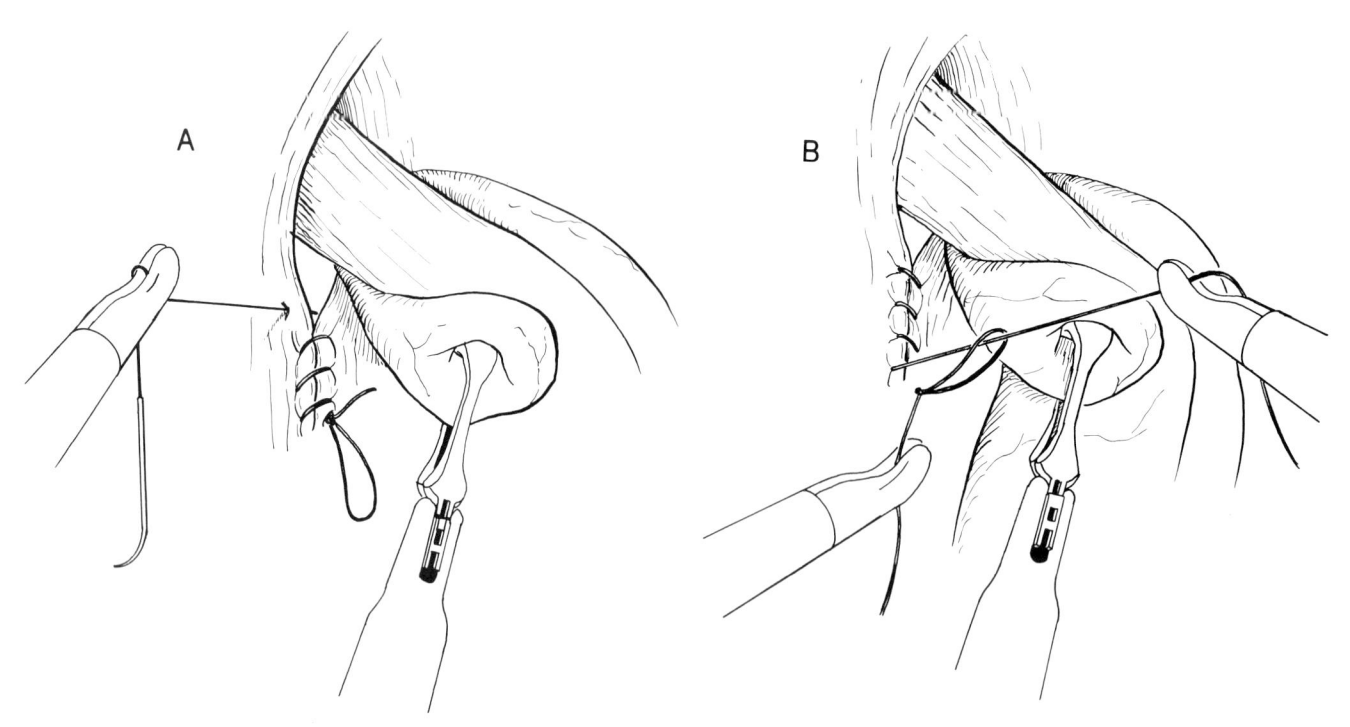

FIGURE 10-11 Large hiatal defects are best closed with a running suture, which starts with a jamming loop knot (A), continues superiorly, and then returns back to its origin where the loop is secured (B).

uses it as the standard operation in patients with reflux disease without hiatal hernia or sizeable hiatal defect. The mobilization is identical to the described for the total wrap. After the fundus has been brought behind the esophagus and medial to the posterior vagus, it is pulled anteriorly and to the left to expose the left crus. With the wrap on the stretch (held by the assistant), the posterior surface of the stomach is sutured to the left crus using two interrupted 2–0 black silk stitches (Fig. 10-12A). The right crus is then sutured to the posterior wall of the stomach using a similar technique (Fig. 10-12B). After fixation to the crura, the two folds of stomach should lie in a symmetric fashion on either side of the esophagus (Fig. 10-12C). Each gastric fold is sutured to the anterolateral surface of the esophagus on either side of the anterior vagus using three interrupted 2–0 black silk sutures (Fig. 10-12D).

ANTERIOR PARTIAL FUNDOPLICATION

This operation was first described by Dor and associates[118] in 1962 and has been slightly modified by Watson.[119] The author uses this procedure only in some patients undergoing laparoscopic cardiomyotomy, that is, those associated with a hiatal defect or who require extensive mobilization of the esophagus (long-standing achalasia). It creates an anterior 180° wrap. The gastrophrenic peritoneum is divided, and the fundus has to be detached from the left crus.

The fundus is then sutured to right margin of the esophagogastric junction in front of the abdominal esophagus and to the right crus starting near its insertion (Fig. 10-13). In general, three interrupted black silk sutures are needed. The modification proposed and used by Watson consists of initial fixation of the esophagus to the repaired crura before the anterior warp is fashioned.

LIGAMENTUM TERES CARDIOPEXY

This operation is indicated in patient with short gastrosplenic ligament or small contracted fundus. The principle of this procedure described by Narbona and colleagues[120] entails the utilization of the teres (round) ligament as a sling around the mobilized esophagogastric junction. The same procedure is conducted laparoscopically.[121] It elongates the intraabdominal segment of the esophagus, restores a HPZ, and accentuates the angle of His. The teres ligament is mobilized from the falciform ligament and fat with preservation of its blood supply from the liver (umbilical fissure). After detachment from the umbilicus, it is rerouted around the esophagogastric junction. The mobilization of the latter is identical to that used in the Rosetti-Hell procedure. The cardiopexy is performed under manometric control. Traction is applied to the sling until the lower esophageal pressure is elevated by 15 to 20 mmHg above zero (gastric). While traction is maintained, the apex

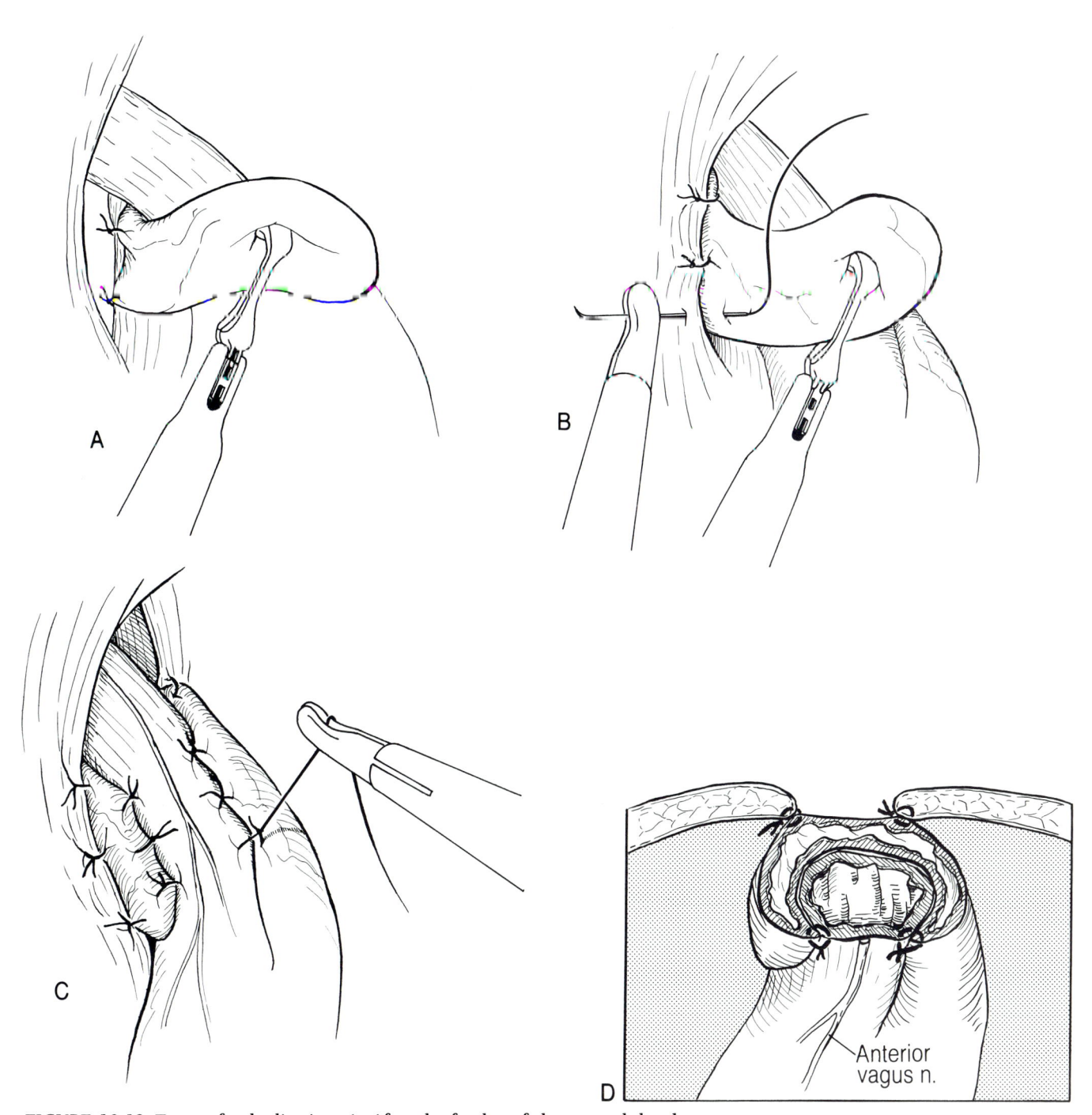

FIGURE 10-12 Toupet fundoplication. A. After the fundus of the stomach has been brought behind the esophagus, the posterior wall of the stomach is anchored to the left crus of the diaphragm with two or three interrupted sutures. B. The wrap is then anchored to the right crus of the diaphragm with two or three interrupted sutures. C. The wrap is completed by anchoring it to the anterior surface of the esophagus on either side of the anterior vagus nerve. D. In cross section, the Toupet is seen to be a 270° wrap with four-point fixation.

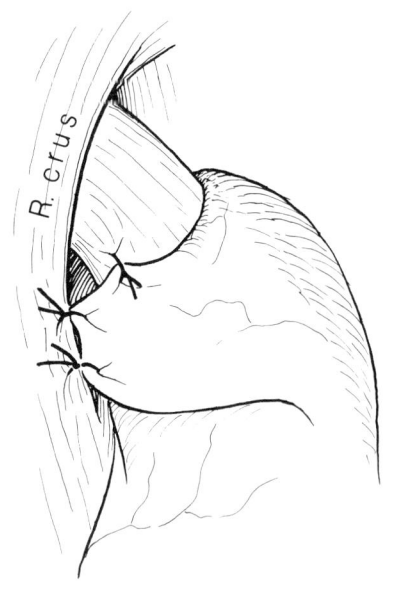

FIGURE 10-13 Anterior 180° fundoplication. This procedure involves mobilization of the left gastrophrenic. Attachments are divided and the anterior fundus is rolled to the right side of the esophagus where it is secured to the esophagus and the right crus of the diaphragm.

of the sling is fixed by a mattress suture to the left side of the junction (Fig. 10-14A). The second suture approximates the fundus of the stomach to the left side of the esophagus above the sling (Fig. 10-14B). The rest of the teres ligament is then fixed to the anterior wall of the stomach parallel to the lesser curve by 3 to 4 interrupted sutures (Fig. 10-14C). In the author's experience, the procedure gives good results in terms of reflux control and healing of the esophagitis and is not accompanied by any adverse sequelae, such as dysphagia and gas bloat.

OUTCOME

Over a period of 3 years, we have performed 72 antireflux procedures in patients with reflux disease. A further 13 patients have been operated on for large incarcerated hernias, usually of the mixed variety. There have been no deaths or serious operative complications. All patients develop mediastinal emphysema, but this is of no consequence and disappears within a few hours. However, two patients developed pneumothorax. Presumably, this is due to unrecognized pleural damage during the dissection of the lower mediastinum. Chest radiography is therefore recommended in the recovery ward soon after the procedure. The other complications encountered have been three instances of chest infections, all in smokers. The average hospital stay is currently 3 days, with a range of 2 to 5. The nasogastric tube is removed the day after the operation.

The results of the laparoscopic antireflux surgery are being reported elsewhere. However, it is clear from our experience that the relief of symptoms and reflux control, as assessed by pH monitoring and endoscopy at 3 months, is of the same order as that achieved by the equivalent open operations.

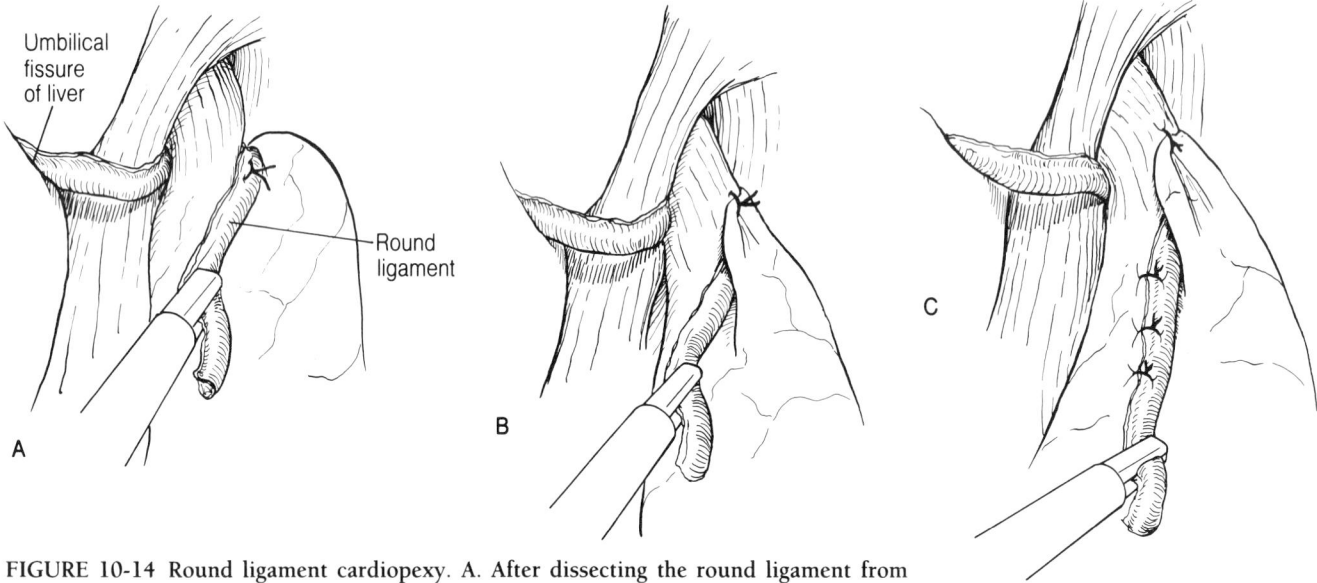

FIGURE 10-14 Round ligament cardiopexy. A. After dissecting the round ligament from the anterior abdominal wall, it is brought from the umbilical fissure of the liver posterior to the esophagus and through the angle of His. The first suture anchors the ligament to the stomach in this position. B. The fundus is then sewn to the esophagus over the round ligament to accentuate the angle further. C. The remainder of the round ligament is secured to the anterior gastric wall parallel to the lesser curvature. Intraoperative manometry is critical if this sling is to provide an adequate physiologic result.

REFERENCES

1. Ellis FH Jr: Controversies regarding the management of hiatal hernia. *Am J Surg* 1980; 139:782–788.
2. Skinner DB: Symptomatic esophageal reflux. *Am J Dig Dis* 1966; 11:771–779.
3. Pearson FC, Cooper JD, Ilves R, et al: Massive hiatal hernia with incarceration. A report of 53 cases. *Can Ann Thorac Surg* 1983; 35:45–51.
4. Willis T: *Pharmaceutice Rationalis*. Oxford, 1674.
5. Gubaroff A von: Ueber den Verschluss des menschlichen Magnes der Cardia. *Arch Anat Ent* 1886; 205:103.
6. Liebermann-Meffert D, Allgower M, Schneid P, et al: Muscular equivalent of the lower esophageal sphincter. *Gastroenterology* 1979; 76:31–38.
7. Magendie F: *A Summary of Physiology*. Translated from the French by John Revere, Baltimore, Coale, 1822.
8. Creamer B: Oesophageal reflux. *Lancet* 1955; 1:279–281.
9. Jackson C: The diaphragmatic pinchcock in so-called cardiospasm. *Laryngoscope* 1922; 32:139–142.
10. Bohnius DI: *Circulus Anatominco-Physiologicus*. Lipsiae, 1710, p 126.
11. Collis JL, Kelly TD, Wiley AN: Anatomy of the crura of the diaphragm and the surgery of hiatus hernia. *Thorax* 1954; 9:175–189.
12. Collis JL, Satchwell LM, Abrams LD: Nerve supply to the crura of the diaphragm. *Thorax* 1954; 9:22–25.
13. Atkinson M, Summerling MD: The competence of the cardia after cardiomyotomy. *Gastroenterologia* 1959; 92:123–134.
14. Peters PM: Closure mechanisms at the cardia with special reference to the phrenoesophageal elastic ligament. *Thorax* 1955; 10:27–36.
15. Bombeck CT, Dilard DH, Nyhus LM: Muscular anatomy of the gastroesophageal junction and the role of the phrenoesophageal ligament. *Ann Surg* 1966; 164:643–654.
16. O'Sullivan GC, DeMeester TR, Joelsson BE, et al: The interaction between distal esophageal sphincter pressure and length of the abdominal esophagus as determinants of gastroesophageal competence. A clinical study. *Am J Surg* 1981; 143:40–47.
17. Bremner CG, Schlegel JF, Ellis FH: Studies of the gastroesophageal sphincter mechanism. The role of the phrenoesophageal membrane. *Surgery* 1970; 67:735–740.
18. Edwards DAW: Progress report. The oesophagus. *Gut* 1971; 12:948–956.
19. Adler RH, Firme CN, Lanigan JM: A valve mechanism to prevent gastroesophageal reflux and esophagitis. *Surgery* 1958; 44:63–76.
20. DeMeester TR, Johnson LF, Kent AH: Evaluation of current operations for the prevention of gastroesophageal reflux. *Ann Surg* 1974; 180:511–525.
21. Fyke FE, Code CF, Schlegel JF: The gastroesophageal sphincter in healthy human beings. *Gastroenterologia* 1956; 86:135–150.
22. Atkinson M, Edwards DAW, Honour AJ, et al: Comparison of cardiac and pyloric sphincters. *Lancet* 1957; 2:918–922.
23. Atkinson M, Edwards DAW, Honour AJ, et al: The oesophagogastric sphincter in hiatus hernia. *Lancet* 1957; 2:1138–1142.
24. Lind JF, Warrian WG, Wanking WJ: Responses of the gastrooesophageal junctional zone to increases in abdominal pressure. *Can J Surg* 1960; 9:32–38.
25. Christensen J, Conklin JL, Freeman BW: Physiologic specialization at the esophagogastric junction in three species. *Am J Physiol* 1973; 225:1265–1270.
26. Christensen J, Freeman BW, Miller JK: Some physiologic characteristics of the esophagogastric junction of the opposum. *Gastroenterology* 1973; 64:1119–1125.
27. Lipshutz W, Cohen S: Physiological determinants of lower esophageal sphincter function. *Gastroenterology* 1971; 61:16–24.
28. Christensen J: Pharmacological identification of the lower esophageal sphincter. *J Clin Invest* 1970; 49:681–691.
29. Goyal RK, Rattan S: Genesis of basal sphincter pressure. Effect of tetrodotoxin on lower esophageal sphincter pressure in opposum in vivo. *Gastroenterology* 1976; 71:62–67.
30. Daniel EE, Taylor GS, Holman ME: The myogenic basis of active tension in the lower esophageal sphincter. *Gastroenterology* 1976; 70:874.
31. Hongo M, Traube M, McAllister RJ, et al: Effects of nifedipine on esophageal motor function in humans. *Gastroenterology* 1984; 86:8–12.
32. Biancani P, Zabinski MP, Behar J: Pressure, tension and force of closure of the human lower esophageal sphincter and esophagus. *J Clin Invest* 1975; 56:476–483.
33. Lind JF, Warrian WG, Wankling WJ: Responses of the gastroesophageal junctional zone to increases in abdominal pressure. *Can J Surg* 1966; 9:32–38.
34. Clark J, Moossa AR, Skinner DB: Pitfalls in the performance and interpretation of esophageal function tests. *Surg Clin North Am* 1976; 56:29–37.
35. Clark J, Hall AW, Cannon JD, et al: Lower oesophageal high pressure zone. Variability in recordings of pressure and length. *Br J Surg* 1978; 65:367–368.
36. Dent J, Holloway RH, Toouli J, et al: Mechanisms of lower oesophageal sphincter incompetence in patients with symptomatic gastro-oesophageal reflux. *Gut* 1988; 29:1020–1028.
37. Ogilvie AL, Atkinson M: Influence of the vagus nerve upon reflex control of the lower oesophageal sphincter. *Gut* 1984; 25:253–258.
38. Dent J, Dodds WJ, Friedman RH, et al: Mechanism of gastroesophageal reflux in recumbent asymptomatic subjects. *J Clin Invest* 1980; 65:256–267.
39. Dent J, Dodds WJ, Sekiguchi T, et al: Interdigestive phasic contractions of the human lower esophageal sphincter. *Gastroenterology* 1983; 84:453–460.
40. Dodds WJ, Dent J, Hogan WJ, et al: Mechanisms of gastroesophageal reflux in patients with reflux esophagitis. *N Engl J Med* 1982; 307:1547–1552.
41. Mittal RK, McCallum RW: Characteristics and frequency of transient relaxations of the lower esophageal sphincter in patients with reflux esophagitis. *Gastroenterology* 1988; 95:593–599.
42. Mittal RK, McCallum RW: Characteristics of transient lower esophageal sphincter relaxations in humans. *Am J Physiol* 1987; 252:G636–G641.
43. Wyman JD, Dent J, Heddle R, et al: Belching: A clue to understanding of pathological gastroesophageal reflux. Abstracted. *Gastroenterology* 1984; 86:1303.
44. Holloway RH, Hongo M, Berger K, et al: Gastric distension: A mechanism for postprandial gastroesophageal reflux. *Gastroenterology* 1985; 89:779–784.
45. Martin CJ, Patrikios J, Dent J: Abolition of gas reflux and transient lower esophageal sphincter relaxation by vagal blockade in the dog. *Gastroenterology* 1986; 91:890–896.
46. Holloway RH, Dent J, Wyman RB: Impairment of belch reflex in achalasia: Evidence for neural mediation of transient lower esophageal sphincter (LES) relaxation. Abstracted. *Gastroenterology* 1986; 91:1055.
47. Csendes A, Oster M, Moller JT, et al: Gastroesophageal reflux in duodenal ulcer patients before and after vagotomy. *Ann Surg* 1978; 188:804–880.
48. Mann CV, Hardcastle JD: The effect of vagotomy on the human gastroesophageal sphincter. *Gut* 1968; 9:688–695.

49. Mazur JM, Skinner DB, Jones EL, et al: Effect of trans-abdominal vagotomy on the human gastroesophageal high pressure zone. *Surgery* 1973; 73:818–822.
50. Temple JG, Goodall RJR, Hay JD, et al: The effect of highly selective vagotomy on the lower oesophageal sphincter. *Gut* 1981; 22:368–370.
51. Thomas PA, Earlam RJ: The gastro-oesophageal junction before and after operations for duodenal ulcer. *Br J Surg* 1973; 60:717–719.
52. Csendes A, Oster M, Brandsborg O, et al: Effect of vagotomy on human gastroesophageal sphincter pressure in the resting state and following increases in intra-abdominal pressure. *Surgery* 1979; 85:419–424.
53. Wallin L: The effect of parietal cell vagotomy on gastro-oesophageal function in duodenal ulcer patients. *Scand J Gastroenterol* 1981; 16:97–102.
54. Laitinen ST, Larmi TKI: Lower esophageal sphincter and the gastroesophageal anti-reflux mechanism. *World J Surg* 1981; 5:845–853.
55. Khan TA: Effect of proximal selective vagotomy on the canine lower esophageal sphincter. *Am J Surg* 1981; 141:219–221.
56. Angorn IB, Dimopoulos G, Hegarty MM, et al: The effect of vagotomy on the lower oesophageal sphincter: A manometric study. *Br J Surg* 1977; 64:466–469.
57. Crispin JS, McIver DK, Lind DK: Manometric study of the effect of vagotomy on gastroesophageal sphincter. *Can J Surg* 1967; 10:299–303.
58. Gotley DC, Ball D, Cooper MJ: Peptic activity in the refluxate of patients with uncomplicated gastro-oesophageal reflux (GOR). Abstracted. *Gut* 1988; 29:A1451.
59. Clark J, Cuschieri A: The effect of truncal and highly selective vagotomy on oesophageal function and the lower oesophageal high pressure zone. *Br J Surg* 1980; 67:829–830.
60. Rattan RK, Goyal S: Neural control of the lower esophageal sphincter. Influence of the vagus nerves. *J Clin Invest* 1974; 54:899–906.
61. Orlando CR: Esophageal epithelial resistance. *J Clin Gastroenterol* 1986; 8(suppl):12–16.
62. Hopwood D, Logan KR, Milne G: Mucosubstances in the normal esophageal epithelium. *Histochemistry* 1977; 54:67–74.
63. Hopwood D, Ross PE, Logan KR, et al: The light and electron microscopic distribution of acid phosphatase activity in normal human oesophageal epithelium. *Histochem J* 1978; 10:159–170.
64. Orlando RC, Bryson JC, Powell DW: Mechanisms of H^+ injury in rabbit esophageal epithelium. *Am J Physiol* 1984; 246:G718–G724.
65. Bass BL, Schweitzer EJ, Harman JW: H^+ back diffusion interferes with intrinsic reactive regulation of esophageal mucosal blood flow. *Surgery* 1984; 96:404–413.
66. Eriksen CA, Sakek SA, Cranford C, et al: Reflux oesophagitis and oesophageal transit: Evidence for a primary oesophageal motor disorder. *Gut* 1988; 29:448–452.
67. Baldi F, Corinaldesi R, Ferrarini F, et al: Gastric secretion and emptying of liquids in reflux esophagitis. *Dig Dis Sci* 1981; 26:886–889.
68. Flook D, Stoddard CJ: Gastro-oesophageal reflux and oesophagitis before and after vagotomy for duodenal ulcer. *Br J Surg* 1985; 72:804–807.
69. Gotley DC, Ball D, Cooper MJ: Peptic activity in the refluxate of patients with uncomplicated gastro-oesophageal reflux (GOR). Abstracted. *Gut* 1988; 29:A1451.
70. DeMeester TR, Johnson LF, Joseph GJ, et al: Patterns of gastroesophageal reflux in health and disease. *Ann Surg* 1976; 184:459–470.
71. Atkinson M, van Gelder A: Esophageal intraluminal pH recording in the assessment of gastroesophageal reflux and its consequences. *Dig Dis* 1977; 22:365–370.
72. Jolley SG, Johnson DG, Herbst JJ, et al: An assessment of gastroesophageal reflux in children by extended pH monitoring of the distal esophagus. *Surgery* 1978; 84:16–24.
73. Lichter I: Measurement of gastro-oesophageal acid reflux: Its significance in hiatus hernia. *Br J Surg* 1974; 61:253–258.
74. Habibulla KS, Ammann JF, Collis JL: Effects of posture in hiatus hernia as studied by oesophageal pH measurement. *Thorax* 1971; 26:689–695.
75. Gillison EW, DeCastro VAM, Nyhus LM, et al: The significance of bile in esophagitis. *Surg Gynecol Obstet* 1972; 134:419–424.
76. Chung RSK, Magri J, Shirazi S, et al: Pathogenesis of acid esophagitis. *Gastroenterology* 1974; 66:675.
77. Goldberg HI, Dodds WJ, Gee S, et al: Role of acid and pepsin in acute experimental esophagitis. *Gastroenterology* 1969; 56:223–230.
78. Bateson MC, Hopwood D, Milne G, et al: Oesophageal epithelial ultrastructure after incubation with gastrointestinal fluids and their components. *J Pathol* 1981; 133:33–51.
79. Lillemoe KD, Johnson LF, Harman JW: Alkaline esophagitis: A comparison of the ability of the gastroduodenal contents to injure the rabbit esophagus. *Gastroenterology* 1983; 85:621–628.
80. Skinner DB: Symptomatic esophageal reflux. *Am J Dig Dis* 1966; 11:771–779.
81. Ismail-Beigi F, Horton PE, Pope CE: Histological consequence of gastroesophageal reflux in man. *Gastroenterology* 1970; 58:163–169.
82. Kaboyoshi S, Kasugai T: Endoscopic and biopsy criteria for the diagnosis of esophagitis with a fiberoptic endoscope. *Dig Dis* 1974; 19:345–353.
83. Goran DA, Shields HM, Bates ML, et al: Esophageal dysplasia: Assessment by light microscopy and scanning electron microscopy. *Gastroenterology* 1984; 86:39–50.
84. Barrett NR: The lower esophagus lined by columnar epithelium. *Surgery* 1957; 41:881–894.
85. Naef AP, Savary M, Ozzello L, et al: Columnar lined lower esophagus: An acquired lesion with malignant predisposition. *J Thorac Cardiovasc Surg* 1975; 70:826–835.
86. Starns VA, Adkins RB, Ballinger JF, et al: Barrett's esophagus. *Arch Surg* 1984; 119:563–567.
87. Dahms BB, Rothstein FC: Barrett's esophagus in children: A consequence of chronic gastroesophageal reflux. *Gastroenterology* 1984; 86:318–323.
88. Chobanian SJ, Cattau EL Jr, Winters C Jr, et al: In vitro staining with toluidine blue as an adjunct to the endoscopic detection of Barrett's esophagus. *Gastrointest Endosc* 1987; 33:99–101.
89. Gillen P, Keeling P, Byrne PJ, et al: Barrett's oesophagus: pH profile. *Br J Surg* 1987; 74:774–776.
90. Gillen P, Keeling P, Byrne PJ, et al: Implication of duodenogastric reflux in the pathogenesis of Barrett's oesophagus. *Br J Surg* 1988; 75:540–543.
91. Paul G, Yardley JH: Gastric and esophageal *Campylobacter pylori* in patients with Barrett's esophagus. *Gastroenterology* 1988; 95:216–218.
92. Trier SJ: Morphology of the epithelium of the distal esophagus in patients with mid-esophageal stricture. *Gastroenterology* 1970; 58:441–461.
93. Gillen P, Keeling P, Byrne PJ, et al: Experimental columnar metaplasia in the canine oesophagus. *Br J Surg* 1988; 75:113–115.
94. Thompson JJ, Zinsser KR, Enterline HT: Barrett's metaplasia and adenocarcinoma of the esophagus and gastroesophageal junction. *Hum Pathol* 1983; 14:42–61.

95. Peuchmauer M, Potet F, Goldfain D: Mucin histochemistry of the columnar epithelium of the esophagus (Barrett's esophagus): A prospective biopsy study. *J Clin Pathol* 1984; 37:607–610.
96. Mangla JC, Schenk EA, Desbraillets L, et al: Pepsin secretion pespsinogen and gastrin in Barrett's esophagus. *Gastroenterology* 1976; 70:669–676.
97. Dayal Y, Wolfe HG: Gastrin producing cells in ectopic gastric mucosa of developmental and metaplastic origins. *Gastroenterology* 1978; 75:655–660.
98. Berensen MM, Herbst JJ, Freston JW: Esophageal columnar epithelial beta-galactosidase and beta-glucuronidase. *Gastroenterology* 1975; 68:1417–1419.
99. Garewal HS, Gerner EW, Sampliner RE, et al: Ornithine decarboxylase and polyamine levels in columnar upper gastrointestinal mucosa in patients with Barrett's esophagus. *Cancer Res* 1988; 48:3288–3291.
100. Garewal HS, Sampliner R, Gerner EW, et al: Ornithine decarboxylase activity in Barrett's esophagus: A potential marker for dysplasia. *Gastroenterology* 1988; 94:819–821.
101. Skinner DB, Walther BC, Riddell RH, et al: Barrett's esophagus: Comparison of benign and malignant cells. *Ann Surg* 1983; 198:554–565.
102. Tamura H, Schulman S: Barrett-type esophagus associated with squamous epithelium. *Chest* 1971; 59:330–333.
103. Cameron AJ, Ott BJ, Payne WS: The incidence of adenocarcinoma in columnar-lined (Barrett's) oesophagus. *N Engl J Med* 1985; 313:857–859.
104. Spechler SJ, Robbins AH, Rubins HB, et al: Adenocarcinoma and Barrett's esophagus: An overrated risk? *Gastroenterology* 1984; 87:927–933.
105. Griffin M, Sweeney EC: The relationship of endoscopic cell dysplasia and carcinoembryonic antigen in Barrett's mucosa to adenocarcinoma of the esophagus. *Histopathology* 1987; 11:53–62.
106. Urschel HC, Paulson DL: Gastroesophageal reflux and hiatal hernia. Complications and therapy. *J Thorac Cardiovasc Surg* 1967; 53:21–32.
107. Skinner DB, Belsey RHR: Surgical management of esophageal reflux and hiatal hernia. Long term results with 1030 patients. *J Thorac Cardiovasc Surg* 1967; 53:33–50.
108. deCaestecker JS, Blackwell JN, Brown J, et al: The oesophagus as a cause of recurrent chest pain. *Lancet* 1985; 2:1143–1146.
109. Vantrappen G, Janssens G, Ghillebert G: The irritable oesophagus: A frequent cause of angina-like pain. *Lancet* 1987; 1:1232.
110. DeMeester TR, Wernly JA, Pellegrini CA, et al: Technique, indications and clinical use of 24 hour esophageal pH monitoring. *J Thorac Cardiovasc Surg* 1980; 79:656–670.
111. Armstrong D, Monnier P, Nicolet M, et al: Endoscopic assessment of oesophagitis. *Gullet* 1991; 1:63–67.
112. Toupet A: Technique d'ocsophago-gastroplastie avec phrenogastropexie appliquée dans la cure radicale des hernies hiatales et comme complément de l'opération d'Heller dans les cardiospasmes. *Mem Acad Chir* 1963; 89:384–389.
113. Cuschieri A: Laparoscopic ligamentum teres (round ligament) cardiopexy, In Berci G (ed): *Problems in General Surgery*, Philadelphia, JB Lippincott, 1991, pp 378–386.
114. Rosetti M, Hell K: Fundoplication for the treatment of gastroesophageal reflux in hiatal hernia. *World J Surg* 1977; 1:439–444.
115. Cuschieri A: Tissue approximation, in Berci G (ed): *Problems in General Surgery*. Philadelphia, JB Lippincott, 1991, pp 366–377.
116. Cuschieri A, Shimi S, Nathanson LK: Laparoscopic reduction, crural repair and fundoplication of large hiatal hernia. *Am J Surg* 1992; 163:425–430.
117. Boutelier P, Jonsell G: An alternative fundoplicative maneuver for gastroesophageal reflux. *Am J Surg* 1982; 143:260–264.
118. Dor J, Humbert P, Dor V, et al: L'intérêt de la technique de Nissen modifiée dans le prevention du reflux après cardiomiotomie extramuqueuse de Heller. *Mem Acad Chir* 1962; 27:877–882.
119. Watson A: A clinical and pathophysiological study of a simple and effective operation for correction of gastro-oesophagial reflux. *Br J Surg* 1984; 71:A991.
120. Narbona B, Olavarietta L, Iloris J: Hernia hiatal reflux gastro oesophagico. Rehabilitacion nofegica y resultados con la pexia del ligamento redondo. *Cir Espanol* 1979; 33:487–495.
121. Nathanson LK, Shimi S, Cuschieri A: Laparoscopic ligamentum teres (round ligament) cardiopexy. *Br J Surg* 1991; 78:947–951.

Chapter 11

Surgical Access for Enteral Nutrition

William Sangster / John G. Hunter

The first used method of access for long-term enteral nutrition was the nasogastric tube. For long-term nutrition, these tubes have many disadvantages; they clog up easily and are quite uncomfortable and unsightly. In addition, gastroesophageal reflux, and subsequent stricture, pulmonary problems, and frequent tube dislodgment add to the consensus that nasoenteric feeding is not a good solution for long-term enteral support.

The gastrostomy tube was first introduced in the early 19th century but was plagued with complications of intraperitoneal leakage until Verneuil in 1876 recognized the necessity to coapt the visceral and parietal peritoneum with silver wire.[1] While there were modifications of the Verneuil principle, such as the Stamm, Witzel, and Janeway gastrostomies, there were few significant advances in enteral feeding until the description of percutaneous endoscopic gastrostomy (PEG) in 1981.[2]

In situations where the stomach cannot be used for enteral feedings or when gastroesophageal reflux and aspiration complicate the clinical history, jejunostomy is indicated. The first open jejunostomy tube was placed in 1879 by a French surgeon,[3] and while there were small technical adaptations that occurred, no major changes in technique occurred over the next century. Shortly after the development of PEG, methods were described for passing tubes through the stomach into the jejunum, and occasionally, it was possible directly to cannulate the jejunum using the PEG technique. The major advance in jejunostomy has been the technique of laparoscopic jejunal tube placement.[4]

In this chapter, we will focus on two techniques, PEG and the laparoscopic jejunostomy. The adaptations of these procedures for percutaneous endoscopic jejunostomy and laparoscopic gastrostomy will be mentioned briefly.

PERCUTANEOUS ENDOSCOPIC GASTROSTOMY

Indications

The two largest groups of patients undergoing this procedure are patients who cannot swallow because of neurologic dysfunction (e.g., severe head injury, stroke, or postoperative cervical nerve injury) and those with oropharyngeal cancer.[5] While nasoenteric tube feedings are an effective bridge for patients expected to recover quickly, most physicians and families have recognized and are dissatisfied with their shortcomings within several weeks of placement. It is in these patients that PEG is truly indicated.

Contraindications

Contraindications to PEG include subtotal gastrectomy (yet one should not assume that every patient who has had partial gastrectomy has insufficient stomach left for PEG placement), ascites, portal hypertension, high-dose steroid dependency, immunosuppression (i.e., ongoing chemotherapy), or obstruction to passage of the upper endoscope. The most frequently overlooked contraindication to PEG is either an extremely short life expectancy or a low quality of life. Before placing a PEG in these patients, discussion with the family or the hospital ethics committee (if the family is not available) should emphasize the costs, both monetary and emotional, of a futile attempt to extend life. PEG is the most common last procedure performed on Americans before death; so we must learn to be more selective in determining patients who will truly benefit from this procedure.

Procedure Notes

PATIENT PREPARATION

Before performing PEG, informed consent must be obtained from the family or the patient. The patient should fast for 12 hours before the procedure. Oral anticoagulants should be stopped 5 days preoperatively, and parenteral anticoagulants (heparin) must be stopped at least 6 h before PEG placement. An examination of the patient should focus on the presence or absence of abdominal scars, which may indicate previous gastric surgery or, at least, intra-abdominal adhesions. Additionally, in patients with head and neck cancer, dierct laryngoscopy may be helpful to assess the status of the hypopharynx. In patients with esophageal cancer, a barium swallow should help predict the likelihood of success. Evidence of other contraindications, including portal hypertension, ascites, or poor wound healing, should be sought. A review of the medication record will frequently reveal long-standing orders for subcutaneous heparin and other long since forgotten medications. Essential laboratory testing includes hematocrit, platelet count, and prothrombin time. In these malnourished hospitalized patients who are receiving broad-spectrum antibiotics, disorders of clotting are not infrequent and would be hazardous if not detected.

PATIENT POSITIONING

The PEG is performed in the endoscopy suite with the patient in a supine position. Because intravenous sedation is usually sufficient, it is wise to restrain the patient's hands and feet to prevent contamination of the operative field. It is helpful to place the patient at a slightly sitting angle, both for the patient's comfort and as an aspiration precaution (Fig. 11-1). Preoperative prophylactic antibiotics are administered if the patient has not previously been receiving antibiotics.

TECHNIQUE

A wide abdominal preparation centered on the left upper quadrant is performed. Sterile drapes, masks, caps, and gowns are advisable for the operating members of the team to prevent contamination of the operative field. While the field is being prepared, the endoscopist performs a standard esophagogastroduodenoscopy to evaluate the patient for other pathology and ensure that there are no esophageal varices, severe esophagitis, or gastric outlet obstruction. After confirmation that the patient has no contraindication to PEG, the endoscope is retracted into the stomach and the stomach, maximally insufflated. The anterior gastric wall is transilluminated in its midportion, and the room lights are darkened so that the surgeon can look for the light (Fig. 11-2). If it is not immediately visible, with a single finger, the surgeon may palpate around the left upper quadrant until a smooth prominent indentation in the stomach is appreciated by the endoscopist. The sterile PEG kit is opened at this point, and its components are arranged on the back table. If neither transillumination or indentation can be achieved, the procedure is aborted.

Then the endoscopist positions an opened snare over the indentation made by the surgeon's palpating finger. The surgeon infiltrates the chosen site with local anesthetic and makes a transverse incision twice the diameter of the tube to be placed. This additional incision length allows for drainage around the gastrostomy tube should heavy contamination of the fascia occur from bacteria picked up during passage of the gastrostomy tube through the oro-

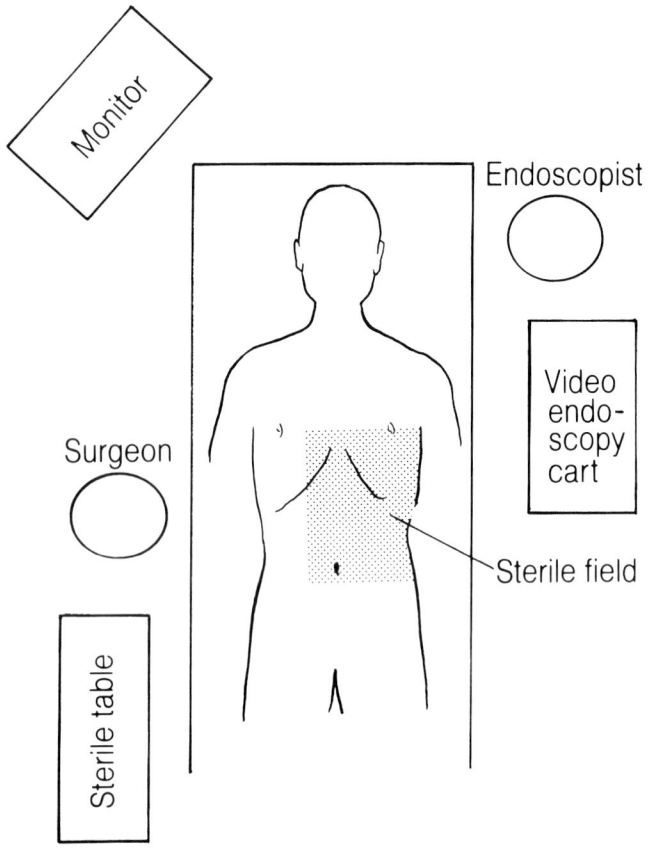

FIGURE 11-1 The patient is placed supine on the operating table. The left upper quadrant is sterilely prepared and draped. The endoscopist stands to the left of the patient near the head. The video monitor is placed where both participants can view it. The surgeon stands on the patient's right, with a sterile table adjacent.

pharynx. After the incision, a 16- to 18-gauge, thin-walled needle is thrust into the stomach and through the snare. Timid advances result in incomplete penetration and risk laceration of serosal vessels and displacement of the stomach from the abdominal wall. The endoscopist then tightens the snare around the needle. The surgeon threads the suture or guide wire through the needle into the stomach. The wire is snared by the endoscopist, and the wire, scope, and snare are pulled out of the mouth as a single unit.

The most popular type of PEG currently in use utilizes an over-the-wire, or push method, of tube placement.[6] This requires the endoscopist to push the PEG tube with its attached 1-m long plastic tapered dilator over the guide wire while the guide wire is held taut by the endoscopy assistant and surgeon. When the dilator starts to emerge through the abdominal wall, the surgeon grasps it and pulls until all of the dilator and half of the gastrostomy tube has been pulled across the abdominal wall. The endoscopist replaces the endoscope and watches the tube to ensure perfect positioning as it is pulled further into the stomach.

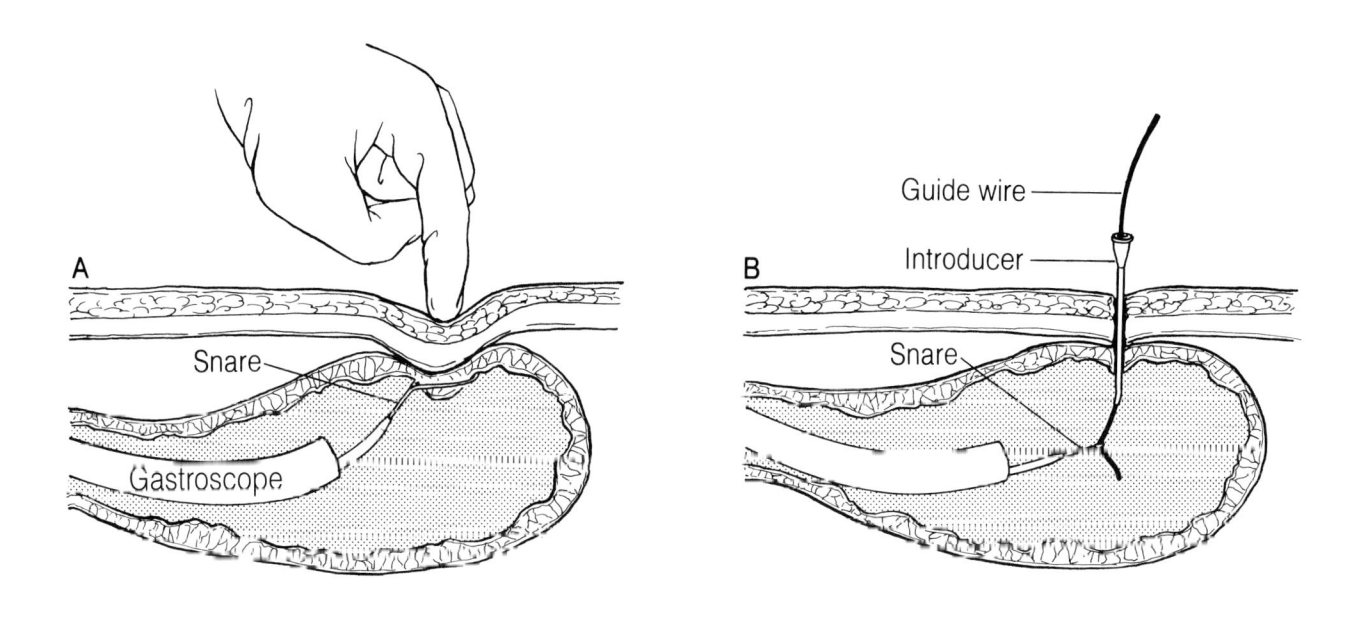

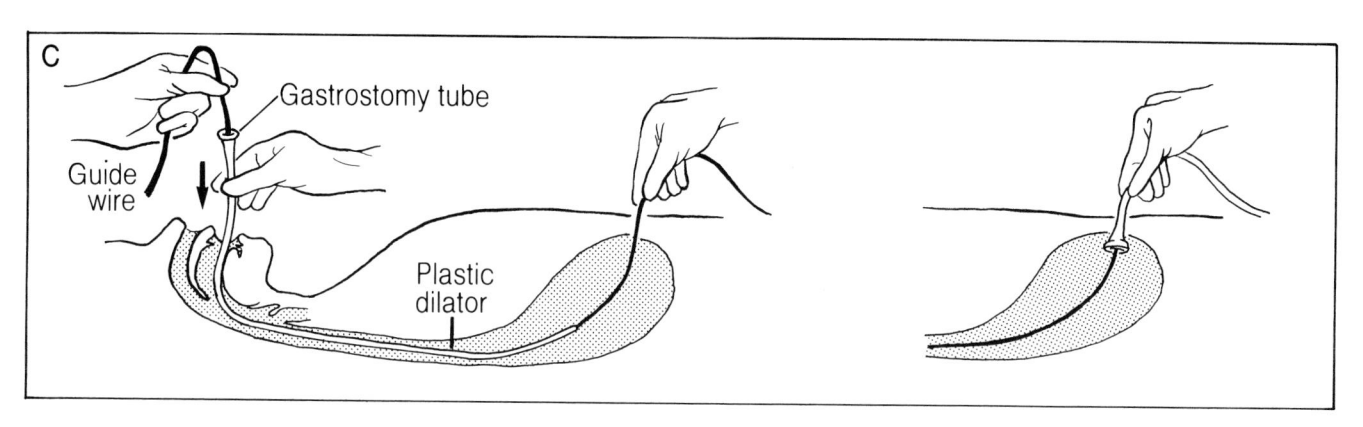

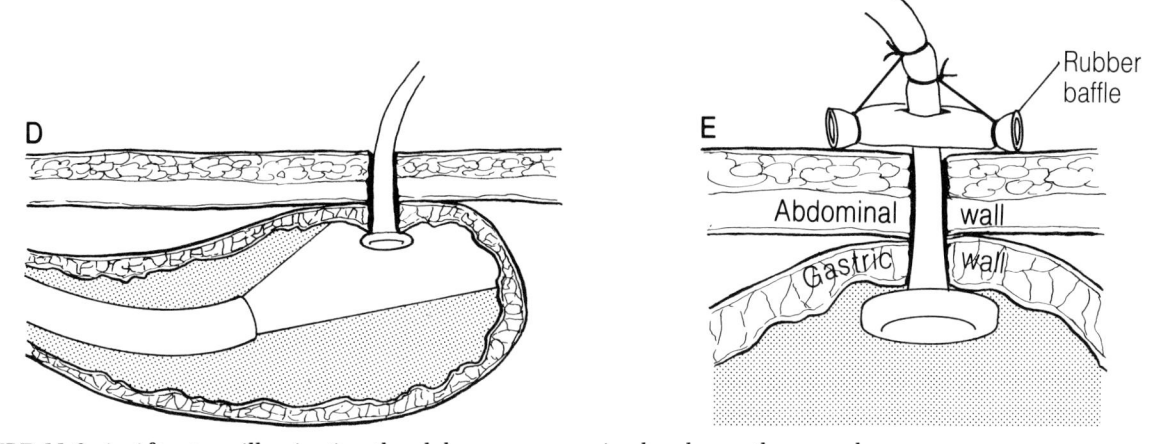

FIGURE 11-2 A. After transilluminating the abdomen, a snare is placed over the mound created by the surgeon's index finger. B. An intravenous catheter is thrust into the abdomen, the needle removed, and a flexible guide wire placed through the plastic sheath. The snare is slid off the end of the plastic catheter, and the wire is firmly snared. The guide wire, snare, and scope are pulled out as a single unit. C. In a push method of percutaneous endoscopic gastrostomy, the gastrostomy tube with its long plastic dilator is passed over the guide wire and through the mouth. The endoscopist pushes the catheter until the tapered dilator appears through the skin, at which point the surgeon grasps and pulls the entire unit through the abdominal wall. D. The tube is guided into place under endoscopic vision to bring the tube up against the gastric wall without tension. E. Distal migration is prevented with a transverse baffle. The baffle and tube are secured in place with two to three stout sutures.

The internal flange of the tube should be close to the gastric wall but under no tension. The stomach is then evacuated of all air, and the endoscope is removed. A transverse baffle is slid down over the gastrostomy tube, externally, and placed in loose coaptation with the abdominal wall. The baffle and tube are secured to the skin.

While there are many sutureless methods of skin approximation, nothing prevents tube dislodgement as effectively as three heavy sutures. The tube exit site is then covered with a sterile dressing, and the bulk of the tube is rolled up under this dressing so that the patient has nothing to grab. If the connector is left ouside the dressing, a nurse can connect the tube for early feeding without exposing the tube to accidental dislodgement.

Postoperative Care

The most important feature in postoperative care is thorough instruction of the patient and family about tube care and the feeding regimen. With a good educational program, PEG can safely be performed on an outpatient basis. The patient resumes liquids when pharyngeal anesthesia has worn off and is started on tube feedings the next day. It is generally advisable to check gastric residual volumes during the first 24 h after initiating tube feedings to make sure that the stomach is emptying normally. If residuals are low, a blenderized diet can immediately be instituted. The exit site is inspected for evidence of cellulitis the day after tube placement, and a light dressing is replaced. The sutures are removed 1 to 2 weeks postoperatively because a good tract should be formed by this time. The tube is replaced on a 3- to 12-monthly interval, depending upon the manufacturer's recommendations. Latex tubes require frequent changing (every 3 months), and silicone tubes may be left in for as long as 1 year without degradation.

Complications

The most serious complications of PEG are intraperitoneal leakage and early tube dislodgement.[7] A Gastrografin study through the tube will generally make the diagnosis of a leak and determine whether the leak is contained. If severe peritonitis or a large fistula is noted, immediate laparotomy is mandatory. Occasionally, a small leak of gastric contents will cause localized peritonitis around the exit site. This latter problem can generally be treated with antibiotics and observation, reserving laparotomy for the patient who fails to improve while receiving antibiotics.

Early tube extrusion is rare if the tube is adequately secured to the abdominal wall. Should this occur immediately post-PEG, it is the judgment of this author that exploration is warranted. If the tube becomes dislodged between 2 and 7 days postoperatively, it may be acceptable to manage the patient with nasogastric decompression and intravenous antibiotics, observing for the development of peritonitis. When the surgeon believes that a tract may have formed, usually greater than 5 days postoperatively, he or she may elect to try passing a Foley catheter gently into the stomach. Under these circumstances, it is essential that a Gastrografin study be obtained before initiating tube feedings. After 2 weeks, a well-formed tract will be present in all patients, except those with severe immunologic or nutritional deficiencies.

The most common postoperative problems are relatively benign. Postoperative pneumoperitoneum is a frequent finding, is rarely symptomatic, and generally should be treated only with reassurance.[8] Exit site infection occurs in 30 percent of patients if antibiotic prophylaxis is omitted and 7 percent of patients if antibiotics are used.[9] Necrotizing fasciitis has been reported and requires tube removal and wide local debridement.[10] Intense peristomal pain often indicates a subfascial abscess, which usually requires tube removal and drainage to heal. Another rare complication of PEG is tube migration down the gastrointestinal tract, with resultant small bowel obstruction. This can be avoided by keeping an external baffle on the gastrostomy tube at all times and making sure that all elements of the tube are removed at the time of tube change or extraction.

Alternate Techniques

The most common radically different approach to PEG utilizes a Hickman catheter-type introducer set to place the tube directly in the stomach.[11] In this procedure, the stomach is inflated, a needle and guide wire are percutaneously placed in the stomach, and the tract is dilated to allow placement of a 20-French peel-away sheath. The dilator and guide wire are removed, a Foley catheter is passed through the sheath, and the sheath is peeled away. The balloon is inflated and pulled into gentle apposition with the gastric wall. The major disadvantage of this technique is that attempts to dilate the percutaneous tract may push the stomach away from the abdominal wall, rendering the procedure more technically difficult.

Despite the theoretic hazards of pharyngeal contamination, the transoral route of tube placement is preferred by the majority of surgeons and gastroenterologists.

PERCUTANEOUS ENDOSCOPIC JEJUNOSTOMY (PEJ)

There are many situations under which jejunostomy is preferable to gastrostomy. These indications have been discussed previously. Various manufacturers have developed coaxial systems that allow gastric decompression through a large PEG tube and enteral nutrition through a small mercury-weighted feeding tube that is passed through the PEG, out of the stomach, and into the small bowel. While it was initially thought that these tubes would help prevent frequent episodes of aspiration occurring in this patient population, it soon became apparent that aspiration was just as frequent during jejunal feeding as during gastric feeding.[12,13] Furthermore, it became apparent that vomiting frequently resulted from the jejunal tube retracting into the stomach.

In the author's experience, the best indication for PEJ is the alert, otherwise functional patient with severe postoperative gastric atony, frequently resulting from pancreatic cancer, pancreatoduodenectomy, or vagotomy.

LAPAROSCOPICALLY GUIDED ENTERAL FEEDING ACCESS

Until recently, the only alternative to percutaneous enteral access was to create a gastrostomy or jejunostomy through a laparotomy incision. Laparoscopic techniques can accomplish the same results as these open procedures, but they are associated with little pain, a short ileus, and few infections. Methods are available to place temporary and permanent gastrostomies laparoscopically and to do jejunostomies.

Laparoscopically Guided Feeding Jejunostomy

Gastrostomy feedings carry the risk of reflux and aspiration. In addition, it is difficult to advance patients rapidly to an optimal level of enteral nutrition because of the variable ability of the stomach to accept feeding. Recent work seems to show improved recovery of head-injured patients when jejunostomy feedings are used instead of gastrostomy feedings.[14] For these reasons, jejunostomy may offer an advantage over PEG. The PEJ has been used but has not been reliable in permanent placement of the tube into the jejunum. Recent series have demonstrated tube migration in 15 to 35 percent of cases.[12,13] Frequently, the tube curls back into the stomach, and one is left with an elaborate PEG. Operative jejunostomy incurs the problems of ileus, infection, and pain, as outlined previously. Laparoscopic jejunostomy allows enteral feeding without the risk of reflux and aspiration, and without the drawbacks of open procedures.

TECHNIQUE

After administration of a preoperative dose of a broad-spectrum antibiotic, patients are brought to the operating room and placed under general anesthesia. Standard methods are employed to create a pneumoperitoneum. A 10-mm laparoscopic port is placed through the umbilicus, and a video laparoscope is inserted. The peritoneal cavity is inspected to ascertain that the left upper quadrant (LUQ) and proximal jejunum is free of pathologic findings and suitable for placement of a jejunostomy tube. After this is done, additional ports are placed, a 5-mm port in the upper midline and a 10-mm port in the right lower quadrant (RLQ). The laparoscope is then moved to the RLQ position, and the umbilical port becomes the primary operating site (Fig. 11-3). The surgeon is positioned on the patient's right and operates via a video monitor on the patient's left; the assistant works in an opposite fashion from the patient's left side. The ligament of Treitz is identified by "walking" along the small bowel with grasping forceps, and a suitable site in the jejunum 12 to 18 in distal to the ligament is brought up to the abdominal wall in the LUQ.

The jejunum is then anchored to the abdominal wall in one of two ways. The assistant may pass a silk suture through the abdominal wall on a straight needle, which the surgeon grasps inside the abdomen and passes through the bowel and back out through the abdominal wall. The assistant then ties the suture on the outside. Alter-

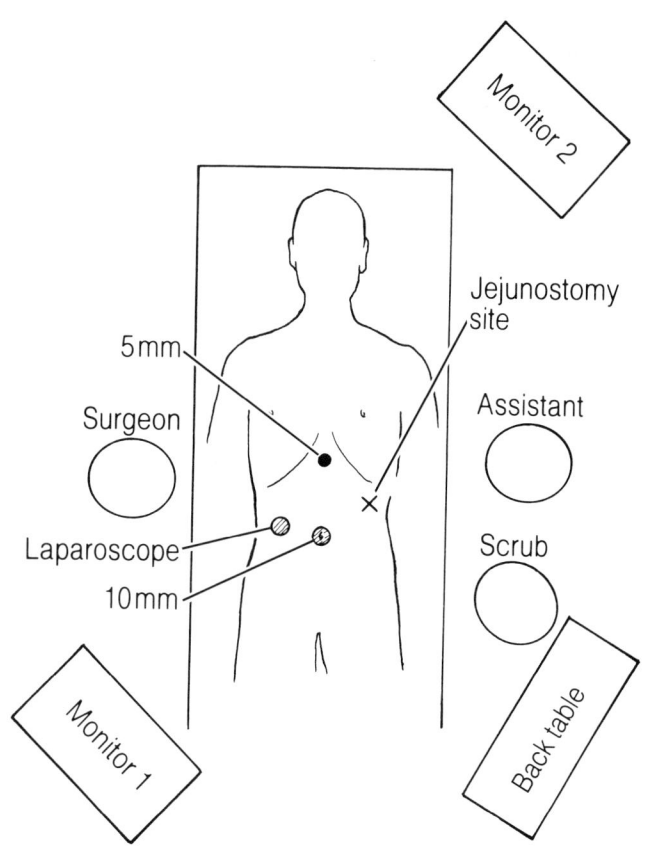

FIGURE 11-3 Port position for laparoscopic jejunostomy. The surgeon stands on the patient's right and the first assistant, on the patient's left. After the pneumoperitoneum is obtained, the telescope is placed in the right lower quadrant 10-mm port.

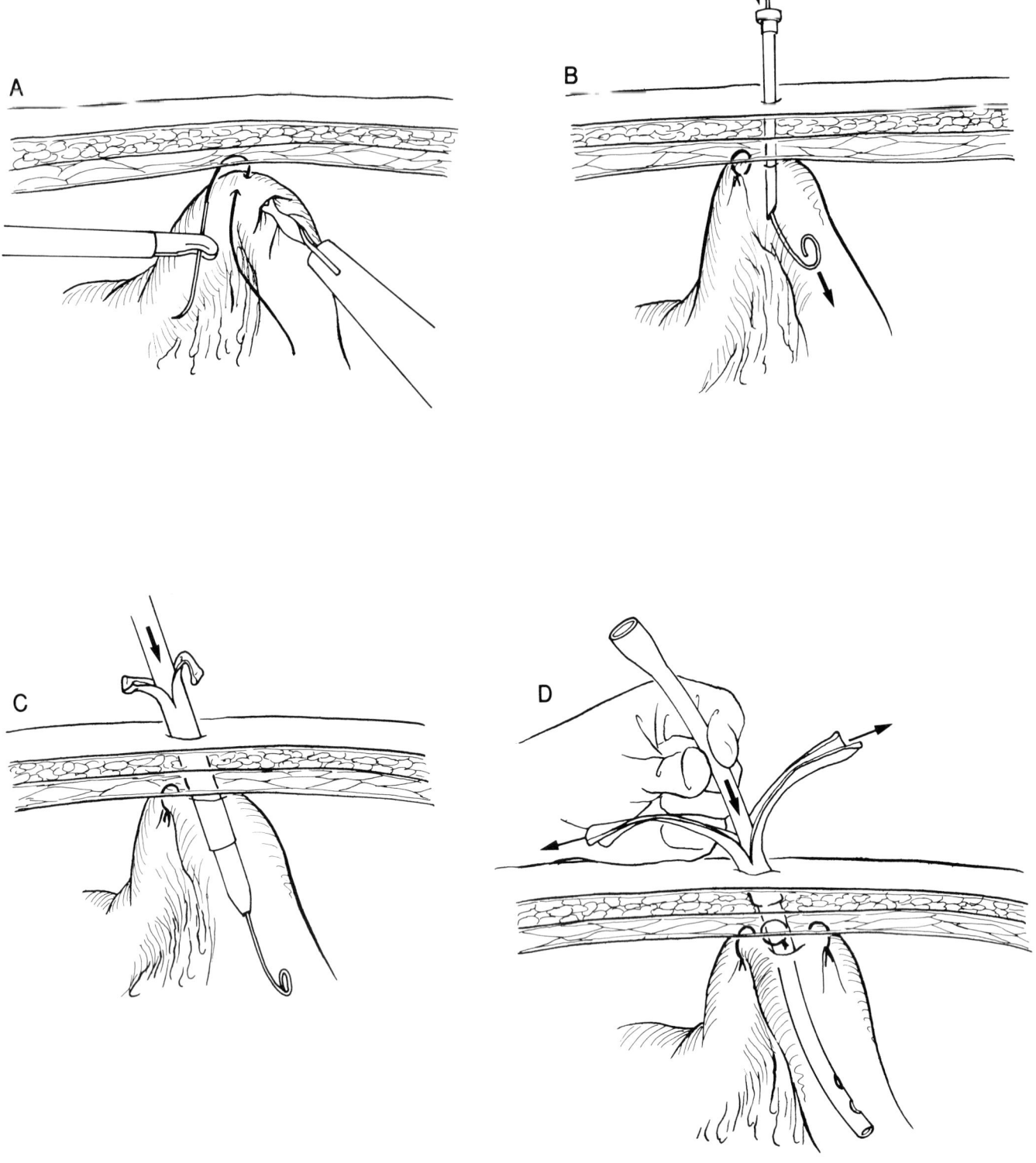

FIGURE 11-4 A. The small bowel may be secured to the abdominal wall with a single interrupted suture placed through the peritoneum from the inside and secured with a knot tied extracorporeally and pushed into place. B. The jejunostomy tube is placed in three steps. A needle is passed transcutaneously into the small bowel, and a floppy-tipped guide wire is placed through the needle. C. The needle is removed, and a 10-French peel-away catheter and dilator are passed over the wire into the small bowel. D. The dilator is removed, an 8-French red rubber catheter is passed through the peel-away catheter, and the sheath is then removed. Additional sutures are placed between the jejunum and peritoneum to add additional security to the jejunostomy.

natively, a suture may be placed internally to the underside of the abdominal wall, securing the jejunum to it (see Fig. 11-4). After the jejunum is securely anchored to the underside of the wall, a standard 12-French venous introducer kit is used to gain access to the jejunum. The needle from the kit is passed through the abdominal wall so that it enters the jejunum just medial to the previously placed suture. The guide wire is then placed through the needle into the lumen of the bowel, and the needle is removed. The dilator and introducer are subsequently placed over the guide wire. A 12-French red rubber catheter can then be placed through the introducer and guided distally in the jejunum by the surgeon. The peel-apart introducer is removed, leaving the catheter in place. The surgeon tacks the jejunum to the peritoneum with several sutures of 3–0 Maxon or its equivalent, which can be tied either intra- or extracorporeally. This ensures a good seal of jejunum to abdominal wall and helps prevent pulling away of the bowel from the wall. The tube is externally secured to the abdominal wall, incisions are closed, and dressings are placed. Feedings may be begun immediately.

RESULTS

Twenty-three patients with inability to feed themselves as a result of either oropharyngeal malignancy or neurologic dysfunction underwent laparoscopic feeding jejunostomy placement using this technique.[4] The procedures lasted an average of 1 hour, and the later procedures were performed in less than 45 minutes. Two patients had superficial skin abscesses near the tube or transabdominal suture. These were easily treated with incision and drainage and appropriate antibiotics. This complication is probably caused by passage of a contaminated Keith needle through the abdominal wall and did not occur in the last six patients, in whom the anchoring suture was placed intraabdominally. All patients advanced rapidly to full nutritional support within 1 or 2 days. None of the patients suffered reflux or aspiration. No other complications were noted.

Laparoscopically Guided Gastrostomy

Laparoscopic-guided gastrostomy tubes may be placed at the same time as jejunostomy. The gastrostomy is performed in a fashion analogous to the method reported previously, using a Russell PEG kit (Wilson-Cook, Bloomington, IN). This allows placement of a 16-French Foley catheter in the stomach. The stomach is held up to the abdominal wall and is entered via a needle passed through the abdominal wall. The guide wire, dilators, and introducer are inserted into the stomach, followed by the tube. Because the Foley catheter has a balloon on it, no sutures are necessary to anchor the stomach to the abdominal wall. Others have reported a similar technique but with a purse-string suture placed in the stomach in the manner of a Stamm gastrostomy.[15]

The development of endoscopic staplers (Endo-GIA, US Surgical Norwalk, CT) has made it possible to perform a permanent (Janeway) gastrostomy. After a pneumoperitoneum is created and a laparoscope is inserted, two 5-mm ports are placed in the left and right midclavicular lines at the level of the umbilicus (Fig. 11-5). The site for the gastrostomy tube in the LUQ is selected by palpating the LUQ of the abdomen and lifting the stomach with grasping forceps to determine the location which will not require excessive tension. A 12-mm port is then placed at this location. The endoscopic stapler is inserted and the stomach held by the graspers so that the stapler can be applied across the front wall of the stomach near the greater curvature. In this way, a 2.5-cm gastric tube is created when the instrument is fired. If a longer tube is desired, the stapler may be reapplied and refired (Fig. 11-6). A 5-mm grasper is then passed down the 12-mm port, and the gastric tube is pulled up into the port. The port and tube are then pulled out to the skin. The pneumoperitoneum is released to a pressure low enough to allow the anterior stomach wall to come up against the peritoneum. The gastric tube is opened and sutured to the skin. A 24-French gastrostomy tube is inserted, the bulb inflated, and the tube pulled up until the bulb is felt to be against the underside of the abdominal wall. Incisions are closed and dressed in the usual manner. Lathrop and colleagues[16] report two patients successfully treated in this manner.

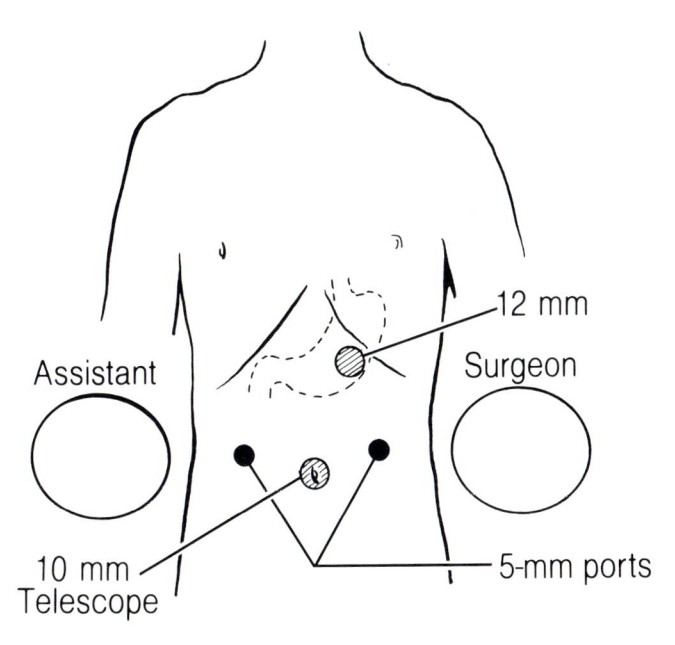

FIGURE 11-5 Port placement for Janeway gastrostomy. In this situation, the surgeon stands on the patient's left and the first assistant on the patient's right.

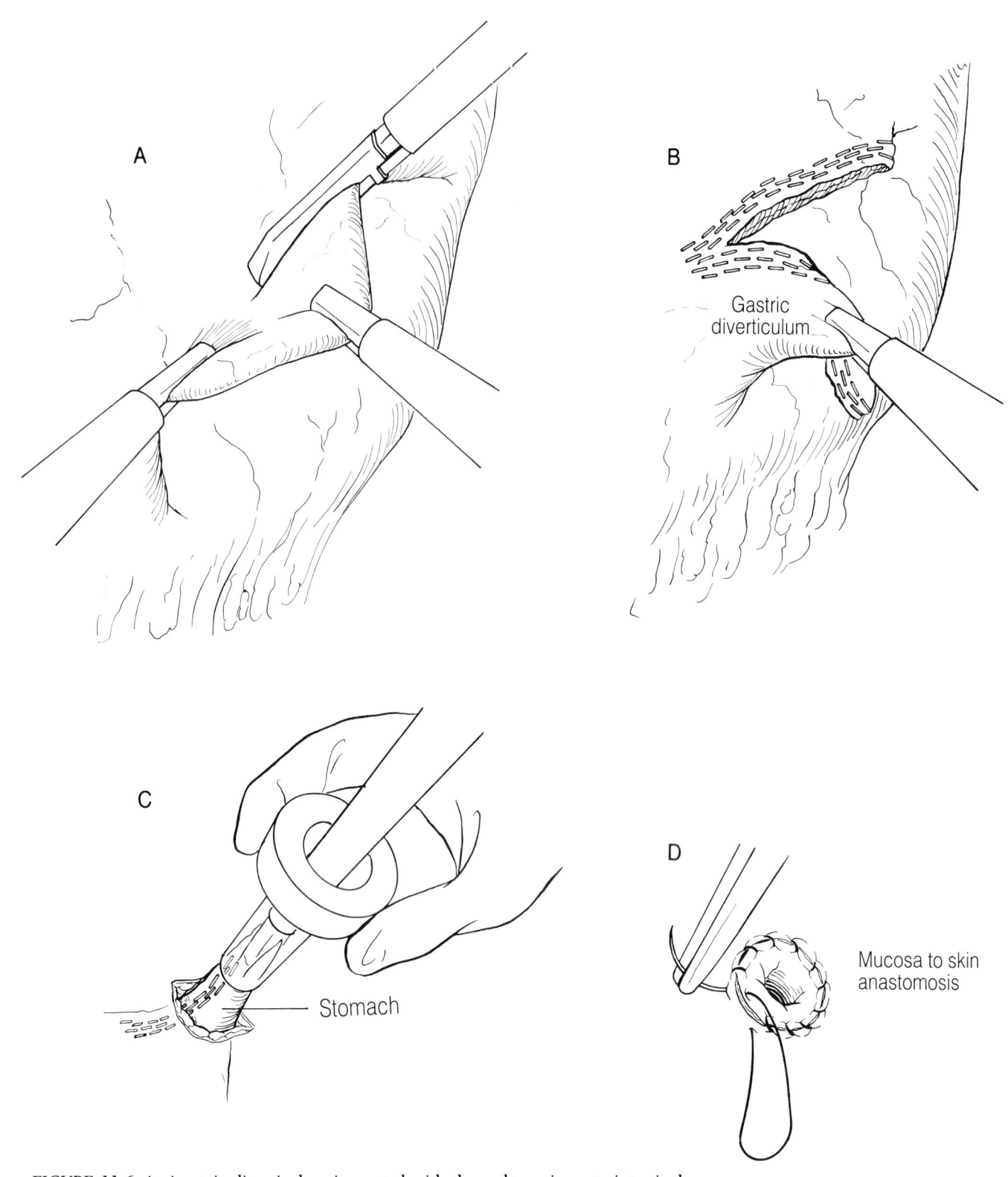

FIGURE 11-6 A. A gatric diverticulum is created with the endoscopic gastrointestinal stapling device. B. Firing of the stapler creates a gastric diverticulum. C. The diverticulum so created is pulled out through the 12-mm port, the port is removed, the diverticulum is opened. D. The diverticulum is sutured securely at the cutaneous level. A tube is placed through the stoma and into the stomach during the initial postoperative period to decompress the stomach.

REFERENCES

1. Shellito PC, Malt RA: Tube gastrostomy. *Ann Surg* 1985; 201:180–185.
2. Ponsky JL, Gauderer MWL: Percutaneous endoscopic gastrostomy: A nonoperative technique for feeding gastrostomy. *Gastrointest Endosc* 1981; 27:9–11.
3. Albert E: Eine neue Methode der Jejunostomie. *Wien Med Wochenschr* 1894; 44:57–59.
4. Sangster W, Swanstrom L: Laparoscopic feeding jejunostomy. *Surg Endosc*, in press.
5. Hunter JG, Laurentano L, Shellito PC: Percutaneous endoscopic gastrostomy in head and neck cancer patients. *Ann Surg* 1989; 210:42–46.
6. Kelsey PB: Percutaneous endoscopic gastrostomy. The "push" technique, in Ponsky JL (ed): *Techniques of Percutaneous Gastrostomy*. New York, Igaku-Shoin, 1988, pp 33–38.
7. Ponsky JL: Percutaneous endoscopic stomas. *Surg Clin North Am* 1989; 69:1227–1236.
8. Gottfried EB, Plumser AB, Clair MR: Pneumoperitoneum following percutaneous endoscopic gastrostomy: A prospective study. *Gastrointest Endosc* 1986; 32:397–399.
9. Jain NK, Larson DE, Schroeder KW, et al: Antibiotic prophylaxis for percutaneous endoscopic gastrostomy. *Ann Intern Med* 1987; 107:824–828.
10. Martindale R, Witte M, Hodges G, et al: Necrotizing fasciitis as a complication of percutaneous endoscopic gastrostomy. *JPEN J Parenter Enteral Nutr* 1987; 11:583–588.
11. Russell TR, Brotman M, Norris F: Percutaneous gastrostomy: A new simplified and cost-effective technique. *Am J Surg* 1984; 148:132–137.
12. DiSario JA, Foutch PG, Sanowski RA: Poor results with percutaneous endoscopic jejunostomy. *Gastrointest Endosc* 1990; 36:257–260.
13. Wolfsen HC, Kozarek RA, Ball TJ, et al: Tube dysfunction following percutaneous endoscopic gastrostomy and jejunostomy. *Gastrointest Endosc* 1990; 36:261–263.
14. Pennings J, Borzotta A, Bohley M, et al: Nutritional support in closed head injury: The role of jejunal feeding. Presented at the Annual Meeting of the Oregon Chapter of the American College of Surgeons, Sept, 1991
15. Reiner DS, Leitman IM, Ward RJ: Laparoscopic Stamm gastrostomy with gastropexy. *Surg Laparosc Endosc* 1991; 1:189–192.
16. Lathrop JC, Felix EJ, Lauber D: Laparoscopic Janeway gastrostomy utilizing an endoscopic stapling device. *J Laparoendosc Surg* 1991; 1:335–339.

Chapter 12

Laparoscopic Treatment of Peptic Ulcer Disease

Namir Katkhouda / Jean Mouiel

It is estimated that more than three to four percent of the Occidental population will eventually develop peptic ulcer disease, representing, therefore, a significant public health concern. The medical treatment for this disease is presently well standardized and very successful in a large number of patients. However, there are cases in which certain ulcers are refractory to medical management, causing considerable disability and impairment in the quality of life of these patients. The development of laparoscopic surgical techniques has expanded the therapeutic options available to the modern physician.

The first vagotomy was performed by Jaboulay in 1901 in Lyon. Subsequently, Latarjet and Wertheimer[1] evaluated gastric denervation in dogs and humans and reported their results in a large clinical series. Their work led to a proposal by Dragstedt and Owen[2] in 1943 for truncal vagotomy in cases of chronic duodenal ulcers; however, after the observation that the division of the vagus nerve frequently led to gastric stasis, a drainage procedure was added. The drainage procedures, including gastroenterostomy and pyloroplasty, frequently resulted in dumping syndrome, diarrhea, and other complications.

Other selective vagotomies were developed by Jackson[3] and others in an effort to control the acid-producing mucosa while avoiding stasis. These techniques were accompanied by the same problems of dumping and diarrhea that were associated with truncal vagotomy and included infarction of the lesser curvature of the stomach. As a result, a highly selective vagotomy was developed by Johnston[4] to fashion a more anatomically pleasing procedure. The results of this procedure have subsequently been questioned, however, with authors reporting a high ulcer recurrence rate after 10 to 15 years.[5] Furthermore, the dissection of the anterior fibers of the vagus nerve is time consuming and not well suited to the laparoscopic approach.

The technique of posterior vagotomy with anterior seromyotomy achieves the same goals as highly selective vagotomy and relies on the fact that branches of the vagus nerve run immediately beneath the serosa, for 1 to 2 cm from the lesser curvature.[6] This procedure achieves effective control of duodenal ulcer disease in a majority of patients[7-9] and seems to equate with a low incidence of dumping or gastric atony.[8-10]

Since the early 1970s, another treatment for peptic ulcer disease has been the use of H_2 blockers, and these pharmaceutical agents have limited the number of peptic ulcer operations performed.[11] Most cases of peptic ulcer disease currently are controlled by medical management, with the surgeon only intervening when bleeding, obstruction, or perforation is present.[12]

The benefits of the laparoscopic approach in the treatment of other disease processes became evident and were applied to the treatment of peptic ulcer disease. This was done by the author (NK) for the first time in Nice in 1989.[13] This chapter will address both the elective treatment of peptic ulcer disease in the acute setting in the presence of perforation and peritonitis.

ELECTIVE TREATMENT BY VIDEO LAPAROSCOPY OF PEPTIC ULCER DISEASE REFRACTORY TO MEDICAL MANAGEMENT

The procedure of choice in this setting is the posterior truncal vagotomy with an anterior seromyotomy. Other authors have performed laparoscopic vagotomy and pyloromyotomy[14] as well as thoracoscopic and highly selective vagotomy.[15] However, it is evident that the anterior seromyotomy is ideally suited to the laparoscopic approach. The operating room setup, the positioning of the surgeon and team, and the necessary equipment for this technique will be described.

Posterior Truncal Vagotomy with Anterior Seromyotomy

PREPARATION OF THE PATIENT

Before surgery, the risks and benefits of the procedure are explained to the patient, and an informed consent is obtained. It is of prime importance to obtain an upper gastrointestinal (GI) endoscopy and a barium upper GI study. The purpose of these studies is to identify the ulcer, document the gastric morphology, and eliminate certain contraindications, such as an associated pyloric stenosis. Gastric pH studies, with basal and maximal acid output, are obtained, as are gastric stimulation tests using pentagastrin or insulin. A gastrin level is required to rule out Zollinger-Ellison syndrome. In addition, the patient is informed of the necessity of postoperative endoscopy, including additional upper GI endoscopies during follow-up to assess the long-term success of the technique. The patient is admitted the day before or the morning of the procedure and fasts after midnight. No preoperative antibiotics are necessary. A Foley catheter is generally not required, but it is important to ensure that the patient voids immediately before surgery.

OPERATING ROOM SETUP

With the patient placed in the supine position and both legs in stirrups, the surgeon stands between the legs of the patient with the first assistant to the right. The second assistant stands to the left of the surgeon. The monitor and insufflation pump are placed to the right of the head of the patient so that the surgeon has a good view of the screen. With this positioning, the surgeon is able to operate using both hands. This would not be feasible if the surgeon were in a lateral position. Ideally, a second monitor should be placed to the left of the head of the patient to allow the assistant on the left also to have a good view of the procedure. The patient is prepared similar to a full laparotomy because, in the event that the laparoscopy is aborted, the procedure can be converted to a laparotomy. A nasogastric (NG) tube is inserted to empty the stomach.

EQUIPMENT

As in open cases, only the necessary instruments should be present on the instrument table. It is imperative to have a 0° 10-mm telescope (Storz, Tutlingen, Germany). It may also be helpful, although not necessary, to have a 30° forward oblique telescope, which will be very useful when the surgeon needs to obtain an acute viewing angle. The camera should be of good quality and high definition and connected to an adequate light source. It is also beneficial to use a sophisticated insufflation pump that can rapidly insufflate up to 9.9 L/min into the intraabdominal cavity. As a rule, the surgeon will use the left hand to grasp the tissue and the right hand to operate. For this reason, it is essential to have a selection of atraumatic graspers, with or without teeth but generally without any ratchet, to permit maximum mobility in the intraabdominal cavity. Three graspers, including an endoscopic Babcock grasper, are sufficient to perform this procedure. The surgeon should also have available coagulating endoscopic scissors and an electrocautery hook.

Five trocars are necessary for this procedure. Three 5-mm trocars, one 10-mm trocar, and one 12-mm trocar that can be reduced to a 5- or 10-mm size multiple- or single-clip applier are also useful in this laparoscopic technique. In addition, a 3- or 5-mm needle holder and 15-mm ski-shaped needle with a 15-cm Prolene thread are recommended.

CREATION OF THE PERITONEUM AND POSITION OF THE TROCARS (FIG. 12-1)

After an umbilical puncture, employing the usual safety maneuvers, a pneumoperitoneum is created. The first trocar (10 mm) is inserted to accommodate the scope and is placed 3 cm above and to the right of the umbilicus. This position allows a full abdominal exploration first to assess the feasibility of the procedure. The second trocar (5 mm) is placed in a subxiphoid position and is used to insert the grasper and the irrigation–aspiration device. Two additional trocars, the lateral trocars, are used to insert the atrau-

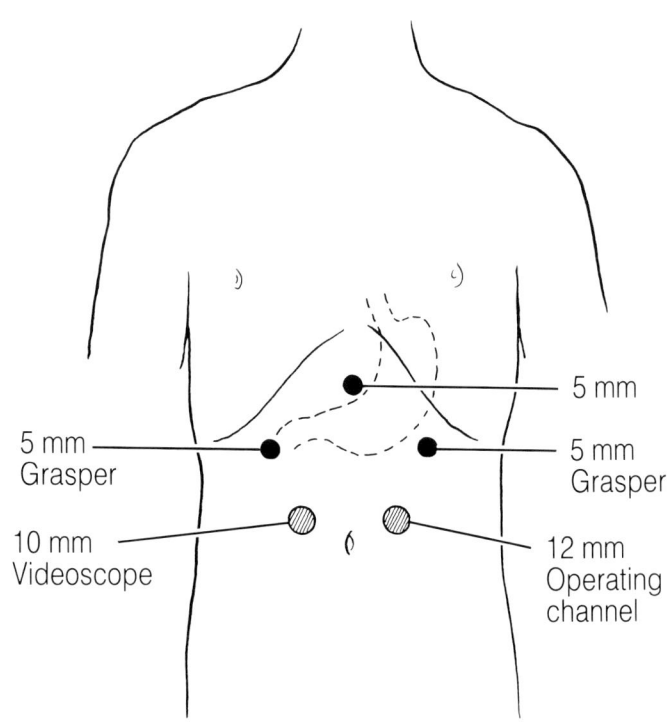

FIGURE 12-1 Position of trocars. 10-mm videoendoscope. 12-mm operating channel. 5-mm graspers. 5-mm palpation or irrigation device. 5-mm grasper.

matic graspers into the abdomen. The last trocar is the operative trocar (12 mm), which will be used for the insertion of the other instruments. This trocar is placed in a position symmetric to the scope trocar or 3 cm above and to the left of the umbilicus. After all are in position, the trocars will form a polygon. These sites of insertion are the same as those used for laparoscopic fundoplication procedures.

PROCEDURE

Posterior truncal vagotomy It is essential at the outset to identify the key landmarks in the region and quickly expose the hiatus. The first step is to retract the left lobe of the liver upward and locate the avascular plane (Fig. 12-2). The left hand of the surgeon grasps the avascular portion with an atraumatic grasper. Using a coagulating scissors, this tissue is divided. To the left of the liver, the right diaphragmatic crus is identified and will be the third anatomic landmark. The crus is grasped with an atraumatic grasper, and the periesophageal peritoneum is carefully opened. Occasionally, it is necessary to mobilize or manipulate the NG tube to identify the position of the esophagus. In some instances, the introduction of a gastroscope is beneficial. The peritoneum is now fully opened, and the anatomic space between the internal aspect of the right diaphragmatic crus and the left side, next to the right aspect of the esophagus, is uncovered. At the upper portion of this space, the right, or posterior, vagus will be located. In most cases, the right vagus is a single trunk that is directly on the wall of the esophagus or on the internal aspect of the right diaphragmatic crus. It is easily identified because of its size, consistency, and resistance to traction. It also has an unmistakable pearly-white color. After this trunk is identified, the surgeon searches for secondary branches, which coexist in about 5 to 10 percent of cases.

Next, the posterior truncal vagotomy is performed (Fig. 12-3) by resecting a 1-cm portion of the nerve between two clips to accomplish perfect hemostasis. The excised portion of the vagus is sent for histologic identification. One should confirm that the hiatal region has not been anatomically modified and the competency of the cardia has been maintained. This must be verified to avoid the creation of an iatrogenic hiatal hernia.

Anterior seromyotomy The anterior seromyotomy includes longitudinal section of the anterior gastric seromuscular layer, taking extreme care not to incise the gastric mucosa. This maneuver indirectly performs a hyperselective vagotomy of the anterior aspect of the stomach.

A seromyotomy is based on the anatomic principle that the anterior vagus nerve undergoes secondary gastric branching at regular intervals on the anterior aspect of the stomach. The secondary branches stem from the major trunk and dive progressively into the gastric wall. Anterior seromyotomy must be performed under strict guidelines. The incision is started at the posterior aspect of the angle of His and continues to about 1.5 cm from the lesser curvature to a region corresponding to the first branch of the *crow's foot*. This end point is located approximately 6 cm from the pylorus.

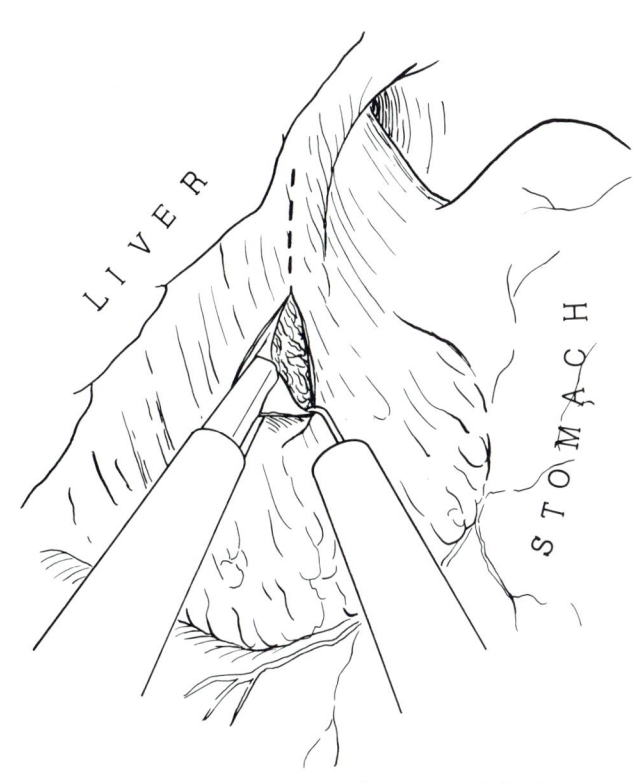

FIGURE 12-2 Opening the avascular aspect of the lesser sac.

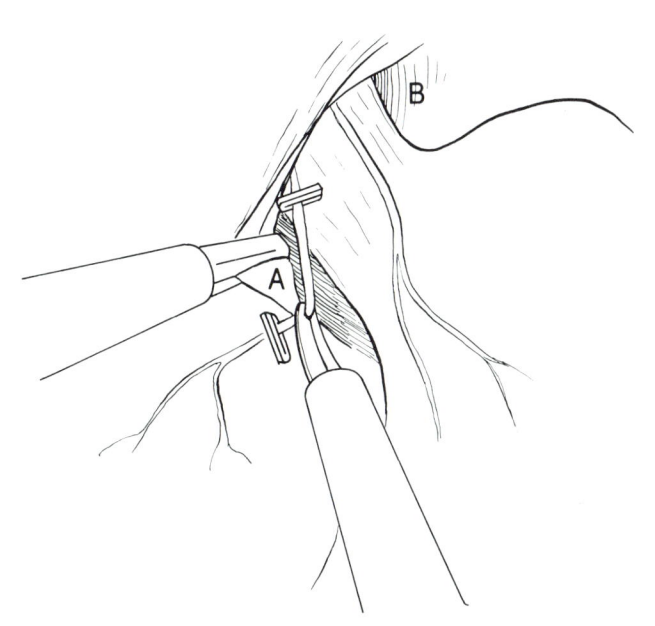

FIGURE 12-3 Right truncal vagotomy. A. Right crus. B. Left crus.

Consistently, the surgeon will encounter three different vessels running on the anterior aspect of the stomach that will need to be controlled. The first step is to mark the anterior aspect of the stomach with the electrocautery hook (Valleylab, Boulder, CO; 25 W for section and 50 W for coagulation). After the trajectory of the seromyotomy has been marked, three or four vascular structures on the anterior aspect of the stomach can be found, dissected, and clipped. This will prevent potential hemorrhage from occurring as a result of injury to these vessels (Fig. 12-4).

Next, the surgeon holds the right grasper with the left hand, and the first assistant elevates the stomach with a grasper. The surgeon uses the right hand to perform the seromyotomy, which should be performed with an electrocautery hook. The gastric mucosa will have a characteristic bluish color that is easily recognizable. Should the mucosa be incised, it should be investigated at the time of intervention by inserting methylene blue into the stomach and carefully observing any leak, which, if identified, should be closed with sutures. The seromyotomy is then extended to the first branch of the crow's foot, which should be included in that section. The seromuscular groove is closely checked with a telescope from its upper to its lowest aspects. A small seromuscular bridge may be identified, which will require sectioning. Completion of the procedure will be signified by the presence of bulging mucosa between the edges of the seromyotomy, as seen during a mucosal pyloromyotomy.

The seromyotomy should then be closed with an overlap repair (Fig. 12-5). A suture will ensure that perfect hemostasis is achieved. An overlapping closure of the edge of the seromyotomy will prevent a possible regeneration of the secondary branches that have just been transsected. It should be noted, however, that such regeneration has never been scientifically proved. At the outset of this series, the closure was performed with a running suture that was only locked twice (Fig. 12-6). We now prefer to close the seromyotomy using a clip applier (Ethicon) to shorten the operating time (Fig. 12-7).

The closure of the seromyotomy requires two layers of sutures. The surgeon introduces an 18-mm ski-shaped needle with an 18-cm suture of 3–0 Prolene. The suturing is accomplished using two needle holders, 3 and 5 mm, introduced via the 5-mm trocars. If the surgeon decides to close the seromyotomy using a stapling device, this should be introduced via a 12-mm trocar in the left periumbilical region. The edge of the stomach is grasped and approximated as the staple is placed in the appropriate position. Approximately 10 staples are necessary to obtain good closure.

At the end of the procedure, the hiatal region and the area of the seromyotomy are irrigated with an antiseptic saline. The solution is then totally aspirated, and hemostasis is checked again. The abdomen is deflated, and all the trocars are removed. The trocar incision sites are then closed with simple sutures.

Two other techniques, although not favored at our institution, will be described: the bilateral truncal vagotomy with forced balloon dilation and the posterior truncal vagotomy with an hyperselective anterior vagotomy.

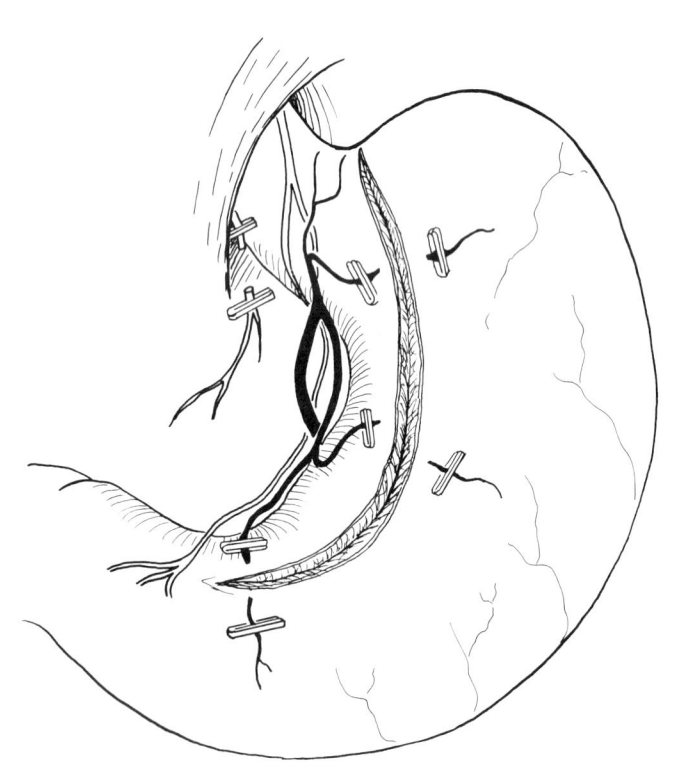

FIGURE 12-4 Anterior lesser curve seromyotomy.

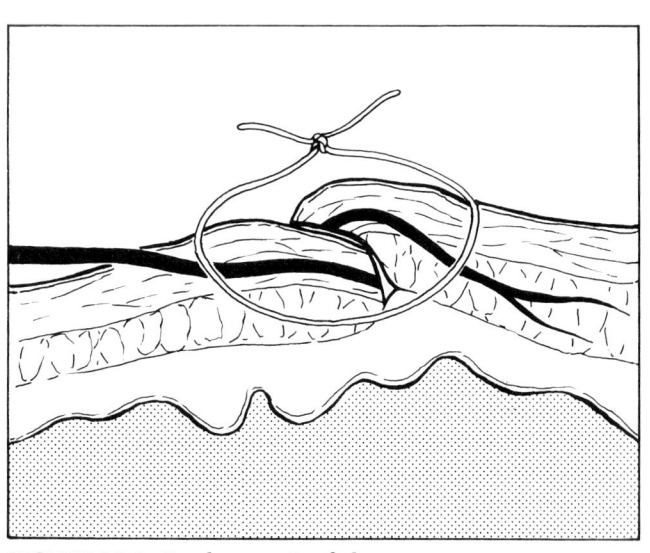

FIGURE 12-5 Overlap repair of the seromyotomy.

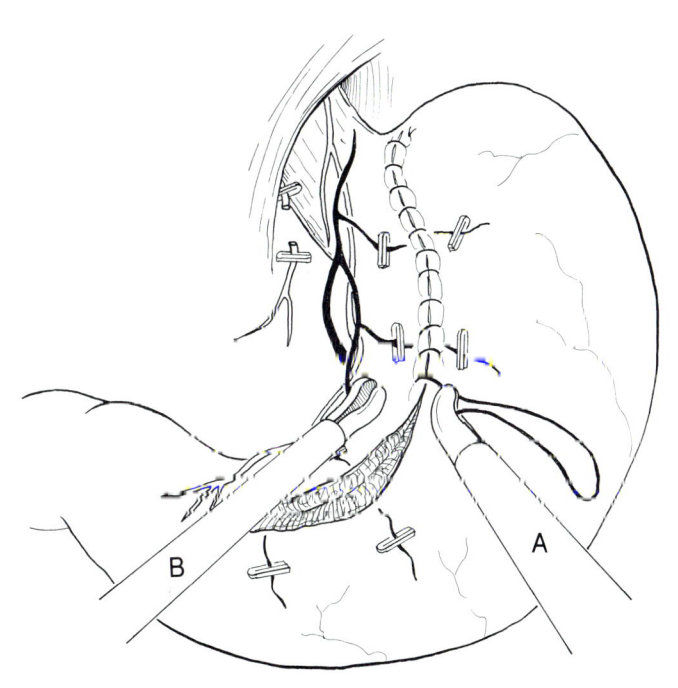

FIGURE 12-6 Suture of the seromyotomy A. 5-mm needle holder B. 3-mm needle holder.

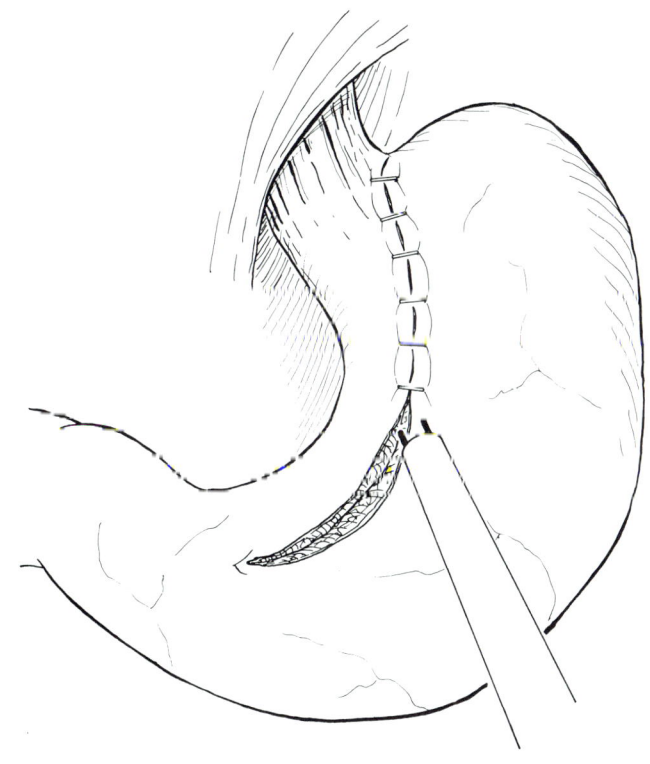

FIGURE 12-7 Closure of the seromyotomy with staples.

Bilateral Truncal Vagotomy with Forced Pyloric Endoscopic Balloon Dilation (Fig. 12-8)

The posterior truncal vagotomy was detailed in the previous section; therefore, it will not be described here. The anterior truncal vagotomy is begun by denuding about 5 cm of the anterior aspect of the gastroesophageal junction. The procedure is started in the hiatal region next to the left crus of the diaphragm. It is imperative that the esophagus in this area be "rolled away" to identify all the secondary neural branches, in particular the *criminal nerve of Grassi*, which is found on the left lateral aspect of the esophagus, or occasionally on the posterior aspect. To roll the esophagus, the NG tube should be removed because it will stent the esophagus too tightly. Under no circumstances should the esophagus be held by the laparoscopic grasper. It should be pushed away or pulled with the grasper in the closed position to avoid potential iatrogenic tears. The various neural branches can be easily identified with the magnified view provided by the telescope. It is of primary importance to obtain good visualization of the left lateral aspect of the esophagus by using a 30° forward oblique telescope.

After the bilateral truncal vagotomy is complete, the pyloric dilation is performed. The pyloric muscle is dilated for 45 s using a balloon introduced under laparoscopic control. This maneuver is repeated several times. The patient should be informed that, in 20 percent of cases, some degree of pyloric stenosis will result. Such endoscopic dilation is not as successful as a surgical pyloroplasty and will probably require repetition during the postoperative

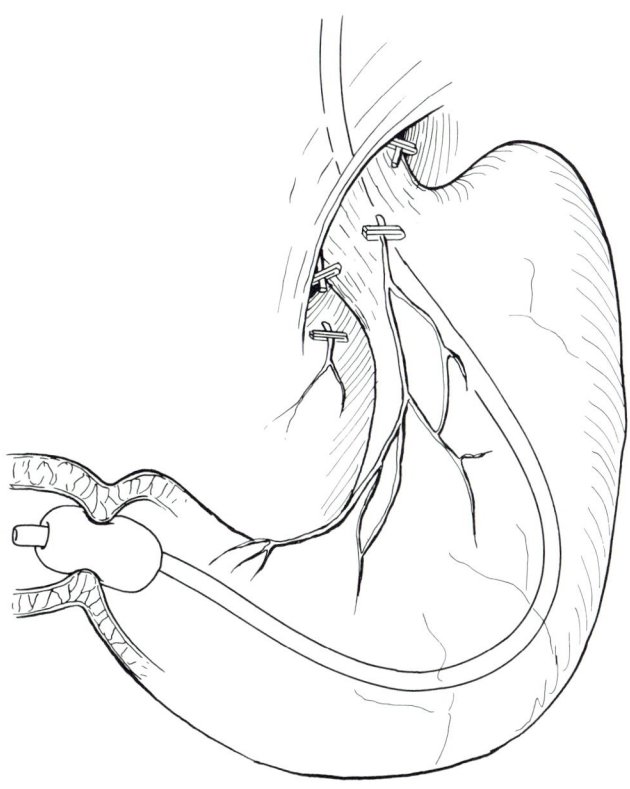

FIGURE 12-8 Bilateral truncal vagotomy and balloon pyloric dilatation.

period. Additional side effects of the bilateral vagotomy, such as diarrhea and the dumping syndrome, have prevented this procedure from becoming the treatment of choice for peptic ulcer disease.

Posterior Truncal Vagotomy with Hyperselective Anterior Vagotomy

In this procedure, an anterior hyperselective vagotomy is added to the truncal vagotomy described earlier (Fig. 12-9). This is done by first identifying the crow's foot and placing the greater curvature under tension by introducing a large-bore NG tube that spreads the gastric pouch. The lesser curvature can then be freed at the level of the first branch of the crow's foot. The dissection is carried proximally, ligating all the vessels traveling with the anterior nerve of Latarjet. This should be done bimanually with the left hand using a holding grasper and the right hand using the electrocautery hook or the dissecting scissors. All the secondary neural branches are selectively clipped. It is imperative to free the anterior aspect of the esophagus and expose the posterior aspect of the angle of His to identify and divide the nerve(s) of Grassi, if present. This is a long and difficult dissection, particularly if a sudden hematoma should occur, causing injury to the anterior vagus, in which case the equivalent of an iatrogenic bilateral truncal vagotomy would be required.

TREATMENT OF PERITONITIS FROM A PERFORATED ANTERIOR DUODENAL ULCER

Suspected intraperitoneal perforation of an anterior duodenal bulb ulcer is a good indication for laparoscopic diagnostic repair.[16] Laparoscopy can confirm the diagnosis by visualization of the perforation, which is generally located on the anterior aspect of the duodenum. Occasionally, numerous inflammatory adhesions will be found that seal either the ulcer with omentum or the gallbladder. First, peritoneal irrigation of the abdominal quadrants, including the pouch of Douglas, should be performed. Then the NG tube is placed in the appropriate position to empty the stomach. In some cases, it may be worthwhile to include definitive treatment of the peptic ulcer disease, that is, posterior truncal vagotomy and anterior seromyotomy.

Technique (Fig. 12-10)

After insertion of the telescope at the umbilicus, the subxiphoid 5-mm trocar is placed to introduce a manipulator to explore the intraabdominal cavity above the transverse colon. A second trocar, to be used for a grasping forceps, is inserted below the right subcostal margin. A final trocar is situated three fingers above and to the left of the umbilicus for passing the various dissecting instruments (scissors, hook, and needle holders).

First, the anterior aspect of the duodenum is identified

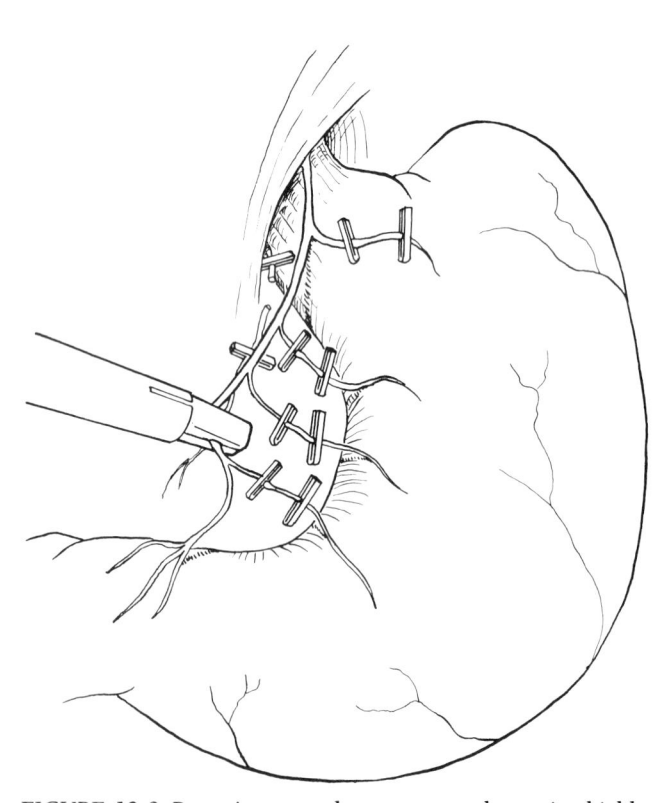

FIGURE 12-9 Posterior truncal vagotomy and anterior highly selective vagotomy.

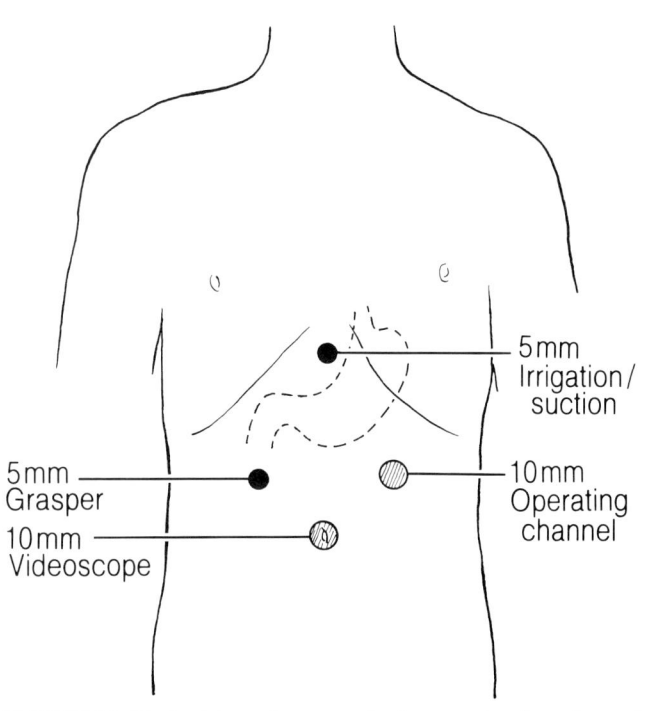

FIGURE 12-10 Position of trocars during repair of perforated ulcers. 10-mm umbilicus (videoendoscope). 10-mm operating channel. 5-mm irrigation suction probe. 5-mm grasper.

as well as the inferior aspect of the liver. Generally, the perforation is immediately obvious on the anterior aspect of the duodenal bulb. Ideally, in cases of postpyloric perforation and to minimize potential pyloric stenosis, the perforation is simply sutured with an omental patch. Then, the suture line can be reinforced with the application of biologic glue (Tissucol, Immuno, Vienna, Austria). The surgeon should refrain from applying this glue with an air-powered gun because there is a significant risk of creating an air embolus. The procedure is completed with extensive intraperitoneal irrigation via the subxiphoid trocar. Large volumes, 9 to 10 L, of sterile saline should be used.

A drain may be placed in Morrison's pouch, which is then brought out in the right flank. Postoperatively, the NG tube is left in place for 2 days, and the patient receives antibiotics for 1 week. A surveillance upper GI endoscopy is performed to ascertain complete healing of the ulcer.

Twenty patients have been treated in this manner, resulting in no postoperative complications and 100 percent resolution of their duodenal ulcers. The mortality rate was zero.

Indications

Duodenal perforation is the best indication for laparoscopic treatment of peritonitis in this setting. The delay between the onset of the perforation, the patient's last meal, and the admission under the care of the surgeon should be less than 12 hours. In addition, the patient should not be in septic shock. This procedure is, therefore, reserved for chemical peritonitis. It should be noted that age is not a contraindication; our oldest patient was 77 years old.

RESULTS OF ELECTIVE TREATMENT OF GASTRODUODENAL ULCER BY POSTERIOR TRUNCAL VAGOTOMY AND ANTERIOR SEROMYOTOMY

Currently, we have treated over 60 patients, the majority of whom were young (average age, 33 years). All these patients had a duodenal ulcer refractory to medical treatment. In the first postoperative month, a surveillance upper GI endoscopy demonstrated resolution of the ulcer in the majority of cases, and an 80 percent decrease of gastric acid output was seen. At 6 months, 58 patients showed no recurrence of their ulcers, with continued gastric output reduction. Two patients were found to have scarring at the site of the ulcer but no evidence of active disease. At 2 years, only one patient was found to have a recurrence of peptic ulcer disease. In this series, there were no deaths, and morbidity consisted of a pneumothorax, three bezoars, and one gastroesophageal reflux in a psychiatric patient. This reflux, however, may have been present before the surgery but was undiagnosed.

CONCLUSION

Posterior vagotomy and anterior seromyotomy is an elegant and effective treatment for chronic peptic ulcer disease refractory to medical treatment. It is a quick and simple procedure with easily reproducible results. Furthermore, surgeons can be well trained in the technique using porcine models. On the other hand, hyperselective vagotomy or posterior truncal vagotomy with hyperselective anterior vagotomy is a longer and more difficult procedure particularly in obese patients, who will be exposed to a higher recurrence rate as a result of technical difficulties. In addition, the results of these latter laparoscopic techniques have not been proved to be superior to the open procedures. Thus, we recommend posterior truncal vagotomy with anterior seromyotomy in the elective management of chronic duodenal ulcer.

Furthermore, interventional laparoscopy can be an excellent surgical therapeutic modality in the treatment of perforated duodenal ulcers. It should be stressed that these procedures are advanced laparoscopic techniques, requiring previous training to minimize complications. It is significant to note that if multicenter studies eventually confirm these initial positive clinical results and a significant long-term cost savings, interventional laparoscopy may be an alternative therapeutic modality in the management of chronic duodenal ulcer.

ACKNOWLEDGMENT

The editors would like to thank Philippe Jean Quilici, M.D., for his excellent translation of this chapter.

REFERENCES

1. Latarjet A, Wertheimer P: L'eneration gastrique. *J Med Lyon* 1921; 5:1289.
2. Dragstedt LR, Owen F: Subdiaphragmatic section of the vagus nerves in the treatment of duodenal ulcer. *Proc Soc Exp Biol Med* 1943; 53:152.
3. Jackson RC: Anatomic study of vagus nerves with a technique of transabdominal selective resection. *Arch Surg* 1948; 96:409.
4. Johnston D: Operative mortality and postoperative morbidity of highly selective vagotomy. *BMJ* 1975; 4:545–547.
5. Hoffman J, Olesen A, Jensen HE: Prospective 14 to 18-year follow-up study after parietal cell vagotomy. *Br J Surg* 1987; 74:1056–1059.
6. Taylor TV: Lesser curve superficial seromyotomy: An operation for chronic duodenal ulcer. *Br J Surg* 1979; 66:733–737.
7. Taylor TV, Gunn AA, MacLeod DAD, et al: Mortality and morbidity after anterior lesser curve seromyotomy with posterior truncal vagotomy for duodenal ulcer. *Br J Surg* 1985; 72:950–951.
8. Barclay GR, Finlayson NDC, Taylor TV: Dumping syndrome following anterior lesser curve seromyotomy with posterior truncal vagotomy. *Br J Surg* 1987; 74:285.
9. Taylor TV, Holt S, Heading RC: Gastric emptying after anterior

lesser curve seromyotomy and posterior truncal vagotomy. *Br J Surg* 1985; 72:620–622.
10. Oostvogel HJM, Vroohoven van TJMV: Anterior lesser curve seromyotomy with posterior truncal vagotomy versus proximal gastric vagotomy. *Br J Surg* 1988; 75:121–124.
11. Kurata JH, Haile BM: Epidemiology of peptic ulcer disease. *Clin Gastroenterol* 1984; 13:289–307.
12. Kurata JH, Honda GO, Frankl H: Hospitalization and mortality rates for peptic ulcers: A comparison of a large HMO and US data. *Gastroenterology* 1982; 1008–1016.
13. Kathkouda N, Mouiel J: A new technique of surgical treatment of chronic duodenal ulcer without laparatomy by videocelioscopy. *Am J Surg* 1991; 161:361–364.
14. Pietrafitta JJ, Schultz LS, Graber JN, et al: Laser laparoscopic vagotomy and pyloromyotomy. *Gastrointest Endosc* 1991; 37:338–343.
15. Dubois F: Laparoscopic vagotomies, in Berci G, Cuschieri A, Sackier JM (eds): *Problems in General Surgery: Laparoscopic Surgery*. Philadelphia, JB Lippincott, 1991, vol 8, pp 348–357.
16. Nathanson LK, Easter DW, Cuschieri A: Laparoscopic repair: Peritoneal toilet of perforated duodenal ulcer. *Surg Endosc* 1990; 4:232–233.

Chapter 13

Laser Therapy in Rectosigmoid Tumors

J. M. Brunetaud / V. Maunoury / D. Cochelard / B. Boniface
A. Cortot / J. C. Paris

Lasers are now commonly used in digestive endoscopy for tumor destruction.[1-4] From December 1979 to July 1991, 657 patients were treated at the Lille Laser Center for rectosigmoid tumors, including advanced cancers,[2] small cancers,[2] villous adenomas,[1,5] and rectal polyps after total colectomy.

TECHNIQUE OF RECTOSIGMOID TUMOR LASER THERAPY

Three types of lasers are used for gastrointestinal endoscopic treatment at Lille.

1. The argon laser (770 Lasersonics, Santa Clara, CA).
2. The Nd:YAG laser (YM 101 CILAS, Marcousis, France).
3. The frequency doubled Nd:YAG (Multilase 2500, Technomed International, Lyon, France).

The argon laser has a 10-W maximum power output, and its wavelength is well absorbed by tissue. It is used at a power of 8 W and a spot size of 1 mm (power density, 1000 W/cm^2) for vaporization of superficial tumors with a continuous beam, until a flat surface is obtained. Delayed necrosis is negligible after argon laser vaporization.

The Nd:YAG laser has an 80-W maximum power output. Its wavelength is less absorbed by tissue than the argon wavelength. The volume of delayed necrosis occurring after Nd:YAG vaporization can be difficult to predict from the macroscopic aspect of the tissue during treatment.[1,2] Therefore, the Nd:YAG laser is used at Lille only for coagulation (blanching) of the tumor, and an interval of 2 to 3 days between treatments allows the coagulated parts of the tumor to slough off. Reproducible effects were obtained at 70 W with 2-mm spot size (2000 W/cm^2) and 0.7-s exposure time.

Since March 1990, we have used a frequency doubled Nd:YAG laser. This laser gives either 100 W at 1.06 μm or 18 W at 0.532 μm. The yellow–green 0.532 μm wavelength was found to have almost the same effect of vaporization as the blue–green argon light. This laser has two advantages over the previous association of argon and Nd:YAG lasers as follows: (1) the higher optic power in the green light shortens the treatment time and (2) the switch from infrared to green light is easily obtained by pushing a button, without having to remove the fiber from the endoscope.

The technique of using both argon and Nd:YAG lasers (or 0.532-μm Nd:YAG) is innovative. The use of green light in gastrointestinal endoscopy is not widespread, probably because the purchase of a second laser is too expensive for most gastroenterologists. Until recently, the multidisciplinary use of lasers[6] enabled gastroenterologists to share expenses with other specialists and, hence, provided an availability of appropriate laser wavelengths for particular lesions. For example, an argon laser might be preferred in the treatment of some tumors for its safety features—absence of delayed effects, low risk of perforation, and limited thermal stenosis[7]—compared with the higher risks associated with Nd:YAG laser treatment. The green light option with the new Nd:YAG lasers should increase the number of green-light users in digestive endoscopy.

The best technique for endoscopic use of the 1.06-μm Nd:YAG laser is also controversial. Some investigators vaporize the tissue with a very high power density (over 10,000 W/cm^2)[8] or they coagulate small lesions and vaporize the larger ones.[9,10] We prefer to coagulate with a lower power density (between 1500 and 2000 W/cm^2) and wait until the coagulated areas slough off.[1,2,5] Others have stressed the increased safety of coagulation of cancer strictures compared with vaporization treatment.[11]

Our treatment technique of using both argon (or 0.532-μm Nd:YAG) and 1.06-μm Nd:YAG lasers and limiting the 1.06-μm Nd:YAG laser effects to coagulation is safe. No complications occurred in patients with small cancers or rectal polyposis. Our complication rates for advanced rectosigmoid cancers (2.4 percent) and villous adenomas (2 percent) are significantly lower than the 10 percent of Mathus-Vliegen and coworker,[9,10] who use a high-power Nd:YAG for vaporization and coagulation.

Procedure Notes

Patients are treated on an outpatient basis, without sedation. They are prepared with a small enema at the Laser Center before treatment. Patients with advanced cancers are treated once or twice a week until there is total destruction of the exophytic part of the tumor. Then they undergo repeat endoscopy and are retreated every 1 to 2 months. Patients with small cancers, villous adenomas, and rectal polyps are treated until complete destruction of the tumor and followed every 2 weeks until complete reepithelialization has occurred. They are followed every 3 to 6 months thereafter and retreated if a recurrence or new lesions occur.

The main disadvantage of laser photoablation is the lack of material available for histologic study of the tumor. Before treatment, multiple biopsy specimens must be obtained. For large tumors, a partial snare electroresection is performed, if possible. Snare resection debulks the tumor and decreases laser treatment time. More biopsies are performed during follow-up examination.

Laser photoablation can be performed in two different ways: (1) coagulation necrosis of the tumor with delayed slough or (2) vaporization with immediate destruction. Coagulation necrosis also occurs at the border of the vaporized area, but the amount depends on the laser wavelength used.

After endoscopic examination of the cancer size and location, coagulation of the entire tumor surface is performed in a proximal-to-distal fashion. The fiber tip is maintained at a distance of 5 to 10 mm from the tissue during treatment. The fibers are protected by a Teflon sheath, through which nitrogen gas flows at a rate of 2 L/min to protect the fiber tip. It also maintains a neutral gas atmosphere in the rectum and prevents possible explosions when high temperature occurs during treatment. With endoscopy, care must be taken to avoid rectocolonic overdistention. It is painful and reduces the thickness of the rectocolonic wall, thus increasing the risk of perforation. To evacuate the gas, a cannula is introduced in the rectum alongside the endoscope during treatment, and suctioning more proximally with the endoscope is performed at the end of treatment. Tumor necrosis and slough occur in 3 to 5 days. Treatments are performed once or twice a week until control of the tumor mass and/or reepithelialization occurs.[2]

For lesions in the lower third of the rectum, rigid anoscopy is preferable to flexible endoscopy if the patient can tolerate the knee–chest position. A suction cannula evacuates necrotic tissue and blood with this technique. Alternative techniques for transanal therapy of rectal lesions are discussed in Chapter 18.

RESULTS OF LASER THERAPY

Rectosigmoid Cancer

PATIENT COHORT

Two hundred fifty patients were treated for rectosigmoid cancers. The average age of the patients was 77 years (range, 33 to 96 years). Two hundred thirty-two patients had advanced tumors. Tables 13-1 and 13-2 give the reasons for treatment and the tumor localizations. The most common complaints at the beginning of treatment were abnormal rectal discharge (80 percent) and obstructive symptoms (20 percent). Eighteen patients had small lesions. A small lesion was defined as a tumor less than 3 cm in length, with a circumferential extension of the base less than one third of the circumference, without signs of infiltration, and having a purely exophytic configuration

TABLE 13-1 Reasons for treatment in patients with advanced and small rectosigmoid cancers

Reasons for Treatment	Advanced cancers No.	%	Small cancers No.	%
Nonsurgical (*)				
Without metastasis	132	57	14	78
With metastasis	51	22	0	0
Colostomy and abnormal discharge	25	11	0	0
Recurrence after surgery	17	7	2	11
Refusal of surgery	7	3	2	11
Total	232	100	18	100

*Nonsurgical candidate because of severe medical or surgical problem making the risk of surgical resection unacceptably high in the opinion of the consulting surgeons and internists.

TABLE 13-2 Localization of advanced and small rectosigmoid cancers

Localization	Advanced cancers No.	%	Small cancers No.	%
Rectum	130	56	11	61
Rectosigmoid junction	57	25	2	11
Sigmoid	45	19	5	28
Total	232	100	18	100

without ulceration. Circumferential extension (anular size of the tumor base) was estimated by comparing the circumferential portion of the bowel lumen occupied by the tumor base with the complete luminal circumference (Fig. 13-1).

For patients with advanced cancers, treatment was judged successful by subjective improvement of the patient and relief of symptoms, as determined by the disappearance of mucous discharge, easy stool passage, no more than two bowel movements per day without nocturnal stools, absence of constipation, and no more than two bloody stools per week. In patients with small cancers, treatment was considered successful when complete local destruction of the lesions and negative biopsy specimens were obtained. Four factors were studied in determining the initial and long-term results as follows: the reason for treatment, the primary symptom at the beginning of treatment, the tumor location, and the circumferential extension of the cancer. (C_1, less than ⅓ of the circumference; C_2, less than ⅔ of the circumference; and C_3, greater than ⅔ of the circumference.) The Fisher exact probability and chi-square tests were used to analyze the immediate results, and life-table analysis with the Mantel test were used for the long-term results.

OUTCOME

The results of treatment in patients with advanced cancers are illustrated in Figure 13-2. One hundred ninety-five patients (84 percent) improved after an average of 15 days of initial treatment (average number of treatments, 2.5). Sixteen percent of patients with advanced cancers failed to improve. Thirty-three patients are still being followed, remaining functionally improved during an average period of 13.5 months after initial treatment (range, 1 to 86 months).

Treatment was discontinued in 162 patients, and the average duration of improvement was 10.3 months (range, 1 to 54.4 months). Among these 162 patients, treatment

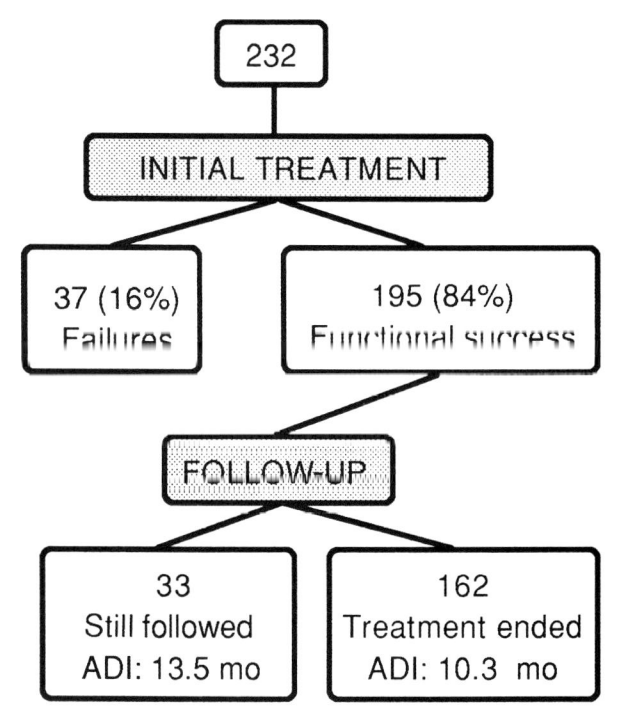

FIGURE 13-2 Diagram of the results in advanced cancers. ADI is average duration of improvement.

was interrupted in 8 because the tumor was too bulky, in 11 as a result of patient intolerance, in 22 who required a colostomy, and in 9 in whom radiation therapy of an anal extension was more appropriate than laser treatment; 12 were lost to follow-up. One hundred patients remained improved until they died; 77 patients expired from the cancer, and 23 patients from another cause.

By the life-table analysis method, 61, 40, and 16 percent of patients with initial success remained improved at 6, 12, and 24 months (Fig. 13-3). Improvement duration was affected by the reason for treatment (longer duration of improvement than for patients without metastases than

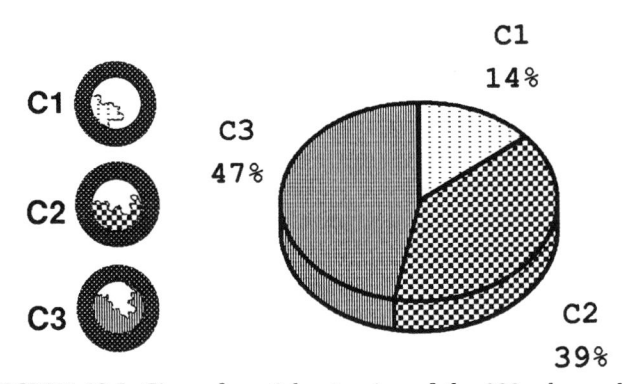

FIGURE 13-1 Circumferential extension of the 232 advanced rectosigmoid cancers. Less than ⅓ of the circumference was C1, between ⅓ and ⅔ was C2, and more than ⅔ was C3.

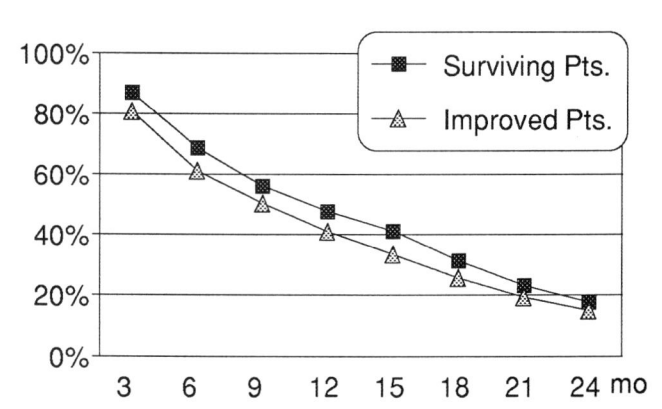

FIGURE 13-3 Survival and improvement rates of 195 patients with a functional success by life-table analysis.

patients with metastases, $P < 0.001$) and circumferential extension (longer duration of improvement for patients with Stage C1 cancer than those with C2 [$P < 0.02$] and for patients with Stage C1 cancer than those with C3 [$P < 0.005$]), but it was unaffected by primary symptom at the beginning of treatment or location.

All Stage C1 cancers were considered advanced stage because they did not fit the criteria for small lesions. However, negative biopsies were obtained in 6 of the 32 patients (19 percent) with Stage C1 tumor. During follow-up, one patient died from liver metastasis 3 months after the end of treatment, one died from another cause after 28 months of follow-up, two had local recurrences 16 months and 2 years after treatment, and one was lost to follow-up after 27 months. The sixth patient, followed for 56 months, had no local recurrence or metastasis.

Complete local destruction with negative biopsy results was obtained in all 18 patients with small cancers. Among them, five died from another cause, four were lost to follow-up, and one had a local recurrence 3.7 years after treatment. Eight patients had no local recurrence or metastasis for an average period of 53 months (range, 30 to 96 months).

Five complications occurred after 2586 laser treatment sessions in patients with advanced rectosigmoid carcinoma (2.1 percent of these patients). There were two perforations at the rectosigmoid junction (one fatal), one perirectal abscess, and two rectovaginal fistulae.

DISCUSSION

Palliative laser therapy is aimed at maintaining the highest quality of life in nonsurgical patients with advanced cancers and limited life expectancy. Symptoms were controlled by laser therapy in 84 percent of our patients after a mean treatment duration of 0.5 months. Other authors have reported similar efficacy with laser therapy.[9,12,13] Immediate success rates were 93, 100, and 82 percent, respectively, for hematochezia and 83, 67, and 75 percent, respectively, for obstructive symptoms.

At Lille, the initial results were affected by three factors as follows: (1) the reason for treatment (more failures in the recurrence after a non-laser treatment and initial colostomy group than in the other patients, $P < 0.05$); (2) the primary symptom at the beginning of treatment (more failures in the occlusive symptoms group than in the group with abnormal rectal discharges, $P < 0.05$); and (3) circumferential extension of the tumor base (more failures in the Stage C3 group than in the Stage C1 and C2 group, $P < 0.05$). The initial results were unaffected by location. An additional factor of poor prognosis in another study was recurrence after a nonlaser treatment.[14]

The average duration of improvement after endoscopic laser treatment was 10.3 months in our series, and functional improvement lasted along with survival in most patients. During follow-up, the duration of improvement was longer in nonsurgical patients without metastases than in the nonsurgical patients with metastases ($P < 0.001$). This can be explained by a shorter survival and, consequently, a shorter duration of improvement in patients with metastases. The duration of improvement was longer also for patients with Stage C1 cancer than for those with C2 ($P < 0.02$) and C3 cancer ($P < 0.005$). This is likely the result of differences in tumor evolution at the time of initial treatment.

The probability of remaining improved was higher in the 195 patients of our series than in the 84 patients of another study[13]: 61 and 40 percent at 6 and 12 months, versus 45 and 15 percent, respectively. In a third study of 88 patients,[14] the percentage of patients who remained symptomatically improved by laser treatment decreased from an initial 82 percent to 51 percent at 6 months and 25 percent at 18 months. Two reasons may account for this disparity between the third study and our results as follows: (1) their patients who failed to improve after initial treatment were not excluded from the follow-up study, as they were in our study, and (2) the retreatments were less frequent (one treatment every 4.7 months) than in our study (one treatment every 1 or 2 months). It is more difficult to explain the difference between the second study and our results. The treatment and evaluation methods were similar; however, their study resulted in a higher prevalence of advanced severe and end-stage malignancy than in our series.

Nonsurgical treatment has been widely used for the curative treatment of small rectal carcinomas. Other groups have used endoscopic lasers to obtain local destruction without difficulty in 12 of 13[8] and 13 of 13[12] treated patients. These two series and our data show that small rectosigmoid carcinomas can successfully be destroyed without complication by endoscopic laser treatment, but the criteria for the definition of *small cancer* are very important (Fig. 13-4). The results are totally different when the tumor is more advanced, as in our 32 patients with Stage C1 cancer ($P < 0.01$).

Rectosigmoid Villous Adenoma

PATIENT COHORT

Three hundred eighty-seven patients were treated for rectosigmoid villous adenoma. Their average age was 71 years (range, 32 to 96 years). Indications for laser treatment were (1) nonsurgical patients (152 patients, 39 percent of total); (2) patients for whom rectosigmoid resection appeared to be too drastic for tumors found benign on biopsy (158 patients, 41 percent of total); (3) recurrent tumor after previous nonlaser treatment (74 patients, 19 percent of total); and (4) patients who refused to undergo surgery (3 patients, 1 percent of total). The localization and circum-

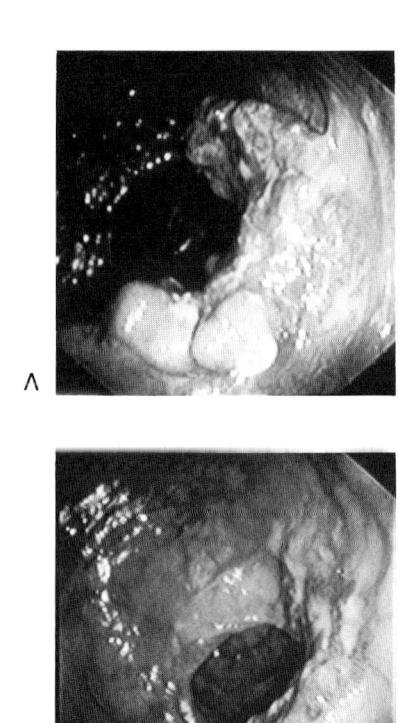

FIGURE 13-4 Palliative treatment of a Stage C2 bleeding rectal cancer in a 61-year-old patient with diffuse liver metastasis. A. Endoscopic view before treatment. A complete ablation of the tumor (with persistent malignant tissue) and a perfect functional result was obtained after two Nd:YAG laser sessions. B. Same patient as in previous figure. Endoscopic view 2 months after the end of initial treatment. A small layer of exophytic malignant tumor can be noticed. The patient was then retreated every 2 months and he remained symptom-free until he died from liver metastasis 13 months after initial laser treatment.

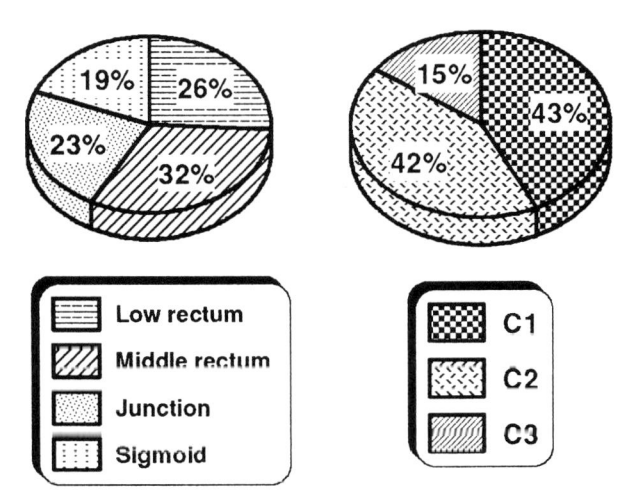

FIGURE 13-5 Location and circumferential extension of the 387 villous adenomas. C1 indicates <⅓ circumference, C2 indicates between ⅓ and ⅔ circumference, C3 indicates >⅔ circumference.

ferential extension of the tumor base (from Stage C1 to C3) are given in Figure 13-5. The material for histology was obtained during pretreatment evaluation by diathermic resection of large particles in 25 percent of patients and by forceps biopsy in 75 percent. A tumor was considered benign when the neoplastic tissue did not penetrate the muscularis mucosae. We used a two-grade system for classification of dysplasia.[5] Low-grade dysplasia was observed in 309 patients (80 percent) and high-grade dysplasia, in 78 patients (20 percent). New biopsies were performed at the end of treatment and whenever, macroscopically, there was a question of malignancy.

Patients with villous adenoma were treated in almost the same way as patients with cancer except that the argon laser was preferentially used to vaporize superficial parts of the tumor and the patients were treated twice a week until complete tumor destruction.[1,5]

Treatment was not completed in 44 patients. Twenty patients were lost to follow-up, 15 died from another cause during treatment, and 9 are still undergoing therapy. The results in the remaining 343 patients are schematized in Figure 13-6.

Invasive carcinoma was detected on biopsy specimens obtained during laser treatment in 22 patients (6.4 percent). The average delay between beginning of treatment and diagnosis of cancer was 5.7 months (range, 1 to 16

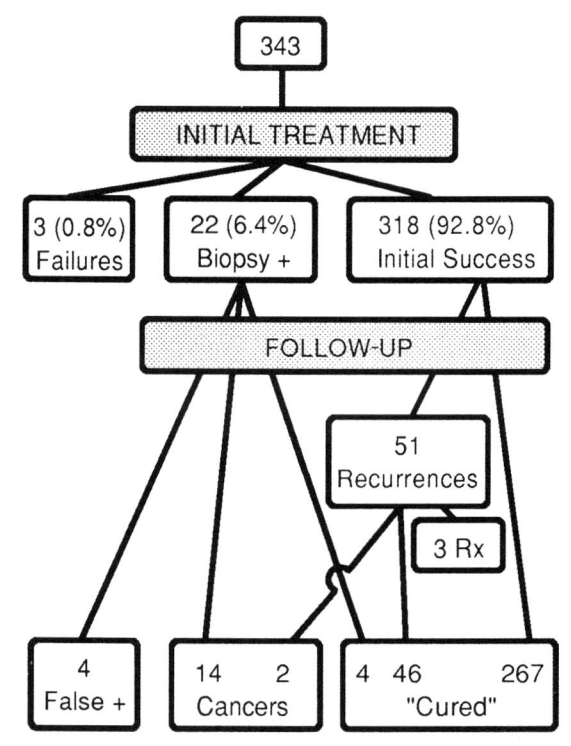

FIGURE 13-6 Diagram of the results from laser treatment in 343 patients with a rectosigmoid villous adenoma. Rx is treatment of the recurrence not completed.

months). Twelve patients underwent surgery (three segmental resections and nine abdominoperineal resections). Histologic examination of the surgical specimen revealed high-grade dysplasia in four patients. Therefore, true carcinoma developed in only 18 patients (5.2 percent). Following Astler-Coller's classification, the extension of cancer in eight operated patients was Stage A in two, B2 in two, C1 in three, and C2 in one. Ten patients with positive biopsies could not tolerate surgery. Nine continued to receive laser treatment for palliation of symptoms. However, complete destruction of the tumor, with negative biopsies and without local recurrence or metastasis, was obtained in four patients during a 35-month average follow-up (range, 12 to 60 months). Among the five others, one died from a bronchogenic cancer, two died from their rectal cancers 6 and 15 months later, and two patients are still being followed for palliation. The final patient was successfully treated by local radiation.

Three patients (1 percent) could not successfully be treated. All had Stage C3 lesions previously treated by nonlaser procedures. The previous treatment in two patients had been electrocoagulation, which resulted in very tight stenoses, making endoscopic treatment impossible. Therefore, only diverting colostomies could be performed. The third patient had been treated by surgical transanal resection. After Nd:YAG laser treatment, he developed a stenosis, which, though not tight enough to require a colostomy, prevented endoscopic treatment.

OUTCOME

Three hundred eighteen patients were successfully treated after an average of 5.7 treatments during an average period of 3.7 months (range, 0.2 to 21 months). This represents 92.8 percent of the patients whose treatment was completed. The average follow-up of the 318 initially successfully treated patients was 30.6 months. Among them, 221 are still being followed during an average period of 35 months (range, 1 to 110 months) (Fig. 13-7). Fifty-nine were lost to follow-up after an average period of 19 months (range, 1 to 98 months), and 38 died from another cause after a follow-up of 24 months (range, 1.7 to 63 months). Among these 318 patients, 51 had recurrences (16 percent). By the life-table analysis method, the recurrence rate

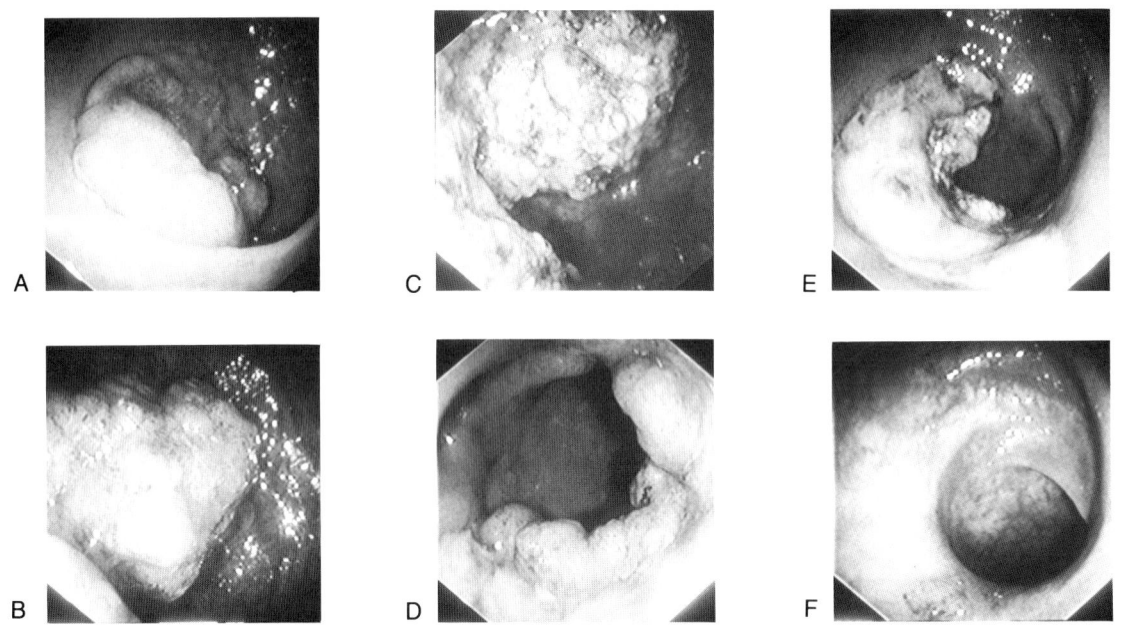

FIGURE 13-7 A. Curative treatment of a Stage C2 villous adenoma of the rectosigmoid junction in a 73-year-old patient. B. Endoscopic view of the lower part of the tumor, which is almost obstructing the bowel (the endoscope cannot pass by). C. Immediate aspect after first laser treatment in same patient. Notice the white color of the surface of the tumor from laser coagulation. D. Endoscopic view after three Nd:YAG laser sessions in same patient. Most of the tumor has been eradicated, and villous tissue persists only at the distal part. E. Endoscopic view immediately after the fourth session in same patient. Notice the large ulceration after the previous three sessions and the coagulation of the distal part after the fourth session. Two more sessions were needed (six in total), and a complete destruction with negative biopsies was obtained 1 month after the first laser session. F. Endoscopic view of a control 3 months after the first laser session. Only a small white scar can be seen. This patient remains tumor-free after a 13-month follow-up.

was 10 percent at 12 months and 19 percent at 24 months (Figure 13-8).

Most recurrences were detected during the first 2 years, and the average delay between the end of initial treatment and the detection of a recurrence was 18.6 months. Nine patients had two recurrences, and two patients had three recurrences. All recurrences were easily retreated in 46 patients during an average of 2.2 treatments. Three patients with recurrences are still being treated.

In the last two patients, cancer was detected by biopsy. The first patient was referred for laser treatment because of a recurrence 6 months after transanal resection. No malignancy was found in the resection specimen nor in the biopsies performed on the first recurrent lesion. A second recurrence of villous adenoma occurred 16 months after laser treatment and was found to be malignant. The second patient had a recurrence, with positive biopsies 1 year after initial laser treatment. Both patients were treated by abdominoperineal resection. Following the Astler-Coller's classification, the extension of the cancer was Stage C1 in the first patient and B1 in the second patient. These two patients are well at 14- and 22-months follow-up.

Treatment was generally well accepted by patients, and only 5.1 percent were lost to follow-up after initial treatment. During treatment with Nd:YAG laser, some patients experienced warmth in the rectum when the tumor was close to the anus. In those cases, the argon or 0.532-μm Nd:YAG laser was used, instead, which was well tolerated. For 2 or 3 days after a laser session, patients often had spotting, with blood and evacuation of necrotic tissue. Three patients had fevers to 38°C for 2 days, not associated with pain, and this spontaneously abated. Asymptomatic stenosis developed in eight patients, without further consequence. No fistulae occurred. Nine complications (2.3 percent) occurred. One patient experienced a hemorrhage, requiring transfusion, which was related to a traumatic ulceration by a thermometer in the laser-treated area (in France, body temperature is taken by rectum). Symptomatic stenoses requiring endoscopic dilatations developed in seven patients. A final complication was a perforation requiring surgical treatment that occurred 12 hours after 0.532-μm Nd:YAG laser vaporization of a Stage C1 tumor in the sigmoid. Since this accident, we have reduced the power when using the 0.532-μm Nd:YAG. We now use 10 W (4000 W/cm^2) instead of 15 W (6000 W/cm^2).

DISCUSSION

Circumferential extension was the only accurate predictor in the determination of three factors: (1) frequency of true cancer during initial treatment (Stage C1 and C2 versus C3, $P = 0.0001$); (2) treatment duration until reepithelialization ($P < 0.0001$); and (3) stenosis development requiring dilatation (Stage C1 and C2 versus C3, $P = 0.001$, Table 13-3).

Recurrence rate after initial treatment, calculated by life-table analysis, was affected by three factors: (1) initial histologic findings (more recurrences in the low-grade dysplasia group than in the high-grade dysplasia group, $P < 0.016$); (2) reason for treatment (more recurrences in the recurrence after a previous nonlaser treatment group than in the others, $P < 0.001$); and (3) location (more recurrences in the lower and middle rectum group than in the high rectum and sigmoid group, $P < 0.012$). The recurrence rate was unaffected by circumferential extension of the tumor base.

We estimated the direct charges, including hospital costs, doctor's fees, and ambulance transportation, for a patient living in the Lille area and treated in our hospital for Stage C1, C2, and C3 tumors. The laser costs included, respectively, 3.2, 7.8, and 13.5 laser treatments; 2, 3, and 4 control endoscopies without treatment; and corresponding ambulance transportation. Surgical costs included 6, 10, and 14 days, respectively, of hospitalization. Results

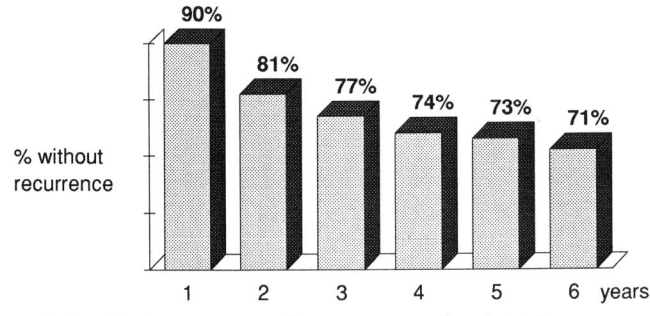

FIGURE 13-8 Frequency of recurrences after initial success in 318 patients with initial success. The frequency of recurrences was calculated by life-table analysis during the first 6 years follow-up period. The numbers indicate the percentage of patients free of recurrence.

TABLE 13-3 Influence of circumferential extension on outcome of villous adenoma treatment

Extension	Cancer Rate (%)	Treatment duration (mo).	Stenosis (%)
C1		2.3	
C2		4.4	
C1 + C2	3.0		0.3
C3	20.0	7.8	20.0
Total	5.2	3.7	2.2

Note: The effect of circumferential extension on the incidence of cancer during initial treatment, treatment duration, and stenosis development requiring dilatation.

showed that laser charges in Lille constituted 28, 37, and 40 percent, respectively, of surgical charges. For the UCLA Center for the Health Sciences (Los Angeles, CA), estimated direct laser care costs were 31, 52, and 69 percent of surgical charges for Stage C1, C2, and C3 tumors, respectively (Dennis Jensen, MD, personal communication).

Four series on endoscopic laser treatment for villous adenoma, including a total of 269 patients,[10,15–17] have been reported since our early results were published in 1985.[1] The initial success rates were 88 percent,[15] 89 percent,[17] 92 percent, and 72 percent.[10,16] Hemorrhage, stenosis, perforation, and fistulae, without fatal consequence, were reported as rare complications. The complication rates were, 2.3 percent in our series, 6 percent,[16] 12.5 percent,[10] 14 percent,[17] and 15 percent.[15] However, in the last series, six of eight complications were listed as stenoses without mention of whether they were symptomatic. This may account for the disparity in other series in which only symptomatic stenoses were reported. Our lower complication rate can also be explained by location of the treated tumors. Three series having higher complication rates than ours treated villous adenomas above the rectosigmoid.[10,16,17] In our series, the indications were limited to the rectum and sigmoid because an increased danger of perforation and delayed thermal stenosis above the rectosigmoid. In our opinion, the risk–benefit ratio is acceptable for locations in the rectum and the sigmoid colon but not acceptable for locations above the sigmoid colon.

The recurrence rate was given as the percentage of recurrences detected during the average follow-up period (16 percent during a 30-month average follow-up in our series) or calculated by the life-table analysis method (10 percent at 1 year, 19 percent at 2 years, and 29 percent at 6 years in our series). In other series, it was 3.8 percent during an 8.4-month follow-up,[15] 25 percent for 18 months,[16] 37.5 percent for 16.5 months,[10] and respectively, 27 percent and 46 percent at 1 and 2 years.[17] Most recurrences were successfully retreated, except in one series,[10] where 66 percent of the recurrences failed retreatment.

The major problem with laser management of villous adenoma is that no specimen is available for complete histologic study,[1] and consequently, a tumor with an undetected invasive cancer could be inappropriately treated. The risk of missing an invasive carcinoma in the pretreatment biopsy should not be overestimated. In the laser series, rates of undetected cancers were either lower than the 5.8 percent of our series (0 percent[15,16] and 2.5%[17]) or higher (15%).[10] Among our 18 patients with undetected cancer, 10 were nonsurgical candidates, and treatment was inappropriate in 8 patients, delaying surgery for a few months.

The major advantage of transanal, transsacral, or transabdominal resection is total histologic examination of the tumor, but postoperative complications and recurrences do occur. The complication rate was 21 percent in two large series,[18,19] including a 2.5 percent death rate. The recurrence rates after surgery range from 3.6 percent to 42 percent,[10–21] with the highest rates occurring after transanal surgery.

Rectal Polyposis

PATIENT COHORT

Twenty patients were treated for rectal polyposis. The average age was 30 years (range, 11 to 46 years). Ten of the patients belonged to four families. Fifteen had familial polyposis, and five had Gardner's syndrome. All of them had undergone surgery with ileorectal anastomoses before rectal laser treatment. The delay between colectomy and endoscopic laser treatment was variable. Five patients were treated by electrocoagulation during an average period of 15 years before laser treatment (range, 8.7 to 22.6 years). In the other 15 patients, the delay was 1.7 years (range, 0.1 to 5 years).

Our technique is to vaporize small polyps which cannot be removed by snare electrosurgery. Argon laser is primarily used. During initial treatment, patients undergo endoscopy twice a month until complete disappearance of all polyps. During follow-up, patients undergo endoscopy twice a year if no recurrence is detected, or every 3 months if new treatment is needed.

OUTCOME

These results are illustrated in Figure 13-9. During initial treatment, destruction of all polyps was unsuccessful in two patients. The number of new polyps becoming visible at each treatment session was too high. An ileoanal anastomosis was performed in one patient, and the second was successfully treated with sulindac.

Complete destruction of all polyps was obtained in the remaining 18 patients after an average of 3.9 months (range, 0.5 to 12.5 months) and 3.4 treatment sessions (range, 2 to 7). During follow-up, one patient died from metastasis related to a Dukes Stage C colonic cancer found at the time of initial total colectomy. A rectal cancer was detected in another patient 5 years after colectomy. An abdominoperineal resection was performed, revealing a Dukes Stage C invasion. The patient died 4 years later. Five patients were lost to follow-up. The other 11 patients were followed for an average of 5.9 years (range, 1.5 to 12.4 years). Repeated treatments were needed to treat new polyps, but no malignancy was detected. No complications occurred in this group of patients.

The management of patients with familial polyposis after ileorectal anastomosis is not easy. The risk of malignancy, even in patients regularly treated, is not negligible. One of our patients developed a carcinoma despite frequent

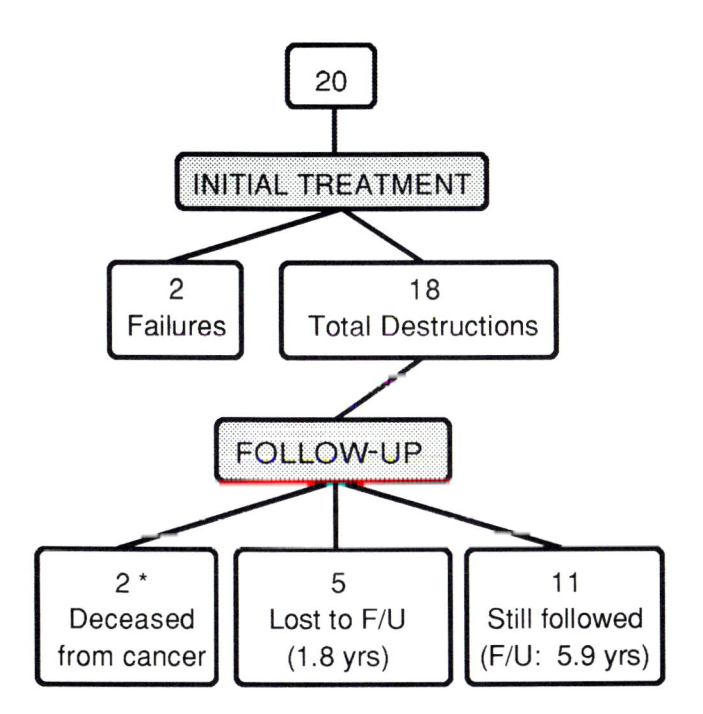

```
           ┌────┐
           │ 20 │
           └────┘
              │
      ┌───────────────┐
      │ INITIAL TREATMENT │
      └───────────────┘
          │        │
   ┌──────────┐  ┌──────────────┐
   │    2     │  │      18      │
   │ Failures │  │ Total Destructions │
   └──────────┘  └──────────────┘
                       │
               ┌──────────────┐
               │  FOLLOW-UP   │
               └──────────────┘
            ┌──────┬──────┬──────┐
   ┌──────────┐ ┌──────────┐ ┌──────────────┐
   │   2 *    │ │    5     │ │      11      │
   │ Deceased │ │Lost to F/U│ │Still followed│
   │from cancer│ │ (1.8 yrs)│ │(F/U: 5.9 yrs)│
   └──────────┘ └──────────┘ └──────────────┘
```

* One of them had a Dukes C cancer at colectomy

FIGURE 13-9 Diagram of the results in rectal polyposis.

control endoscopies. Therefore, in this type of palliative therapy, laser treatment incurs the same limitations as electrocoagulation, but its primary advantages over electrocoagulation are rapidity[7] and good healing quality without scarring, as demonstrated by Mathus-Vliegen and associates.[10]

SURGERY OR ENDOSCOPIC LASER THERAPY?

The cost of any new treatment is a major, worldwide problem, and attempts to assess the amount are inconclusive. Each country has different cost accounting and health insurance systems, rendering absolute cost comparisons difficult. Therefore, we preferred to estimate the relative cost of laser treatment and surgery. We estimated the direct costs (hospital, doctor, and ambulance transportation fees) and found them to be in favor of laser treatment for all three types of tumors (Stage C1 to C3). If indirect costs were included (e.g., loss of time from work, disability, and complications), laser treatment was even more cost effective, especially for Stage C1 tumors, which require only a small number of laser treatments.

Surgery is more expensive, has more complications (some being fatal), and results in more recurrences (at least for transanal surgery) than endoscopic laser treatment. On the other hand, endoscopic laser requires multiple treatments for complete destruction therapy of tumor and car-

ries the risk of missing an undetected carcinoma. However, these should not be considered competitive techniques but, rather, complementary. Patients with Stage C3 tumors should be referred for laser treatment only if they are not candidates for surgery. Laser treatment is too lengthy, and the risks of undetected cancer and stenosis that are induced by the treatment are too high. For patients with Stage C1 and C2 tumors, the risk of surgical complications should be balanced against the risk with laser treatment of delayed detection of a carcinoma. Proposed treatments must be discussed with patients on a case by case basis.

Our treatment of ambulatory patients without premedication or special diet beforehand is well adapted to the elderly population. In addition, ambulatory but repeated endoscopic laser treatment is safer for an elderly fragile patient, whereas a younger healthier patient may prefer a single surgical procedure. Because the higher complication rate with transsacral or transabdominal surgery, villous adenoma should be treated with laser therapy. However, the risks of complication and disturbance caused by a total colon preparation preclude, in our experience, good laser treatment for lesions above the rectosigmoid.

CONCLUSION

Endoscopic laser treatment is a safe and effective technique for the treatment of benign sessile rectosigmoid tumors and for palliation of symptoms from malignant tumors. Two major disadvantages of laser therapy are the high purchase price and lack of total histologic examination, particularly with villous adenoma and familial polyposis. The first problem can be mitigated with multidisciplinary shared use.[6] The second problem requires careful histologic investigation before, during, and after treatment and a good selection of patients, where the risk of malignancy must be balanced against the risk of surgery. Patients with biopsy-proven adenocarcinoma should be selected for palliation only if they are not candidates for surgery.

REFERENCES

1. Brunetaud JM, Mosquet L, Houcke M, et al: Villous adenomas of the rectum: Results of endoscopic treatment with argon and Nd:YAG lasers. *Gastroenterology* 1985; 89:832–837.
2. Brunetaud JM, Maunoury V, Ducrote P, et al: Palliative treatment of rectosigmoid carcinoma by endoscopic laser photoablation. *Gastroenterology* 1987; 92:663–668.
3. Fleischer D: Lasers and colon polyps: Technique and pathology: The courtship continues. *Gastroenterology* 1987; 90:2024–2025.
4. Jensen DM: Lasers in the GI cancer war and on other fronts. *Gastroenterology* 1984; 87:974–976.
5. Brunetaud JM, Maunoury V, Cochelard D, et al: Endoscopic laser treatment for rectosigmoid villous adenoma: Factors affecting the results. *Gastroenterology* 1989; 97:272–277.
6. Brunetaud JM, Mosquet L, Bouren J, et al: Organization of a

multidisciplinary laser center, in Fleisher D, Jensen D, Bright-Asare P (eds): *Therapeutic Laser Endoscopy in Gastrointestinal Diseases.* Boston, Martinus Nijhoff, 1983, pp 167–172.

7. Dixon JA, Burt RW, Roetering RH, et al: Endoscopic argon laser photocoagulation of sessile polyps. *Gastrointest Endosc* 1982; 28:162–165.
8. Lambert R, Sabben G: Photodestruction par laser des tumeurs colorectales: Résultats précoces, abstracted. *Gastroenterol Clin Biol* 1983; 7:59A.
9. Mathus-Vliegen EM, Tytgat GN: Nd:YAG laser photocoagulation in gastroenterology: Its role in palliation of colorectal cancer. *Laser Med Sci* 1986; 1:75–80.
10. Mathus-Vliegen EM, Tytgat GN: Nd:YAG laser photocoagulation in colorectal adenoma: Evaluation of its safety, usefulness, and efficacy. *Gastroenterology* 1986; 90:1865–1873.
11. Jensen DM: Palliation of esophagogastric cancer via endoscopy. *Gastroenterol Clin Biol* 1987; 11:361–363.
12. Escourrou J, Delvaux M, Frexinos J, et al: Traitement du cancer du rectum par le laser neodyme YAG. *Gastroenterol Clin Biol* 1986; 10:152–157.
13. Naveau S, Brajer S, Poynard T, et al: Endoscopic Nd-YAG laser therapy for palliative treatment of colorectal adenocarcinoma: A multivariate prognosis analysis. *Lasers in Med Sci* 1989; 4:251–257.
14. Van Cutsem E, Boonen A, Geboes K, et al: Risk factors which determine the long-term outcome of neodymium-YAG laser palliation of colorectal carcinoma. *Int J Colorectal Dis* 1989; 4:9–11.
15. Escourrou J, Delvaux M, De Bellisen F, et al: Traitement par laser Nd:YAG des tumeurs villeuses rectales: Expérience de 57 cas, abstracted. *Gastroenterol Clin Biol* 1987; 11:276.
16. Naveau S, Zourabichvili O, Brunie F, et al: Traitement par le laser Nd:YAG des tumeurs villeuses colo-rectales. *Gastroenterol Clin Biol* 1988; 12:604–609.
17. Souquet JC, Sabben G, Chavaillon A, et al: Traitement laser des tumeurs villeuses rectales. *Ann Gastroenterol Hepatol* 1987; 23:311–314.
18. Malafosse M, Roge P: Surgical management of villous tumors of the colon and rectum. *Dig Surg* 1984; 1:168–171.
19. Thompson JP: Treatment of sessile and tubulovillous adenomas of the rectum: Experience of St Mark's Hospital. *Dis Colon Rectum* 1977; 20:467–472.
20. Chiu YS, Spencer RJ: Villous lesions of the colon. *Dis Colon Rectum* 1978; 21:493–495.
21. Delile P, Marche C, Edelman G: Les tumeurs villeuses du colon et du rectum. Problémes diagnostiques et thérapeutiques. *Ann Chir* 1977; 31:829–842.

Chapter 14

Laparoscopic Suturing and Tissue Approximation

Zoltan Szabo

THE RELEVANCE OF MICROSURGERY TO LAPAROSCOPIC SURGERY

Tissue division, excision, and reapproximation are crucial maneuvers in surgery; therefore, important rules have evolved to guide these manipulations. The underlying principles were described by Halsted[1] in the late 1800s, establishing the basis of modern surgery. At the turn of the century, Carel and Guthrie[2] developed suturing methodology for the precise maneuvers required in vascular surgery. As other branches of surgery evolved, each specialty developed its own tissue approximation and suturing methods that were relevant to the target anatomy. Finally, it was the development of microsurgery that brought precision surgery, in particular atraumatic tissue handling and suturing techniques, to its current high level. During this process, many technical questions were settled and new standards established.[3-5]

Besides precision, the other important issue influencing the outcome of surgery was method of access. Microsurgery improved the precision of repair as long as tissues could easily be accessed. Similarly, minimizing the trauma of accessing target tissues provided patient care improvement. Therefore, the combination of microsurgical precision technique with laparoscopic minimal access was a logical evolutionary step in surgery. No union, however, is without its disadvantages, and the challenges presented are the focus of this chapter.

TISSUE APPROXIMATION METHODS

Choices

Reapproximating tissue edges has been a challenging task since ancient times. Thrusting a pin across both edges and wrapping thread under and around this pin was the earliest method used. This evolved into a single device that combined both needle and thread. Attempts were made at gluing[6] and stapling, but neither was a universally adaptable solution.

Suturing dominated traditional open surgery for centuries until stapling devices[7] gained popularity. As long as the tissues and devices were employed in an open approach and manipulated directly by the human hand, good results were obtainable. The surgeon has limited access, however, in the laparoscopic approach, where tissue visualization and manipulation are indirect. Although some staplers have been adapted for laparoscopic use, the adequacy of tissue approximation by this method was called into question. The use of traditional suturing in laparoscopic procedures was difficult and discouraging, too, resulting in a need for alternate methods of approximation.

Preference

Despite its technical challenges, intracorporeal laparoscopic suturing became the preferred technique. Instrumentation and suture materials were already available; suturing was universally adaptable, flexible, and economical. The greatest obstacle in suturing was the lack of skill, but this could be overcome by proper technique, training, and instrumentation.

Laparoscopic suturing (Fig. 14-1) can be learned with proper thorough training. Key factors to success include motivation, willpower, and discipline. As one surgeon noted, the challenge is similar to an athletic event (Wolfe BM. Personal communication, August 1991). To develop a competent confident technique, one must approach training to perform intracorporeal suturing in a manner similar to training for athletic competition. This includes develop-

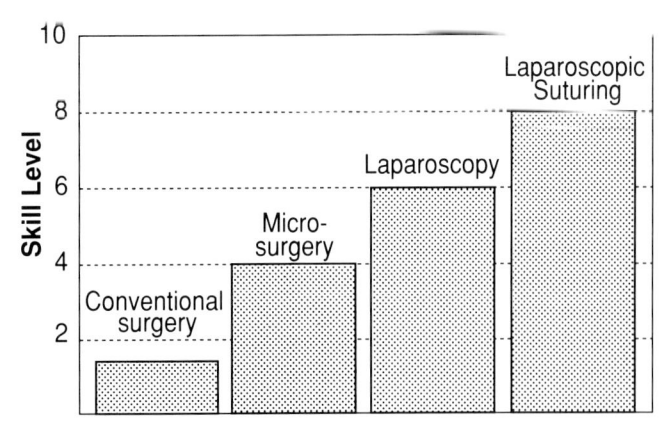

FIGURE 14-1 A relative comparison of skill level required for various surgical modalities.

ing a "feel" for the goal and achieving optimal physical and mental condition, with dietary concern for harmful stimulants. Ongoing advances in instrumentation combined with skill development make this challenging technique less formidable. Although other methods of tissue approximation exist,[8] this chapter will focus on the techniques most likely to be clinically applicable and endurable.

BASIC CONCEPTS IN LAPAROSCOPIC SUTURING AND TISSUE APPROXIMATION

Instrumentation and Sutures

Basic laparoscopic equipment includes the trocars and suture materials.

TROCARS

The ideal trocars are just a little longer than the thickness of the abdominal wall. If too long, the trocar interferes with instrument mobility and function. It can prevent the opening of instrument jaws and generally minimize instrument movement within the abdomen. A means of temporary fixation to the abdominal wall is desirable to prevent the trocar from slipping out of the puncture site. The preferred diameter is 10 to 11 mm, permitting passage of curved needles and a variety of instruments. A frequent problem is reducer caps, often requiring two hands to remove and replace while changing instruments or passing a needle through.

SUTURE

Considerable redesign is needed to develop ideal suture materials suited for all procedures. Although there are some common needs, each surgical procedure requires specific needle configurations and needle and thread combinations. When ideal needles have not been available, they often have been modified from existing ones. For example, early experimental work[9] involved the use of a partially straightened half-circle needle on a 6–0 monofilament nylon thread. Its placement was arduous and the knot tying difficult because of the ill-suited needle and suture combination.

Early suturing performed by Semm[10] and others[11] was accomplished with a large straight needle that could be passed through the trocar and grasped with the early needle driver. In today's complicated maneuvers, however, correct needle and suture materials are needed for intracorporeal suturing. The physical properties of suture and needle geometry can affect the surgeon's performance. Tissue response is another concern. When selecting the suture, the following considerations are important.

Handling characteristics The scooping motion of tissue entrance and exit bites ensures adequate inclusion and penetration of tissue layers, which is necessary for tissue approximation and reconstruction. These movements mandate a curved needle geometry and specific length. The straight needle, while easier to grasp and pass through the trocar, requires extensive help from the assisting grasper. The ski-shaped needles currently available combine the favorable characteristics of both, offering a reasonable solution. The ideal needle should have a bicurve geometry. By changing these curvatures, the handling and scooping characteristics of a needle can be adapted to particular tissues and their access requirements. For example, the ideal configuration of needle curvature is radically different for suturing a gastric seromyotomy than for anastomosing the bladder neck to the urethra.[11a]

The tip Needle tip geometry controls the tissue penetration characteristics and the size and shape of the tunnel cut (tissue defect made by the needle). Other standard configurations include the triangular profile with cutting in all directions (e.g., skin needles), the so-called reverse cutting tip, the spatulated, and the tapered vascular tip. For laparoscopic suturing, the ease of penetration is important to minimize tissue defect (i.e., without cutting a large hole). The tapered needle with a small cutting tip, popular among microsurgeons, might also be the best solution in laparoscopic suturing.

The diameter and profile of the needle Another important factor is how the needle is held in the jaws of the needle driver and assisting grasper instrument. When the needle profile and inside jaws of the needle driver are matched well, the result is a secure hold without brute force. This refined grip is an important component of precision suturing technique. Thicker tissue layers require stronger sturdier needles; more delicate tissues require smaller thinner needles.

The suture material The selection of suture material is based on favorable tissue response, handling characteristics, and visibility. While the suture industry has established multiple coloring schemes for various suture materials, such differentiation is useless when visibility is limited, as in laparoscopic surgery. A pitch-black or fluorescent white (PTFE or Gore-tex) color are the unanimous favorites.

The bending and folding characteristics of suture material are an important consideration because the "memory" can be a favorable or unfavorable factor. Based on practical experience, 2–0 and 3–0 silk is the easiest to see, handle, and tie into a secure knot. If it had a little more memory, it would be the ideal suture material for laparoscopic suturing. The handling of woven suture material appears easier than its monofilament counterpart, but its disadvantage lies in the wet field, where woven material has a tendency to become limp.

Hand Instruments

In open surgery, direct contact by the human hand plays an important role in tactile feedback (diagnosis) and general accessing (manual retraction and finger dissection).[12] Suturing and specific tissue retraction are more dependent on hand instruments. Traditional needle drivers (often called needle holders) and assisting graspers were designed in the last century and have been simple, effective, and economical to manufacture.

The role of the needle driver is to grasp and hold the needle securely during needle passage, specifically while making entrance and exit bites in tissues. These instruments hold the needle by sheer force. They lock and unlock using a ratchet located immediately adjacent to the ringed handles. These instruments exert great pressure and require considerable palm-grip force. The ratchet can be closed reasonably smoothly; however, it is the reopening that can be jarring. The necessity for redesign in laparoscopic instruments has become apparent. Some of the more important and desirable features will be discussed.

When microsurgical techniques were developed in ophthalmology, innovations were made in needle holding and driving. Because maximum yet delicate control of the fine needles was required, the needle driver was redesigned for finger control, easy rotatability, and smooth action with a writer's precision pencil grip.[13] One of the best designs to emerge has been the Castroviejo needle driver.

The first laparoscopic needle drivers were traditional graspers. The tip and stem were coaxial. However, the handle was bent in a pistol grip angle, and the fingers were thrust into the rings at the end of the handle.[12] This design was suitable for allowing the surgeon a view parallel to and above the instrument. While useful in allowing manipulation of tissues in a tight channel, it restricted complex instrument tip movement and rotation needed during suturing. Such restrictions in instrument tip mobility have largely accounted for the lack of progress in laparoscopic suturing, hampering development of more sophisticated laparoscopic procedures. Intracorporeal suturing has, for most surgeons, remained an exotic and intimidatingly difficult technique.

The first significant step in the evolution of laparoscopic instruments was the mating of the microsurgical handle to the laparoscopic instrument, permitting freer movement and full rotatability. Also important was the introduction of two-handed suturing techniques and the design of instruments as a matched pair (Szabo-Berci needle holders, Karl Storz Endoscopy-America, Culver City, CA), with each performing its specific role of needle driving or assisting grasper. The first prototypical modification was made by bending the handle of an otolaryngology alligator grasper straight and welding a round handle in place of the ring handles. A pair of these prototypes was fabricated by the author to facilitate intracorporeal suturing and knot tying.[14] Specifically designed tips were required for the needle driver and assisting grasper and were incorporated into the prototypes.

The primary role of the needle driver is handling the needle, although suture and tissue grasping are also part of its functions. A slight spooning curvature is the preferred shape of the tip. The assisting instrument mainly handles tissues and sutures, provides counterpressure, and performs a minimal role in needle driving. In special cases, the assisting grasper can also hold and drive the needle, particularly when this approach provides the easiest or only available alternative for a given setup (ambidextrous approach). For grasping tissue and looping suture, the tip must be able to reach in almost any direction. This is best accomplished with an aggressively curved or angled tip, for example, a flamingo beak-shaped tip.

Visual Perception

In open surgery, direct observation of tissues provides an excellent means of visual clues to guide the surgeon's hand and allow crucial decision making. When loupes or the surgical microscope is used, the resulting magnified surgical field facilitates a more precise, delicate repair. However, this enhanced visual perception results in an eye–hand coordination imbalance that must be compensated. In laparoscopy, the basic principles of operating in a magnified microsurgical field[15] can be applied to remedy this imbalance. Magnified visual perception differs from unaided vision primarily in the presentation of a larger image with greater details; however, the disadvantages are increased speed of movement (proportionate to the magnification factor) and reduced depth and size of the field.

Macular vision, where accurate vision takes place, requires much concentration and constant shifting of attention. It is noteworthy that the human brain will create an image from the least amount of available visual information. The remainder of the image is made up of visual memory developed during training. The importance of proper training is obvious because building up a good visual memory and concurrent reasoning allows the surgeon to read poor quality visual clues correctly.

Good visual health, correction to 20/20 vision, and rested eyes are components of the ideal physical and mental conditioning required in laparoscopic suturing. It has been observed during microsurgical training that slight visual flaws that did not disturb surgeons during open surgery became problematic when looking at the magnified surgical field. A visit to the ophthalmologist is recommended before taking a laparoscopic course or proceeding to operate with the aid of magnification.

Video Magnification

Video magnification is the preferred method for laparoscopy, although the image quality is less than ideal. A well-tuned high-quality setup will provide a video picture that is adequate for most suturing procedures.

Sustained concentration on the video screen can cause eye strain, therefore, adjusting the image for sharpness and clarity is vital. The camera assistant is instrumental in providing the best visual image because holding and guiding the camera is one of the most difficult roles performed by the operating team. The camera assistant must know exactly what the primary surgeon needs to see and provide that view accordingly, making certain that the image is always focused and the objective lens is clean. This concentration is difficult to maintain for more than 30 min, particularly when the procedure is not going smoothly. It is helpful for the assisting surgeon, whose role is to retract tissues, and the camera assistant to rotate jobs from time to time to maintain proper concentration. There is much need for a camera holder, such as the First Assistant (Leonard Medical, Huntingdon Valley, PA) or the Lapo Tract M.I.S. Support System (Omni-Tract Surgical, St. Paul, MN).

Although video magnification, as measured on the video screen, can range from 1× to 15×, the most frequently used magnification range is approximately 3× to 4×. This relatively low level of magnification is equivalent to the low range of the surgical microscope and the working range of loupes. In microsurgery, this requires only moderate adaptation in surgical technique. In laparoscopic surgery, the length of the instrumentation multiplies the degree of difficulty, and proportionately greater adaptation is needed.

Eye–Hand Coordination in the Magnified Surgical Field

In minimal-access surgery, magnification and the use of long instruments calls for special techniques to adapt the open procedures and duplicate those results in the laparoscopic modality. One of the greatest challenges confronting this approach is the distorted eye–hand coordination balance.[16]

Reestablishing this balance is accomplished by slowing one's movements significantly. Ideally, one should slow down proportionately to the magnification factor, or until proper control is reestablished. There will be some variation in the speed of movements during a procedure as the scope is pulled back and forth to change magnification and the size of the field.

To place a stitch precisely, the laparoscope is brought in closely; when tying the knot, the laparoscope is pulled back to provide a greater field of view. When an important decision is required during the procedure, magnification is increased and focused on that particular part of the field, with the surgeon's movements slowed down even further, always inversely proportional to the magnification. Reducing speed of movement not only restores eye–hand coordination balance but also allows the brain to compose and calculate the most informative image possible, all of which is needed to proceed correctly in making decisions such as whether to accept a current position or change it. On the other hand, if the surgeon rushes, the current position may be accepted for the sake of expediency, which can result in error. Error is manifested in reduced precision, increased trauma, and wasted time spent making a correction. The ultimate goal for the surgeon is to develop a *flawless technique*.

Reducing speed can dramatically lengthen operating time, which, of course, is counterproductive, considering anesthesia time and operating costs. A means of increasing efficiency can be found in two important principles: the combination of an *economy-of-motion principle* with a *choreography-of-movements technique*. For example, knot-tying movements have been studied and choreographed into the least number of necessary movements that flow into one another smoothly.[16,16a]

In intracorporeal suturing and knot tying, precise control in movement of the instrument tip is vital. Considering the possibility of iatrogenic injury, learning to control the tip is essential, necessitating training, supervised practice, and proper frame of mind. The tips of the needle holder and assisting grasper must work in an orchestrated fashion, like a duet, with each tip utilizing its ideal function and range. Depending on the task, each instrument is called into action, either taking turns or working simultaneously. Such choreography is an important time- and effort-saving technique that should be learned by novices and will be appreciated by experienced surgeons. Obviously, it is better to grasp the suture carefully once than to make several fruitless attempts.

Besides choreography, another necessity is accurate targeting and placement of instrument jaws because sutures, needles, and tissues need to be grasped repeatedly. Such accuracy is a significant challenge when working in a two-dimensional visual field. Nothing wastes more time and causes more frustration than groping about and missing the intended target. The remedy is to slow down significantly, try to touch the target to confirm its location, and avoid confusion caused by misleading clues in the two-dimensional field. To grasp accurately, the instrument jaw is opened and the lower jaw slowly positioned just under the target; when confirmed, the jaws are closed. It should be the goal of the surgeon to avoid missing the intended target even once during the entire procedure to maintain a flawless technique.

This slowed choreography requires considerable patience and fresh energy. It is recommended that one abstain from caffeine and other stimulants and be in perfect health, that is, top physical and mental condition. At the beginning of a procedure, a surgeon has a limited amount of energy for precision surgery. This limit can be increased by a sportsman-like life style, conditioning, and discipline. It is also vital to avoid mental and physical distractions in the operating room and other factors that dilute concentration.

Tissue Handling

In intracorporeal tissue approximation, a major concern is the handling of tissues. Because tissue handling involves long leveraged instruments, collateral trauma can easily occur, leading to adhesion formation, increased scarring, and overall poorer postoperative results. One of the main considerations is retraction. Often performed by less experienced assistants, tugging and pulling of tissues is unavoidable; however, frequent handling of this sort with instruments can result in battered tissues.

Most currently available instruments have jaws with small foot pads that can exert considerable pressure. Traditional bowel clamps, for example, the Allis, Babcock, and similar designs, are necessary because these instruments provide greater grasping surface, reduced leverage, and thus, less pressure per square inch. The result is less crushing and ripping injury. Although it might seem desirable to have universal laparoscopic instruments that could handle tissue, needles, and sutures with equal effectiveness, no such instrument is possible. The more diverse the functions that are required of an instrument, the poorer each function will be performed.

Retractors perform best at their intended function. Although a needle driver could grasp tissue, it was not intended for that purpose, and its powerful short leveraged jaws could easily crush and lacerate tissue in an unintended move. The jaws of the assistant grasper were designed to grasp suture, tissue, and occasionally, the needle. When handling tissue with locking instruments, activation of the locks and ratchets can be especially dangerous because this can place excessive force on tissues.

The need for delicate tissue handling cannot be overstressed. Tissues need to be handled as gently as possible, especially when being positioned for needle passage. Counterpressure should be provided immediately adjacent to the point of needle entrance or exit by the jaws of the assisting grasper. Minor adjustments and initial testing of tissue can be made with the tip of a needle firmly held in the grip of the needle driver (Fig. 14-2).

A good setup facilitates the entire procedure. If tissue edges to be approximated are brought within close proximity of each other and positioned well, suturing can be a fairly straightforward process. Another set of "hands" may be needed to create the optimal setup; whether they are in the form of another instrument or device can be decided by the surgeon. Future devices may include retractors and clamps that can be passed down through the 10- to 11-mm trocar, deployed, and retrieved again. Such devices would enable more complicated tissue approximation techniques and conduit anastomoses.

BASIC TECHNIQUES

Setup and Angles of Approach

In challenging tissue approximation procedures, the proper setup of trocars can make a significant difference. While

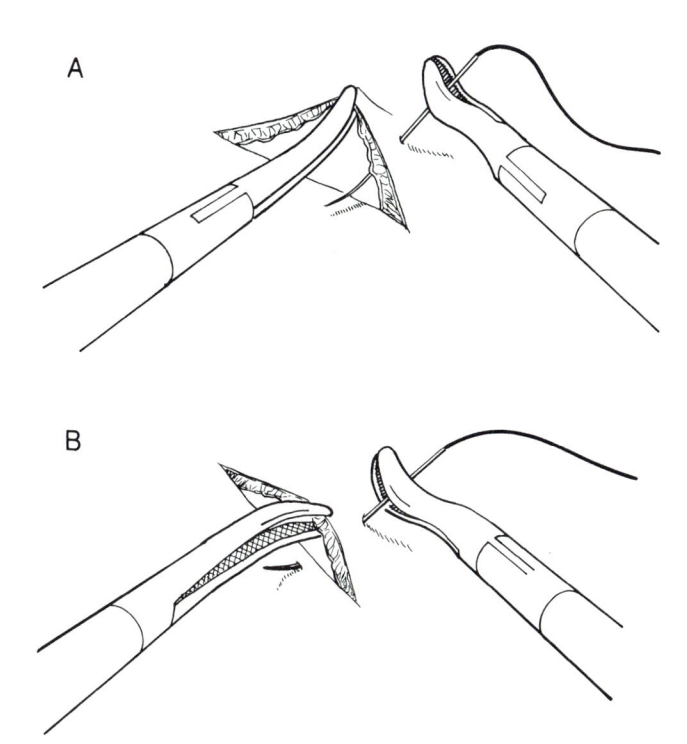

FIGURE 14-2 A. The needle is positioned firmly in a needle driver, and countertraction is applied with the assisting grasper by lifting the tissue edge near the entrance point. B. For the exit bite, counterpressure is applied by gently lifting and folding back the corresponding tissue edge. In each case, the needle tip is driven head-on (perpendicular) against the tissue surface, requiring rotation of the needle driver, similar to a scooping motion.

many advanced procedures are feasible, they must also be practical for use in a clinical setting. Therefore, every possible advantage should be sought without compromising the outcome of the procedure.

LAPAROSCOPE AND CAMERA LOCATION

Positioning the camera through the umbilicus is sufficient for most procedures, although it can be changed to accommodate the need for special access.

INSTRUMENT LOCATIONS

The relation of the suturing instruments (needle driver and assisting grasper) to the camera position is important, especially when considerable suturing is required. Also important is the position of the surgeon in relation to the patient.[18] Positioning can follows two models: (1) the natural position of the surgeon, left hand, viewing port, right hand, where viewing is centered and the needle driver and assisting grasper are on either side of the laparoscope or (2) an offset position with the instrument pair located on one side of the laparoscope or the other. In the latter case, the ports should be far enough apart, 6 to 7 in, to avoid a chopstick effect. After mastering the suturing skill, either position is adequate, including an upside-down setup, although this positioning never feels completely natural. A mirror-image setup is the only near-impossible proposition, carrying too great a risk for serious error.

Ideally, the needle driver should be lined up parallel to the proposed suture line so that the needle is held perpendicular in the instrument jaws and perpendicular to the suture line. The assisting grasper should be offset at least 45° to 90° and set 6 to 7 in apart (Figs. 14-3 and 14-4).

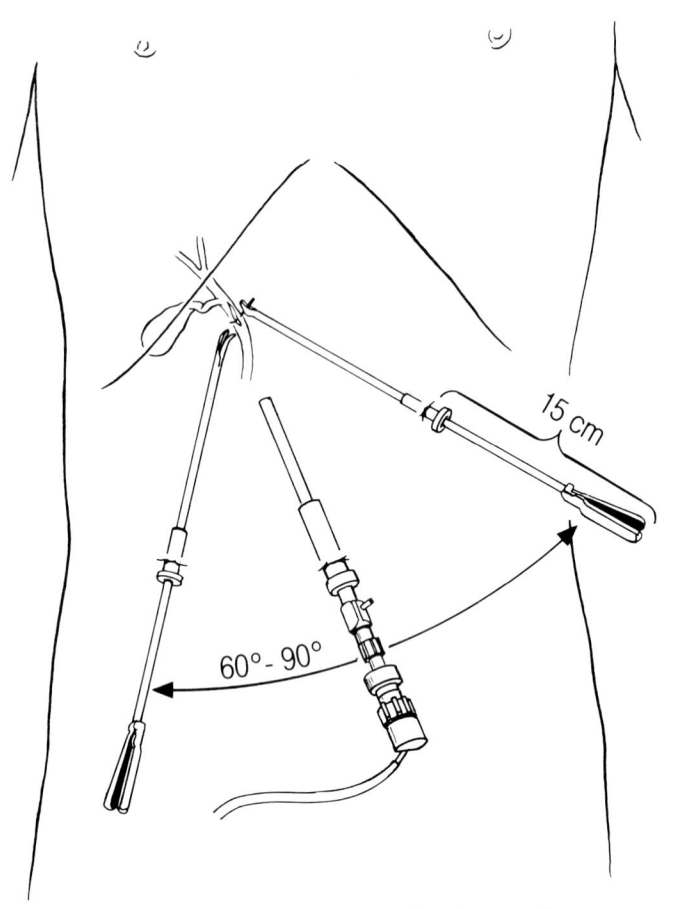

FIGURE 14-4 The ideal port position for closure of a choledochotomy spreads the needle holder and assisting forceps by 60° to 90° with one half of the instrument (15 cm) in the patient and one half out.

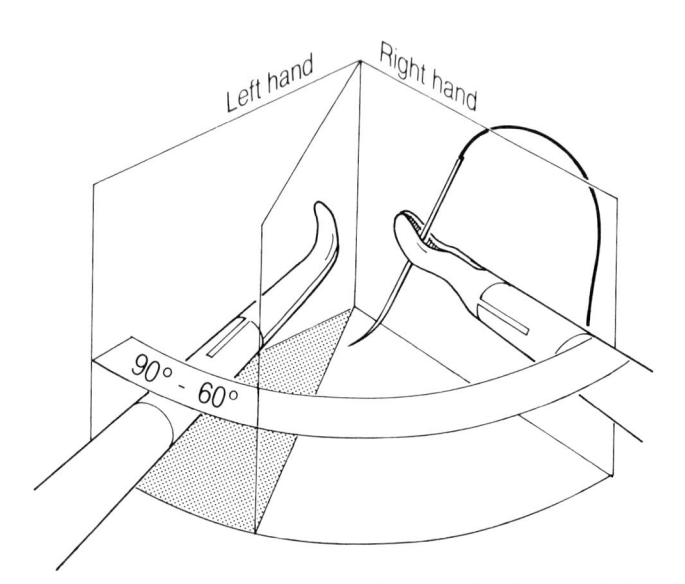

FIGURE 14-3 Ideal positioning of the needle driver and the assisting grasper is a 60- to 90-degree angle.

Needle Control

GRASPING AND LOADING IN THE NEEDLE DRIVER

The needle is brought through either a needle introducer (5-mm reducer) or passed directly through the trocar (10 to 11 mm). The reducer cap is removed from the trocar, and the needle driver is threaded through. Then, grasping the thread about 1 in behind the needle, it is inserted into the trocar, and the reducer is replaced. Once in the field, the needle is identified and pulled all the way in. The full length of the suture should not exceed 6 to 7 in in length; otherwise it tangles up and becomes unmanageable. The next task is to load the needle into the needle driver. This is done first by grasping the thread about 1 in from the needle with the assisting grasper. Then it is dangled in a fashion so that the tip of the needle touches the tissue surface (Fig. 14-5). The needle is rotated and pivoted until it lines up in the exact direction needed; it is then grasped with the needle driver. The surgeon is now ready to suture. Difficulties arise when the needle is not lined up precisely or is knocked askew.

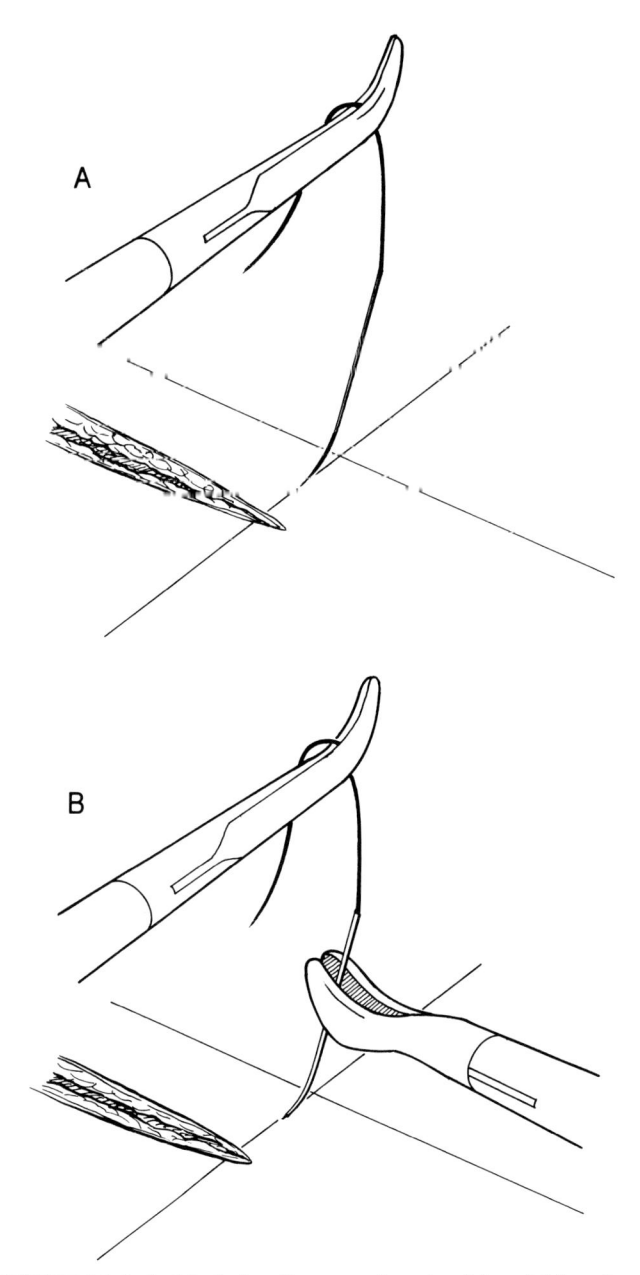

FIGURE 14-5 A. Ideal tip alignment is gained by picking the suture up by the tail and pirouetting the needle on the tissue surface. B. Grasping is done with the needle holder when proper alignment is achieved.

ADJUSTING THE NEEDLE

Beginners will attempt to reposition the needle by handing it back and forth between the assisting grasper and needle driver, hoping to adjust it in the process. This technique might seem logical; however, it requires considerable skill and can turn into a frustrating "catch me if you can" situation. A better method also requires skill and concentration but is quicker and more practical. This involves a trick maneuver of hooking the needle tip into the tissue just lightly enough to fix it, loosening the grip on the needle without actually letting it go, then pushing, pulling, or rotating the needle driver to pivot the needle into the desired position. Another method is grasping the needle lightly and brushing it backward against adjacent tissues. This movement will sweep the point of the needle exactly opposite of the direction it is pushed. After the ideal position is reached, the grip on the needle is tightened to lock it into position, and the needle is lifted up and positioned with the tip perpendicular to the tissue surface it is to penetrate.

NEEDLE DEFLECTION AND REMEDY

The plane of the needle, from tip to end, should be perpendicular to the shaft of the instrument, and the needle should be positioned perpendicular to the suture line (Fig. 14-6). The needle tip should be rotated until it is perpendicular to the tissue, which is achieved by rotating the instrument counterclockwise (see Fig. 14-8B). The needle is then hooked into the tissue at the entrance point and the precise alignment checked (Fig. 14-7). If satisfactory, counterpressure is provided, and the needle is slowly driven into the tissue, making sure that the direction of penetration is maintained head-on against tissue resistance (Fig. 14-8). Small adjustments can be made, as necessary, by pushing or pulling on the needle to alter its direction slightly. Although this maneuver is quite challenging at first, it promotes good habits and self-confidence in precision-control techniques.

A common problem is that, when the needle is pushed

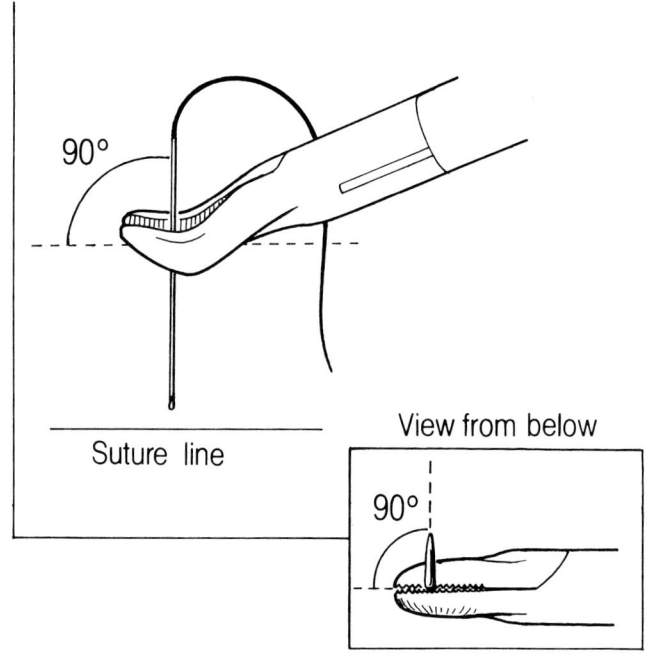

FIGURE 14-6 The needle is aligned at right angles to the needle holder in two planes.

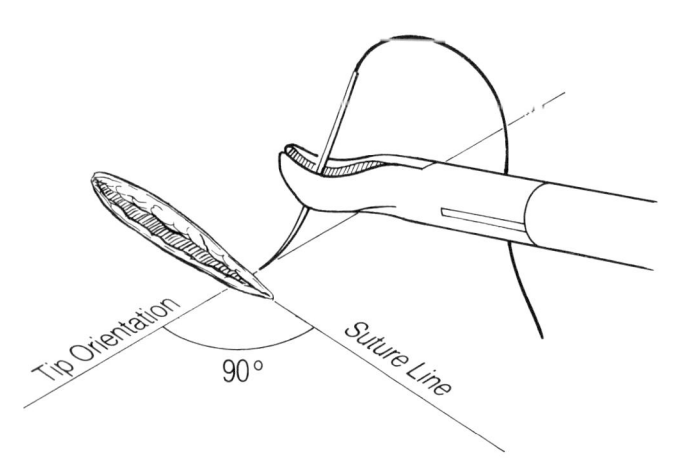

FIGURE 14-7 The properly positioned needle is brought to the tissue defect, ready to begin the entrance bite.

into the tissue, it will deflect to the side. This results from deviating from the principle of pushing the needle head-on against tissue resistance. Proportional to the angle of deviation, the driving force will be applied sideways to the needle, causing rotation (Fig. 14-9). The solution is to drive the needle slowly so that, if deflection begins to occur, the direction of penetration can be corrected or the needle adjusted in the previously described manner. A logical, although dangerous, solution to this problem is to use the needle driver with a rock-solid grip. The problem with this approach is that it can lead to tearing of tissues because the rigidly held needle will act like a knife during an accidental movement. The softer grasping technique is, therefore, preferred, particularly in the early phases of learning the needle-driving technique.

Entrance and Exit Bites

SELECTION OF ENTRANCE POINT

When using a single-armed needle, the direction of passage for an entrance bite is from outside the tissue to inside, rendering it more difficult than an exit bite, where the needle passes from inside to outside. Therefore, in certain cases, double-armed suturing, where both the entrance and exit bites are executed in the same manner (i.e., two exit bites), is recommended because this is easier and safer.

Selecting the first entrance point will set the stage for the remainder of the stitches and should be carefully calculated to create a suture line ideal for the reconstruction. For example, the point of the entrance bite is different when reapproximating a peritoneal incision than during anastomosis of the bowel. With the former, the goal is merely to reapproximate the edges to re-create continuity. When anastomosis of the colon is done, there are more critical concerns, such as watertight suture line and inverted edges. Therefore, the points of entrance and exit as well as the size of bite must be selected accordingly. Mistakes are often

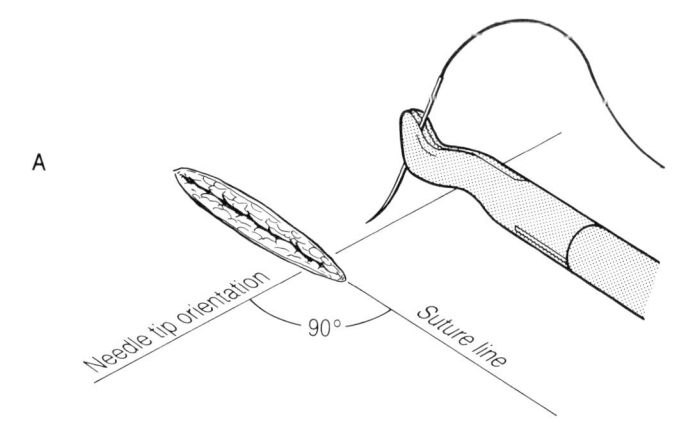

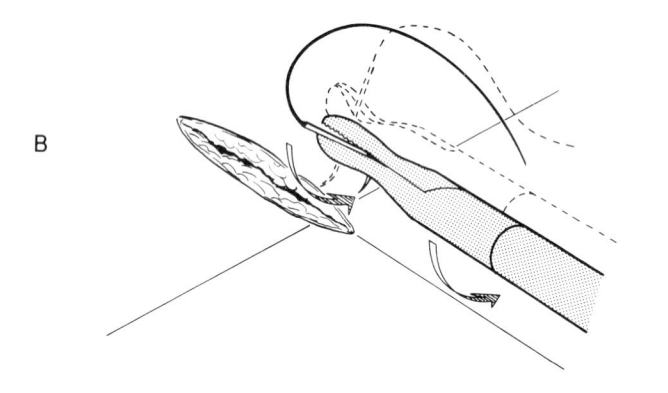

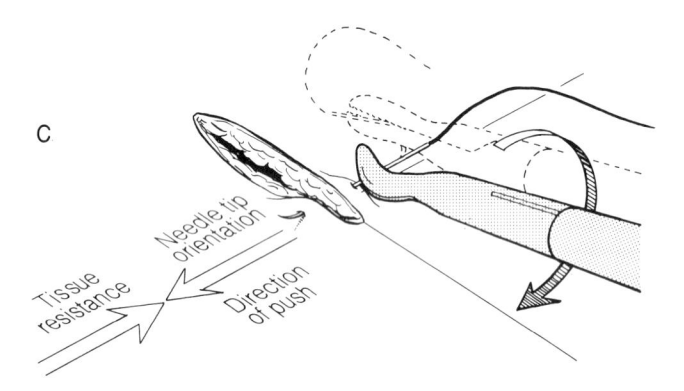

FIGURE 14-8 A. The needle driver is to be rotated counterclockwise in preparation for the entrance bite. B. In this position the needle tip is to be hooked into the tissue with the tip perpendicular to the suture line (C) in a scooping motion.

made in selecting an entrance bite that is either too small or too large, or in using a combination of the two, resulting in a tortuous suture line.

AMOUNT OF BITE

The selection of entrance and exit bites will control how much tissue will be bunched together in the suture loop.

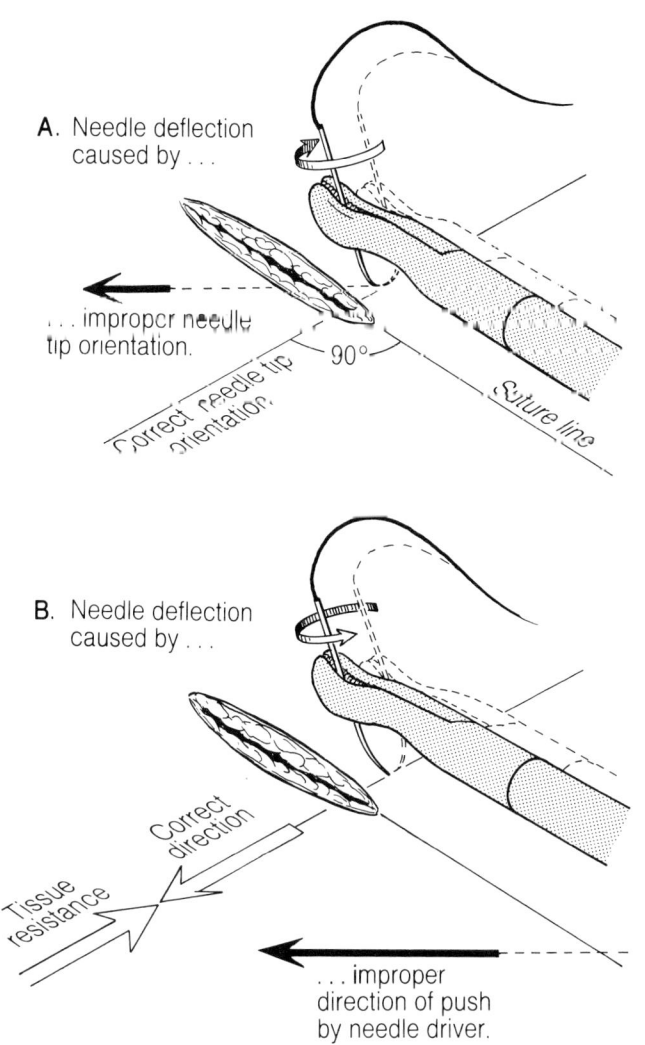

FIGURE 14-9 Two causes of tip deflection. A. Improper tip orientation with correctly directed needle driving. B. Proper tip orientation with incorrectly directed needle driver.

Too little may not provide adequate seal or strength, requiring the placement of many more stitches than necessary, thereby wasting time and inflicting additional trauma. Too large a bite will gather excessive tissue, resulting in a bulky suture line, possibly narrowing the lumen of a conduit, and perhaps resulting in tissue necrosis. The amount of bite needs to be precisely calculated for each structure, keeping in mind the function and reconstructive goal.

EXIT BITE

The exit bite is an easier pass to make than the entrance bite; therefore, double-armed suturing is encouraged where two exit bites could complete the stitch. This is especially advantageous during anastomosis of conduits. This technique involves cannulation of the lumen with each needle tip individually.

To locate the proper exit point, the needle tip is turned upward (external direction), creating an upward tenting of the tissue. The correct point of exit is estimated, and if the bite appears too large or small, adjustments can be made. Depending on the amount of bite, a certain length of needle tip shows, and if it is too short, the needle can be regrasped further back and pushed forward. This tip can then be grasped either with the assisting grasper or the needle driver. In either case, the needle is pulled out, carefully adjusting it to minimize trauma.

INTRACORPOREAL KNOT-TYING TECHNIQUES

In laparoscopic suturing, intracorporeal knot tying has been a formidable challenge, so much so that it has taken a back seat to extracorporeal knot tying and the use of substitute devices. The latter are limited in their application, and a need still exists for intracorporeal knot tying because, without it, advanced laparoscopic surgical techniques are hampered in their progress.

The ability to confidently and competently tie knots intracorporeally with laparoscopic instruments is an essential and fundamental skill because it is based on time-honored universally adaptable methods that can utilize readily available materials. When sophisticated devices fail, or if practicing in locations where economic conditions deem such devices unfeasible, what remains is surgeons and their skills. Furthermore, intracorporeal suturing and knot tying need not be an overwhelming challenge because all that is necessary is the proper approach and technique, in particular, the choreographed knotting technique presented subsequently.

Square Knot

First, the ideal knot needs to be selected, one that will be simple to tie, hold securely, and be adaptable for multipurpose use. Such a knot is the traditional square knot, familiar to most surgeons, with this added feature. It can be converted into a slip knot that is adjustable and reconvertible into the locking configuration (square knot) numerous times. This permits the employment of slip knot suspension technique,[19] a practical method of conduit anastomosis. The choreographed sequence that is presented in the figures must be practiced precisely to achieve the time- and effort-saving benefits of this approach.

After the knot-tying movements are analyzed and broken down into their basic movements, they can be reassembled into a teachable sequence, choreographed into the least number of required movements (8 steps), and standardized for predictable results. The breakdown of movements also allows the sequence to be recognizable and permits slow meticulous execution in the limited-access magnified surgical field (Fig. 14-10).

A. Make C-loop with right hand.

B. Wrap with right hand.

C. Grab short tail... ...and pull through

Intracorporeal Square Knot

D. Lay down first flat knot.

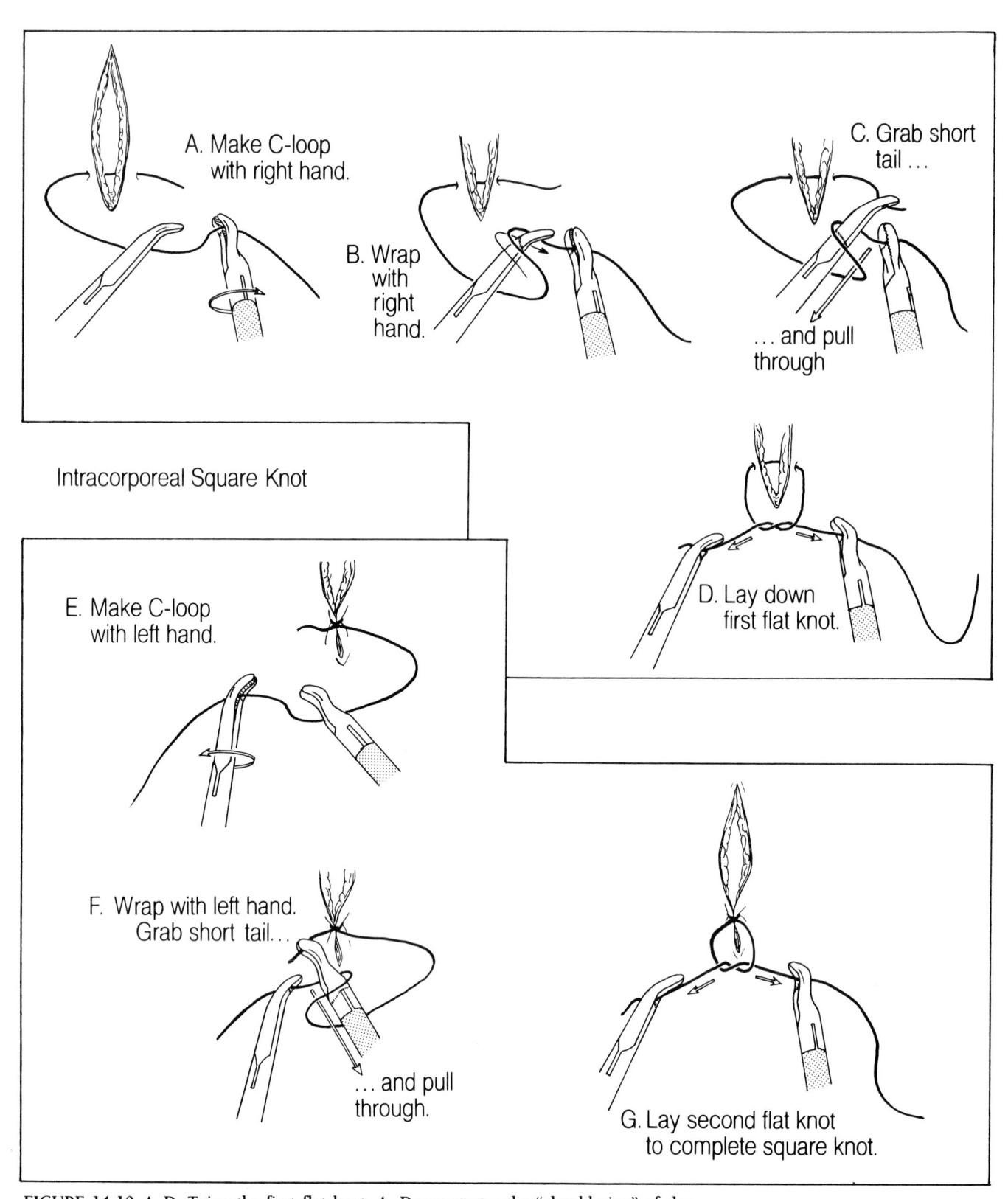

E. Make C-loop with left hand.

F. Wrap with left hand. Grab short tail... ...and pull through.

G. Lay second flat knot to complete square knot.

FIGURE 14-10 A–D. Tying the first flat knot. A. Demonstrates the "shouldering" of the thread, that is, rotating the instrument holding the thread forward to cause it to buckle and form a shoulder, which facilitates the looping of the thread. B. A "knitting technique" is employed, that is, the instrument tips maintain constant contact, so that the tips slide on one another similar to knitting. C. The short (1 to 2 cm) tail is grasped. D. The knot is set down flat. E–G. Tying the second opposing flat knot, resulting in a square knot. E. A C-loop and shoulder are created. F. The tail is grasped. G. The second knot is placed down squarely. H. Beginning conversion from square to slip knot. I. Conversion to the slipping configuration. J. Sliding the slip knot. K. Cinching the slip knot down in its final position. L. Reconverting the slip knot to the square knot. M. Square knot re-created.

Chapter 14 Laparoscopic Suturing and Tissue Approximation 151

Conversion of Square Knot to Slip Knot

H. Grab suture loop... ...and long tail.

I. Pull in opposite directions.

J. Slide knot to tissue.

K. Cinch slip knot.

L. Pull ends in opposite directions.

M. Square knot recreated.

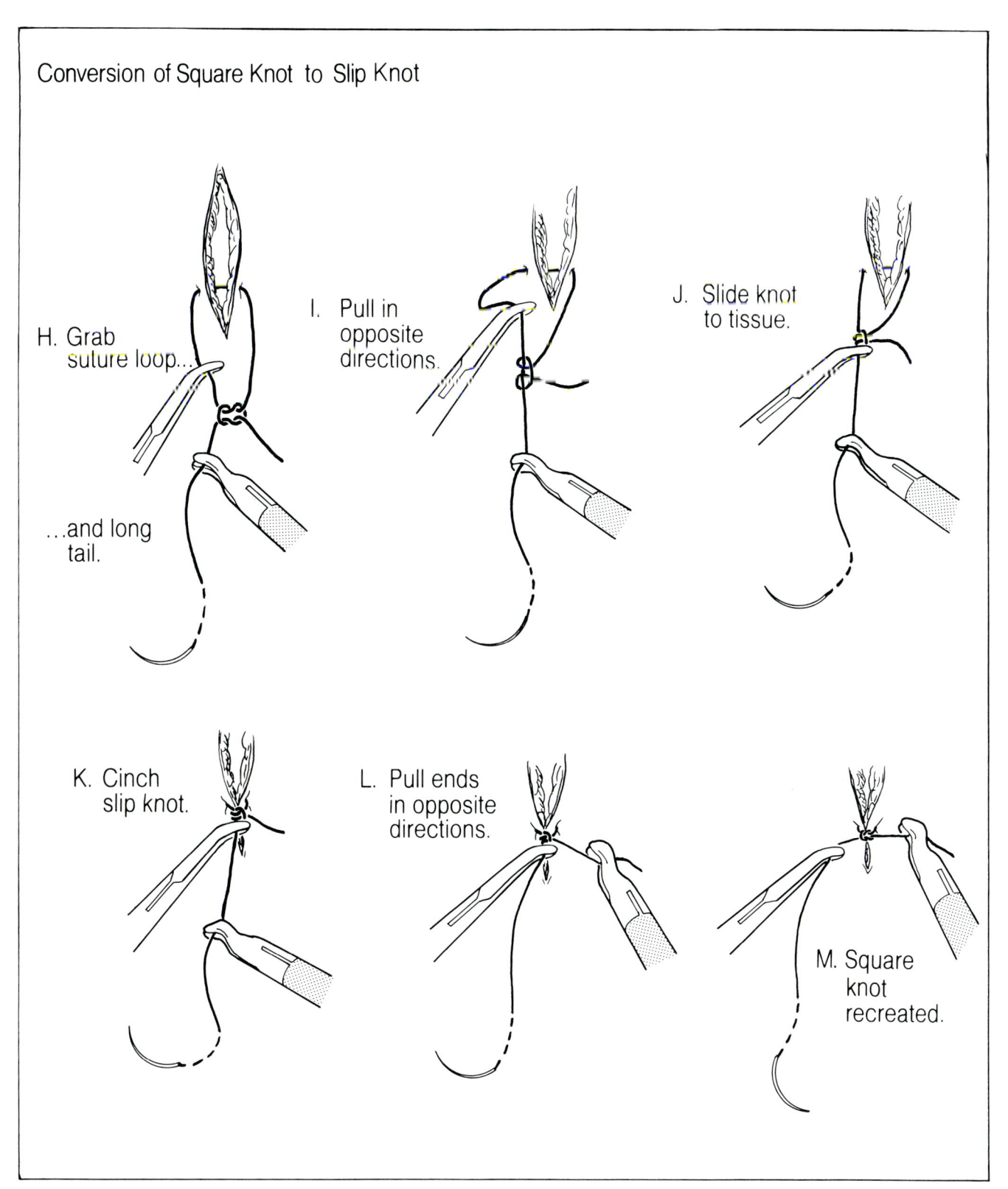

FIGURE 14-10 (Continued)

Selection of suture material is critical for this knot-tying technique. The ability to use instruments to handle suture material with memory and elastic deformation characteristics is essential. A stiff thick monofilament suture is difficult to work with because it bends and springs unpredictably, does not deform to lock the knot in place, and requires multiple hitches to secure. On the other end of the spectrum is a flimsy braided suture, which becomes limp in the surgical field, shreds when grasped, and when pulled harder, locks the knot irreversibly. The 2–0 and 3–0 braided absorbable and silk sutures seem to be adequate; however, serious efforts are underway to develop both permanent and absorbable suture material.

EXTRACORPOREAL KNOT-TYING TECHNIQUES

Extracorporeal techniques are frequently used by the novice in laparoscopic surgery who has not yet achieved the skills necessary for intracorporeal knotting. However, experienced laparoscopic surgeons occasionally encounter situations in which extracorporeal knotting is very helpful. Two such situations include: (1) in continuity ligature of ductal structures and (2) approximating tissue under tension, where an intracorporeal knot might slip before it could be adequately locked.

The simplest extracorporeal knot is the Röder's knot, a modified tonsil ligature developed in 1918.[20] This knot is very much like a fishing knot and is the knot used for pretied catgut ligatures (Surgi-Tie, AutoSuture, Norwalk, CT, or Endo-Loop, Ethicon, Somerville, NJ; Fig. 14-11).

While the Röder's knot is a convenient knot to know and is valuable for application of gut ligatures, it will slip when made out of monofilament, synthetic materials, such as polyprolylene (Prolene, Ethicon, Inc., Somerville, NJ), nylon, or polyglyconate (Maxon, Davis & Geck, Danbury, CT). This problem can be overcome by the use of a standard square knot and knot pusher.

Extracorporeal square knotting was first used by Semm[11] as a method of performing standard surgical ligatures in a laparoscopic environment. An extracorporeal square knot is shown in Figure 14-12. The technique involves the use of a long (minimum, 30-in) suture, which is passed down a 5- or 10-mm port. If the goal is suturing, the needle mounted on the end of the long suture is passed through tissue and pulled out the same port. If the goal is to ligate in continuity, the suture is passed around the structure to be ligated and again pulled out the same port. A simple overhand knot is created, and a knot pushing-instrument is placed over the knot. Even countertraction is placed on both ends of the suture, and the knot is pushed down through the trocar until it is snug around the structure to be ligated. The knot pusher is then pulled out, a second throw is formed (reversed to the first throw if a square knot is desired), and this knot is then pushed down with the knot pusher in an identical fashion. As many throws as are necessary, depending on the suture material, are applied. A scissors is brought down along the suture or through another port to cut the suture material.

While extracorporeal knotting is rapid and efficient, the major drawback is tissue trauma that occurs when a large amount of suture is pulled through the needle tract or

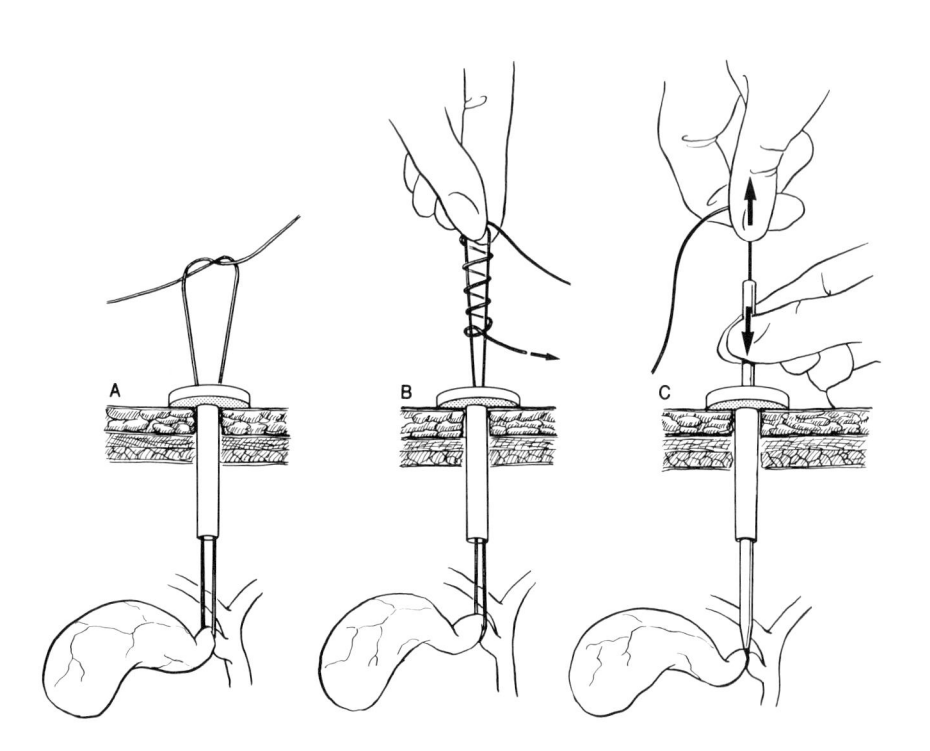

FIGURE 14-11 A. A Röder's knot is constructed by forming an overhand knot and then wrapping the suture tail back around both arms of the loop three times. B. The suture is locked by bringing the tail back through the large loop, between the last two twists of the wrap. C. The knot is slid down with a plastic applicator rod.

around a delicate duct. Also, the weight of the trocar creates torque on the suture, causing further tissue trauma. In addition, some knot pushers are traumatic to suture and may cause the suture to break during creation of a knot. Lastly, the requirement to have suture material traveling through a trocar ensures that there will be a low volume gas leak during the formation of the knot. For all these reasons, the author prefers to use intracorporeal knotting except for the situations mentioned at the outset of this section.

INTRACORPOREAL SUTURING TECHNIQUES

Linear Incisions and Lacerations

INTERRUPTED SUTURING

The intracorporeal suture line is composed of continuous, interrupted, or a combination of both types of stitches. When reapproximating an incision in flat tissue planes, it is referred to as a linear suture line; when approximating conduits, it is called circumferential. Staplers will undoubtedly play a role in constructing these suture lines, and a combination of both staples and suture may be a desirable approach. When constructing either suture line, tissues should be prepared so that the reapproximation can be accomplished with a minimum of tension. Tissues can be positioned by the assistant, or self-retracting devices can be used. There is a need for the development of intracorporeal retractors, clamps, and other related instrumentation to assist with these procedures.

When constructing a linear suture line, the factors involved in creating entrance and exit bites need to be considered. These factors include the length of the incision or laceration, the type of tissue layers to be approximated, and their function. In addition to selecting the needle and thread combination, the length of suture needs to be calculated and trimmed to the shortest necessary length to avoid tangling in the field. The needle driver and assisting grasper trocars should ideally be positioned so that the needle driver instrument is parallel to the suture line; the assisting grasper is offset from the needle driver between 45° and 90°; and the trocars are positioned at least 6 in apart. In preparing the most effective setup, the surgeon should be positioned so that the entrance–exit scooping motion occurs at right angles to the incision line (Fig. 14-4). An ambidextrous approach is desirable, and intracorporeal knot-tying techniques must be second nature.

As the suture line is constructed, interrupted stitches may be placed using a suspension slip-knot technique[19] (see Figs. 14-10H–M) to approximate tissue initially that may be under considerable tension, or where visibility is needed for the placement of subsequent stitches. Stitches should be placed evenly, bringing the tissues together without excessive tension or misalignment of layers. The number of stitches required is based on the number needed to complete a suture line adequately or provide tissue edge alignment. The particular configurations and techniques are discussed in the chapters dealing with specific clinical procedures.

CONTINUOUS SUTURING

In laparoscopic training, interrupted suturing is practiced first to develop necessary eye–hand coordination, basic suturing technique, and proper tissue alignment. The next step is to learn continuous suturing, which is quicker but more difficult to perform correctly.

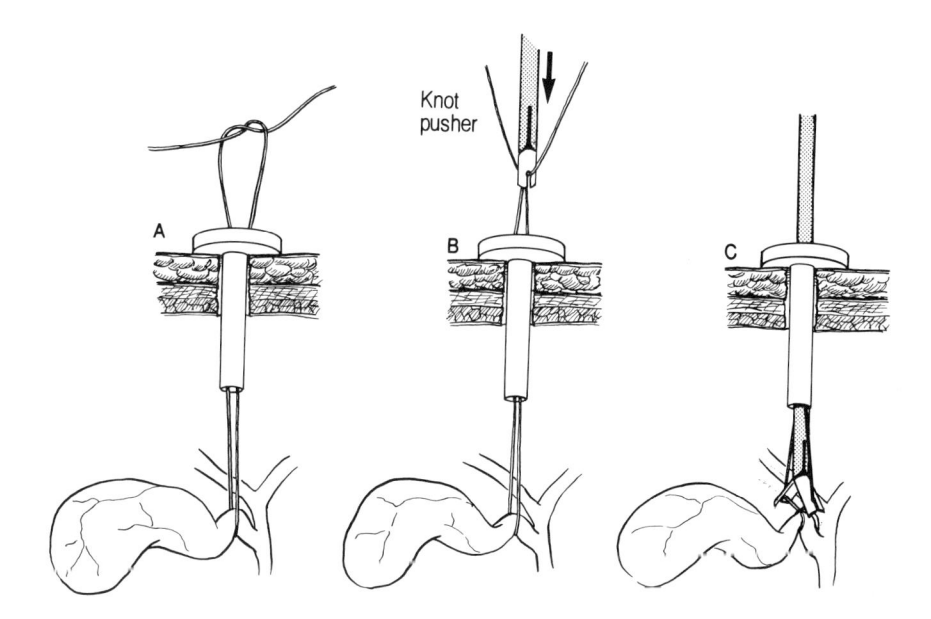

FIGURE 14-12 A. An extracorporeal square knot is also started with an overhand knot, but then a grooved knot pusher (model shown is Gazayerli instrument, Baxter V Mueller, Chicago, IL) is used to slide the knot into place (B). Repeated squared throws prevent suture slippage (C).

The continuous-suturing technique begins and ends in an anchoring knot, the latter of which can be tied to the loop of the last stitch or secured with an Aberdeen knot (see Fig. 15-8).[20a] Because intracorporeal knot tying is unfamiliar to most laparoscopic surgeons, hemoclips, silver beads, and other methods have been used in its place; however, a precisely placed stitch and tied knot is preferred, when possible. During training, one should practice suturing both directions of the suture line, to and fro, left to right, and right to left. An assisting grasper with a flamingo tip is an invaluable tool that is useful in identifying the cut edges, positioning the tissues for entrance and exit bites, and adjusting the tension on the suture loops as the approximation progresses.

The choice of suture material is important because monofilament and braided material behave quite differently. The stiff springy monofilament material run in a noninterlocking fashion promotes speed but may result in an uneven suture line, although it is still sometimes the material of choice. Woven threads, particularly 2–0 and 3–0 silk, have a tendency to drag and lock the suture line, and every stitch has to be adjusted to the necessary tension. Use of a single-armed suture is suitable for linear suture lines; however, double-armed or double-pointed needles can also be used.

Ductal Anastomosis

As laparoscopic use becomes more widespread, techniques, tricks, and clever devices will become popular that will make the methodology easier and more cost effective. Laparoscopic ductal anastomosis is particularly challenging, although its feasibility has been demonstrated.[20a] While vascular anastomosis was perfected around the turn of the century, such demanding technique is, for the moment, beyond the reach of the laparoscopic approach. However, ductal structures with less critical demands could benefit from some of the techniques and principles developed for high-pressure ducts. For example, gastrointestinal tract anastomosis can be accomplished with end-to-end, end-to-side, or side-to-side techniques, and in fact, these anastomoses have already been proved to be practical (Gardiner BN, Wolfe BM, et al. Personal communication September 1991). Although these structures are low-pressure conduits, a watertight seal and proper mucosal reapproximation are necessary. A redesign of current laparoscopic anastomosis technique is necessary to maximize efficiency, considering the difficulty of approach.

END-TO-END ANASTOMOSIS

End-to-end anastomosis is the preferred method of joining equal caliber and wall-thickness conduits. The number of stitches and the amount of bite are calculated for each particular organ, depending on its function. Either interrupted or continuous sutures can be used. Interrupted stitches give greater precision and control; the continuous technique is more rapid, although less forgiving. Assisting devices, such as self-retractors, clamps, or intraluminal stents, can be useful.

END-TO-SIDE ANASTOMOSIS

End-to-side anastomosis allows the union of conduits with disparate lumens and wall-thickness conduits and is technically easier to accomplish than end-to-end anastomosis. It is less invasive than the end-to-end technique because the fenestration on the recipient structure involves only part of its circumference. Conduction of the luminal contents is a concern because it is necessary to turn a corner to advance.

SIDE-TO-SIDE ANASTOMOSIS

Side-to-side anastomosis is similar to end-to-side anastomosis and is frequently employed in the gastrointestinal tract. It provides a convenient joining of conduits that normally lie side by side.

REFERENCES

1. Burket WC (ed): *Surgical Papers of William Stuart Halsted*. Baltimore, Johns Hopkins Press, 1924.
2. Guthrie CC: *Blood Vessel Surgery and Its Application: A Reprint*. Pittsburgh, U of Pittsburgh, 1959, pp 1–69.
3. Serafin D, Buncke HJ (eds): *Microsurgical Composite Tissue Transplantation*. St. Louis, CV Mosby, 1979, pp 111–144, 154–163.
4. Daniel RK, Terzis JK (eds): *Reconstructive Microsurgery*. Boston, Little Brown, 1977, pp 61–115, 670.
5. Troutman RC: *Microsurgery of the Anterior Segment of the Eye*. St. Louis, CV Mosby, 1974, Vol 1, pp 37–205.
6. Casanova R, Herrera GA, Engels BV, et al: Microarterial sutureless anastomosis using a polymeric adhesive: An experimental study. *J Reconstr Microsurg* 1987; 3:201–207.
7. Rubio PA: *Atlas of Stapling Techniques*. Rockville, Aspen Publishers, 1986.
8. Quigley MR, Bailes JE, Kwaan HC, et al. Comparison of bursting strength between suture- and laser-anastomosed vessels. *Microsurgery* 1985; 6:229–232.
9. Estes JM, Szabo Z, Harrison MR: Techniques for in utero endoscopic surgery—a new approach for fetal intervention. *Surg Endosc* 1992; 6:215–218.
10. Semm K: Tissue-puncher and loop-ligation: New aides for surgical therapeutic pelviscopy (laparoscopy): Endoscopic intra-abdominal surgery. *Endoscopy* 1978; 10:119–127.
11. Reich H: Laparoscopic reversal of sterilization (abstract). Presented at the Second World Congress of Gynecologic Endoscopy, Flairemont-Ferrard, France, June 5–8, 1989.
11a. Bowyer DW, Moran ME, Szabo Z: Laparoscopic radical prostatectomy—canine model (video abstract). Presented at the Fourth International Meeting of the Society for Minimally Invasive Therapy, Dublin, Ireland, November 8–10, 1992.
12. Cuschieri A, Berci G: *Laparoscopic Biliary Surgery*. London, Blackwell Scientific, 1990, pp 15–37.
13. Troutman RC: *Microsurgery of the Anterior Segment of the Eye*. St. Louis, CV Mosby, 1974, 37–86.

14. Szabo Z: A new precision control needle holder and assisting grasper for advanced suturing and anastomosis techniques in operative laparoscopy. Proceedings of the 1991 AAGL Annual World Congress on Gynecologic Endoscopy, Santa Fe Springs, in press. (Announced publication: January 1993.)
15. Szabo Z, Burch BH (eds): *Atlas of Microsurgical Techniques.* San Francisco, Microsurgical Research Institute, 1983, pp 1–147.
16. Buncke HJ, Chater NL, Szabo Z: *Manual of Microvascular Surgery.* Danbury, Davis & Geck, 1975, pp 1–21.
16a. Szabo Z: Extra and intracorporeal knotting and suturing technique, in Berci G (ed): *GI Endoscopy Clinics of North America.* Philadelphia, WB Saunders, 1993, in press.
17. First Assistant™. Leonard Medical, Huntingdon Valley, PA.
18. Katkhouda N, Mouiel J: A new technique of surgical treatment of chronic duodenal ulcer without laparotomy by videocoelioscopy. *Am J Surg* 1991; 161:361.
19. Szabo Z, Stellini L, Ellis MS, et al: Slip-knot suspension technique: A fail-safe microanastomosis for small caliber vessels. *Microsurgery* 1992; 13:100–102.
20. Röder H: *Die Technik der Mandelgesundungbestrebungen.* München, Aertzl Rundschau, 1918, pp 169–171.
20a. Shiwli S, Banting S, Cuschieri A: Laparoscopy in the management of pancreatic cancer: Endoscopic cholecystojejunostomy for advanced disease. *Br J Surg* 1992; 79:317–319.

Chapter 15

The Sutured Laparoscopic Gastrointestinal Anastomosis

L. K. Nathanson

Laparoscopic suturing techniques were introduced and utilized by Semm in gynecology in the mid-1970s.[1] The limitation of straight needles and slow internal knotting coupled with the difficulty in acquisition of the right level of expertise with these techniques contributed to their limited appeal to many surgeons. With the development of more efficient techniques of laparoscopic hand suturing, they were evaluated initially in bilioenteric anastomosis and, more recently, in gastrojejunostomy and colonic resection.

The progress in application of these techniques in the broader context of everyday intestinal surgery remains embryonal. Many of the cardinal principles of bowel surgery are skirted in these new techniques. Emphasis is made at this point that if these techniques are applied, for instance, to the opening of obstructed bowel for anastomotic bypass without proximal control of luminal contents, then extensive and dangerous peritoneal contamination will ensue. What may be accomplished using normal bowel does not translate automatically to what may be safely achieved in other pathologic situations.

THE BASIC SUTURED ANASTOMOTIC TECHNIQUE

Instrumentation

GRASPING FORCEPS

Manipulation of bowel around fixed cannula positions requires patience and care. While the instruments themselves may be atraumatic, as soon as the bowel is pulled or pushed, the apex of contact between the forceps and the bowel very easily acts as a point where perforation is induced. Steps to minimize this hazard include the following. Before bowel manipulation, ensure it is free of adhesions and mobile. Patient positioning and tilting of the operating table uses gravity to displace the bowel without the need for repeated manipulation. Both of the operator's hands should be used to improve tactile feedback, and with a third grasper in the hands of the assistant, this allows a stepwise grasping and releasing of bowel to "walk" along the bowel efficiently to the region of interest. (No hesitation should be felt about using a fifth access port if required). The grasper must be kept in the field of view at all times while being moved to minimize the chance of bowel injury. On occasion, the telescope might better be inserted through one of the other ports as far away from the bowel as possible to facilitate an overall view of the proceedings.

The spring-handled atraumatic grasping forceps and Dorsey bowel grasper are the best instruments for bowel manipulation (Fig. 15-1). Frequently, the atraumatic grasping forceps slip when excessive traction is applied, although at times this is irritating, it provides a safeguard against accidental bowel perforation. With due care, dissecting forceps (Fig. 15-1) may be useful to retract bowel when applied to the appendices epiploicae.

NEEDLE HOLDERS AND SUTURES

Basic techniques of endoscopic suturing are covered elsewhere in this text, with mastery of internal knotting by square or reef knots being essential skills. The Semm needle holder system was designed to allow straight needles to be inserted through the nondisposable 5-mm cannula and provide secure manipulation of this round-bodied needle by wedging it at right angles to the shaft of the needle holder in the coarse transverse ridges of the jaws (Fig. 15-2). The 3-mm needle holder was designed to introduce the needle and suture into the suture applicator which then acted as an airtight unit introduced into the 5-mm cannula protecting the suture at the same time from the action of the cannula trumpet valve. The 3-mm needle holder introduced through another port is then used to grasp and

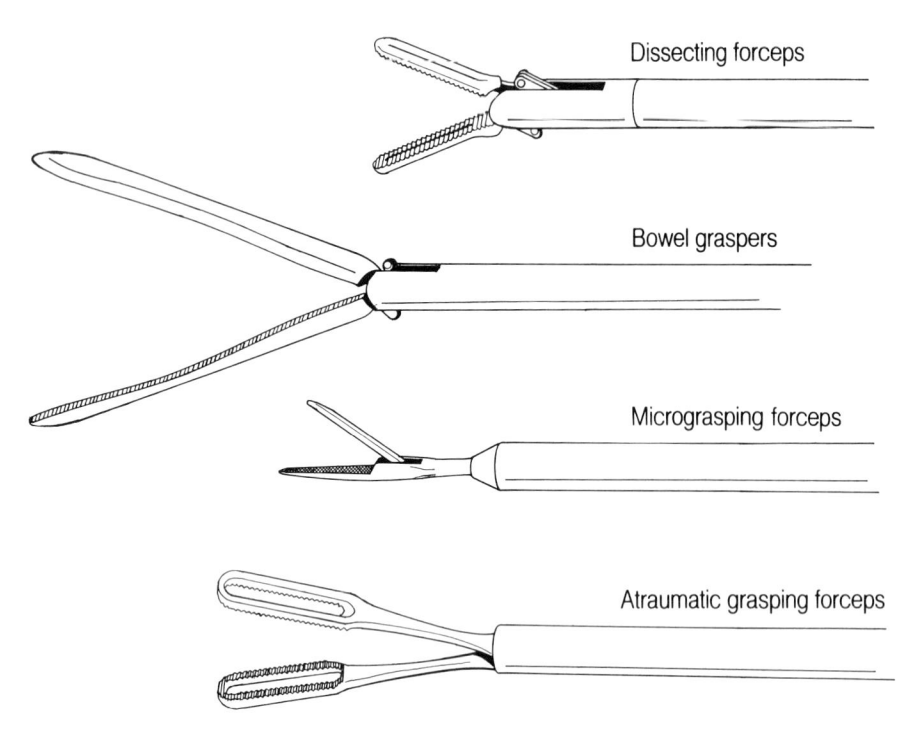

FIGURE 15-1 A variety of graspers are displayed in this panel. (top to bottom) A standard tissue grasper frequently used for laparoscopic cholecystectomy will hold tissue quite firmly but may cause crush injury and may tear tissue as it is dislodged. A Dorsey- or Glassman-type clamp is designed for manipulating the intestine. It is atraumatic and, because of its long length, may provide luminal occlusion when necessary. A fine grasping forceps is useful for picking up the edges of delicate tubular structures, such as the cystic duct or common duct. The spring steel tubal graspers come from a previous generation of gynecologic instruments. Nevertheless, these are valuable for atraumatic handling of delicate tissues (e.g., small bowel) where a Glassman-type clamp is not available.

manipulate the needle. The advantages of the system are that it can operate through 5-mm cannulae, the needle is easily oriented and grasped without the risk of needle rotation (as may occur with the curved needle), and a secure grip of the needle promotes correct passage through tissue. The disadvantages of this system are that the straight round-bodied needle is of limited use with friable tissue and can easily tear tissue at its point of entry. The needle is also not able to be grasped obliquely to the needle holder to facilitate needle insertion in the correct plane relative to the cut edge of the suture line, which becomes important when the needle holder shaft does not run parallel to the suture line. In areas where space is confined, the straight needle is also somewhat more difficult to insert and complete its pass through the tissue.

Second-generation needle holders are illustrated in Figure 15-3. The improved jaw design of the Ethicon, Cook, and Wolfe instruments allows much more secure grasping of standard flattened needle shafts, and so, they have paved the way for the use of standard curved needles. Introduction of the curved needle requires the diameter of the larger 11-mm port. Suture and needle tangling in the port valve mechanism during insertion can be minimized by first backloading the suture and needle into a reducer tube. Once introduced, the orientation of the needle is best achieved by allowing it to drop onto a flat surface below the cannula site and then grasping it with the needle holder. Final orientation and obliquity of the needle shaft is adjusted by pressure applied via the grasping forceps in the surgeon's left hand. The Cook curved needle holder has an altogether different jaw design. It certainly has the advantage of grasping the needle securely but suffers from being a bit awkward to regrasp the needle. It must be exchanged for another grasper to fashion knots internally.

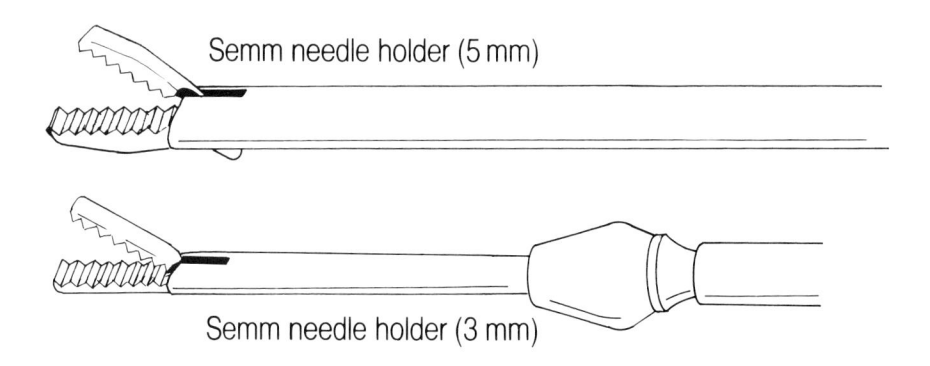

FIGURE 15-2 The Semm needle holder system. A 5-mm needle holder with transverse serrations provides a firm right angle grip. The 3-mm needle holder provides a method for introducing needle and suture through a 5-mm port without getting hung up on the trumpet valve. A suture applicator or 3.5-mm reducer is used with this instrument.

FIGURE 15-3 Second-generation needle holders have assumed a variety of handle and tip configurations. The Wolfe microsurgical needle holder offers universal (diamond-jawed) grip pattern for orienting the needle in any angle the surgeon prefers. The handle also allows more opportunity for needle holder rotation. The Cook needle holder is preferred by many gynecologists and urologists. This needle holder holds a curved needle firmly at right angles to the needle holder. It seems best utilized for driving needles through tough tissue where a less secure grasp of the needle might result in needle rotation. The Ethicon needle holder has a tip configuration most similar to needle holders used at laparotomy, but with an axial handle that allows 360° rotation of the instrument.

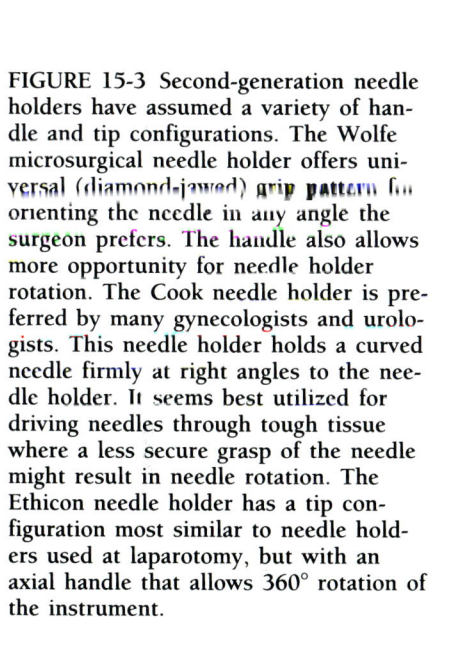

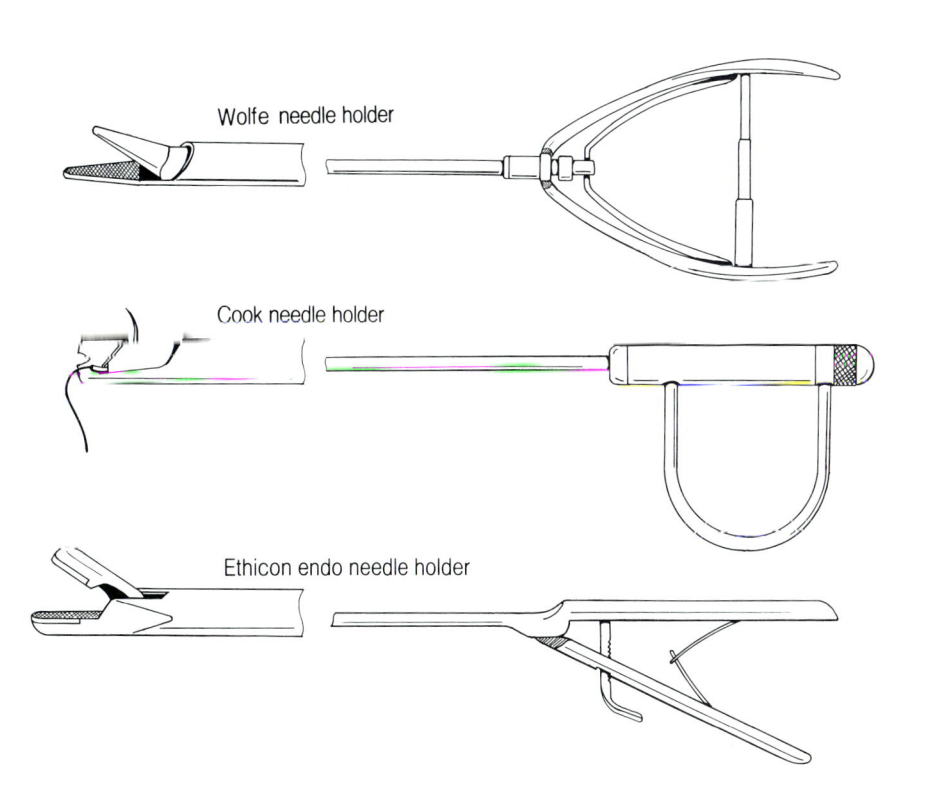

The surgeon's second hand should use tissue grasping forceps, ideally with a curved tip, which allows tissue and needle grasping. The jaw hinge design may be single or twin action but must be engineered so that during internal knotting the loops of the suture wound around the shaft of the forceps during knot formation do not become jammed in the hinge mechanism as the loops of the knot slide down.

Suture-grasping forceps used by the assistant should have a jaw finely engineered so that it grasps fine sutures without slipping but also has rounded edges so that accidental cutting of the suture is avoided as traction is applied. The micrograsping forceps (see Fig. 15-1) are suitable for the task, but the edges of the jaw need to be checked when first used. They should be smoothed and rounded if found to be sharp. Needle designs commonly used are illustrated in Figure 15-4. The straight needle introduced early on as part of the Semm suturing technique has been discussed. The ski-shaped needle, with a standard flattened shaft, and standard curved needles both are well controlled with the jaws of the second-generation needle holders.

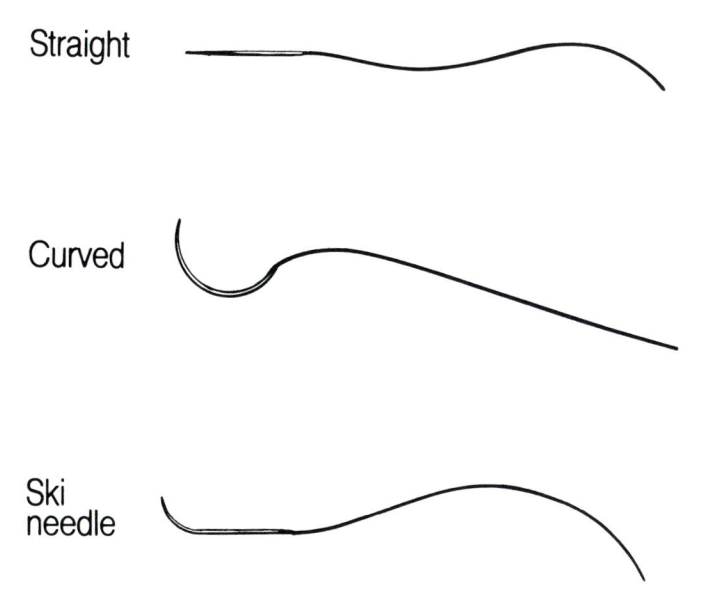

FIGURE 15-4 Laparoscopic suturing may be accomplished with a straight needle as described by Semm, a semicircular (standard curved needle), or a ski-shaped needle with a flattened shaft, which helps orient the ski with the tip up in a second-generation needle holder.

BOWEL OCCLUSION

Instrumentation for proximal and distal control of bowel are not readily available currently. One technique is a sling of silicone or thick suture material, which is passed around the bowel and back out through the abdominal wall, to sling and occlude the bowel lumen. This can be secured in place by an external clamp (Fig. 15-5). The technique has the added advantage of elevating the bowel and providing traction.

Prototype atraumatic bowel clamps are being developed that have a shaft diameter of 10 mm and effective jaw length of 50 mm. The advantage over the sling occlusion method is a more secure clamping of the bowel lumen. However, they occupy the port used to insert them, therefore limiting instrument access, and the jaw length is inadequate to ensure complete cross clamping, especially in the colon. This will no doubt change as further instrumentation becomes available.

INSTRUMENTAL ACCESS AND PORT PLACEMENT

The key to suturing with comfort lies with having the shaft of the needle holder (as it emerges from the abdominal wall) run parallel to the length of the suture line. The tissue-grasping forceps in the left hand should approach in such a way that it arrives at the suture line at right angles to the needle holder. The placement of the third instrument (assistant's port) should be out of the way of the other instruments and not block the endoscopic view of the suture line. At least one of the accessory ports should be 11 mm in diameter to allow large shaft instruments to have access if required.

A surgeon's preference of suture materials is traditionally quite personal. The demands on patience and time laparoscopically mandate that some of these choices are adapted to use suture materials with good handling characteristics, such as silk and polyglactin. One should avoid the use of polypropylene or polydioxanone sutures where possible because their "memory" and spring during handling add considerably to manipulation skills required.

The commencement of a continuous suture line can be facilitated by fashioning a jamming loop knot using the steps illustrated in Figure 15-6. This is performed outside the peritoneal cavity using a standard needle holder. The suture with completed jamming loop is then introduced into the peritoneum via the cannula with care to avoid it

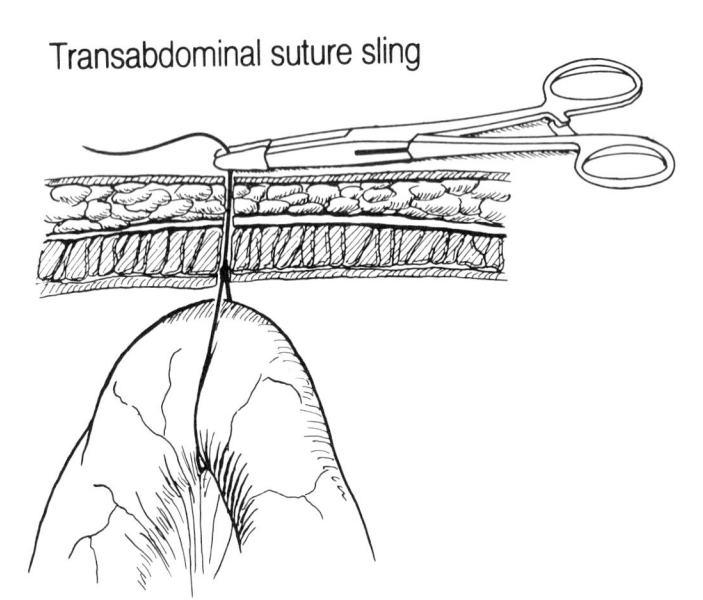

FIGURE 15-5 Bowel occlusion can be attained by passing a thick suture, silicone rubber, or umbilical tape through the abdominal wall on a straight needle, underneath the bowel and back through the abdominal wall. Occlusion and traction can be maintained with a hemostat at skin level.

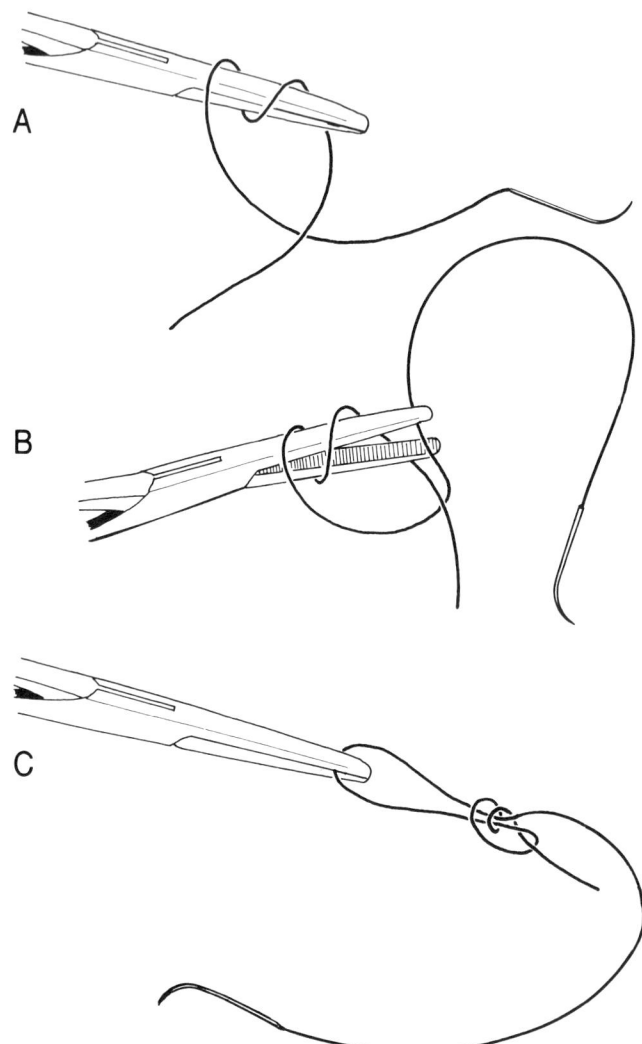

FIGURE 15-6 A jamming loop knot made outside the abdomen facilitates the initiation of a running suture. A. The knot is started by wrapping the tail of the suture around a needle holder. B. The body of the suture 5 cm from the loop is grasped with the tip of the needle holder. C. It is pulled back through the initial wrap to create a loop.

slipping closed as it is introduced. The locking of the jamming loop knot is illustrated in Figure 15-7. On completion of the row of continuous sutures, the suture is knotted by a reef knot or by the instrumentally tied Aberdeen knot, using the steps illustrated in Figure 15-8. Providing a minimum of three locking throws are performed before pulling the tail through the loop, the Aberdeen knot is stronger than a reef knot. The suture tail is trimmed long enough for subsequent grasping to allow accurate suture placement of the last few sutures of the anterior layer of the anastomosis.

CHOLECYSTOJEJUNOSTOMY

Patient Selection

The most common indication by bypass of the biliary tract is malignant obstruction of the lower end of the bile duct by adenocarcinoma of the pancreatic head. Many of these patients will be offered the chance of insertion of endoscopic stents. Perhaps this is a reasonable initial approach, with laparoscopic bypass reserved for those unable to be stented or where difficulty with the stent, dislodgement or blockage occur.

A choice must be made between enteric bypass to the gallbladder or directly to the bile duct. In unselected patients undergoing bypass to the gallbladder, approximately 25 percent will require reoperation for subsequent jaundice caused by malignant encroachment, most often the result of low insertion of the cystic duct into the common bile duct. This is best avoided by intraoperative imaging of the cystic duct and conversion to open bypass directly to the bile duct for those patients seen to have low cystic duct insertion.

At open surgery, bypass of the duodenum by gastroenterostomy was often combined with biliary bypass to anticipate the duodenal obstruction that will occur in approximately 50 percent of patients. In the era of laparotomy access, prophylactic duodenal bypass made sense because a second laparotomy in a frail patient (at a time when the duration of their survival was limited) constituted poor palliation. The case for prophylactic combination of gastroenterostomy with the biliary bypass with laparoscopic exposure seems far more tenous. The morbidity related to a second laparoscopic procedure is minor, the ileus induced is minimal, and most stomas function within 3 days. It therefore is reasonable for gastroenterostomy to be reserved for those with existing or incipient duodenal obstruction. In the patients who subsequently develop obstruction, a laparoscopic gastroenterostomy can simply be performed at that time. This approach will minimize the complications (especially bleeding) and morbidity related to the gastroenterostomy in those who would not need it.

Patient Positioning, Port Placement, and Exposure

The patient is placed supine to facilitate operative cholangiography. The skin is prepared with aqueous povidone-iodine solution, and there is a wide exposure of the abdominal wall, with anchoring of the drapes using a sterile plastic adhesive sheet. The surgeon stands on the patient's left, and the ancillary instrument stand and video monitor is placed at the head of the table opposite the patient's right shoulder. The assistant stands on the patient's right with the scrub nurse on the same side as the surgeon. Port placement is illustrated in Figure 15-9. A minimum of four ports are used. The right upper quadrant port used by the assistant is moved inferiorly when a combined stapled and sutured anastomosis is planned and is 12 mm diameter to

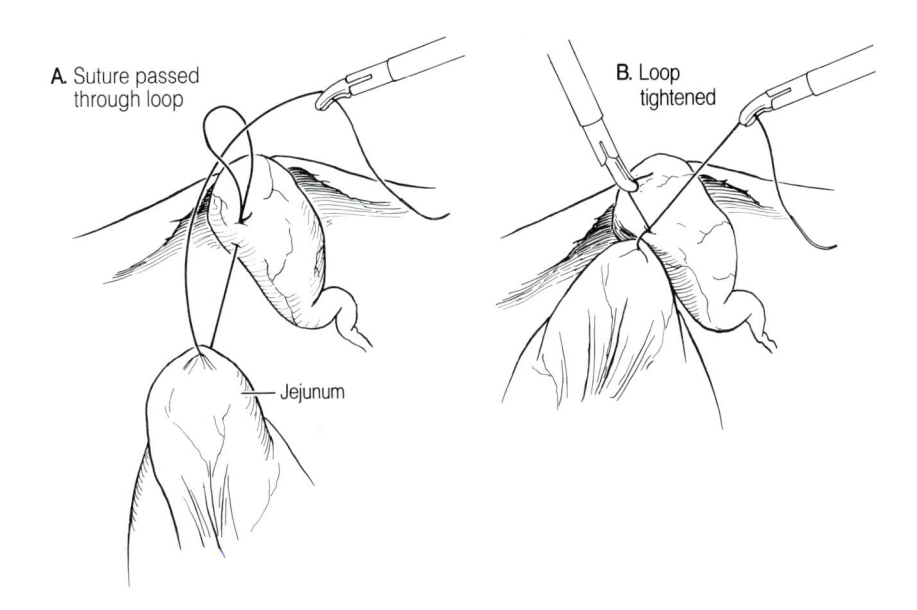

FIGURE 15-7 Intracorporeal use of the jamming loop knot. A. After the needle has been passed through both tissues to be approximated, the body of the suture is brought back through the loop. B. It is tightened by pulling on the body of the suture and the short tail.

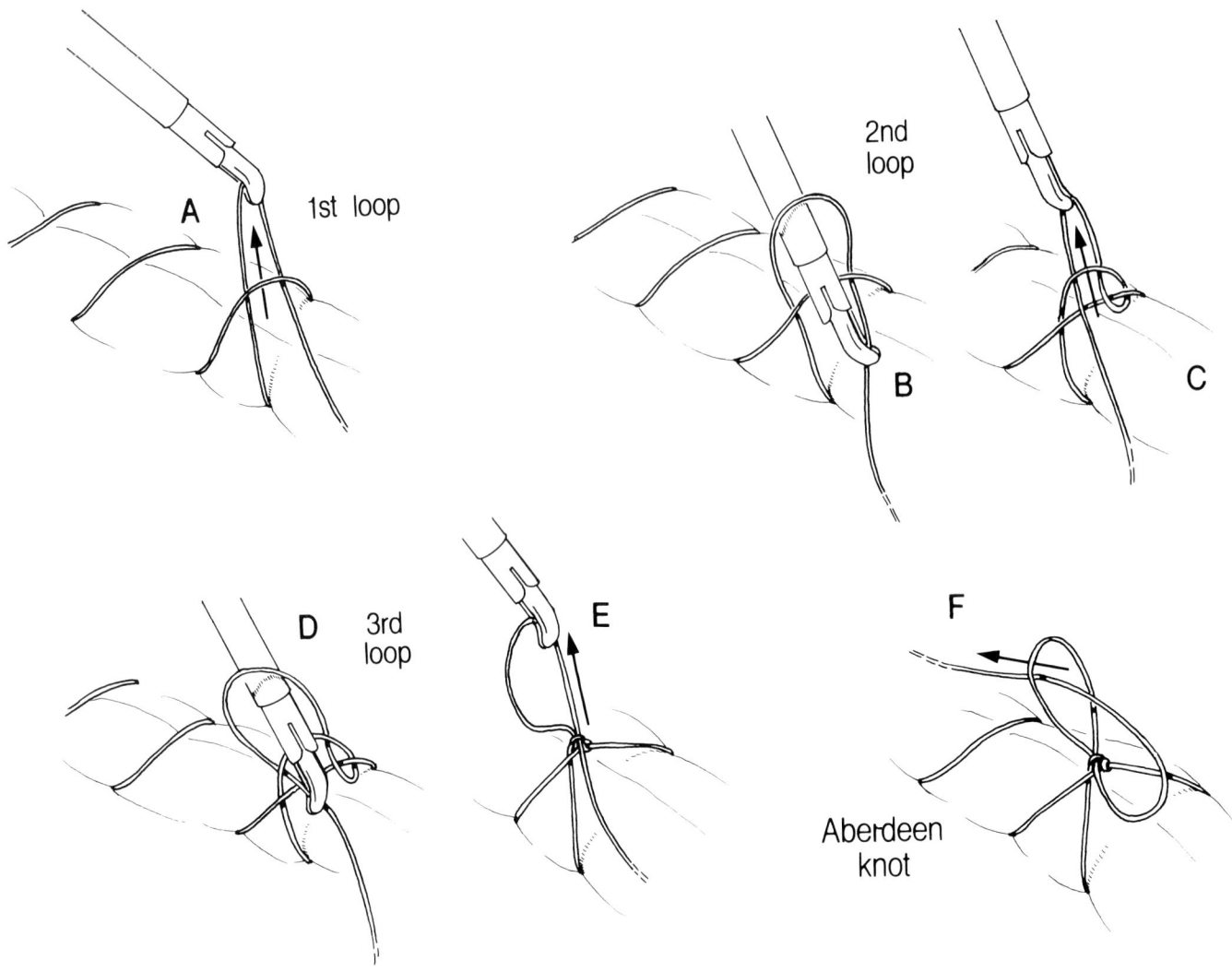

FIGURE 15-8 At the end of a running suture the suture line can be controlled in one of two ways. A square knot may be utilized or an Aberdeen knot (also known as crochet knot or daisy chain) may be used. This knot is made as follows. A. A loop of the suture body is brought under the previous bite. B. A second, (C, D) then third loop of the suture body is brought through the first and second loops. E. The slack is removed from all but the last loop. F. The suture and needle are brought through the last loop to lock up the chain.

accommodate the linear stapler/cutter. The two ports used by the surgeon must be anchored to the skin to prevent displacement and have flapper or silicone valve mechanisms, which improve instrument manipulation, an important factor when suturing.

Laparoscopic exposure of the peritoneum is established with gas presures set at 12 mmHg or less. Accessory ports are placed under direct visual guidance.

Cholangiography

Unless accurate information concerning the site of cystic duct entry to the common hepatic duct is available, this is achieved by introducing contrast into the gallbladder as the first step of the procedure. The Veress needle, introduced through the abdominal wall at the proposed site of the anastomosis to the gallbladder, works well. Bile is aspirated until the gallbladder is at least half empty. Delay in aspiration caused by thick inspissated bile can be more easily removed by the introduction of saline, which is mixed with the bile by gentle agitation, and then aspirated. Contrast is then introduced under image intensifier control to watch filling of the gallbladder and note the precise point of entry of the cystic duct to the common bile duct and the relative position of the carcinoma obstructing the duct distally. Early visualization of the flow of the contrast is important knot (see Fig. 15-6). This is introduced into the peritoneum; the needle is passed through the tissue and then through the loop, which then closes as traction is placed on it. I use a 26-mm standard semicircular ski needle with 3–0 polyglactin about five times the length of the suture line (10 cm). The sutures are placed taking the full thickness of the gallbladder wall and extramucosal bites of the bowel wall. Accurate suture placement takes patience, and after each suture is tightened for correct tissue approximation, this tension is maintained by the assistant grasping the suture with the micrograsping forceps some 2 cm away from the suture line. This "following" of the suture by the assistant is repeated after each pass of the needle.

An alternative technique, often useful when tissue approximation is proceeding with ease, is for the surgeon's left hand to grasp and follow. By traction on the suture at the time of needle insertion, the bites of tissue can be accomplished, and suturing proceeds quickly.

On completion of the posterior layer, the suture is tied either with a reef knot or Aberdeen knot, and the tail is left about 3 cm long. The gallbladder is then opened along the diathermy line and aspirated dry to minimize bile spillage. The bowel then similarly is opened over a 25 mm length. A second suture 10 cm in length with a pretied jamming loop knot is introduced, and with the assistant identifying the apex by traction on the long tail of the posterior suture, the suture line is commenced. Extramucosal or full-thickness bites at 5-mm intervals complete the anastomosis. The area is copiously lavaged with warm Ringers lactate solution, and the paracolic gutters and pelvis are aspirated dry. Routine drainage is not employed.

Stapled and Sutured Anastomosis

The technique employed here uses the 30-mm linear stapler/cutter (Endo GIA, Unitd States Surgical Corporation, Norwalk, CT) to complete the main part of the anastomosis, with closure of the residual defect using sutures. This has been found to be easier than closing the residual defect by triangulation using a second firing of the stapler. The difficulty experienced arises from inability to apply the second firing of the device precisely while, on the one hand, ensuring complete closure of the defect and, on the other, avoiding stenosis of the efferent jejunal lumen.

Port positioning is illustrated in Figure 15-9. Care must be taken with placement of the 12-mm port used to introduce the stapler because this must be sufficiently far away to allow the jaw to open and approach the fundus of the gallbladder at the optimum angle to staple across its fundus. Again the need to align the needle holder parallel to the suture line dictates the position of the left upper quadrant port.

The gallbladder is inspected and a cholecystocholangiogram performed in the same manner as described previously for the entirely hand-sewn anastomosis. The siting

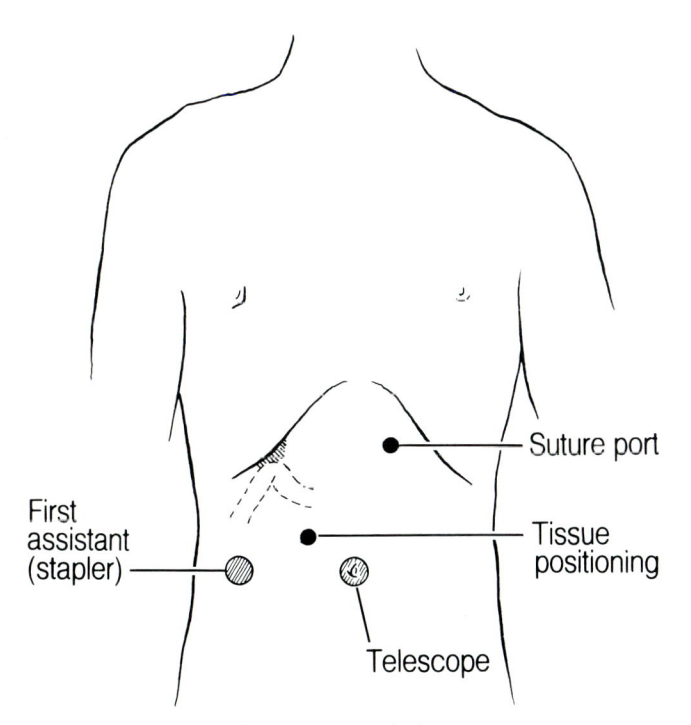

FIGURE 15-9 Port placement for cholecystojejunostomy. A 10-mm port is placed in the umbilicus. The three accessory ports may be 5 mm in diameter unless a stapler is to be used to fashion the anastomosis. In this case, the right upper quadrant port is replaced with a 12-mm port in the right iliac fossa.

because the most accurate information regarding the course of the cystic duct is often available during the initial flow into the common bile duct. After larger volumes of contrast are injected, large dilated ducts overlap on the image, leading to uncertainty in some instances as to the site of cystic duct entry relative to the tumor. Successful mapping of the cystic duct course allows a decision to be made early in the operation about whether the patient is suitable for laparoscopic cholecystojejunostomy or whether an alternative bypass to the common hepatic duct or more proximal ducts should be performed.

Sutured Cholecystojejunostomy

The gallbladder is then emptied of contrast and bile to minimize spillage as the needle is withdrawn. A suitable segment of jejunum, about 50 cm distal to the duodenojejunal flexure, is marked on its antimesenteric border with light diathermy over a 25-mm length, and the same length is marked with light diathermy of the serosa of the fundus of the gallbladder. These lines mark the incision lines, ensure an adequate size of anastomosis, and maintain the surgeon's orientation during suturing.

The suture is prepared as the next step. My preference is to fashion a loop at the tail of the suture with a jamming of the needle puncture in the gallbladder should be such that it coincides with the point selected for the entry of the jaws of the stapler (Fig. 15-10). This should be situated on the gallbladder fundus somewhat laterally to the right to facilitate staple line position at the apex of the fundus. On completion of the cholangiogram, an 8-mm opening in the gallbladder is made, bile aspirated, and a slightly smaller hole made on the antimesenteric aspect of the jejunum. The 30-mm stapler, loaded with the bowel stapling cartridge, is introduced as illustrated with support of the gallbladder and jejunum by the atraumatic grasper. The stapler is closed. Its position is checked, and then it is fired. An alternative method to help anchor the gallbladder to the jejunum before introducing the stapler is by using an internal tacking suture. This has not been as useful to me as initially expected, however. An external anchoring suture is quicker to place and far more useful. It is inserted through the abdominal wall laterally from the right flank, provides traction for insertion of the stapler, and is readily removed before suture of the defect.

Closure of the residual defect is done using an 8-cm 3–0 polyglactin suture with a pretied jamming loop knot. This is commenced with care to include the apex and includes bites of tissue 5 mm apart, incorporating the full thickness of the gallbladder wall and extramucosal layers of the jejunum. Completion of the suture line is by reef or Aberdeen knotting. Routine drainage of the peritoneum is not employed. This combination of stapled anastomosis with closure of the defect by sutures, in my hands, is the most practical method of creating a cholecystojejunostomy currently.

Conversion to Laparotomy

The most common reason for conversion to bypass to the bile ducts would be tumor encroachment to or near to the cystic duct. Laparotomy will be required where the identification of the duodenojejunal flexure has not been achieved, with the risk of incorrect siting of the anastomosis along the jejunum. Uncontrollable bleeding has not been a problem. Bile contamination is common but easily aspirated. Caution is advised in opening the jejunum laparoscopically that is dilated with evidence of distal obstruction. Peritoneal contamination without the use of bowel clamps will be considerable. All patients receive prophylactic antibiotic coverage intraoperatively.

Technical breakdown of equipment may abort an otherwise successful operation but can be minimized by having back-up equipment.

Postoperative Recovery

Patients are encouraged to mobilize and take oral fluids as soon as they have recovered from anesthesia. Postoperative narcotic analgesia requirements are minimized by infiltration of all wounds with 0.25% bupivacaine in combination with 1:200,000 epinephrine and the administration of an indomethacin suppository 1 g in the recovery room. Patients usually tolerate food by the first day after the operation and request discharge by the third postoperative day.

GASTROJEJUNOSTOMY

Patient Selection

Patients with gastric outlet obstruction as a result of chronic peptic ulceration are well suited to undergo laparoscopic gastrojejunostomy. In a proportion of these patients, the extent of fibrosis and distortion around the pylorus will be minimal, allowing a pyloroplasty to be performed if preferred. Another group is those patients having cholecystojejunostomy for malignant distal bile duct obstruction with incipient or established duodenal obstruction. A proportion of patients without duodenal obstruction will develop it and require duodenal bypass later on in the course of their disease. Some patients with pyloric gastric carcinoma and obstruction, where extensive metastatic spread or associated medical illness determine that resection is ill advised, are suitable for palliative bypass.

Patient Positioning and Port Placement

Prophylactic intravenous antibiotics are administered after induction of anesthesia. The patient is supine with nasogastric tube drainage of the stomach. Little in the way of table tilt is required. Port positioning is illustrated in Figure 15-11 with special care to ensure that the port in the left upper quadrant used by needle holder in the surgeon's right hand aligns the needle holder shaft parallel to the suture line on the stomach. A minimum of three accessory ports are required, one of which should be 11 mm in diameter to introduce large instruments or curved needles.

Initial inspection of the peritoneum is completed. If gastric outlet obstruction is as a result of chronic peptic ulceration, a truncal vagotomy is performed before commencing the gastroenterostomy (see Chap. 12).

The duodenojejunal flexure is then identified by carefully grasping the transverse colon and omentum with two atraumatic forceps and elevating it anterior and cephalad to the stomach. The assistant is then able to maintain this position with one atraumatic grasper while the surgeon, using two atraumatic graspers, follows the small bowel up in a hand-over-hand manner until the flexure is reached. The small bowel is then followed down, and a suitable point is chosen for the anastomosis by allowing the transverse colon to fall back into position and bringing the small bowel around it up to the anterior wall of stomach. This is important because there is a tendency to underestimate the length of proximal small bowel required when viewing and handling it endoscopically.

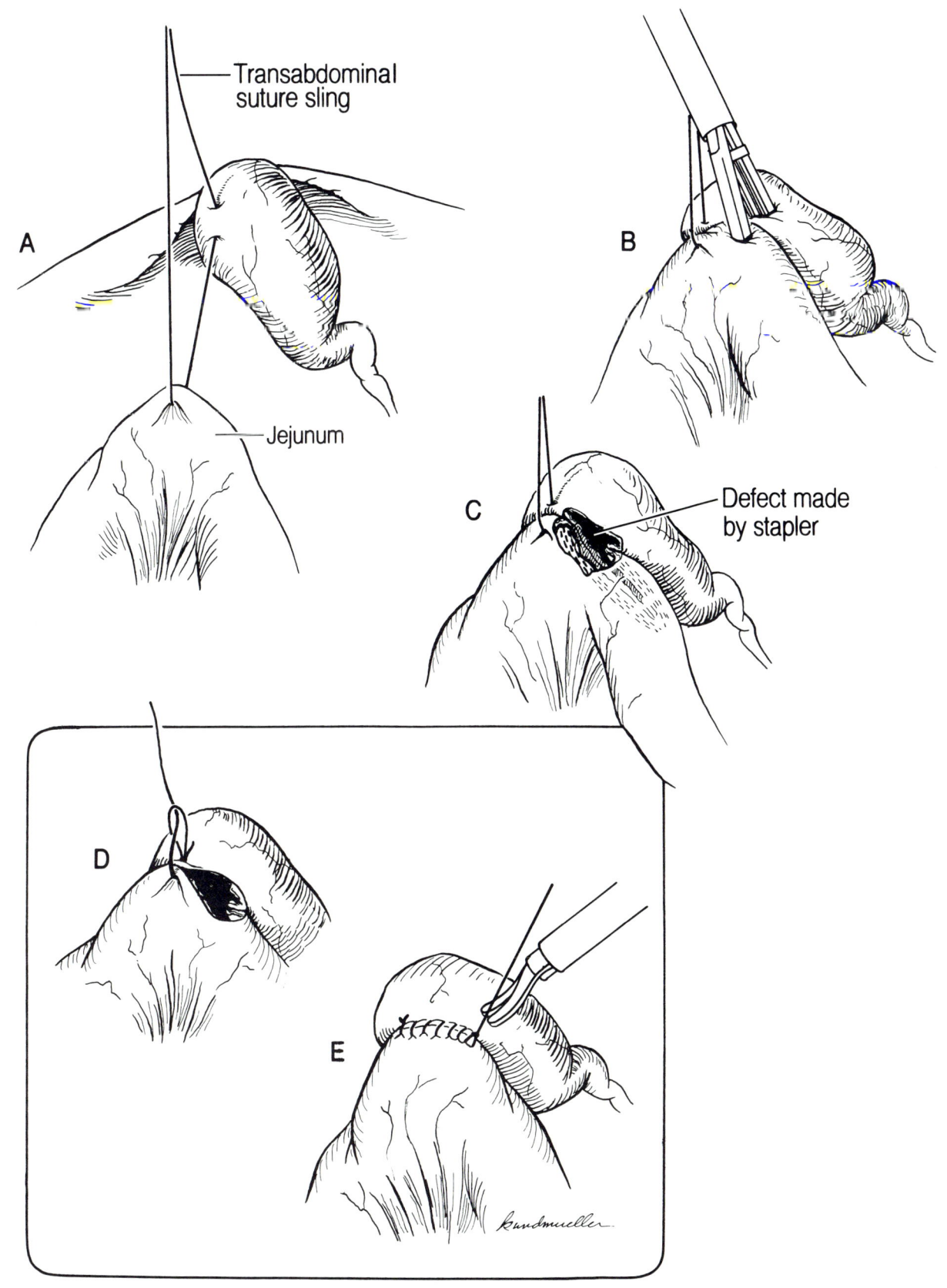

FIGURE 15-10 The stapled and sutured cholecystojejunostomy. A. A suture sling is inserted through the abdominal wall and anchored externally (see Fig. 15-5). B. Small cholecystotomy and enterotomy incisions are made, and a linear cutting stapler is placed in the gallbladder and small intestine. C. The staple line is inspected for hemostasis. D. The enterotomy is closed with a running suture. E. An Aberdeen knot finishes the suture line, and the excess suture is removed.

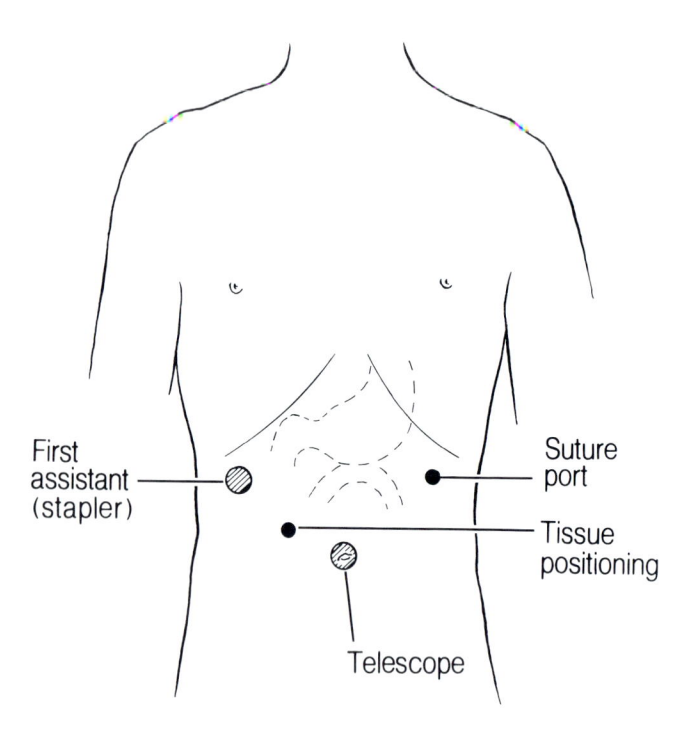

FIGURE 15-11 Port positioning for gastrojejunostomy. The telescope is placed in the umbilicus. A 10-mm port is placed on the right subcostal margin through which a Babcock clamp can be used to bring the small bowel antecolic to the stomach. The 5-mm ports are placed in the left subcostal area for suturing and near the telescope on the right for the surgeon's assisting grasper.

Sutured Anastomosis

The assistant then grasps the bowel at this point, the serosa is scored on its antimesenteric aspect with diathermy for 6 cm, followed by marking a 6-cm line on the antrum of the stomach selected for the anastomosis. The length of the anastomosis must be judged by reference to a calibrated marker because experience during open surgery, repeated again experimentally, shows that this length of suture line heals with a 2- to 3-cm stoma. Shorter anastomoses after healing are inadequate. The diathermy marks, in addition, maintain the orientation of the jejunum and stomach during suturing.

Figure 15-12 illustrates the sequence of the anastomosis. The posterior layer is sutured first. This is achieved with a single layer of continuous sutures, two in number each about 15 cm in length. My preference is to use 3–0 polyglactin on a standard needle. The first suture is introduced with its tail tied with the jamming loop knot (see Fig. 15-6). At this point, instillation of air into the stomach via the nasogastric tube sometimes improves exposure of the anterior wall of the stomach with displacement of the antrum from beneath the left lobe of liver and facilitates suture placement in the stomach. The apex of the suture line is identified, the needle is passed to incorporate the full thickness of bowel wall, and then the loop knot is locked (see Fig. 15-7). With the assistant holding the suture and following after each pass through tissue by the needle, the first suture completes the first half of the posterior layer and is then tied with either a reef or Aberdeen knot (see Fig. 15-8). The second suture is then used to complete the posterior layer. It is tied and, the tail is cut long.

At this point, the bowel is opened. This is initiated by deeper blended diathermy of the serosa and muscle layers to minimize bleeding. The jejunum is then opened with round-nosed scissors and any contents aspirated. Attention is then turned to the stomach, which is emptied of air and gastric juice by suction on the nasogastric tube. Monopolar diathermy is used to open the line of the serosa marked initially. Control of bleeding from the rich blood supply of the stomach is most important to allow accurate suture placement and prevent postoperative suture line hemorrhage. After the mucosa is reached, this can be opened using the dissecting scissors. Elevation of the anastomosis, by traction on the tail of the apical suture by the assistant, minimizes the spillage of gastric content by a combination of gravity and positive pressure of the insufflated CO_2 gas, which often encourages drainage of any gastric juice up the nasogastric tube rather than down into the peritoneum. Care should be taken to ensure complete hemostasis at this time. Aspiration of the cut edges and gastric lumen may be required to obtain a better view of the bleeding points. The anterior continuous layer is then commenced at the apex using the long tail of the posterior apical suture as a guide. Two sutures of 15 cm length are used, each initiated with the jamming loop knot and ended by using the Aberdeen knot. Alternatively, after using the tail of the posterior suture as a guide to the placement of the final few sutures, it can be simply tied to this using a reef knot.

The peritoneum is lavaged with warm Ringers lactate solution and aspirated dry. Peritoneal drainage is not routinely employed.

Comment

The entirely sutured anastomosis has some drawbacks in the context of gastroenterostomy. Because of the long suture line, it takes time and patience to complete. Interrupted, "continuous" sutures over this 6-cm anastomosis are also desirable to prevent loosening of the tension on the tissue caused by alteration in bowel length with shortening of the suture line during peristaltic waves. Adequate hemostatic tension must be maintained after each pass of the needle by the assistant when grasping the suture and elevating it upward. This is especially important with the renowned vascularity of the stomach and its propensity for suture line hemorrhage in the early postoperative period.

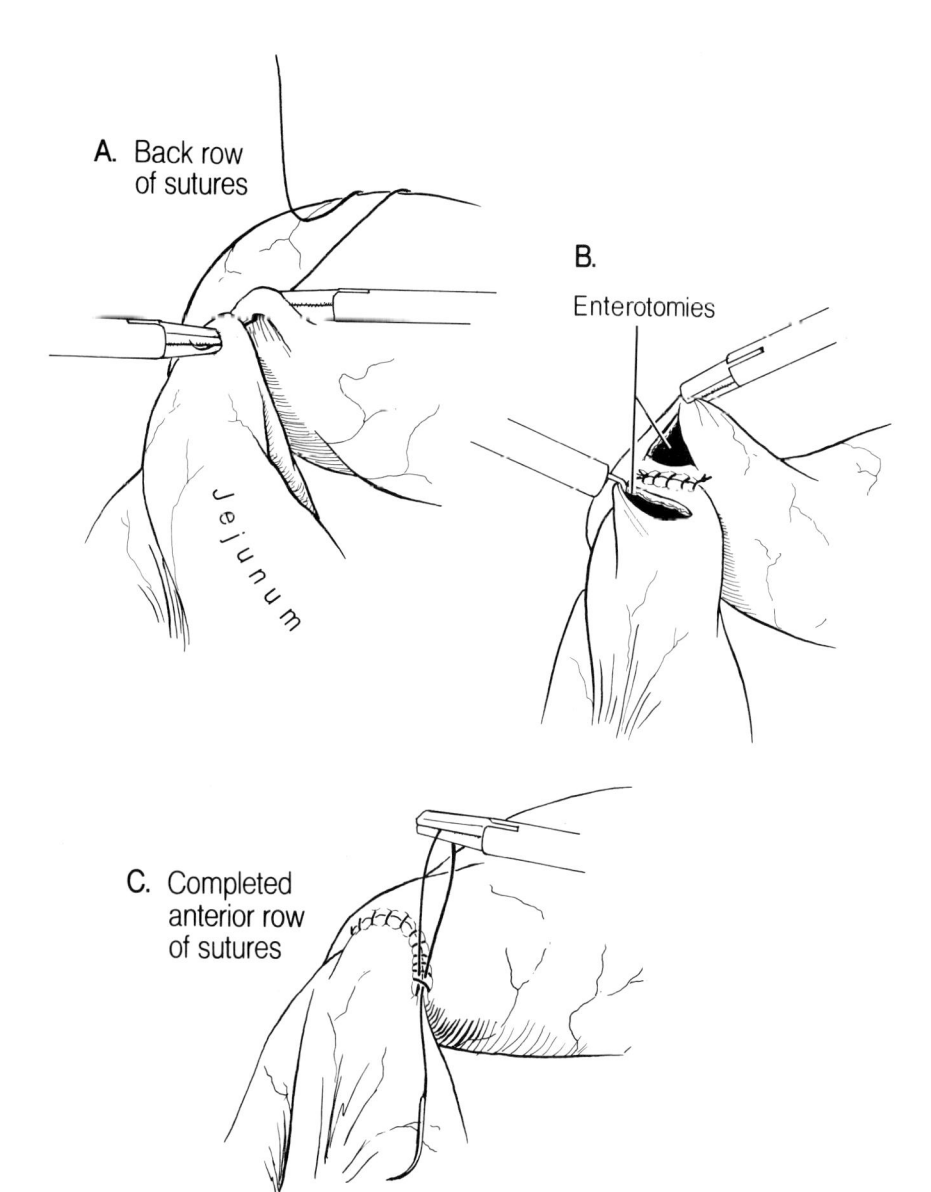

FIGURE 15-12 Technique of sutured gastrojejunostomy. A. The back row suture line is placed with several interrupted sutures or in a running fashion. B. Enterotomies are made, and two further suture lines are placed. Both suture lines are started on the pyloric side of the anastomosis and run toward the greater curvature. The first running suture line incorporates a full-thickness layer of stomach and jejunum posteriorly. The second suture line incorporates a full thickness of the stomach and jejunum anteriorly. C. At the completion of both suture lines, the sutures can be tied to each other or individual Aberdeen knots can be made.

Stapled and Sutured Gastrojejunostomy

The combination of stapling combined with suture closure of the residual defect is attractive in this long 6-cm anastomosis. It allows rapid creation of the stoma, and its only drawback lies with the expense of the disposable stapler and refill cartridge.

The ports are placed as in the sutured anastomosis except the 12-mm port for the stapler is used in the right upper quadrant. The selected portion of jejunum is grasped by the assistant, and an 8-mm enterotomy is made using diathermy and scissors, followed by a similar enterotomy in the antrum of the stomach at the distal end of the proposed anastomosis. An external anchoring suture placed through the stomach and jejunum at the efferent aspect of the anastomosis facilitates retraction and approximation of the jejunum and stomach. The 60 mm linear stapler/cutter is introduced and inserted into the jejunum and then the stomach, parallel to the greater curve, is clamped. Its position is checked, and then it is fired. After removal, the suture line is inspected for hemostasis.

If the 30-mm stapler is used, two firings are required. The first is completed as described for the larger stapler. Once completed, the stapler is removed, and a fresh bowel cartridge is inserted. The reapplication of the stapler to extend the suture line takes care by the surgeon because the apex of the previous two rows of staples must be accurately found and the second firing must continue from this point if a devascularized segment of bowel is to be avoided.

After the stapling has been completed, the defect in the stomach and jejunum is closed with a continuous 3–0 polyglactin suture on a ski-shaped or standard curved needle. A pretied jamming loop knot is used (see Fig. 13-6), and after passing through the apex of the suture line taking full-thickness stomach and jejunal wall, it is locked, tightened, grasped, and then held in traction by the assistant. The sutures are then placed 5 mm apart by incorporating full-thickness bites of stomach and jejunum. Completion of the suture line is with a reef or Aberdeen knot (see Fig. 15-8).

Comment

Practically, the combination of suture closure of the residual defect after establishment of the bulk of the staple line using the stapler works well. Attempt at triangulation of the jejunal and stomach walls to staple closed the residual defect is difficult. In attempting to ensure complete closure, a large portion of jejunal wall is included and results in stenosis at the efferent end of the staple line. This process can likewise take a lot more time than initially estimated and planned suture closure is quicker. Routine peritoneal drainage is not employed.

Measures to minimize the risk of stomal ulceration are taken in all patients who have not undergone concomitant vagotomy. These usually entail the long-term use of alginates or H_2-receptor blockers.

ILEOCOLOSTOMY

Patient Selection

Laparoscopic excision of the right colon with anastomosis by suture within the peritoneal cavity is not performed currently. Extraction of tissue specimens of any appreciable size down the lumen of the colon and out via the rectum is impractical. On the other hand, laparoscopic mobilization of the right colon, assisted by a minilaparotomy just large enough to remove the specimen, is useful. With this achieved, the exteriorized ileum proximally and colon distally are simply anastomosed outside the abdomen. The mesenteric defect is closed and then replaced back into the peritoneum.

For a small number of patients, where indications for palliative bypass of a lesion of the right colon without removal of the colon are present, laparoscopic ileocolic side-to-side anastomosis is useful. Currently, this is best achieved by a combination of staples and sutures, rather than by sutures alone.

Patient Position and Port Placement

The patient is placed supine and will have received prophylactic antibiotics on induction of anesthesia. The left upper quadrant and right iliac fossa ports are used by the surgeon's left and right hands for suturing and should be anchored to the skin to prevent displacement. Preferably they should have flapper or silicone valves. The left upper quadrant port should be 12 mm to convey the linear stapler/cutter.

Exposure and Control of Peritoneal Contamination

After initial laparoscopy confirms the pathologic condition, the suitable point for anastomosis to the colon (usually the transverse colon) is chosen, and omentum is reflected from its surface for 10 cm and displaced superiorly. This portion of the colon must be mobilized enough to allow access to both aspects of its mesentery. This allows 0 Prolene suture on a straight needle, introduced through the abdominal wall in the right upper quadrant, to be passed posterior to the colon via a mesenteric avascular window, proximal to the site of the anastomosis and brought out again through the abdominal wall. A second suture sling distal to the anastomosis provides control of distal colonic contents, with gentle traction on both slings being maintained by artery clips. The isolated portion of colon is emptied by milking as much of its contents distally as possible before traction on the distal sling.

Stapled and Sutured Anastomosis

A suitable segment of ileum is then selected and grasped by the assistant. An 8 mm opening in the antimesenteric aspect of the ileum and colon is made, and the 60-mm stapler is introduced from the left upper quadrant port. The ileum and colon are then threaded over the jaws of the stapler and held in place while the jaws are closed. The stapler position is finally checked by rotation of its shaft, and then it is fired. Care is taken during stapler removal back out of the port to avoid gross contamination of the port. A reducer tube should be used with this port for the rest of the procedure to protect the instruments from contamination. (The externally applied plastic reducer valves do not help in this regard because they do not provide a cover for the contaminated internal surface of the port and flapper valve.) Indeed, it is reasonable to exchange this cannula for a sterile cannula.

The colonic mucosa in the immediate region of the residual defect is then carefully cleaned of macroscopic fecal contents by pledgets introduced down a reducer tube. On completion, the contaminated pledgets, grasping forceps, and reducer tube can be discarded from the sterile field.

The residual defect is closed using a 3–0 polyglactin suture, 10-cm long and mounted on a ski-shaped needle. The continuous suture line is commenced at the apex with the externally fashioned jamming loop knot (see Fig. 15-6) and locked once in place (see Fig. 15-7). Extramucosal bites of the bowel, some 5 mm apart, are taken, and after each pass of the needle, the assistant follows by grasping the suture and maintaining tension on it. The suture line is completed by either a reef or Aberdeen knot (see Fig. 15-8). The external suture slings are removed and the peritoneum copiously lavaged with warm Ringers Lactate and aspirated dry. Routine drainage is not employed.

COLOCOLOSTOMY

Patient Selection

Resection of the sigmoid colon for complications of diverticular disease and carconoma are readily achieved laparoscopically. However, the subsequent suturing of the anastomosis internally in these formal resections is currently impractical. The most useful techniques for removal of the excised colon and subsequent intraluminal stapled anastomosis are covered elsewhere in this text (see Chap. 16). However, sutured anastomosis is the method of choice after colotomy, for instance, for removal of a benign adenomatous polyp with subsequent specimen extraction via the rectum. The most common site for this clinical situation to arise is in the sigmoid colon, but the principles can be applied to more proximal pathologic conditions.

Patient Position and Port Placement

Patients undergo preoperative oral bowel preparation and prophylactic intravenous antibiotics are given on induction of anesthesia. The patient is positioned supine on the operating table with their legs apart and supported with Allen or Lloyd Davis stirrups, taking care when using the latter to ensure that the hips although abducted are not flexed at all. This prevents later difficulties encountered with the patient's flexed thighs preventing free movement of instruments during manipulation through the caudad ports while still allowing the surgeon access to the rectum. The bladder is catheterized, and the patient anchored to the table with secure straps to allow maximum roll and tilt of the operating table. The entire abdomen is prepared and draped. The right iliac fossa port should be of flapper-valve design to facilitate smooth operation of the needle holder, and all ports should anchor to the abdominal wall with spiral locking devices to minimize gas leakage and accidental port displacement.

Localization of Luminal Pathologic Findings

The description of the mobilization here will be for sigmoid polyp removal. The same principles and techniques apply for other sites.

The surgeon stands on the patient's right side facing toward the foot of the operating table with the video monitor opposite. the patient is placed in 40° Trendelenburg tilt with a 20° roll to the right. This allows the small bowel to be lifted up from the pelvis and displaced superiorly without falling back into the operative field.

Crucial to locating the point for incision of the bowel to excise the polyp lies in identifying its position intraoperatively. Preoperative colonoscopic injection of dye into the bowel wall has been used. In my experience, this has not been reliable because it rapidly spreads along the lymphatic drainage and is not well seen on the peritoneal aspect of the colon. Planned intraoperative localization with the colonoscopic is the best technique. It is introduced by the assistant after laparoscopic access has been established. By transillumination, it pinpoints the site of disease, which is then marked on the serosal aspect by application of metal ligating clips. The amount of gas inflation of the colon required by the colonoscopist is minimal and does not interfere with the laparoscopist. Difficulty progressing up the colon lumen can be overcome by laparoscopic manipulation of the bowel. During withdrawal of the colonoscope, colonic gas is aspirated.

Bowel Mobilization

Mobilization of the sigmoid is started by identifying its lateral peritoneal reflection using medial and cephalad retraction on the proximal sigmoid colon by the assistant and the surgeon's left hand distally. The reflection is then divided, and this plane is deepened until the gonadal vessels and ureter are identified. There is a marked tendency with the laparoscopic two-dimensional view to dissect too laterally, and great care must be taken to stay in the corect plane on the sigmoid mesentery.

Proximal Control of the Colon, Specimen Excision, and Extraction

A simple method to occlude and elevate the bowel proximal to the site of elected colotomy is by inserting a sling. This is accomplished using a Prolene suture on a 60-mm straight needle inserted through the abdominal wall of the left lower quadrant, passing posterior to the colon through a mesenteric window and back through the abdominal wall to be anchored externally. Gentle traction on this sling is all that is required to prevent the downward flow of fecal fluid. The upward elevation of the colon also improves exposure. Alternatively, atraumatic bowel-clamp forceps are available that can be introduced via 10-mm ports. The problem with their use is that they then occupy that port site for the duration of the anastomosis, and another port may have to be introduced for the assistant.

A large bore rectal catheter is then introduced. The bowel lumen is washed clean and aspirated dry.

The colon is then incised with cutting electrosurgery, the margins of the base of the polyp identified, and the full-thickness excision completed, maintaining a 5-mm margin of surrounding normal mucosa. Bleeding may be encountered if the base is on the mesenteric aspect; these individual vessels are easily identified and controlled with endoclips. The specimen is then removed by insertion of a round-nosed grasping forceps through an operating sigmoidoscope. The luminal grasping forceps is advanced under visual laparoscopic guidance to the colotomy, grasps the specimen, and extracts it through the rectum.

Sutured Anastomosis

The colotomy is cleaned by suction of blood clots and fluid from the surrounding serosa and mucosa. The anastomosis is achieved with a single-layer extramucosal technique using 3–0 polyglactin sutures mounted on a ski-shaped needle. The 10-cm suture is introduced into the peritoneum with the jamming loop knot having been pretied at the tail end (see Fig. 15-6). The apex is chosen to close the colotomy transversely, the suture placed, and then the jamming loop knot locked and tightened (see Fig. 15-7). The assistant follows the suture by traction with grasping forceps to maintain tension and correct tissue approximation after each pass of the needle by the surgeon. With a long colotomy of almost the full circumference of the bowel, the continuous suture should be only used for 4 cm and then tied with a reef or Aberdeen knot (see Fig. 15-8). Another continuous suture is then commenced and ended in the same way. This technique of interrupted–continuous sutures avoids the concertina effect of a long row of continuous sutures, which may contribute to luminal stenosis.

On completion, the Prolene sling suture is released. The operative field is lavaged with warm Ringers lactate solution and aspirated dry. Routine insertion of a drain is not employed.

CONCLUSION

Many aspects of sutured anastomosis require further instrumentation and refinement to even begin to approach the instrumentation available for open surgery. Simple atraumatic bowel clamps are needed. These should be able to be disconnected from their shaft once applied and so allow ports to be used for other instrumentation. Truly atraumatic bowel-grasping forceps are required, which function with little or no risk of perforating bowel (especially obstructed bowel). On the horizon, are methods of suture fixation other than knots, which can be rapidly applied and will speed up this process greatly.

The capacity to suture competently using the laparoscope adds greatly to a surgeon's ability and confidence. Moreover, it increases the usefulness of the remarkable range of new stapling devices now becoming available.

REFERENCE

1. Semm K: *Operative Manual for Endoscopic Abdominal Surgery.* London, Year Book Publishers, 1987.

Chapter 16

The Diagnosis and Treatment of Acute Appendicitis with Laparoscopic Methods

David W. Easter

Inflammation of the vermiform appendix is the most common surgical emergency encountered in Western countries. Although the typical case is readily diagnosed as acute appendicitis, there remains a substantial number of unnecessary explorations for this condition and some cases that go on to perforation despite adequate access to medical care.

The clinical diagnosis of appendicitis eluded medical knowledge until 1886, when Reginald Heber Fitz of Boston described the clinicopathologic entity formerly known as *typhlitis*.[1] Little in the diagnosis and management of suspected appendicitis has changed in the last century. Although methods for diagnostic laparoscopy have been available to the surgeon since the early 1900s, it remained for Kurt Semm[2] in 1982 to apply laparoscopy to the removal of this organ. Almost a full decade later, general surgeons are only now beginning to embrace and evaluate this "new" technology.

THE DIAGNOSTIC PROBLEM

Approximately 1 of every 14 persons from industrialized countries will develop acute appendicitis during their lifetime.[3] This incidence correlates to more than 200,000 appendectomies performed annually in the United States. Regional variations influence this rate, that is, the incidence and prevalence of this disease is reduced in areas, such as Africa, where meals high in dietary fiber are consumed.

Unfortunately, the variations in clinical presentation, coupled with the various positions of the appendix, often cause diagnostic confusion. Not infrequently, acute appendicitis is mistaken for diseases of the stomach, colon, pelvic organs, and indeed, any organ within the abdomen. Even in the *classic case*—where discomfort and nausea progress to localized abdominal pain with fever and leukocytosis—the incidence of unnecessary celiotomy for the diagnosis of a condition other than appendicitis remains at 10 to 30 percent.[3]

Other than diagnostic laparoscopy, little can be added to the accuracy of a good history and physical examination performed by an experienced clinician. This inaccuracy is not, however, because physicians have not tried over the years to improve upon their diagnostic capabilities. Barium enema has been used to identify a *normal appendix* (one that fills completely without defects) and thus avoid negative laparotomies in the pediatric population. Despite this selective use of barium enema in children with possible acute appendicitis, negative explorations occur in as many as 20 to 30 percent of patients.[4]

Ultrasonography has also been used to verify or exclude the diagnosis of acute appendicitis.[5] However, the requirements of a skilled and dedicated (if not enthusiastic) ultrasound team, and the limitations of ultrasound capabilities around the gas-containing intestines limits its usefulness.

Despite the abilities of skilled clinicians with selective noninvasive testing, the incidence of false-positive diagnosis in women of childbearing age remains 20 to 40 percent.[3,6] Even in men, where pelvic inflammatory disease and gynecologic disorders are not confounding problems, the incidence of negative explorations for appendicitis remains 5 to 20 percent.[3]

Diagnostic laparoscopy can reliably identify which patients have appendicitis and which do not. As importantly, it can accurately be used to explore the remaining abdomen and identify coexisting pathologic conditions without enlarging the incisions. Few laparoscopically trained surgeons will disagree that the viewing capabilities through the laparoscope far exceed that of open exploration through a right lower quadrant incision.

HISTORY OF LAPAROSCOPIC APPENDECTOMY

Disorders of the appendix have been diagnosed laparoscopically since the early days of laparoscopy, when rigid cystoscopes were first introduced into the abdomen.[7] The first specialists to utilize this technology for the removal of the organ were gynecologists, led by Kurt Semm[2] in Germany. For these surgeons, incidental appendectomy was most often performed in conjunction with other pelviscopic procedures. This was considered justifiable to avoid future diagnostic confusion and the possible morbid complications of acute appendicitis.

The incorporation of laparoscopic techniques in the expanding repertoire of the general surgeon followed the introduction of laparoscopic cholecystectomy in Europe and the United States. From 1989 to 1990, surgeons have been able and willing to remove both the acutely inflamed organ and the noninflamed (incidental) appendix; but the specific indications, appropriate exclusions, and the benefits or added risks of laparoscopic appendiceal surgery have yet to be clarified.

Currently, few reports of substantial series size have been published.[8-16] What can be concluded from these reports is that: (1) laparoscopic appendectomy is certainly feasible with currently available methods and equipment; (2) laparoscopy, as the last diagnostic step, may minimize the rate of false-positive abdominal explorations; and (3) laparoscopic appendectomy can be performed safely.

In clinical practice, the laparoscopic management of the appendix can be considered in five situations: the incidental appendectomy, the patient with a possible diagnosis of acute appendicitis, the relatively secure diagnosis of appendicitis, the case of presumed complicated appendicitis, and chronic appendicitis.

Incidental Appendectomy

That the uninflamed appendix can be safely removed during *open* laparotomy has been demonstrated.[17] However, for the rare patient with a complication possibly linked to such an appendectomy (e.g., postoperative wound infection), the seemingly trivial event becomes potentially quite tragic. Furthermore, the possibility of litigation directed at the unnecessary event (appendectomy) reasonably limits the practice of this potentially useful addition. The exception is with those (forward looking or foolhardy?) surgeons who plan ahead for incidental appendectomy and document clearly the frank discussion necessary when performing prophylactic surgery. Given that the incidence of the disease is maximal among young adults, it would very likely not benefit many adult or elderly patients to receive an incidental appendectomy.

This situation is directly applicable to laparoscopic cholecystectomy and pelviscopic surgery. The addition of incidental laparoscopic appendectomy is surgically simple, and probably safe,[17] but for the same reasons as in open surgery of the abdomen, it should be reserved for those cases wherein complete preoperative consent is obtained, and subsequent potential benefits can be argued to exceed the risks.

Unsure Diagnosis of Appendicitis

Laparoscopy as the final step in the diagnosis of acute appendicitis can limit the number of false-positive explorations based on less invasive methods. Whether this diagnostic step eliminates any morbidity is unresolved. Additionally, as the insufflated carbon dioxide gas has local vasodilatory effects on the surface vessels of the appendix, in this author's experience, it can be quite difficult to completely exclude the early stages of appendiceal inflammation.

When the preoperative diagnosis of acute appendicitis is found to be erroneous, the next logical step is to remove the appendix (to avoid subsequent diagnostic controversy) after exploring the abdomen for the responsible pathologic condition. It is probable, although unproved, that laparoscopic exploration is more complete in searching for coexisting pathologic conditions compared with access via a right iliac fossa incision.[14]

Acute and Complicated Appendicitis

When the diagnosis of acute appendicitis is in doubt, laparoscopy can be an extremely useful diagnostic tool. When the diagnosis is firm, arguments can be made regarding the utility of this technique. The best argument in favor of its routine use in this situation is that even the best clinicians with the best adjuvant tests cannot accurately diagnose this disease with 100 percent accuracy. Those with a classic presentation for appendicitis, who harbor pathologic conditions other than acute appendicitis, may be spared a muscle-splitting incision and may have a more thorough abdominal exploration as a result of the preemptive laparoscopy.

Arguments against using laparoscopy when the diagnosis is believed to be sure are—again, without firm objective data—that: (1) the hospitalization for negative appendectomy exploration does not need to be any longer than that for negative laparoscopy, (2) the incision is not substantially larger nor more morbid than the incisions necessary for a thorough laparoscopic exploration, and (3) the rate of rupture of an acutely inflamed appendix may be greater with laparoscopic methods than with open methods. In this last argument, one might be tempted to remove an acutely inflamed or gangrenous appendix with laparoscopic methods and spill or contaminate what could be more safely controlled with an open exploration.

Time and accumulated experience will answer whether these concerns are justifiable. One can only hope that objective trials can be organized that can answer these questions before the wholesale adaptation of one or another method is based on marketing or public pressure demands.

Chronic Appendicitis

This condition is more accurately termed *recurrent acute appendicitis*. Nevertheless, for those who believe in this entity, the laparoscopic diagnosis of chronic appendicitis may present difficulties. One may guess that adhesions involving the appendix represent prior episodes of inflammation. These adhesions, or an awkward location of the organ, may present difficulties for the recently trained laparoscopic surgeon. On the whole, the laparoscopic diagnosis and treatment of this condition most closely parallels that of incidental appendectomy or unsure diagnosis, as described previously.

METHODS OF LAPAROSCOPIC APPENDECTOMY

There are already many variations in the methods of laparoscopic appendectomy. Importantly, the very same operative methods for open treatment can be employed using laparoscopic techniques, but with different instrumentation. That is to say, one can retract, ligate, staple, suture, irrigate–aspirate, electrocauterize, or laser dissect with laparoscopic instrumentation. Therefore, one should not compromise surgical principles because of a change in the method of access through the abdominal wall.

Three to four ports are necessary for laparoscopic appendectomy. In the three-port method, trocars are placed in the umbilicus (10 mm), right upper quadrant (5 mm), and left lower quadrant (5 mm, Fig. 16-1). If a gastrointestinal stapler (e.g., Endo-GIA) is to be used, either trocar may be replaced with a 12-mm trocar. Similarly, if a hemoclip and Roeder knot method is to be used, either 5-mm port may be replaced with a 10-mm trocar. A fourth port in the right lower quadrant may be necessary to provide added appendiceal traction on occasion. A pre-tied Roeder loop passed through this trocar and around the tip of the appendix provides marvelous retraction in difficult cases.

The external knotting technique preceded other methods of laparoscopic ligature and, as such, was one of the first methods used for appendectomy (Fig. 16-2). In this technique, the appendix is visualized, and a loop knot is passed around the tip of the organ to assist in atraumatic manipulation. Windows are then created as necessary through the mesoappendix to pass slip-knot ligatures, in

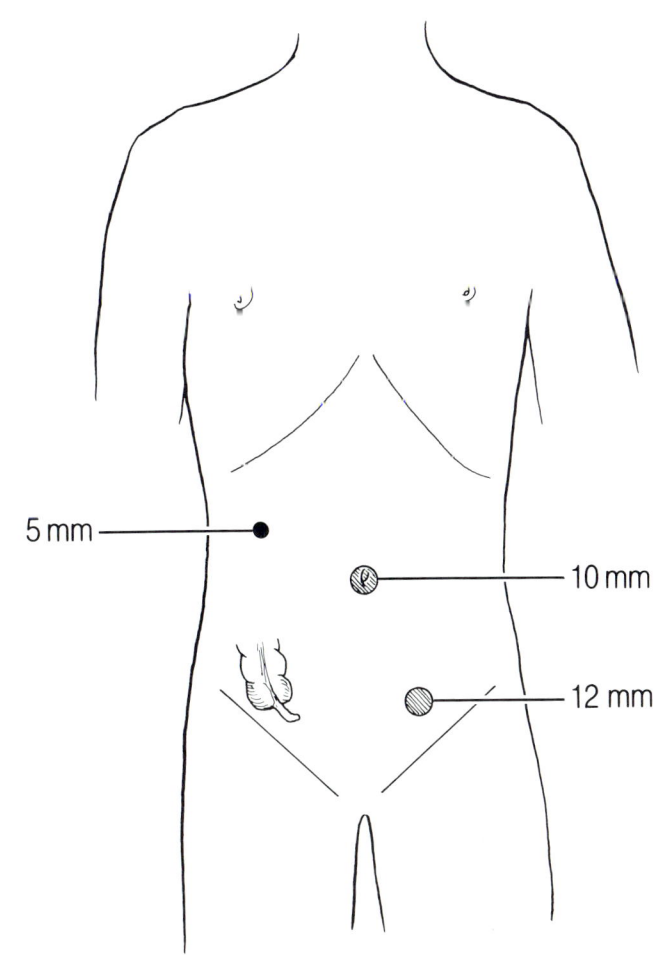

FIGURE 16-1 Port placement for laparoscopic appendectomy. Flexibility in port positioning and port size is paramount. Each of the accessory ports should be 15 cm (half the length of a laparoscopic instrument) from the location of the appendix.

continuity, around the vessels supplying the appendix. It is not usually necessary to ligate the appendix side of these vessels. The mesoappendix is taken off of the appendix with sharp dissection, and three more loops are passed to ligate the base of the appendix doubly at the cecum and control spillage when dividing between ties. The organ is then extracted from the abdomen within the 5-mm reducer tube, shielding the appendix from contaminating the abdominal wall.

With the availability of both reusable and disposable clip applicators, some of these steps have become easier. Clips are used to ligate the mesoappendix before division, but it remains preferable to use loops to tie the base of the appendix securely and provide for an atraumatic holder for the tip (Fig. 16-3).

Recently, a stapling device has been used for appendectomy.[16] Again, a loop ligature is passed around the tip of the organ to assist in atraumatic manipulation. Next, the

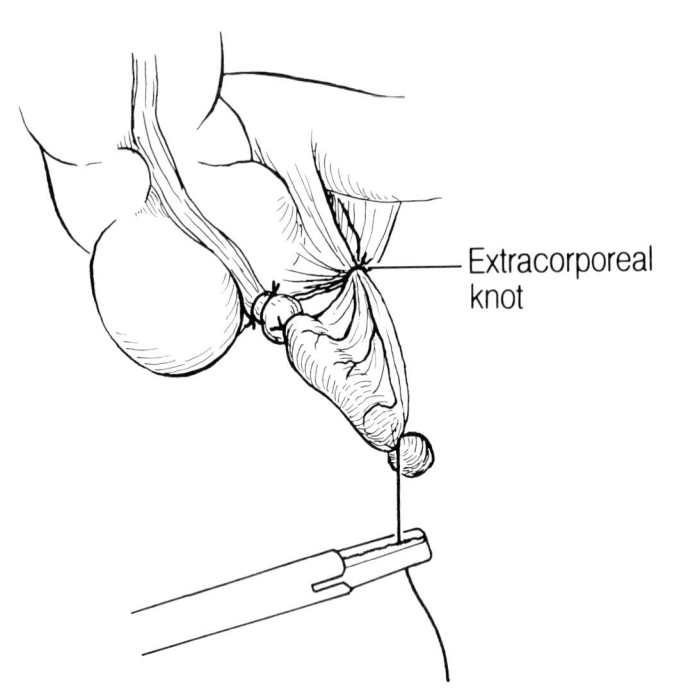

FIGURE 16-2 The appendix is retracted without crushing by a loop around the tip while the mesoappendix vessels are ligated and divided in continuity before the appendix is divided between ties.

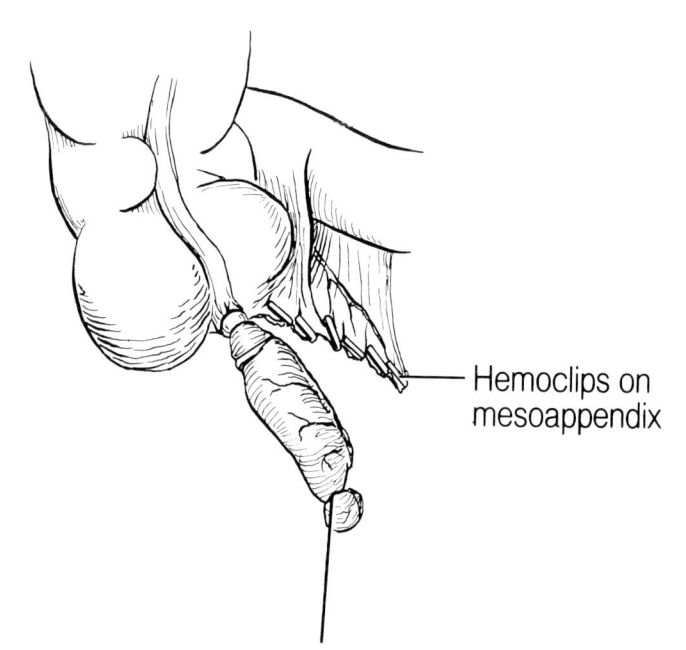

FIGURE 16-3 Clips are placed only on the mesoappendix side, close to the appendix, to minimize the bulk of tissue to be extracted.

mesoappendix is divided using a stapling cartridge that applies vascular staples on either side of a dividing razor. The base of the appendix is then amputated using a second stapler cartridge (Fig. 16-4).

With each of these methods, electrocautery or laser energy can be used for coagulation and cutting, depending on the training and preferences of the surgeon. A word of caution about the use of monopolar electrosurgery (MPES) to amputate the appendix is in order. Stories (but no published reports) of delayed stump leakage after ligature appendectomy have circulated throughout the country. If MPES is used to cauterize the appendiceal stump and the stump is not buried, as it rarely is with laparoscopic appendectomy, there is a very real risk of thermal necrosis of the base of the appendix and slough of the dead tissue with resultant cecal fistula. The mechanism of this injury is easily explainable in biophysical terms. If a ligature reduces the diameter of the appendix by 50 percent, it reduces the cross-sectional area by 75 percent. Electrical energy applied to the divided base of the appendix returns to the ground pad through the appendiceal stump. At the point of ligature, the current density is four times as great as at the point of contact (current density, $\sim$ 1/cross-sectional area, Fig. 16-5). Tissue heating increases as a squared function of current density. Thus, heating of the appendix at the point of ligature is 4^2 or 16 times the heating at the point of contact! Many surgeons unaware of this effect have noted tissue sizzle at the appendiceal ligature points. Surprisingly, few of such conducted cecal injuries have resulted in fecal fistulae. If one desires to invert the tip of the amputated appendix, this can be done using a needle and suture brought through one of the larger cannulae, suturing under direct vision, and either external or internal knotting tech-

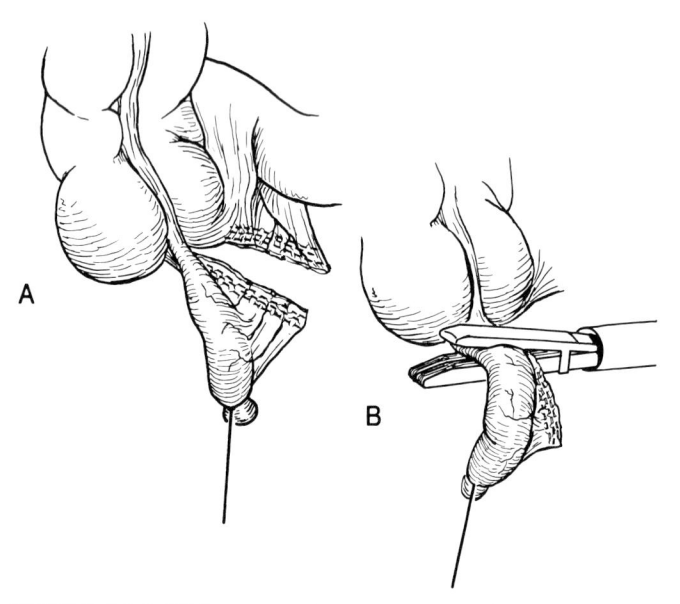

FIGURE 16-4 With atraumatic retraction, A. the mesoappendix is ligated and divided using a vascular cartridge, and B. the appendix base is separated using the gastrointestinal cartridge.

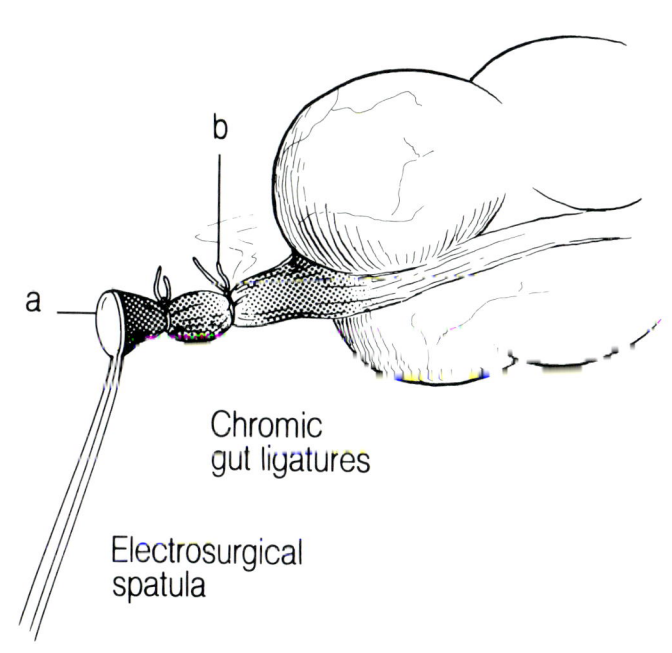

FIGURE 16-5 If an electrosurgical spatula is placed across the base of the amputated appendix, the temperature reached at point b will be 16 times the temperature at point a if the diameter of the appendix at point b is ½ the diameter at point a.

niques. It does not appear that inverting the amputated stump is necessary during laparotomy or laparoscopy.[18]

RESULTS OF LAPAROSCOPIC APPENDECTOMY

Currently, the published series on laparoscopic treatment of both acute appendicitis and incidental appendectomy have been overwhelmingly favorable as a result of the enduring capacity of newly trained laparoscopic general surgeons.

In 1987, Gangal and Gangal[9] reported on their experience with 73 patients requiring both acute and interval appendectomy. The pathologic findings were not stated. With rudimentary instruments and using band applicators (as in female sterilization), they found longer operating times but had more surgical options as a result of improved visual access and a more comfortable postoperative course for their patients.

Gotz and associates,[8] in 1990, reported on 388 cases performed over a 2.5-year period at their institution in Linnich, Germany. They used Roeder loop knots to ligate the base of the appendix after electrocautery dissection of the mesoappendix. Pathologic findings were acute in 85 percent of cases. Only 12 patients required conversion from a laparoscopic to conventional technique. They reported very good patient satisfaction and excellent postoperative mobility of their patients. They suggested that laparoscopic surgery of the appendix is safe and postulated that these new techniques might considerably reduce hospitalization time and costs.

Browne[10] reported in 1990 on 100 consecutive cases of laparoscopic-guided appendectomy from Queensland, Australia. Fifty-eight of his patients had either a normal appendix or fibrous obliteration of the organ. Mild chronic appendicitis was found in 27 with acute appendicitis in only 4 from this group. Although there were no cases of peritonitis and no serious complications, seven patients had wound abscesses. Of particular interest was that the laparoscope was used merely to localize the appendix, and the resection subsequently was performed extracorporeally. Despite these questionable indications and less-than-superb results, he believed that his method was simple, safe, reliable, and effective, especially in the case of chronic appendicitis.

Extracorporeal resection after laparoscopic mobilization was also used by Valla[11] in his report on 465 children undergoing appendectomy in the south of France. In this series, there were five conversions to open appendectomy (one percent). There was a 2.6 percent incidence of intraoperative difficulties, including insufflation of the omentum, visceral injuries (n = 2), and appendiceal rupture (n = 9). Postoperative complications, including hernia, bowel obstruction, and recurrent fever, were seen in three percent of patients.

In 1991, O'Regan[12] reported on 21 patients who underwent laparoscopy for suspected appendicitis. Twelve underwent laparoscopic appendectomy. Alternate diagnoses were readily made at diagnostic laproscopy, for example, perforated duodenal ulcer. The Roeder loop–knot technique was used for appendectomy, with all such patients recovering sufficiently for discharge by the second day after the operation. He suggested that morbidity was reduced, exploration of the abdomen was facilitated, and that wound infection might possibly be eliminated with proper shielding of the appendix on extraction through the abdominal wall.

Pier and associates,[14] updating the experience from Linnich, reported on 625 cases of laparoscopic appendectomy in 1991. In this series, the average operating time was 15 to 20 minutes. Conversion to open appendectomy was required in two percent of the cases. The majority of these cases (70 percent) were performed for acute appendicitis. The complication rate was quite low. Postoperative abscess occurred in only 2 percent and, in only one patient, did a stump leak occur from excessive coagulation. In three cases, bleeding occurred, requiring conversion to open appendectomy.

Laparoscopic appendectomy with the aid of a stapling device was reported by Olsen[16] in 1991. Although results were not given, he suggested that the advantages of such methods included a quicker operation and superior ligature of the base of the appendix compared with loop ligature. He speculated that this and future equipment modifications would make laparoscopic appendectomy the method of choice for most cases of appendicitis.

CURRENT PERSPECTIVE

Currently, there is ample evidence that the diagnosis and treatment of acute appendicitis using laparoscopic techniques is a viable alternative to conventional methods. Proponents of these new methods argue that there are real advantages associated with the laparoscopic approach. This remains to be proved in well-designed trials. At issue is whether or not one method is safer, less expensive, more useful, or less disabling than the other.

It appears that laparoscopic appendectomy is safe, at least in the hands of skilled laparoscopic surgeons who are enthusiastic about the new techniques. It remains to be seen if these results will be duplicated by the scores of general surgeons that are currently learning and practicing the laparoscopic management of other abdominal conditions (specifically, cholecystectomy). It is likely that the safety of laparoscopic appendectomy is only as secure as the intraoperative wisdom of the surgeon, that is, knowing when one's own techical limits have been reached, before they are exceeded!

It is doubtful that laparoscopic management of these patients will significantly reduce hospital costs. The largest predictor of hospital charges is the number of days required in treating the illness. As there is very little or no paralytic ileus associated with the open management of uncomplicated appendicitis, the hospital stay difference between groups of patients will be minimal. One can project that patients with uncomplicated appendicitis or incidental appendectomy for a false-positive clinical diagnosis will remain overnight, have diet rapidly instituted, and be discharged within 36 hours of operation (if so desired or "pushed" by third-party payers). This situation will not likely change with laparoscopic management, but if health care reimbursers begin insisting, both treatment methods could conceivably be shortened to an outpatient stay with close follow-up for the uncomplicated cases.

The laparoscopic access to the abdomen probably has advantages over open access through a right iliac fossa incision. This is immediately clear to surgeons the first time they peer through a laparoscope at a normal appendix. It is a simple matter at that point to explore the remaining viscera of the abdomen in a search for offending pathologic conditions. The converse situation is awkward, at best, when peering through a muscle-splitting incision. To demonstrate with actual results this visual advantage, however, one must have a large series of negative explorations for appendicitis and compare the untoward outcomes from each group of patients. Common sense in this comparison should be more meaningful than cumbersome trials, that is, the visual inspection of the abdomen at laparoscopy is superior to that through a standard appendectomy incision.

Is laparoscopic appendectomy less disabling than open appendectomy? Proponents would argue definitely "yes," but this remains to be demonstrated. For the majority of patients that will be managed without complications, it is likely that the multiple punctures necessary for laparoscopic extraction of an inflamed appendix will be more comfortable than a single muscle-splitting (tearing) incision. A quicker method than (and probably as accurate as) a large prospective randomized trial comparing discomfort would be a poll of surgeons trained in both techniques to ask which method they would prefer for themselves if so stricken! Given the public's response to laparoscopic cholecystectomy, patients will likely prefer laparoscopic methods when available. Furthermore, patients will, given the opportunity and education, actively search for surgeons capable of delivering those methods believed to be advantageous, even if such results remain scientifically unproved.

CONCLUSION

The diagnosis of acute appendicitis frequently baffles the clinician. The recent utilization of laparoscopic techniques by general surgeons has provided new methods in dealing with this illness. The early experience with laparoscopic appendectomy suggests that (1) the diagnosis of acute appendicitis is accurately made or excluded through laparoscopic evaluation, (2) incidental appendectomy via the laparoscope is probably safe when performed by surgeons trained in these methods, (3) current methods allow for safe dissection and delivery of an inflamed (or normal) appendix, and (4) when acute appendicitis is excluded on initial laparoscopic inspection, the visual diagnostic capabilities of laparoscopy exceed those of open operation. In the very near future, general surgeons can be expected to employ laparoscopic techniques routinely in the management of patients with suspected acute appendicitis.

REFERENCES

1. Lyons AF, Petrucelli RJ: *Medicine, An Illustrated History*. New York, Abradale Press, 1987, pp 531.
2. Semm K: Endoscopic appendectomy. *Endoscopy* 1983; 15:59–64.
3. Adiss DG, Shaffer N, Fowler BS, et al.: The epidemiology of appendicitis and appendectomy in the United States. *Am J Epidemiol* 1990; 132:910–925.
4. Gilbert SR, Emmens RW, Putnam TC, et al: Appendicitis in children. *Surg Gynecol Obstet* 1985; 161:261–265.
5. Ceres L, Alonso I, Lopez P, et al: Ultrasound study of acute appendicitis in children with emphasis upon the diagnosis of retrocecal appendicitis. *Pediatr Radiol* 1990; 20:258–261.
6. Whitworth CM, Whitworth PW, Sanfillipo J, et al: Value of diagnostic laparoscopy in young women with possible appendicitis. *Surg Gynecol Obstet* 1988; 167:187–190.

7. Kelling G: Zur coelioscopie. *Arch Klin Chir* 1923; 126:226–229.
8. Gotz F, Pier A, Bacher C: Modified laparoscopic appendectomy in surgery: A report on 388 operations. *Surg Endosc* 1990; 4:6–9.
9. Gangal MT, Gangal MH: Laparoscopic appendectomy. *Endoscopy* 1987; 19:127–129.
10. Browne DS: Laparoscopic-guided appendicectomy: A study of 100 consecutive cases. *Austr N Z J Obstet Gynaecol* 1990; 30:231–233.
11. Valla JS, Limone B, Valla V, et al: Laparoscopic appendectomy in children: Report of 465 cases. *Surg Laparosc Endosc* 1991; 1:166–172.
12. O'Regan PJ: Laparoscopic appendectomy. *Can J Surg* 1991; 34:256–258.
13. Schreiber JH: Early experience with laparoscopic appendectomy in women. *Surg Endosc* 1987; 1:211–216.
14. Pier A, Gotz F, Bacher C: Laparoscopic appendectomy in 625 cases: From innovation to routine. *Surg Laparosc Endosc* 1991; 1:8–13.
15. Leahy PF: Technique of laparoscopic appendectomy. *Br J Surg* 1989; 76:616.
16. Olsen DO: Laparoscopic appendectomy using a linear stapling device. *Surg Rounds* 1991; 14:873–883.
17. Storm PR, Turkelson ML, Stone HH: Safety of incidental appendectomy. *Am J Surg* 1983; 115:819–822.
18. Engstrom L, Fenyö G: Appendicectomy: Assessment of stump invagination versus simple ligation: A prospective randomized trial. *Br J Surg* 1985; 72:971–972.

Chapter 17

Laparoscopic Colon and Rectal Surgery

Jonathan M. Sackier

It was inevitable that the laparoscope would be used to examine diseases of the colon and rectum in the wake of the laparoscopic cholecystectomy revolution. Many of the obstacles that had to be overcome to enable colonic resection to be performed had already been addressed to solve problems for removal of the gallbladder.

Laparoscopy had been employed to evaluate colorectal disorders in a number of scenarios. Most prominent among these was the assessment of the patient with colorectal cancer where the laparoscope could be used to stage the disease; obtain tissue from the liver, peritoneum, and bowel serosa; and plan operative management.[1] The big difference is that currently the laparoscope is also the vehicle by which extirpative therapy may be delivered. Similarly, in patients with inflammatory bowel disease, laparoscopic evaluation has proved valuable in the past, and currently, we may not only look but also divert or resect.

Patients with chronic abdominal pain[2,3] have previously been investigated with the laparoscope. Therapy currently is available (Fig. 17-1).

In the emergency setting, laparoscopy is useful for the patient with abdominal pain. Largely, of course, this has been used for the distinction of appendicitis from other, usually gynecologic, causes.[4] This has been dealt with separately in this volume (see Chap. 16). The patient who presents with diverticulitis may be graded into either noncommunicating (peridiverticulitis) or communicating types.[5] This distinction is extremely important because it will dictate whether urgent surgical intervention is required. Laparoscopy has been useful in the past to evaluate such patients, but currently, of course, definitive treatment may be delivered at the same time. Patients with blunt and penetrating abdominal trauma have also undergone endoscopic assessment with the laparoscope.[6–9] This is a valuable method to distinguish between significant hemoperitoneum or cases where the source of bleeding has stopped, such as a minor mesenteric tear in a deceleration injury (see Chap. 28).

Where the site of penetration from a stab wound is thought to involve the colon, laparoscopy will allow the surgeon to determine whether the knife has, in fact, penetrated the peritoneal cavity. If not, then, of course, injury to a peritoneal organ is impossible. For gunshot wounds, the case is not as clear-cut, and laparoscopy is probably only useful when the patient is obese, the caliber of the weapon is small, and the entrance and exit wounds suggest a tangential course, which has, thereby, missed the peritoneal cavity.[10]

The benefits of laparoscopic surgery are clear and have been summarized in Chapter 1. There is no doubt that similar advantages will accrue to the patient undergoing

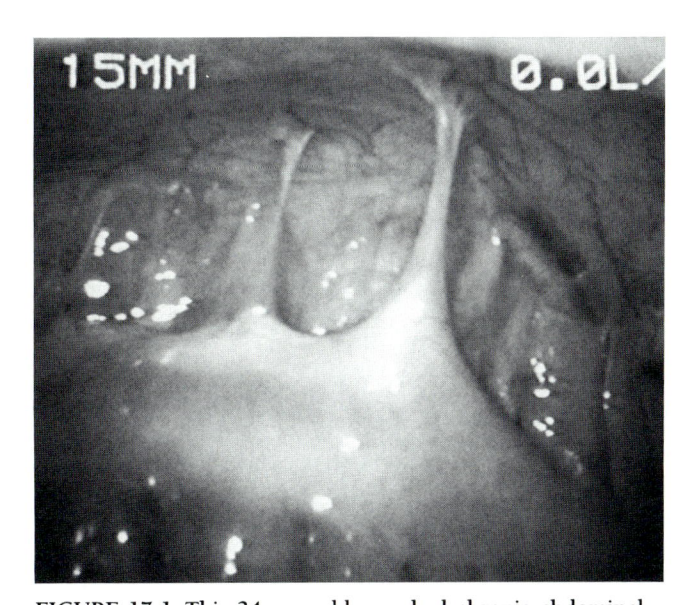

FIGURE 17-1 This 34-year-old man had chronic abdominal pain, and all radiologic investigation findings had been normal, except for some reproduction of his pain at colonoscopy. Laparoscopy revealed congenital bands between the sigmoid colon and the parietal peritoneum. These adhesions were divided.

colonic surgery by the laparoscopic route because such open operations usually take a long time and exposure of the internal milieu to the atmosphere therefore is extensive.

There are, however, certain concerns that must be addressed for laparoscopic colon surgery to become the gold standard. First, whenever the bowel is open, there is the potential for fecal contamination of the abdominal cavity. During open surgery, it is possible to pack off areas using abdominal gauze; obviously, this is not feasible when the only access to the abdomen is through small cannulae. Therefore, systems have to be developed to prevent this. It is vital that any operation for malignancy follows the principles of cancer surgery, that is, to resect with good margins and excise draining lymph nodes and adjacent tissue.

The removal of solid organs from the abdominal cavity during laparoscopy has led to some innovative ideas, such as tissue morcellation.[11] However, this is a potential problem because the pathologist will not be provided with a complete organ and will therefore be unable to give a prognosis for that patient. Additionally, this will lead to a reduction in the amount of knowledge we have about the disease as a whole. Such techniques of extraction also have the potential for seeding the tract with malignant cells.

Laparoscopic operations also take much longer, certainly in the early phases of a surgeon's experience. This will limit the number of operations that any one surgeon can complete during the course of a day and will also affect the availability of operating rooms.

One of the advantages that was originally claimed for laparoscopic cholecystectomy was that it was a great deal less expensive than the open variant due to the savings in the length of hospitalization.[12] However, with the passage of time and the development of evermore complex equipment, these financial advantages hae been lost.[13] With the increased operating time required and the use of numerous pieces of equipment, it is likely that any cost saving for laparoscopic colon resection will similarly be affected.

We are certainly at a very early stage in the evolution of laparoscopic colon surgery, and it is important that we develop our experience and report this in the time-honored fashion, that is, through peer-reviewed journals, at scientific meetings, and in consensus panels. To this end, the moves undertaken by the Society of American Gastrointestinal Endoscopic Surgeons[14] and the American Society of Colon and Rectal Surgery[15] are welcomed. The registers that these two organizations have initiated will doubtless yield much valuable data. Although we should not "just do it" and sacrifice holy cows on the altar of laparoscopic technology, nor should we be so cynical and suspicious as to prevent what seems to be, initially at least, an extremely promising and exciting new era in general surgery.[16]

TRAINING

There is no doubt that laparoscopic colon and rectal procedures are considerably more demanding than laparoscopic cholecystectomy, and therefore the wise surgeon will have accumulated considerable experience removing the gallbladder before commencing any other operations. A degree of proficiency in laparoscopic suturing is mandatory[17,18] (see Chap. 14), and it behooves the surgeon to practice intracorporeal and extracorporeal knots. The use of a training box to develop these skills is recommended.[19]

Unfortunately, the porcine model, which was so useful for learning laparoscopic cholecystectomy, is of little value for colon and rectal surgery because the pig has a spiral, deeply adherent colon.[20] The canine model is preferred, but the long mesentery does not make for a very demanding resection.[21]

EQUIPMENT

The basic hardware that the surgeon will have become familiar with during laparoscopic cholecystectomy are used. A high-flow insufflator, 300-W xenon light source, and a video recorder with static image capture facility are standard. The television screen should be positioned so that it is in line with the surgeon's eyes and hands and the organ under consideration, thereby creating one straight line.

Although the 0° forward-viewing telescope is acceptable for gallbladder surgery, it is not suitable when working on the colonic mesentery or in the pelvis. Here, the 30° or 45° forward-oblique scopes are required, and at least two scopes should be available in the 10-mm size to visualize the mesenteric vessels, as will become apparent during the discussion on laparoscopic colectomy.

As in laparoscopic cholecystectomy, a great deal of discussion still occurs as to the best means of dissecting tissue. Monopolar[22,23] and bipolar cautery,[24] lasers,[25] cavitronic ultrasonic aspirator,[26] harmonic scalpels (Amaral AF. Unpublished data, 1991), and hydrodissection[27] have all been advocated. However, the author prefers to use monopolar electrocautery. To locate vessels in an extremely fatty mesentery, a laparoscopic Doppler probe is a valuable tool (Fig. 17-2).

One of the major anatomic concerns during large bowel surgery is injury to the ureters. During the open operation, we have the advantage of tactile sensation, and this may be enhanced by placing a ureteric catheter before the operation. Obviously, during the laparoscopic procedure, we are not able to feel the ureter nor to see it as clearly. Therefore, it is advantageous to insert an illuminated 6-French ureter probe through a cystoscope into the ipsilateral side as the colonic lesion before the operation. At the appropriate moment, this is connected to a light source, the laparoscope is turned down, and the course of the ureter may be seen in its entirety.[28]

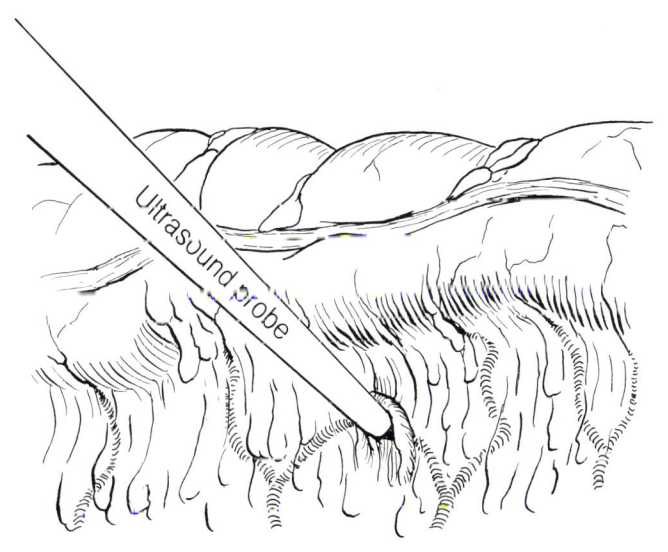

FIGURE 17-2 The laparoscopic Doppler probe may be used to locate vessels in a fatty mesocolon.

PREPARATION

The patient must be prepared for major surgery as in the open operation but with a few modifications. Obviously, the consent form will reflect the laparoscopic approach but must also include open surgery because conversion will occasionally be necessary. Bowel preparation should be thorough, and mannitol should be avoided because it tends to produce a rather gas-filled colon. The anesthesiologist should be asked not to administer nitrous oxide because this may lead to intestinal distention, which interferes with the progress of a laparoscopic procedure. The patient should be placed in the lithotomy or Lloyd-Davis position to allow access to the perineum for perioperative endoscopy and perianal stapling. Otherwise, the preparations are as detailed in the chapter on laparoscopic cholecystectomy (see Chap. 21).

TECHNIQUES

Repair of Injured Bowel

Unfortunately, during the course of other laparoscopic operations, or in penetrating trauma, the large bowel may be injured. The surgeon has a number of choices, and the course of action selected will depend upon personal experience, availability of equipment, amount of peritoneal soiling, and the patient's general condition. The first and obvious option is to convert the patient to open surgery and either exteriorize the bowel as a stoma or repair it with, or without, anastomotic protection. However, even if this is the chosen course, then the patient may benefit from laparoscopy because the incision can be guided and the surgeon may choose to mobilize the bowel for such a laparoscopically assisted repair. The third option involves placing sutures to close the defect, and this should obviously only be done by the experienced laparoscopist for a small injury in a stable patient where there is little peritoneal soiling. Finally, the surgeon may chose to place a Foley catheter inside the injury and bring this out percutaneously (Fig. 17-3). The advantage of this technique is that it is quick and relatively simple and will allow for later evaluation of this controlled fistula.[79] Obviously, lavage of the contaminated abdomen would be the next step.

Repair of Full-Thickness Excision of Bowel Wall

Patients who present with endometriosis are most likely to fall into this category.[30] Two cannulae, in addition to the one accommodating the telescope will be required and should form a triangle over the site of resection. The bowel is firmly grasped, and the diseased wall is excised. Repair of the defect follows the same guidelines described previously. This may also be a valuable adjunct to colonoscopic excision of large polyps with either laparoscopic surveillance or to aid in excision.

Drainage of Abscess

Patients who present with diverticulitis and localized peritonitis may be assessed with a CT scan of the abdomen.

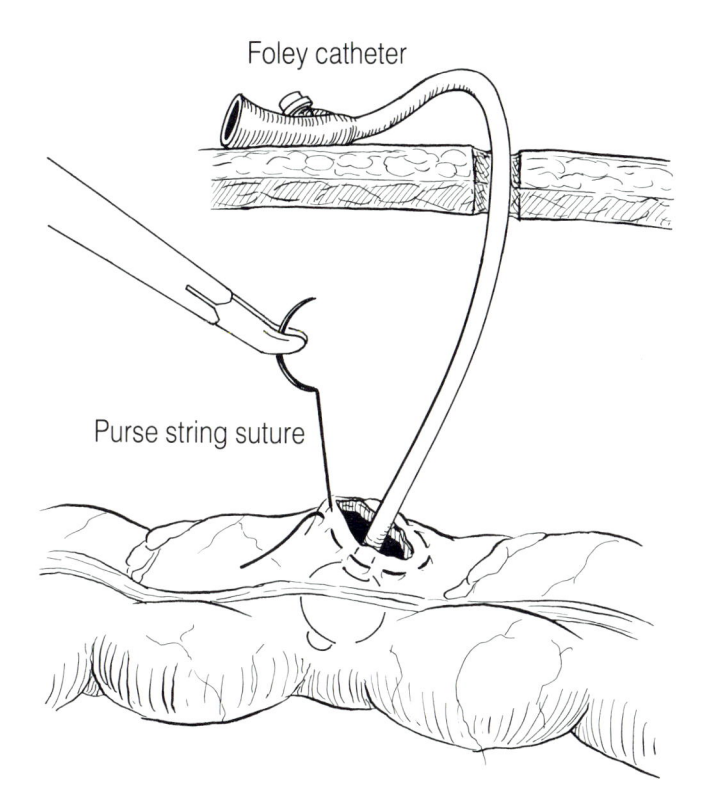

FIGURE 17-3 A small colon injury may be managed with a Foley catheter held in place by inflating the balloon and inserting a purse-string suture.

Occasionally the clinical condition will mandate that surgery be performed. If obstruction is not the presenting feature, then laparoscopy can be used to establish whether the abscess is communicating with the peritoneal cavity or not.[31] If it is deemed appropriate, then a large drain may be brought in through a separate abdominal stab incision, held with laparoscopic graspers, and introduced into the abscess cavity. Copious lavage and aspiration will allow removal of the abscess contents. Of course, a defunctioning proximal stoma may also be fashioned. This will be discussed later.

Ileostomy

Although it is a relatively simple matter to make a gridiron incision to retrieve a segment of small bowel, it is occasionally useful to assess the nature of the abdominal contents, such as in patients with inflammatory bowel disease. After the diagnostic laparoscopy has been completed with the telescope in the umbilical position, a 10-mm cannula is introduced at the preselected stoma site. In the right hypochondrium, an additional 5-mm trocar is introduced, and between these two accessory cannulae, grasping forceps isolate a segment of small bowel. To assess mobility of the ileum, the pneumoperitoneum may be released slowly, and the appropriate tension applied to the bowel. If extra length is needed, the peritoneal surfaces on both sides of the mesentery are scored. A window is then made while one grasper holds the bowel at the appropriate site. Through the preselected stoma site cannula, a cotton tape is introduced and passed from one grasper to another. Then both ends are held by the grasper that passes through the stoma site cannula (Fig. 17-4). The grasper, tape, attached bowel, and cannula are then withdrawn as one, and the bowel is brought to the abdominal wall. The stoma may then be constructed in the usual fashion as either a Brooke[32] or Alexander-Williams[33] type of ileostomy. After the bowel has been secured to the skin, the pneumoperitoneum is slowly reestablished, and the laparoscope is used to evaluate the position of the bowel.

COLOSTOMY

It is beyond the scope of this chapter to detail all the indications for colostomy. The example given will relate to the formation of a loop colostomy,[34] although it will be clear that, by dividing the distal limb and replacing it in the abdomen, an end stoma may be fashioned.

Initially, the diagnosis is confirmed with the telescope in the umbilical position. At the preselected stoma site, a disk of skin is excised, and a 20-mm trocar is positioned (Fig. 17-5). An additional trocar is placed above the pubis for a sigmoid colostomy or in the hypochondrium for a transverse colostomy. As for ileostomy, the bowel is grasped and brought to the abdominal wall. The pneumoperitoneum is

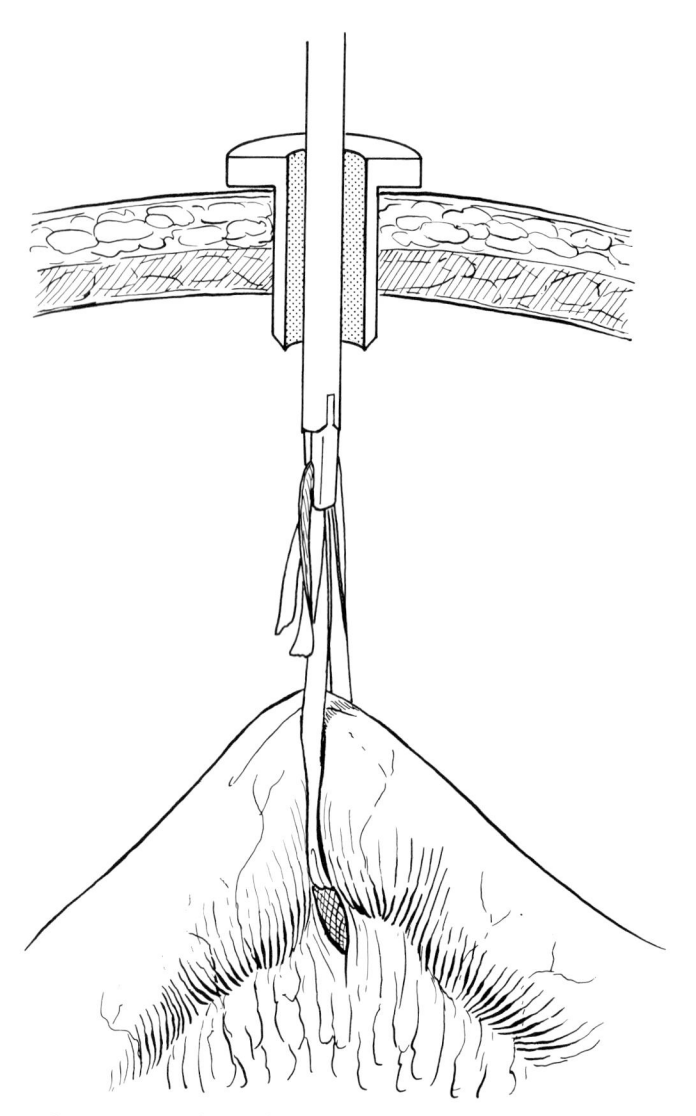

FIGURE 17-4 A loop of ileum is held with a tape passed through a window in the mesentery. The pneumoperitoneum is released, and the bowel is brought out via the cannula at the preselected stoma site.

gently released to ascertain bowel tension. If necessary, extra mobility is gained by incising the peritoneum. For the large bowel, especially when dilated, the use of a red rubber Robinson tube is more effective than cotton tape because this may tend to cut into the bowel wall. Having completed the mucocutaneous attachments, laparoscopy will allow the surgeon to ascertain whether the colon is well positioned and whether any intracorporeal sutures are required to prevent the formation of internal hernias.

Cecopexy

The debate about management of cecal volvulus continues to rage between right hemicolectomy, cecostomy, or cecopexy.[35-37] Certainly, all three operations are feasible lapar-

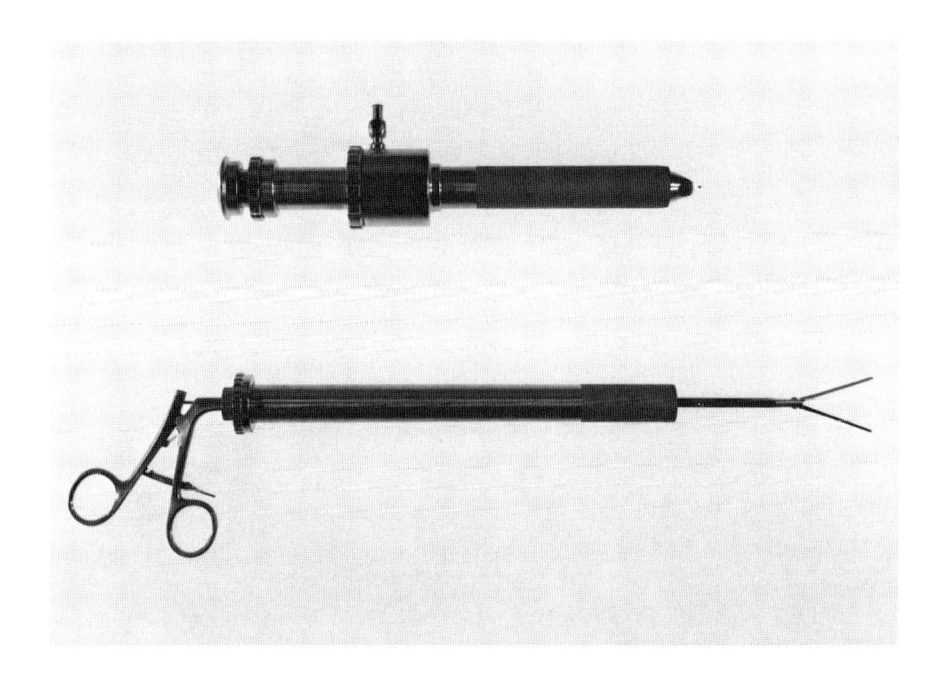

FIGURE 17-5 The 20-mm trocar–cannula and reducer are shown here with a bowel grasper.

oscopically, but the latter, cecopexy, is minimally invasive and may be suitable in certain circumstances.[38] The laparoscope is placed in the normal position, and additional trocars are positioned, one in the right hypochondrium in the midclavicular line and one in the right iliac fossa. Sutures of nonabsorbable material are placed using ski-shaped needles and tied with intracorporeal knots between the taenia coli and the parietal peritoneum. If a cecostomy is desired, this is brought in through an additional trocar. Having placed purse-string sutures in the cecum in the fashion of a Stamm gastrostomy, the cecopexy is completed. To prevent leakage, the cecum is secured to the abdominal wall, using either sutures or staples (Fig. 17-6).

Rectopexy

This procedure is potentially one of the most obvious for the laparoscopic approach because the condition of rectal prolapse, although benign, is common, debilitating, and usually present in elderly patients with coincident disease. Therefore, the minimally invasive approach is more preferable to either open rectal suspension or colectomy. It is interesting to note the vast variety of procedures for the correction of this deformity that have been described in the literature.[39-41] A number of these have been adapted for the laparoscopic technique (Arregui M. Unpublished data, 1991. Cuschieri A. Unpublished data, 1991). In all, the telescope is placed in the umbilical position, and the bowel is grasped via a portal in the midline just above the pubis. Two working ports, one in each iliac fossa, provide access to each side of the rectum to allow for dissection. Having placed the patient in Trendelenburg position, the small bowel is swept toward the upper abdomen. Using a Bab-

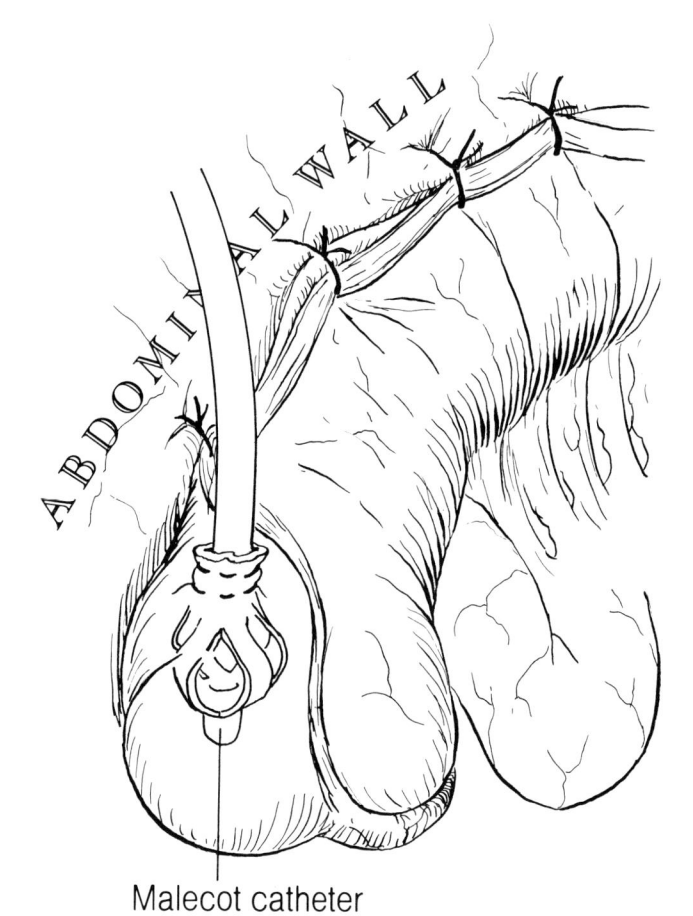

FIGURE 17-6 The freely mobile cecum is sutured at the taenia coli to the parietal peritoneum. A Malecot cecostomy tube is placed and held with two concentric purse-string sutures.

cock forceps, the rectum is elevated toward the anterior abdominal wall and pulled in a cephalic direction. Starting on the anterior aspect of the rectum, the peritoneum is scored, and this is continued laterally to right and left. The plane between the rectum and sacrum is developed until a space exists from right to left. In women, obviously, it is necessary to dissect the rectum posteriorly, from the vagina anteriorly. A speculum placed on the cervix and manipulated by another operator standing between the legs is valuable here. Indeed, if the uterus is large, it may be valuable to place a Keith needle through the abdomen into the uterus and then back out through the abdominal wall, tying the suture on the outside.

Fixation of the rectum to the sacrum may be achieved with Marlex mesh, using a strip approximately 3 × 8 cm. This is fashioned into a roll and introduced into the peritoneal cavity through one of the portals. This may then be secured to the sacrum with sutures or with a laparoscopic sacral tacker, which obviously facilitates the speed of the procedure.[42] Attachment to the rectum is usually by sutures placed through the mesh and into the muscle (Fig 17-7).

One major advantage of laparoscopic colon surgery is that control of hemostasis is usually excellent, and the need for drains is thus obviated.

REVERSAL OF HARTMANN'S PROCEDURE

This operation is frequently challenging to even the most skilled colon and rectal surgeon because of the adhesions and the need to mobilize the proximal bowel. If it is possible to gain entry into the abdominal cavity using either open insertion techniques or ultrasound mapping, then laparoscopic surgery may be beneficial. Having mobilized the colostomy from the abdominal wall, the anvil of the end-to-end stapling device is secured inside the freshened end of the bowel around a purse-string suture (Fig. 17-8). This is dropped into the abdomen, and the wound is closed. Laparoscopically, the proximal bowel may be mobilized from the splenic flexure and the rectum located by placing the end-to-end stapling device in situ. After the small bowel has been cleared from the pelvis, the point of the stapler is advanced through the rectal stump

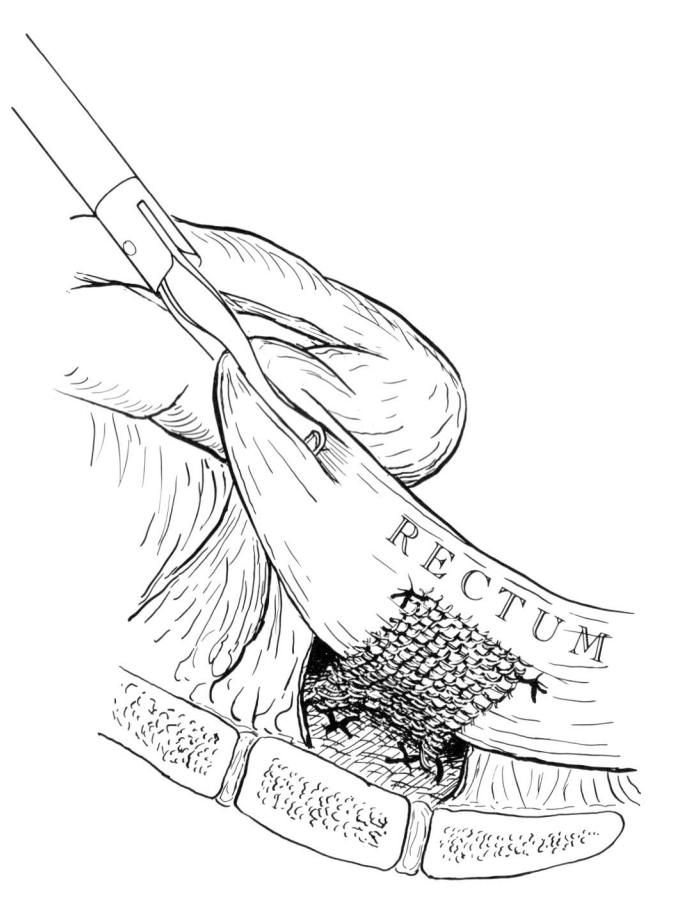

FIGURE 17-7 The sigmoid colon is retracted anteriorly and in a cephalic direction. A space has been created between the rectum and sacrum. A piece of Marlex mesh has been secured to the sacrum and the rectum.

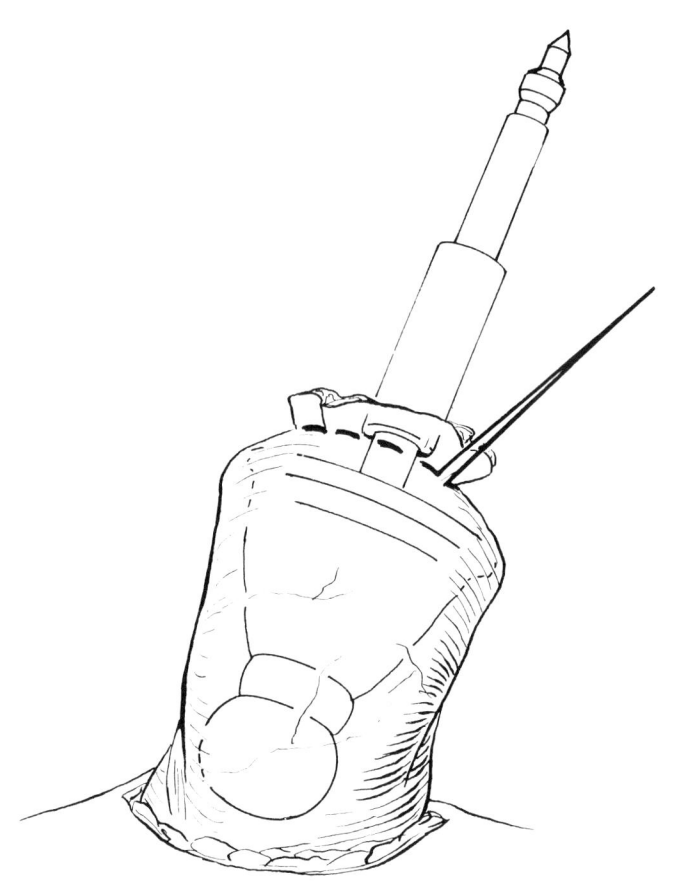

FIGURE 17-8 A purse-string suture is placed in the freshened end of the proximal bowel. The anvil of the end-to-end stapling device is positioned in the colon.

and attached to the anvil in the proximal bowel. Having completed the anastomosis, the mesenteric defect is closed under laparoscopic control.

LAPAROSCOPIC COLECTOMY

This is really the ultimate challenge of laparoscopic colon and rectal surgery and, broadly speaking, falls into two categories. The first is laparoscopic-assisted colectomy,[43] where the dissection and mobilization are done under laparoscopic control, but the resection and anastomosis are completed outside, through a small incision. Laparoscopic control is then reinstituted and utilized to assess the integrity of the anastomosis and to survey the abdomen. Currently, this is the only acceptable technique for right hemicolectomy and is used to remove large left-sided lesions. Pure laparoscopic colectomy[44] is the method in which the entire procedure is done without any incisions larger than for a trocar, and the specimen is retrieved through the anus.

Right Hemicolectomy

The surgeon stands to the patient's left and the assistant, to the patient's right. The surgeon watches the television screen on the patient's right. The telescope is introduced through the umbilicus and accessory trocars are positioned (Fig. 17-9). The patient is rolled with the right side up and head down, and the small bowel is encouraged to fall toward the left side of the abdomen. The dissection commences with the small bowel, and this is elevated with a Babcock grasper. A window is made in the mesentery through which a cotton tape is passed and tied to provide a point for graspers. The mesentery is then scored, and the lateral attachments of the colon are incised to reflect the bowel toward the left. The ureter will be detected with the illuminated probe as previously described.[28] If the duodenum is not immediately obvious, a gastroscope can be inserted and manipulated past the pylorus. If it is not possible to see the vessels in the mesentery clearly and a laparoscopic Doppler probe is not available, then the surgeon should pass a second telescope in through a laterally placed cannula and transilluminate the mesentery by turning down the umbilical telescope light source.

After the mesentery has been mobilized to its root and the major vessels have been secured and divided between clips or ties, the hypochondrial trocar insertion sites mark the position through which the bowel is brought for resection, anastomosis, and closure of the mesenteric defect. The bowel is replaced into the abdomen, the incision closed, and thorough irrigation and aspiration are performed.

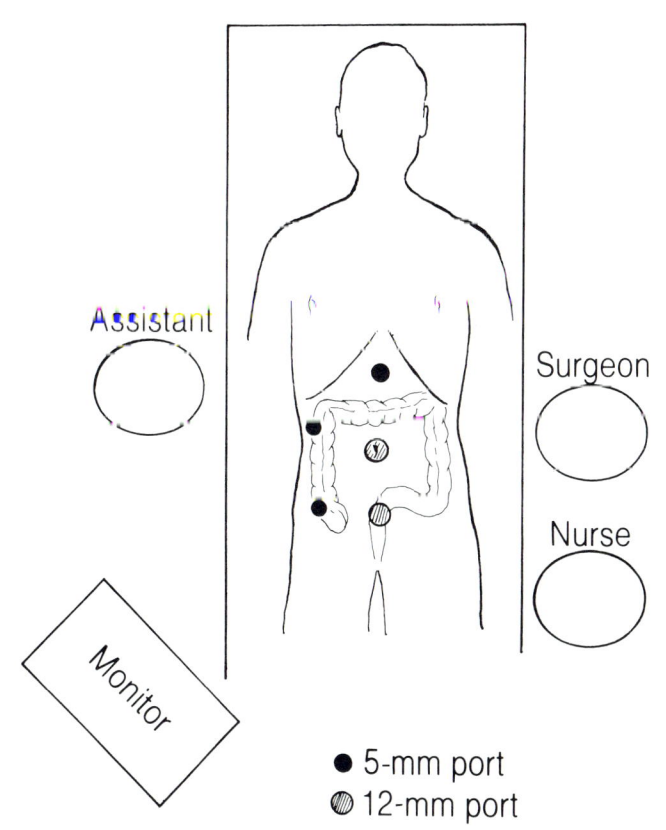

FIGURE 17-9 For right hemicolectomy, the surgeon stands to the patient's left, and the television is placed opposite. The cannulae positions are illustrated.

Left Hemicolectomy

The surgeon stands to the patient's right and watches the procedure on the television screen on the patient's left. The cannulae are positioned (Fig. 17-10). Through the umbilical portal, the surgeon directs the procedure. The bowel is elevated through graspers placed via the hypochondrial and suprapubic graspers. If the lesion in question is not obvious on the serosal surface of the bowel, a colonoscope is introduced per anus, and the position of the lesion is established. It is important to occlude the proximal bowel with a Glassman clamp, or the insufflated gas will cause the colon to become unmanageably distended. After the lesion has been found, indentation on the exterior with a laparoscopic instrument, coupled with transillumination from the interior will locate the serosal position. This may then be marked by scoring the bowel or placing a suture (Fig. 17-11). After the limits of resection have been chosen, a window should be made in the mesentery and cotton tapes placed and stapled across to act as graspers. Alternatively the bowel may be divided with the linear stapler–cutter.

Broadly speaking, the most important issue is the technique of anastomosis that will be utilized. This will dictate how the operation continues.

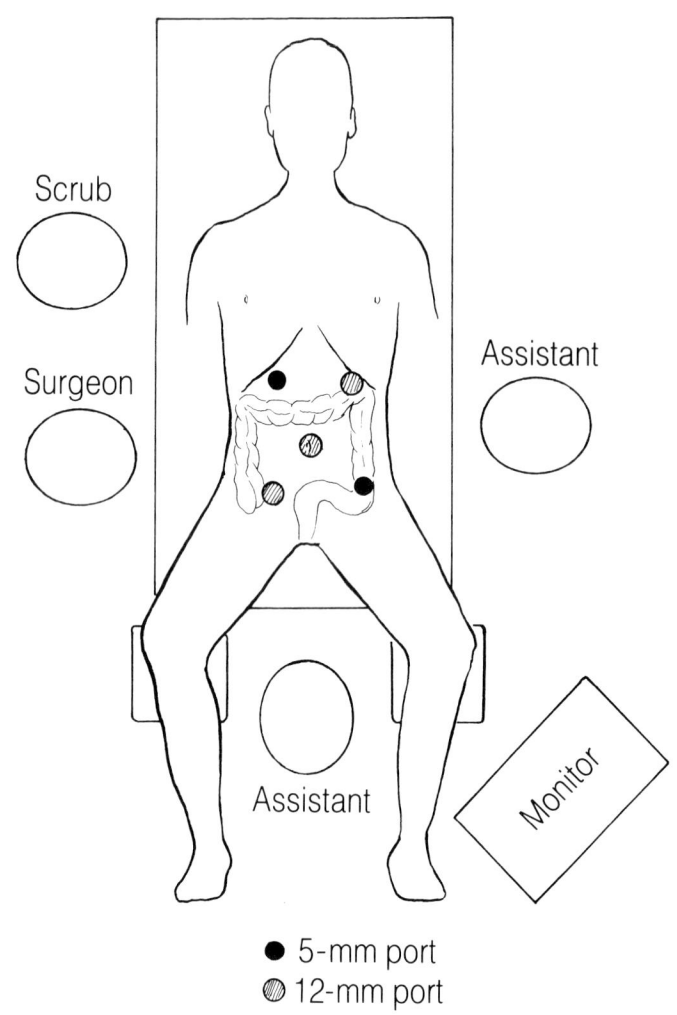

FIGURE 17-10 For left hemicolectomy, the lithotomy position allows an assistant surgeon access to the perineum for colonoscopy and stapling. The surgeon stands to the patient's right, and the television is on the patient's left. The cannulae positions are demonstrated.

For a laparoscopically assisted operation, one will merely mobilize the bowel as for a right hemicolectomy and bring it out through a mirror-image gridiron incision in the left groin. The bowel may then be resected and anastomosed. The mesenteric defect may be closed, and the bowel returned to the abdominal cavity as before.

Alternatively, a 20-mm trocar may be placed in the left iliac fossa and the proximal bowel brought out through this after it has been divided from the distal bowel. Into this open lumen, the anvil of the stapler is placed with a hand-sutured purse string (see Fig. 17-8). This is then replaced in the abdomen, and the diseased bowel may be either brought out through this incision by stapling across the rectosigmoid, or by simply cutting across this junction, it may be retrieved at the anus with ring forceps. To complete the stapled anastomosis, the pointed anvil may be passed through the staple line or a purse-string suture may be positioned. By manipulating the anvil down to the rectum, a standard stapled anastomosis can be fashioned.

Another alternative is to divide the bowel, withdraw the specimen from the anus, and then fashion a hand-sutured anastomosis. This is technically challenging and time consuming (see Chap. 15).

Yet another approach is to use the biofragmentable anastomotic ring (BAR), which has recently been demonstrated to be of value in open surgery.[45,46] This has been used in laparoscopically assisted left hemicolectomy.[47] Recent modifications have allowed for its placement for colon resection by laparoscopy.[48] First, it is necessary to place a purse-string suture, and initially, these were hand sutured, which is a frustrating facet of the operation. The modified Judd forceps[49] and specially designed laparoscopic purse-string device may solve this problem.[50] After resection of the bowel and removal through the anus, purse-string sutures are placed on both proximal and distal bowel. An applicator for the BAR is passed per anus and the purse-string suture on the anus is then tightened (Fig. 17-12). The proximal bowel is brought down over the BAR and tightened, and the device is then fired in a similar fashion to the end-to-end stapling gun. This pressure anastomosis is just as safe and efficacious as staples or sutures.[51]

When withdrawing the specimen from the anus, it is wise to place it inside a plastic bag, which is brought into the abdomen through one of the cannulae. One might think that withdrawing the specimen through the rectum would lead to immediate loss of pneumoperitoneum. However, the anterior and posterior walls of the rectum stay together similar to a valve and prevent loss of gas.

It is likely that other anastomotic techniques such as glues[52] and laser welding[53] may be appropriate to colonic anastomosis but such tactics are currently experimental (see Chap. 33).

ABDOMINOPERINEAL RESECTION OF THE RECTUM

Indications for this operation include extremely low carcinoma of the rectum or anal carcinoma, which has proven intractable to radiotherapy and chemotherapy. Additionally, patients with incurable fecal incontinence may be better served by abdominal incontinence through a colostomy than perineal incontinence into their underwear.

The laparoscope is positioned through the umbilicus, and the patient is placed head down and left side up to allow the small bowel to fall toward the head and right side, thus exposing the sigmoid colon. The cannulae positions are the same as in a left hemicolectomy. The point of division is chosen, and a window is made in the mesentery and divided with the linear stapler–cutter. The mesentery is divided, securing vessels with clips, ligatures, or electrocau-

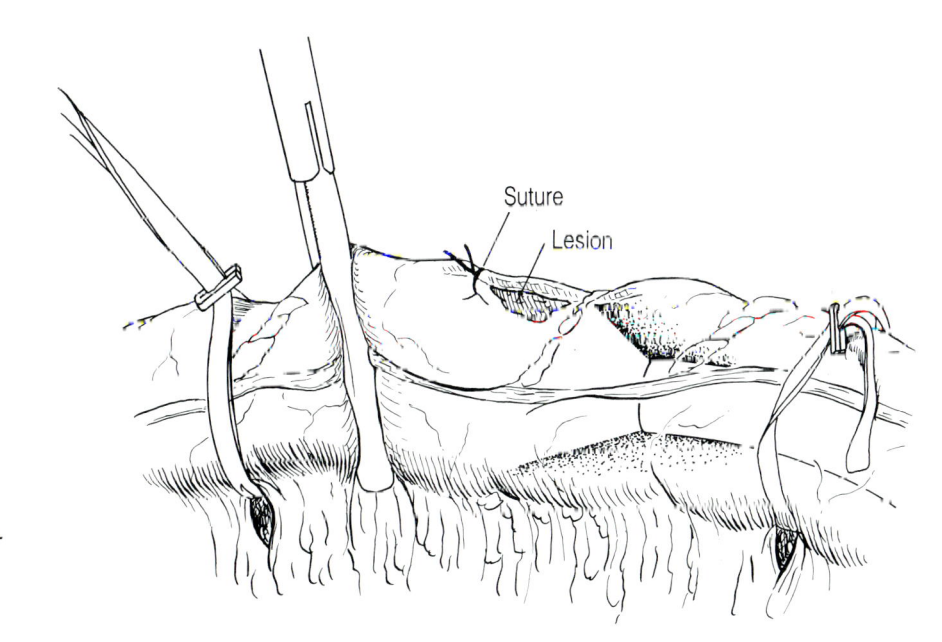

FIGURE 17-11 The proximal colon is occluded with a Glassman clamp, and the sites of division are selected. A colonoscope is used to locate the lesion, and a stitch marks its position on the serosal surface of the bowel.

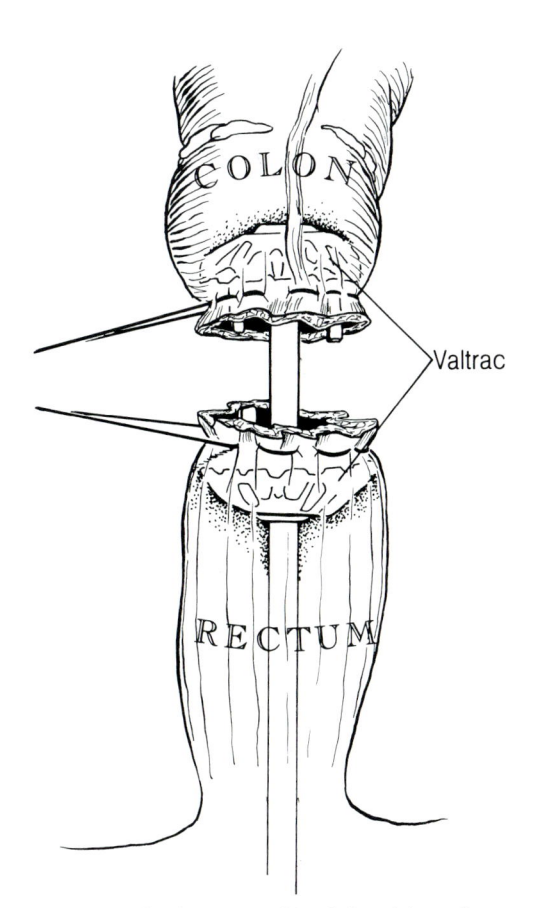

FIGURE 17-12 In both proximal and distal bowel, a purse-string suture has been placed, and the specimen has been withdrawn from the anus. The BAR is introduced from below, the purse strings are tightened, and a pressure anastomosis is fashioned.

tery as required. The rectum is mobilized from the sacrum similar to rectoplexy, and having closed the anus with a purse-string suture, perianal dissection continues in the normal fashion.

After the finger of the perineal operator is seen, the laparoscopic operator may continue the dissection around the sphincteric muscles, dividing the lateral stalks of the rectum as required. At the preselected stoma site, a circle of skin is excised, a 20-mm trocar is introduced, and the bowel is brought up to the abdominal wall, releasing pneumoperitoneum as required. After the bowel has been brought through, a gas seal may be maintained with a petroleum jelly-soaked gauze swab to allow reevaluation of the abdominal cavity. Drains will be placed through the perineum, and these may be viewed laparoscopically. After the perineum has been closed and the pneumoperitoneum reestablished, copious lavage and aspiration will be possible.[54]

Total Abdominal Colectomy

This laparoscopic procedure is really a combination of right and left hemicolectomy and does not merit any specific discussion of technique. One extremely good indication for total colectomy is in patients with ulcerative colitis or familial polyposis coli. A recent prospective trial[55] demonstrated that, although laparoscopically assisted total colectomy was feasible, the length of time was significantly longer, and it did not seem to have any immediate benefits for the patient compared with standard laparotomy. There is currently insufficient data to merit any further description of this operation. At the moment, it is sufficient to state that this is a tour de force with no obvious application to general surgical practice. Additionally, the ileoanal reservoir itself is a highly specialized procedure that should be performed only in centers with a special interest in this operation.

REFERENCES

1. Greene FL: Laparoscopy in malignant disease. *Surg Clin North Am* 1992; 72:1125–1138.
2. Sackier JM, Berci G, Paz-Partlow M: Elective diagnostic laparoscopy. *Am J Surg* 1992; 161:326–331.
3. Nagy AG, James D: Diagnostic laparoscopy. *Am J Surg* 1989; 157:490–493.
4. Patterson-Brown S, Eckersley JRT, Sim AJW, et al: Laparoscopy as an adjunct to decision making in the acute abdomen. *Br J Surg* 1986; 73:1022–1024.
5. Hinchley EJ, Schall PGH, Richards GK: Treatment of perforated diverticular disease of the colon. *Adv Surg* 1978; 12:85–109.
6. Gazzaniga AB, Slanton WW, Bartlett RH: Laparoscopy in the diagnosis of blunt and penetrating injuries to the abdomen. *Am J Surg* 1976; 131:315.
7. Cuschieri A, Hennessy T, Stephens R, et al: Diagnosis of significnt abdominal trauma after road traffic accidents: Preliminary results of a multicenter clinical trial comparing minilaparoscopy with peritoneal lavage. *Ann R Coll Surg Engl* 1988; 70:153–155.
8. Du Priest RW Jr, Rodriguez A, Khaneja SC, et al: Open diagnostic peritoneal lavage in blunt abdominal trauma victims. *Surg Gynecol Obstet* 1979; 148:890–892.
9. Sackier JM: Laparoscopy in the emergency setting. *World J Surg* 1992; 16:1083–1088.
10. Sosa JL, Sims D, Martin L, et al: Laparoscopic evaluation of tangential abdominal gunshot wounds. *Arch Surg* 1992; 127:109.
11. Clayman RV, Kavoussi LR, Soper JN, et al: Laparoscopic nephrectomy: Initial case report. *J Urol* 1991; 146:278–282.
12. Graves HA, Ballinger JF, Anderson WJ: Appraisal of laparoscopic cholecystectomy. *Ann Surg* 1991; 213:655–664.
13. Voyles CR: The laparoscopic dividend. *JAMA* 1992; 267:1469.
14. Berman IR: Frontiers in general surgery: Pioneers, cowboys and desperadoes. *Surg Endosc* 1992; 6:82–83.
15. American Society of Colon and Rectal Surgeons: Policy statement. *Dis Colon Rectum* 1992; 35:5A.
16. Schrock TR: The endosurgery evolution: No place for sacred cows. *Surg Endosc* 1992; 6:163–168.
17. Ko ST, Airan MC: Therapeutic laparoscopic suturing techniques. *Surg Endosc* 1992; 6:41–46.
18. Soper NJ, Hunter JG: Suturing and knot tying in laparoscopy. *Surg Clin North Am* 1992; 72:1139–1152.
19. Sackier JM, Berci G, Paz-Partlow M: A new training device for laparoscopic surgery. *Surg Endosc* 1991; 5:158–159.
20. Getty R: *The Anatomy of the Domestic Animals*. Philadelphia, WB Saunders, 1975, vol 2, pp 1281–1282.
21. Sackier JM: Training for minimal access surgery. *Curr Pract Surg* 1992; 4:227–234.
22. Voyles CR, Meena AL, Petro AB, et al: Electrocautery is superior to laser for laparoscopic cholecystectomy, editorial. *Am J Surg* 1990; 160:457.
23. Hunter JG: Laser or electrocautery for laparoscopic cholecystectomy? *Am J Surg* 1991; 161:345–349.
24. Olsen DO, Corbitt JD, Edelman DS, et al: Clinical experience using a bipolar electrosurgical device for laparoscopic cholecystectomy. *Surg Endosc* 1992; 6:104.
25. Reddick EJ, Olsen DO: Laparoscopic laser cholecystectomy. *Surg Endosc* 1992; 6:104.
26. Wetter LA, Payne J, Kirschenbaum G, et al: The ultrasonic dissector (CUSA) facilitates laparoscopic cholecystectomy. *Arch Surg*, in press.
27. Nezhat C, Nezhat FR: Safe laser endoscopic excision or vaporization of peritoneal endometriosis. *Fertil Steril* 1989; 52:149–151.
28. Sackier JM: Visualization of the ureter during laparoscopic colon resection. *Br J Surg*, in press.
29. Birns MT: Inadvertent instrumental perforation of the colon during laparoscopy: Nonsurgical repair. *Gastrointest Endosc* 1989; 35:54–56.
30. Reich H, McGlynn F, Budin R: Laparoscopic repair of full-thickness bowel injury. *J Laparoendosc Surg* 1991; 1:119–122.
31. Sackier JM: Perforated diverticulitis, in Carter C, Russell RCG, Fielding LP (eds): *Rob and Smiths Operative Surgery*. London, Butterworth-Heinemann, 1993.
32. Brooke BN: The management of ileostomy. *Lancet* 1952; 2:102–104.
33. Alexander-Williams J: Loop ileostomy and colostomy for faecal diversion. *Ann R Coll Surg Engl* 1974; 54:141–148.
34. Lange V, Meyer G, Schardey HM, et al: Laparoscopic creation of a loop colostomy. *J Laparoendosc Surg* 1991; 1:307–312.
35. Todd GJ, Forde KA: Volvulus of the cecum: Choice of operation. *Am J Surg* 1979; 138:632–634.
36. Howard RS, Catto J: Cecal volvulus: A case for nonresectional therapy. *Arch Surg* 1980; 115:272–277.
37. Ostergaard E, Halvorsen JF: Volvulus of the cecum: An evaluation of various surgical procedures. *Acta Chir Scand* 1990; 156:629–631.
38. Shoop SA, Sackier JM: Laparoscopic cecopexy for cecal volvulus. *Surg Endosc*, in press.
39. Ripstein CB: Surgical care of massive rectal prolapse. *Dis Colon Rectum* 1965; 8:34–38.
40. Wells C: New operation for rectal prolapse. *Proc R Soc Med* 1959; 52:602–603.
41. Corman ML: Rectal prolapse, in *Colon and Rectal Surgery*, ed 2. Philadelphia, JB Lippincott, 1987, pp 209–248.
42. Berman IR: Sutureless laparoscopic rectopexy for procidentia. *Dis Colon Rectum* 1992; 35:689–693.
43. Fowler DL, White SA: Laparoscopy assisted sigmoid resection. *Surg Laparosc Endosc* 1991; 1:183–188.
44. Jacobs M, Verdeja JC, Goldstein HS: Minimally invasive colon resection (laparoscopic colectomy). *Surg Laparosc Endosc* 1991; 1:144–150.
45. Hardy TG, Pace WG, Maney JW, et al: A biofragmentable ring for sutureless bowel anastomosis: An experimental study. *Dis Colon Rectum* 1985; 28:484–490.
46. Hardy TG, Aguilar PS, Stewart WRC, et al: Initial clinical experience with a biofragmentable ring for sutureless bowel anastomosis. *Dis Colon Rectum* 1987; 30:55–61.
47. Sackier JM, Slutzki S, Wood CB, et al: Laparoscopic endocorporeal mobilization followed by extracorporeal sutureless anastomosis for the treatment of carcinoma of the left colon. *Dis Colon Rectum*, in press.
48. Sackier JM, Jessup G, Easter DW: Laparoscopic colon and gastroenteric anastomosis with the biofragmentable anastomotic ring. *Surg Endosc*, in press.
49. Bessler M, Treat MR: Laparoscopic Judd forceps for placement of purse-string sutures. Presented at the Society of American Gastrointestinal Endoscopic Surgeons (SAGES) Annual Scientific Session, Washington DC, April, 1992.

50. Sackier JM, Jessup G: A device for placing purse-string suture in laparoscopic surgery. *Br J Surg,* in press.
51. Bubrick MP, Corman ML, Cahill CJ, et al: Prospective, randomized trial of the biofragmentable anastomosis ring. *Am J Surg* 1991; 161:136–143.
52. Cuschieri A: Tissue approximation. *Prol Gen Surg* 1991; 8:366–377.
53. Sauer JS, Hinshaw JR, McGuire KP: The first sutureless laser-welded, end-to-end bowel anastomosis. *Lasers Surg Med* 1989; 9:70–73.
54. Sackier JM, Berci G, Hiatt JR, et al: Laparoscopic abdominoperineal resection of the rectum. *Br J Surg* 1992; 79:1207–1208.
55. Wexner SD, Johanson OB, Nogueras JJ, et al: Laparoscopic total abdominoperineal colectomy. *Dis Colon Rectum* 1992; 35:651–655.

Chapter 18

Endoluminal Therapy of Rectal Tumors: Transanal Endoscopic Microsurgery

Gerhard Buess / Marco Maria Lirici

Endoscopic surgery for rectal neoplasms is based on principles of local rectal excision that were developed by Kraske, Mason, and Parks.[1,2] The oncologic and pathologic benefits of wide local excision of rectal cancers have been reported by various authors,[3-5] and the local excision of sessile adenomas and early rectal cancer, especially Stage pT1 low-risk carcinoma (Hermanek classification) is currently endorsed.[5]

In 1983, transanal endoscopic microsurgery (TEM) was brought into clinical use by Buess and associates[6] for local excision of such tumors. This technique of local rectal surgery has resulted in a postoperative complication rate lower than either the Kraske or Mason procedures and a recurrence rate lower than the Parks operation.[7,8] It offers a cost-effective and minimally invasive approach to surgery for rectal tumors.[9]

TEM

Equipment

The technology for TEM was developed by Buess and associates.[6,7,10] A 40-mm diameter rectoscope (Richard Wolf, Rosemont, IL), 12 or 20 cm in length, depending on the location of the tumor, is utilized (Fig. 18-1A). A double ball-and-socket mechanical arm is used to fix the rectoscope to the operating table after the proper position is obtained.

An insert provided with five ports is mounted on the basic element of the rectoscope. One port is for the optic, and as many as four other surgical instruments can be introduced through sealing elements into the other ports (Figs. 18-1B, C).

A recycling insufflation unit provides pressure-controlled gas dilatation of the rectum with CO_2. The suction rate of a roller pump integrated into the unit is lower than the insufflation rate to preserve the gas distention of the cavity.

A stereoscopic telescope, angulated at the end and tip, is introduced through the optic port and provides the surgeon with a three-dimensional magnified view. The telescope is also outfitted with a second optical channel. This additional optic is used as a semiflexible teaching attachment or as a rigid optic for video monitoring, thus allowing the assistant to participate in the operation via the video screen. A channel for optic lens rinsing is integrated into the system.

The endoscopic instrument set facilitates precise surgical resection, coagulation of bleeding points, and closure of the defect by continuous suture technique. Instruments include a high-frequency (HF) knife, a monopolar electrode connected with the electrosurgical unit, right- and left-angled endoscopic forceps and scissors, a needle holder, and a suction–coagulation probe. The tips of these endoscopic instruments are tilted slightly downward to reach the sacral concavity of the rectum better. A specially designed device applies a silver clip onto the thread, thus securing the running suture.

Procedure Notes

INDICATIONS

Sessile adenomas and early carcinomas are the lesions best approached with TEM. Among malignant neoplasms, five types of lesions approachable with TEM can be defined as follows.[5]

1. Stage pT1 low-risk carcinoma (submucosal well-to-moderate differentiation). In this group, the operation has a high probability of being curative.

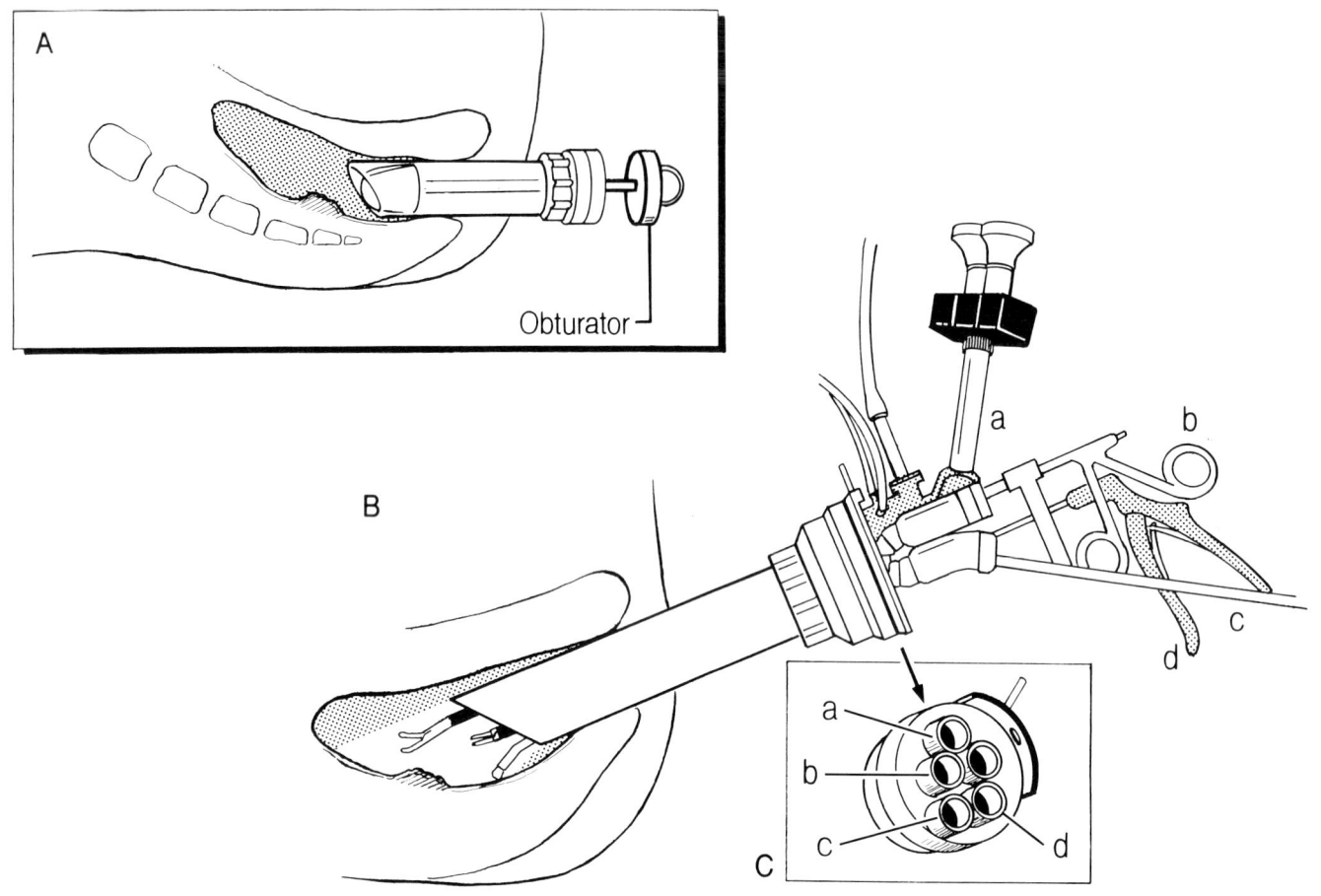

FIGURE 18-1 A. The 40-mm rectoscope (12 or 20 cm long) is introduced into the rectum. B and C. An insert with five ports is mounted on the scope to accommodate the telescope and up to four instruments.

2. Stage pT2 low-risk carcinoma (muscle involvement). In this group, the operation has a limited probability of being curative.
3. Stage pT3 carcinoma (transmural).
4. Palliative operations for advanced cancers.
5. Unsuspected or previously undetected cancers.

The last group is the largest because large adenomas contain areas of malignancy in up to 20 percent of cases and preoperative diagnosis is extremely difficult. These lesions are usually in situ or stage pT1 carcinoma, and a full-thickness TEM excision is usually curative.[11,12] Ulcus simplex of the rectum (solitary rectal ulcer), single rectal diverticulum, non-Hodgkin lymphoma, and rectal carcinoid are less frequent indications for TEM.

PREOPERATIVE ASSESSMENT

Careful preoperative staging is mandatory before endoluminal rectal surgery is performed. Digital rectal examination, rectoscopy with multiple biopsies, and endoluminal ultrasonography are included in the routine examination. Rectoscopy with a rigid endoscope allows definition of the exact location and extent of the neoplasm. The assessment of tumor position relative to rectal circumference is important for the correct positioning of the patient on the operating table (Fig. 18-2).

Endoluminal ultrasonography (EUS, transrectal/transvaginal probe, Diagnostic Sonar, Cambridge, OH) is used in the preoperative staging of rectal carcinoma to obtain as much information as possible about the depth of infiltration. Conventional EUS utilizes a water balloon to inflate the rectum and provide acoustic coupling. The disadvantage of this method is that it pushes sessile polyps and early carcinomas into the rectal wall, preventing a precise evaluation of infiltration.

A new waterproof system (Kretz Company) is currently used in EUS staging of patients undergoing TEM procedures.[13–15] Before the examination, the rectum is filled with a saline solution via the ultrasonic probe. The probe has three transducers with different frequencies (5, 8, and 10 MHz). The frequency can be changed during the examination. The assessment of the mucosa and submucosa is usually carried out with the 10-MHz transducer. The 8-MHz transducer is used to investigate the perirectal tissue and lymph nodes. The 5-MHz probe is utilized in assessing deep areas of the rectum and colon. In this technique, the entire polyp is floating in water during the examination, and therefore, compression of the lesion is avoided.

PREOPERATIVE MANAGEMENT AND ANESTHESIA

Informed consent to explain the nature of the possible complications after TEM is obtained from the patient. Preparation includes a bowel lavage with 10 L of Ringers solution given over 2 h via a nasogastric tube and perioperative antibiotic prophylaxis using metronidazole and a second-generation cephalosporin. The operation is performed under general or regional anesthesia. If the patient is positioned in the prone position, TEM must be performed under general endotracheal anesthesia. In our series at Tuebingen, regional anesthesia was utilized in 25 percent of cases.

PATIENT, TEAM, AND OPERATING ROOM SETTING

Depending on the location of the tumor, the patient is positioned in the prone, lithotomy, or lateral position. As a result of the angulation of the optic, the lesion must be situated at the bottom of the field (see Fig. 18-2). Skin disinfection and patient draping are performed in the same manner as for transanal procedures and transurethral resection. The surgeon sits and operates with the stereoscopic rectoscope. The assistant sits on the surgeon's left, with the scrub nurse on the right and behind. The video and camera equipment is positioned to the right of the surgeon and the endo- and electrosurgical units to the left of the assistant.

OPERATIVE PROCEDURE

Rectoscopy, utilizing an instrument with a glass window and manual insufflation, is performed to locate the tumor. Correct positioning of the rectoscope is completed by attaching its basic element to the mechanical arm.

At the beginning of the operation, the surgeon defines the margin of clearance around the tumor. The margin should exceed 5 mm in small adenomas and 10 mm in large adenomas or in carcinomas. It is easily marked with coagulation dots using the electric HF knife (Fig. 18-3A).

The depth of excision depends on the type, location, and extension of the lesion. The mucosectomy technique is performed in cases of small adenomas and exophytic tumors lying above the peritoneal reflection, with the full-thickness technique utilized in cases of large sessile adenomas or carcinomas. In patients with proven carcinomas, the retrorectal fat up to the fascia of Waldeyer can be excised. Lymph node dissection may also be performed in these cases.

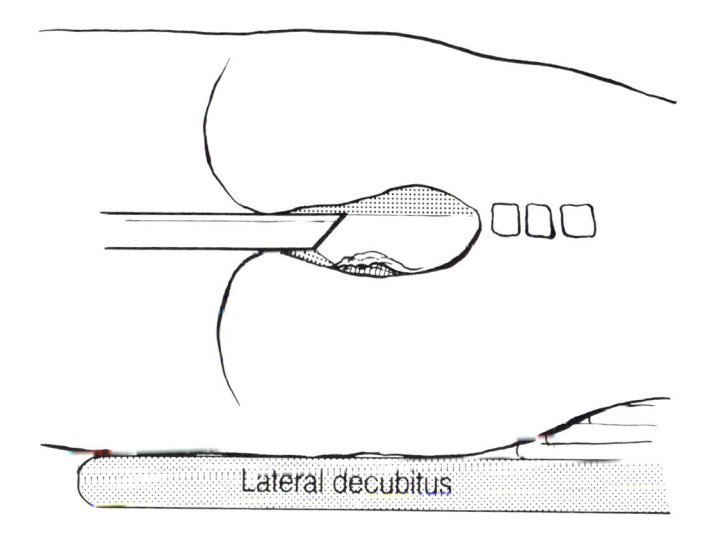

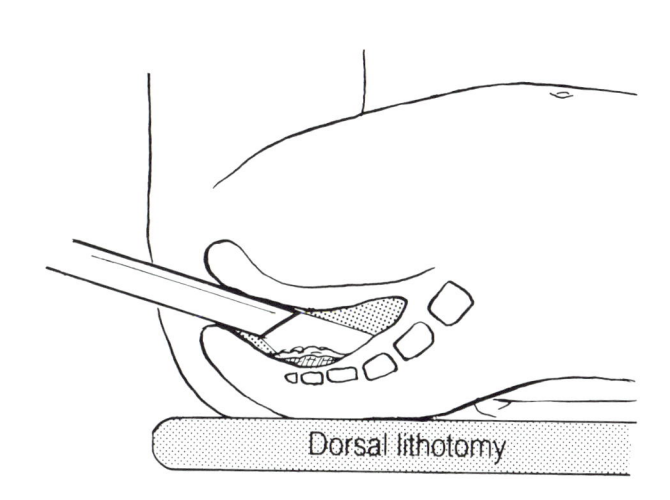

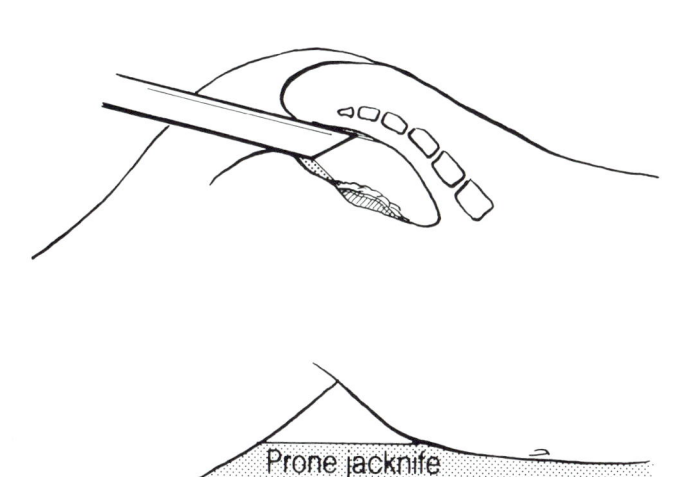

FIGURE 18-2 Because of the angulation of the rectoscope and the need for the lesion to be situated at the bottom of the field, careful positioning of the patient is vital.

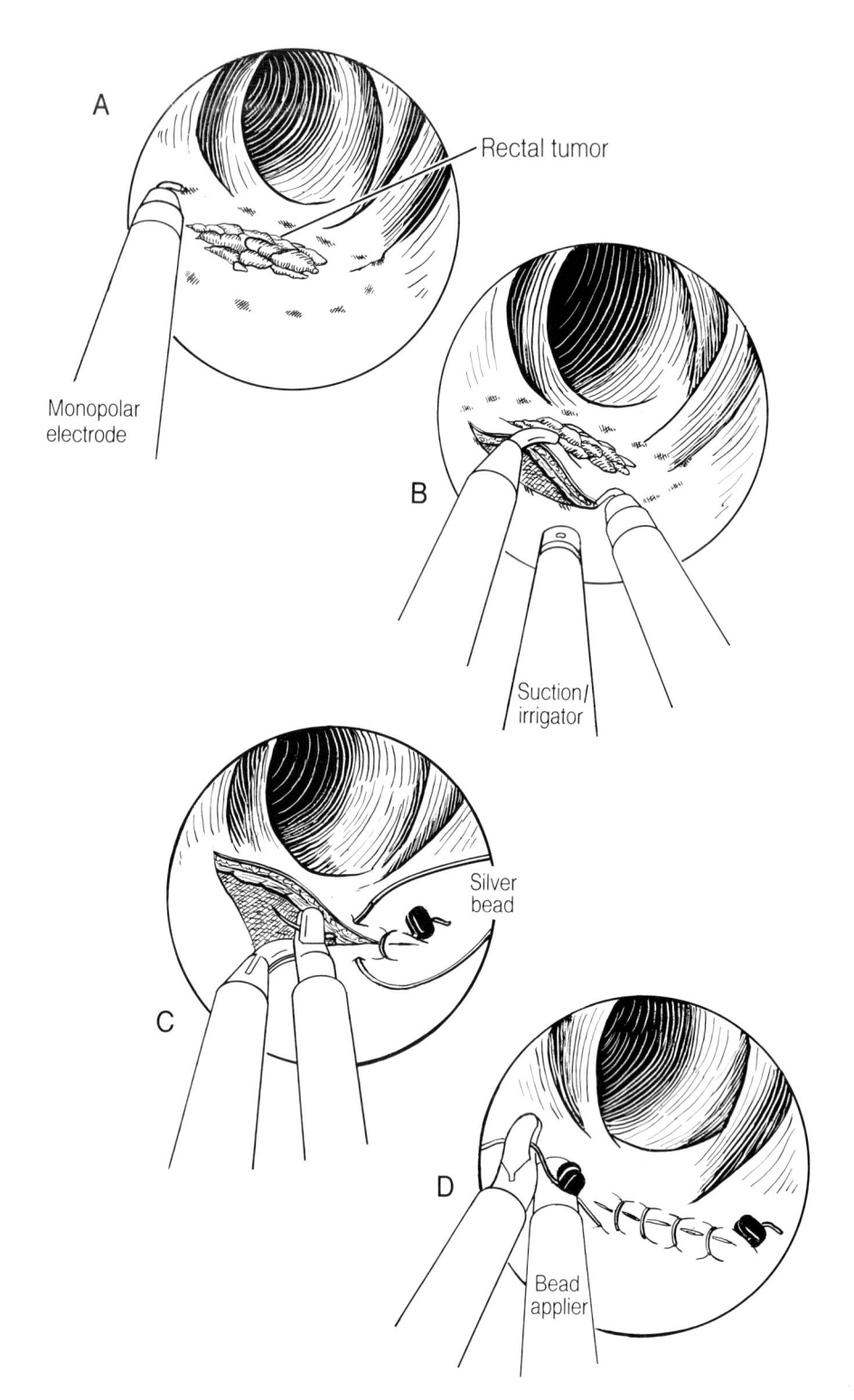

FIGURE 18-3 A. The margins of excision around a rectal lesion are marked with "dots" burned onto the mucosa by monopolar electrosurgery. B. Dissection of the lesion commences at the distal border. The lesion is elevated, electrosurgery is utilized and a suction–irrigation probe maintains a clear field. C. The defect is closed transversely. A silver clip obviates the need for tying knots. D. The running stitch is completed with another silver clip.

A segmental full-thickness resection is possible only in the middle third of the rectum. Rectal segments up to 8 or 10 cm in length can be removed using this technique. Full-thickness excision, an effective treatment of early cancer, is feasible by TEM only in the extraperitoneal part of the rectum, approximately 12 cm anteriorly to 20 cm posteriorly from the dentate line and related to the location of the neoplasm (anterior, left or right lateral, or posterior). When a segmental resection involves the intraperitoneal section of the rectum, a partial-thickness excision must be performed. Even in cases of neoplasms close to the dentate line, partial-thickness excision is the surgical method of choice to avoid injury to the sphincter.

Dissection of the lesion begins at the distal border (Fig. 18-3B). The bowel wall is divided using the HF knife, with immediate coagulation of bleeding vessels as they are encountered. After mobilization of the distal border, the incision is carried along the lateral aspects and then proximally, with careful control of the bleeding points. The transsected margins are lifted, and excision of the base is performed. The resected polyp is removed via the rectoscope, the operative field is checked, and residual bleeding is controlled.

Suturing of the defect is performed using a short monofilament thread (Polydioxanone 3–0) with a special silver clip pressed onto its end (Fig. 18-3C). A transverse running suture is carried on and, when completed, fixed by pressing a second silver clip onto the thread (Fig. 18-3D). To close extended or circular defects, up to four 8-cm PDS threads can be used. In these cases, the wound edges are first approximated with several interrupted stay stitches. The specimen is stretched and pinned onto a cork plate for macroscopic evaluation and sent to the pathologist for histologic examination.

The technique of TEM requires manual dexterity and proper training before clinical practice. For very large adenomas which require an extended excision or segment resection, TEM should be reserved for the surgeon with a great deal of TEM experience.[16,17] Training for TEM is available as a 5-day course in Germany, but programs are beginning to be established in the United States.

POSTOPERATIVE MANAGEMENT

After mucosectomy, patients are given liquids on the first postoperative day and a regular diet on the second day. They may be discharged after the third postoperative day. After full-thickness excision, the patient receives liquids intravenously for 2 days. A full liquid diet is possible on the third day, with regular meals on subsequent days; the patient may be discharged after the fourth postoperative day.

Results

In a series of 386 TEM techniques performed at the University Hospitals of Cologne, Mainz, and Tuebingen from 1983 to 1991, 283 procedures were for rectal adenoma and 96 for cancer. A full-thickness technique was performed in 70 percent of patients with adenomas operated on in Mainz and Tuebingen, with mucosectomy or partial-thickness excision in the remainder. A segmental resection or retrorectal fat dissection was performed, respectively, in five percent and four percent of cases. In the group of carcinoma patients operated on in Mainz and Tuebingen, a full-thickness technique was performed in 85 percent of cases; dissection of the retrorectal fat was additionally carried out in 22 percent of cases. The mean operating time ranged from 36 minutes for a mucosectomy to 90 minutes for a full-thickness technique or 120 minutes for a segmental resection.

Excision can generally be performed up to a length of 8 cm without problems related to suturing of the wall defect. Postoperative complications are usually related to tension. In a series of 191 TEM procedures for adenomas, dehiscence or fistula occurred, respectively, in 5 and 3 cases. When the defect is large, a temporary colostomy is required for prompt recovery. Local wound healing problems led to stenosis in five other cases, all responding to bougienage. Other complications included bleeding, a full-thickness excision above the peritoneal reflection that required anterior resection, and one case of pulmonary embolism.

The postoperative complication rate for TEM is approximately 9 percent, and the mortality rate is 0.5 percent. Postoperative pain is generally absent if the excision does not involve the dentate line. Strict follow-up is mandatory after transanal local resection. The recurrence rate of adenoma after TEM is about three percent, and treatment usually involves excision by means of snare resection or hot biopsy forceps.

When TEM is performed for carcinoma, postoperative staging and grading of the neoplasm must be carefully evaluated to recommend to the patient either radical reintervention or close follow-up. Patients suffering from Stage pT2 or more advanced tumors are advised to undergo radical procedures when cure is a possibility.

In patients with Stage pT1 high-risk tumors (Hermanek classification), TEM is less curative than in those with Stage pT2 low-risk carcinomas.[11] In the Buess report, 55 patients with cancer (between 1985 and 1991) underwent TEM without further immediate surgical treatment. Thirty-five of the patients were operated on for Stage pT1 tumors. In those patients with Stage pT1 low-risk cancers (30 cases), the recurrence rate was three percent. In five patients with Stage pT1 high-risk neoplasms, the recurrence rate was 40 percent. Sixteen patients suffering from Stage pT2 low-risk carcinomas refused to undergo radical reintervention. In this group, the recurrence rate at follow-up was six percent.

As a result of tumor stage, some patients have undergone radical reoperation immediately after TEM resection of a carcinoma. Residual cancer has not been found in any of the operative specimens from these patients.

TRANSANAL ENDOSCOPIC RECTOPEXY (TER)

Moderate and reducible rectal prolapses can be treated using TER. Because this technique is under clinical evaluation, TER is not recommended currently for the treatment of extended prolapses.[10]

The operating room setup and equipment are similar to that described for TEM. With the patient in the lithotomy position, the longer rectoscope is introduced up to the middle rectum. The posterior wall of the middle third of the rectum is opened transversely, and the presacral structures are exposed with dissection in the presacral space to the upper third of the rectum.

The procedure involves fixing the upper third of the rectum to the presacral fascia by means of U-shaped stitches (Fig. 18-4A). After the sacral promontory is exposed and the sacral curvature palpated with the aid of the suction probe, the posterior wall is divided, and the retrorectal fat is transsected upward for a length of at least 5 cm. After exposure of the presacral fascia, the first stitch is passed. The stitch, secured with a silver clip, comes from the luminal side, runs through the presacral fascia, and returns to the luminal side, where it is fixed by means of a second clip (Fig. 18-4B). Up to three U-shaped stitches are passed in a similar manner, and after accurate control of the bleeding points, the rectal incision is sutured using the technique described for TEM.

CONCLUSION

Further developments in TEM technology will enable combined laparoscopic–rectoscopic procedures for endoscopic resections of the left colon and rectosigmoid. In these procedures, the bowel is prepared laparoscopically and the anastomosis, performed rectoscopically. These innovative techniques have been tested during a 1-year in vivo study. Currently, a clinical trial is underway at the University of Tuebingen.

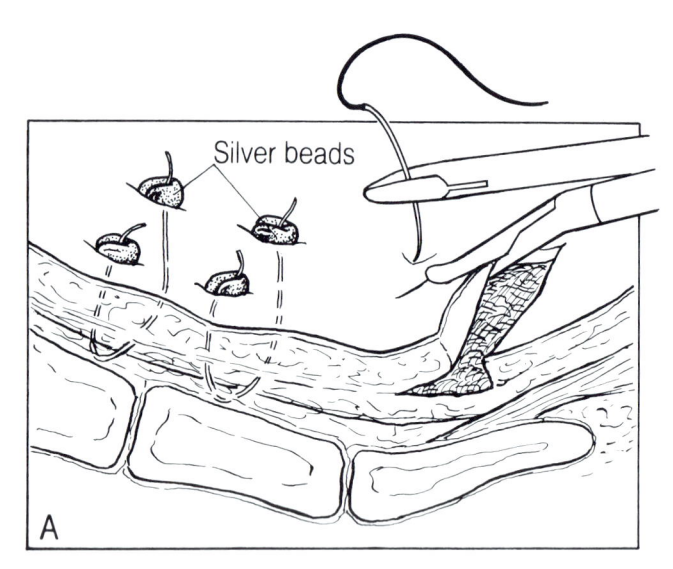

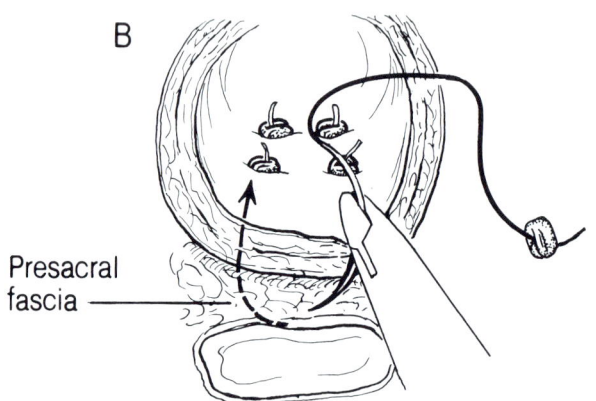

FIGURE 18-4 A. Transanal endoscopic rectopexy commences with a transverse incision in the upper third of the rectum and U-shaped sutures are utilized. B. The sutures pass from the rectum to presacral fascia and back again, where they are secured with silver clips. The rectal defect is then closed.

REFERENCES

1. Kraske P: Zur Exstirpation hochsitzender Mastdarmkrebse. *Verh Dtsch Ges Chir* 1885; 14:464–474.
2. Mason AY: Surgical access to the rectum: A transsphincteric exposure. *Proc R Soc Med* 1970; 63:91–94.
3. Gall FP, Hermanek P: Cancer of the rectum: Local excision. *Surg Clin North Am* 1988; 68:1353–1365.
4. Graham RA, Garnsey L, Milburn Jessup J: Local excision of rectal carcinoma. *Am J Surg* 1990; 160:306–312.
5. Hermanek P, Gall FP: Early (microinvasive) colorectal carcinoma. *Int J Colorectal Dis* 1986; 1:79–84.
6. Buess G, Theiss R, Guenther M, et al: Endoscopic operative procedure for the removal of rectal polyps. *Colo-Proctology* 1984; 5:254–261.
7. Buess G, Kipfmueller K, Hack D, et al: Technique of transanal endoscopic microsurgery. *Surg Endosc* 1988; 2:71–75.
8. Buess G, Kipfmueller K, Ibald R, et al: Clinical results of transanal endoscopic microsurgery. *Surg Endosc* 1988; 2:245–250.
9. Buess G: Mikroskopische endoskopische Tumorchirurgie: Was ist moeglich? *Langenbecks Arch Chir* 1989; Suppl II: 553–559.
10. Buess G: Endoluminal rectal surgery, in Cuscheri A, Buess G, Perissat J (eds): *Operation Manual of Endoscopic Surgery*. New York, Springer Verlag, 1992.
11. Buess G, Kipfmueller K, Ibald R, et al: Transanale endoskopische Mikrochirurgie beim Rektumcarcinom. *Chirurg* 1989; 60:901–904.
12. Buess G, Mentges B, Manncke K, et al: Minimal invasive surgery in the local treatment of rectal cancer. *Int J Colorectal Dis* 1991; 6:77–78.
13. Heintz A, Buess G, Frank K, et al: Endoluminal untrasonic examination of sessile polyps and early carcinomas of rectum. *Surg Endosc* 1989; 3:92–95.
14. Heintz A, Buess G, Frank K, et al: Endoluminal sonography in follow-up of rectal carcinoma. *Surg Endosc* 1989; 3:199–202.
15. Heintz A, Buess G, Junginger T: Endorektale Sonographie zur praeoperativen Beurteilung der Infiltrationstiefe von Rektumtumoren. *Dtsch Med Wochenschr* 1990; 115:1083–1087.
16. Kipfmueller K, Buess G, Narhun M, et al: Training program for transanal endoscopic microsurgery. *Surg Endosc* 1988; 2:24–27.
17. Kipfmueller K, Buess G: Ausbildung zur transanalen endoskopischen Mikrochirurgie. *Akt Chir* 1989; 24:27–31.

Chapter 19

Radiologic Procedures in the Management of Biliary Disease

Franklin J. Miller

Radiologic procedures in the biliary tree were primarily of diagnostic use until the 1970s when biliary obstructive disease was relieved by fluoroscopically guided catheter drainage using only local anesthetics and sedation.[1] A wide variety of percutaneous biliary procedures have been developed since that time and continue to develop. Endoscopic placement of biliary drainage tubes has stolen the limelight from many of the percutaneous techniques. Recently, laparoscopic cholecystectomy has made a much needed major advance in the treatment of gallstones. This chapter will review the current percutaneous radiologic techniques available to manage patients with biliary disorders when other techniques either fail or are unavailable.

STENTING OF BILE DUCT STRICTURES, BENIGN AND MALIGNANT

Most patients with advanced periampullary cancer, whether pancreatic, duodenal, bile duct, or metastatic in origin, undergo attempts at retrograde placement of plastic endoprostheses for palliation.[2,3] These stents usually 10-French in size (Fig. 19-1). and are routinely changed every 3 months to avoid the likelihood of complete occlusion by inspissated bile or tumor.

In some instances, retrograde placement is not possible unless a wire is placed percutaneously through the liver and out the major papilla. Using a combined radiologic and endoscopic procedure, a 600-cm 0.038-in guide wire is placed from a hepatic duct into the duodenum where the endoscopist can snare the wire and pull it out the patient's mouth. A duodenoscope is passed over the wire, and a 10-French plastic stent is passed through the scope, over the wire, and pushed into position in the usual fashion. This technique is cumbersome, however, because additional personnel are utilized, and the patient's position is changed during the examination. When the retrograde approach fails, the transhepatic approach is an alternative to draining the left, right, or both hepatic ducts radiologically.[4–6]

Before hepatic puncture, the prothrombin time must be checked and should be within 2 s of normal. The partial thromboplastin time should be within 10 to 12 s of control and platelet count should be more than 80,000/mm^3.

Using continuous monitoring of oxygen saturation, electrocardiography, blood pressure, fentanyl and midazolam are used for conscious sedation. Morphine sulfate may be substituted for fentanyl because the latter has only a short duration of action.

We have used celiac ganglion blocks in half our patients during the past 2 years for added comfort. The anterior abdominal approach for the block is quick, easy, and safe using the L1 pedicle on the right as a target, pulling back 2 cm from the pedicle, and injecting 30 to 40 mL of 0.5 mL lidocaine with 1:200,000 epinephrine. In addition, we also block three intercostal nerves adjacent to the puncture site with 2% lidocaine. Antibiotics are routinely begun using 2 g of an intravenous cephalosporin before the procedure, and antibiotics are continued for 5 days after the procedure. The antibiotic is adjusted if necessary based on culture results.

The liver is approached either from the right or from the left hepatic duct (the left is marked with ultrasound) with a 21-gauge needle and a 0.018-in guide wire for access (Fig. 19-2). The key to safe access is using a thin needle and wire, staying within the liver substance, and accessing a peripheral duct. Entry with large needles into central ducts is more likely to lead to complications, in-

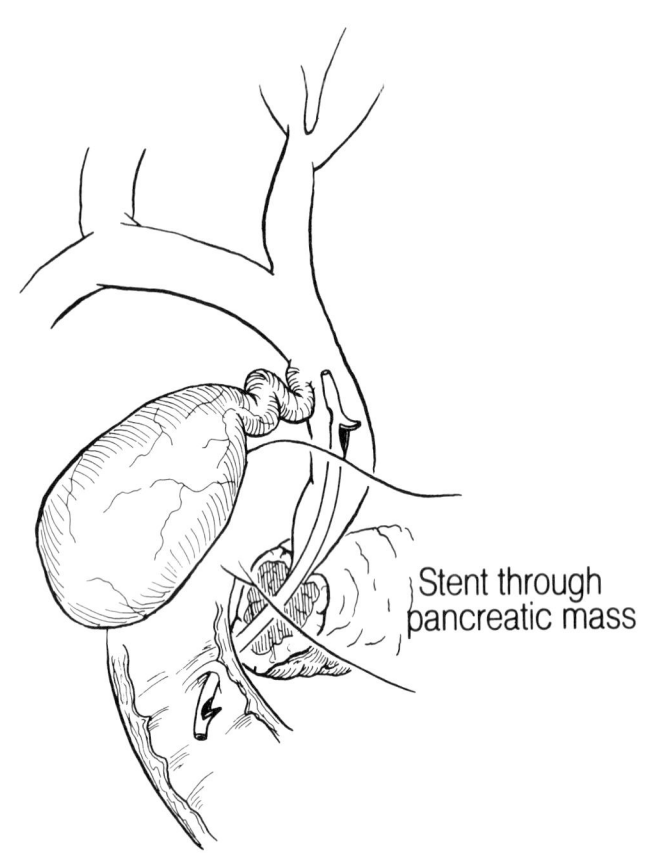

FIGURE 19-1 A 10-French stent endoscopically placed across pancreatic cancer.

cluding pseudoaneurysm with hemorrhage. A small left lobe can be troublesome in advancing catheters and may lead to increased complications, including bleeding.[6] From the right side, access is gained from above the 11th rib to avoid the pleural space, the penetration of which could cause biliary empyema.

After the small wire is within a duct, preferably pointed toward the common hepatic duct, an 0.038-in Coons wire (Cook, Inc) is placed alongside the 0.018-in wire through a special access kit (Accustix, Medi-tech; Neff Kit, Cook, Inc.). The 0.038-in wire then allows placement of a 6-French directable catheter to help steer through benign and malignant strictures. If the wire can be placed into the duodenum at the first sitting (90 percent of cases), an 8- or 10-French soft drainage catheter is placed for external–internal drainage (Fig. 19-3). In those cases where initial efforts fail to cross the obstruction, a second attempt after 1 to 2 days of external drainage will usually be successful. On rare occasions (less than one percent) we will be unable to cross the lesion because a completely transected duct is present after iatrogenic injury. Bile specimens are sent for cultures and Gram staining routinely.

All patients undergo external drainage until bilirubin levels are noted to be falling and cholangitis is under control. The catheters are irrigated with 10-mL of saline each shift initially, and the family is instructed in the technique, which is carried out daily at home.

Although patients with cancer and plastic catheters require tube changes every 3 months and episodes of cholangitis require antibiotic treatment, most patients are content with plastic internal or external tubes, and few require metal stents. Although metal stents are more convenient for the patient (and physician), when occlusion occurs, removal is not possible, and recanalization is, at best, a lengthy and difficult procedure. The art is to know which patient will die of their disease before the metal stunt occludes.

Metal stents for biliary cancer are available and certainly play a role in treating some patients with obstructive jaundice.[7,8] The stents include those manufactured by Johnson & Johnson (Palmaz, Fig. 19-4A), Pfizer (Wallstent, Fig. 19-4B), and Cook (Gianturco, Fig. 19-4C). Tumor ingrowth can be a problem with all of them but especially with the Gianturco (Cook) because the struts are widely spaced. The wide spaces in the Gianturco stent are an advantage, however, for treating benign disease.

To place a metal stent, access is gained as described previously. With the wire into the duodenum an 11.0- or 9.0-French sheath is first placed across the obstruction before inserting the Gianturco or Palmaz stent, respectively. At least two stents should always be used because a single stent (3.0 cm) alone is not long enough to ensure complete stricture stenting.

The Wallstent is preferred by us because of the smaller sheath required (7 French), its flexibility, and the availability of two lengths, 68 and 42 mm. The Wallstent is self-expanding to 10 mm. The other two stents require balloon expansion.

An external safety catheter is left for 1 to 2 days to ensure that the metal stent is functioning properly. Antibiotics are recommended for 5 days or until evidence of clinical infection has cleared. No maintenance is needed as with external plastic stents, but recanalization of an occluded metal stent is difficult. Recently, argon laser probes have been used to open stents.[9] Usually, an external plastic stent is placed when occlusion occurs. The metal stent cannot be removed easily even with surgical techniques. A second stent may be placed through the first stent if dislodgement occurs (Fig. 19-5).

Although metal stents are a technical advance, the ideal stent should remain patent for many years, at least as long as the remaining years of the patient's life. This stent does not exist currently.

Malignant Strictures

Cholangiocarcinoma is the most common primary malignancy of the bile ducts. It has been associated with sclerosing cholangitis, ulcerative colitis, liver fluke disease, gall-

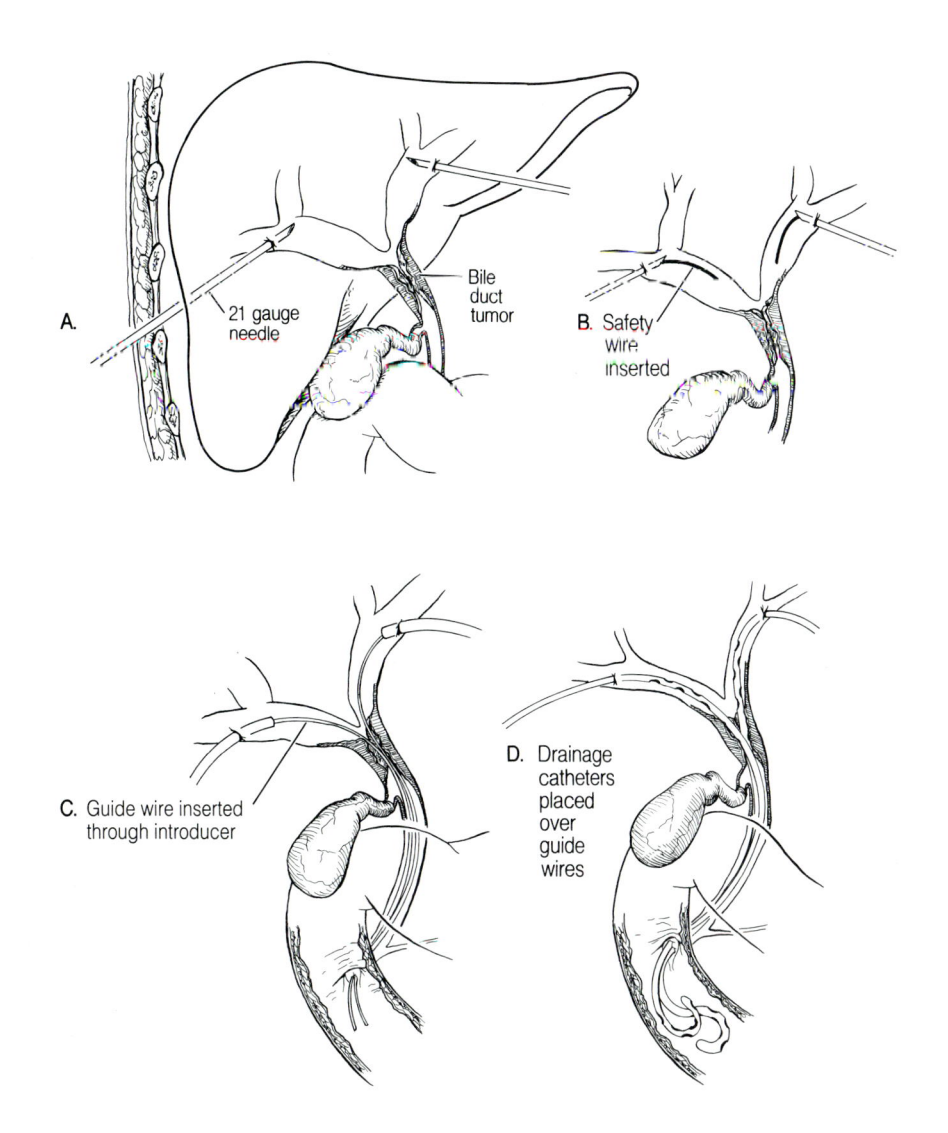

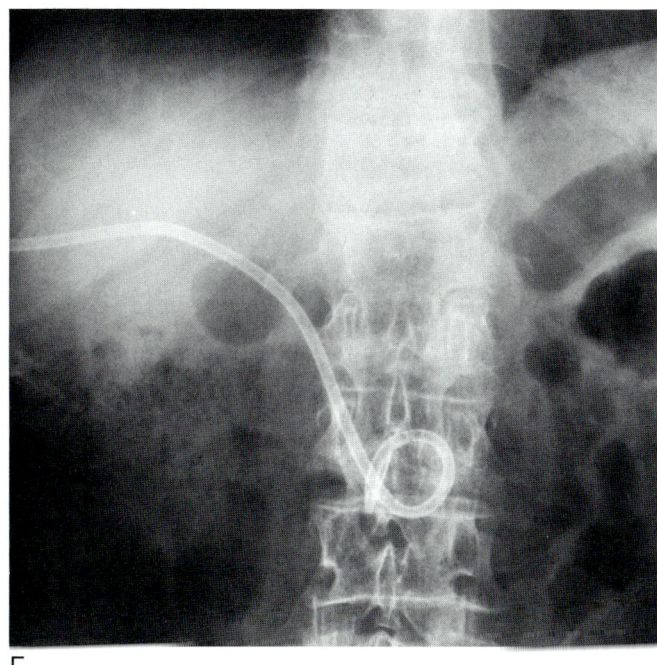

FIGURE 19-2 A. The thin-needle approach into the liver parenchyma to engage the appropriate duct. B. A small wire is passed to gain access to the duct. C. A plastic catheter is passed over the small guide wires and a heavier gauge guide wire is passed through the obstruction. D. Left and right bile duct tubes for external–internal drainage are placed over the guide wire. E. The radiograph of an external–internal catheter.

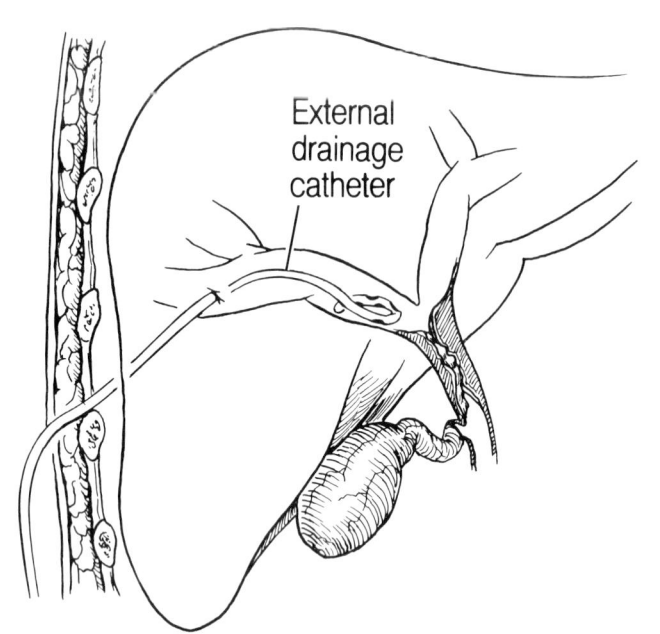

FIGURE 19-3 Diagram of external drainage used when access to the duodenum not possible on the initial procedure.

stones, and choledochal cysts. These lesions arise in the larger bile ducts, occurring in the proximal extrahepatic ducts in approximately 50 percent of cases.

Most commonly, cholangiocarcinoma is an infiltrating sclerotic mass. Less commonly, these tumors present either a bulky exophytic mass or a polypoid intramural tumor, for example, papillary cholangiocarcinoma.

Surgical resection remains the best method to achieve cure for this disease. Unfortunately, most patients we see have sclerosing tumors at the bifurcation of the common hepatic duct (Klatskin tumors), making resection difficult.

Our approach to these patients has been transhepatic biliary drainage of both the left and right ducts if an endoscopic approach fails. We prefer the transhepatic approach because we use Iridium-192 seeds for palliative therapy in addition to external beam irradiation.[10] Working with short percutaneous tubes and radioactive Iridium-192 seeds is technically easier than through long nasobiliary tubes. For suspected Klatskin tumors, we usually drain both lobes at the same time if feasible and maintain antibiotic coverage for 5 days based on the culture and sensitivity reports.

Confirming a bile duct tumor is accomplished by placing a Portney-Kolpe catheter system (Cook, Inc.) into the ducts for brushing and biopsy. Recently, we have used a 3-French biopsy forceps (Cook Urologic) via the Portney-Kolpe catheter. Biopsy sites are selected on the basis of their radiologic appearance after 2 to 3 days of drainage to avoid areas where bile sludge may give the appearance of tumor. More recently, we have also used small, 8- and 10.5-French

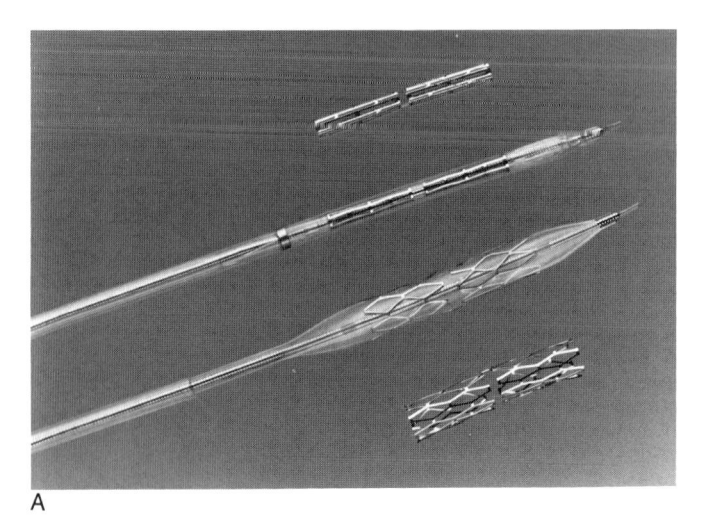

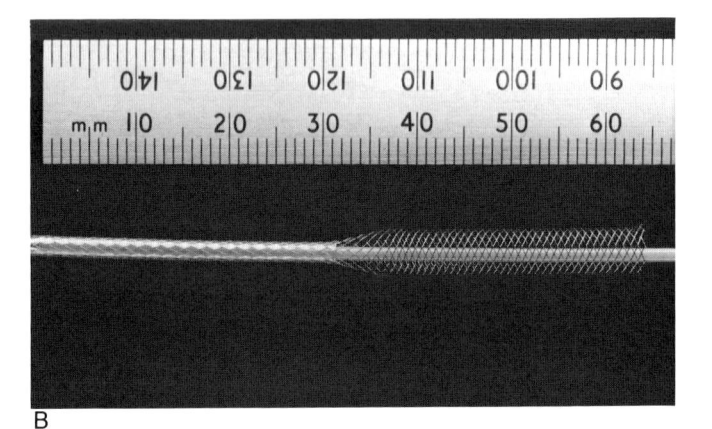

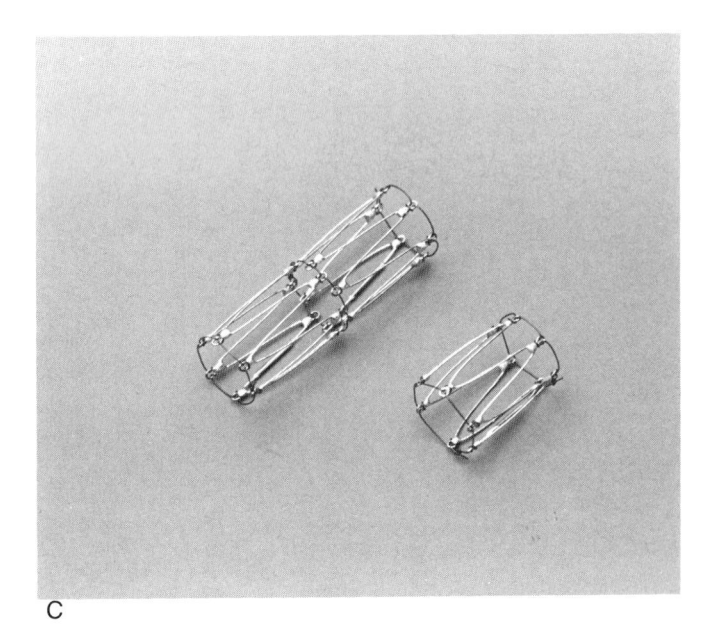

FIGURE 19-4 A. The Palmaz stent shown in the nonexpanded and expanded states. B. Wallstent. C. Gianturco stent.

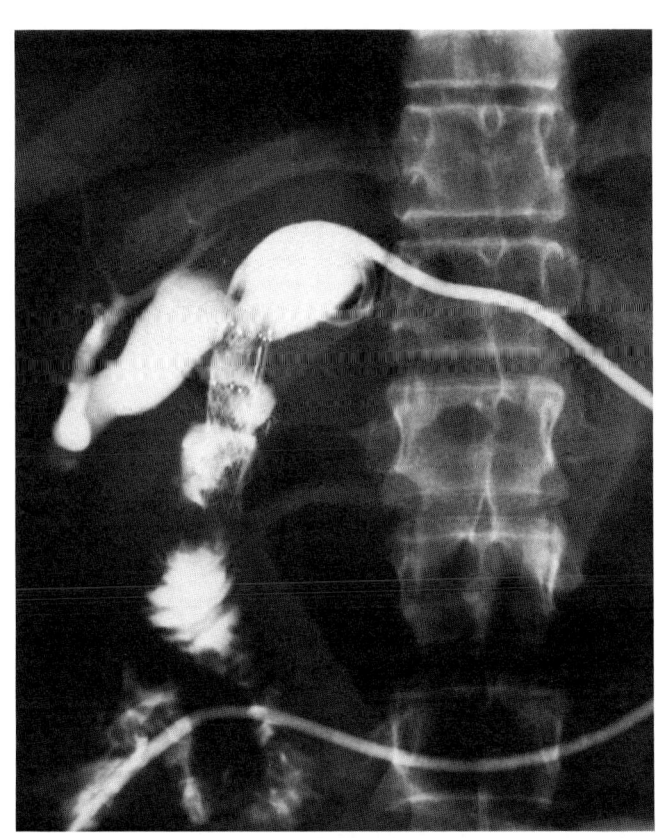

FIGURE 19-5 Benign stricture secondary to Caroli's disease. The first stent (Gianturco) became dislodged into the Caroli sac and a second stent (Palmaz) was then placed inside the first one. Then both were repositioned through the stricture.

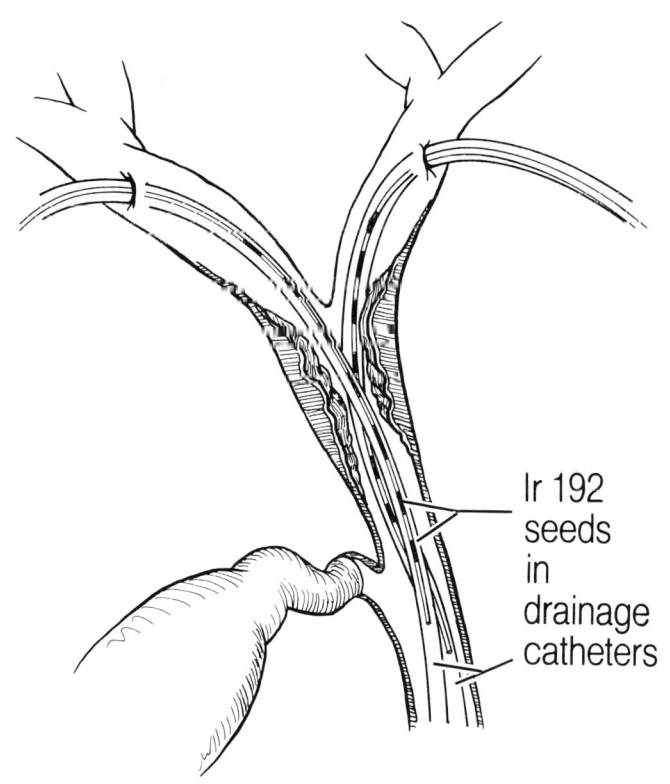

FIGURE 19-6 Placement of Iridium-192 seeds through the left and right bile ducts for additional radiation. External radiation therapy is also given usually for a total of 7000 to 8000 Gy.

flexible ureteroscopes to enter the percutaneous tract, and a biopsy of the tumor is done under direct visualization. If all these methods fail (20 to 25 percent will yield no diagnosis), we then will use a Simpson 8-French atherectomy catheter (Peripheral Vascular Systems) (see Chap. 31), which can yield material for hematoxylin and eosin sectioning. The anatomy is sometimes not favorable for biopsy with the Simpson device because the cutting chamber is rigid and could result in a through-and-through biopsy of the duct, especially if attempting biopsy on the curved portion of a duct. Obviously, in instances where we see this potential risk, the biopsy with this instrument is abandoned. Open biopsy is occasionally required for diagnosis. Regardless of the biopsy technique used, bile for cytologic examination is collected during the 8-h nursing shift after tube insertion or biopsy.

The bile drainage catheters are prepared for Iridium-192 seed placement by placing two 6-French catheters (0.038-in wire size) into the duodenum (Fig. 19-6). These catheters are irrigated daily and left for external drainage for the first week after placement. Cholangitis after placement is common during the first week. The radiotherapy team places the Iridium-192 seeds across the tumor using fluoroscopy and cholangiography for selection of final seed placement.

The drainage catheters are plastic and allow easy irrigation and routine changes every 3 to 4 months on an outpatient basis. Elective tube removal is occasionally possible 4 to 6 months after radiotherapy, provided no stricture remains.

The increasing use of metal stents and internal plastic stents is often based on patient refusal to wear an external catheter. Although much has been written about external tubes that the patient sees and feels, we rarely treat a patient who insists on external–internal tube replacement with a metal or plastic internal stent. In our experience with cancer patients, replacing an occluded external plastic tube is an easy outpatient procedure in comparison to redraining a patient or attempting recanalization of an occluded metal stent. Replacing endoscopic plastic stents is also an outpatient procedure and readily accomplished.

Carcinoma of the head of the pancreas continues to be a disease with a poor prognosis. Transhepatic biliary drainage is a reasonable alternative to surgical drainage,[6,11] but both procedures have been supplanted with endoscopic placement of plastic stents. More recently, metal stents for palliation are used in some of these patients.[12] Although surgery continues to be used to place a Roux-en-Y loop in selected cases, many can be treated with stenting unless gastric or duodenal obstruction occurs.

Those patients with gastric outlet obstruction usually require surgical bypass of both the bile duct and the stomach or duodenum. We have managed a few frail patients with endoscopic biliary stents and feeding jejunostomy tubes placed percutaneously. This latter nonsurgical approach is acceptable to some patients with the diagnosis of widespread carcinoma of the pancreas and a limited life expectancy.

For pain control, a celiac plexus block with chemolysis can also be performed. It is usually done from the posterior oblique approach by an anesthesiologist.

Benign Strictures

The benign bile duct strictures we treat currently are usually iatrogenic, frequently at a biliary–enteric anastomoses. Occasionally, they may result from inflammation, from common bile duct stones, and sclerosing cholangitis.

The preferred therapy for postoperative benign strictures is surgical reconstruction when feasible. However, in the elderly patient and in those in whom the stricture is high in the common hepatic duct, repeated surgical procedures have increased morbidity and mortality. In these patients, less invasive procedures are appropriate.[13] In sclerosing cholangitis, balloon dilatation and stenting will slow the development of biliary cirrhosis.[14–16] In some patients, palliation with balloons and stents may delay liver transplantation for several years. The technique of percutaneous biliary dilatation is as follows.

Access to the stricture may be through a previous T-tube tract or through a percutaneous approach. Using fluoroscopy, an 0.035-in guide wire is placed across the stricture. Although the number of dilatations, duration of balloon inflations, and the use of long-term stenting after the dilatation remain controversial, agreement on using high-pressure balloon dilators is accepted (Fig. 19-7). We dilate each stricture for 4 to 5 min and perform long-term (6 to 12 months) stenting with 12 to 14-French plastic stents. Metal stents are also being used currently, and small series have been published.[17] We have used the Gianturco stent for benign strictures. When stents are used, we prefer this latter type because the space between struts is wide, unlike the other two available stents, and they are less likely to occlude with sludge.[18,19] The stent is placed via an 11.0-French sheath, and a minimum of two stents are always used (a single stent is too short and tends to slip through the stricture).

Our concern over using a metal stent for benign disease is management after occlusion occurs. Simple removal is not possible, and recanalization is cumbersome and not always successful even with the use of argon laser probes. We empirically order ursodeoxycholic acid therapy for patients with benign strictures and metal stents to help decrease stone formation from cholesterol deposits.

An external–internal plastic stent is used when attempts at opening occluded metal stents for benign stricture are unsuccessful. If liver failure intervenes, liver transplantation is an option for some patients.

Another method to permit access to a choledochojejunostomy anastomotic stricture for repeated balloon dilatation is through the efferent jejunal limb where it has been sutured to the abdominal wall and peritoneum and marked with surgical staples, making percutaneous access feasible. Although this method has been available since the mid-1980s,[20] this surgical modification has not been widely used. Until long-term patency for metal stents is documented, most choledochojejunostomy procedures for benign strictures should have this added feature for easy percutaneous access (Fig. 19-8). In these instances, access and simple balloon dilatation may be accomplished in an outpatient setting, and dilatation may be repeated as needed without the concern of metal stents occluding. We could also apply this technique to malignant disease, allowing easy access, if desired, when tumor has invaded the anastomosis. The disadvantage to this procedure is scarring which will make transplantation more difficult.

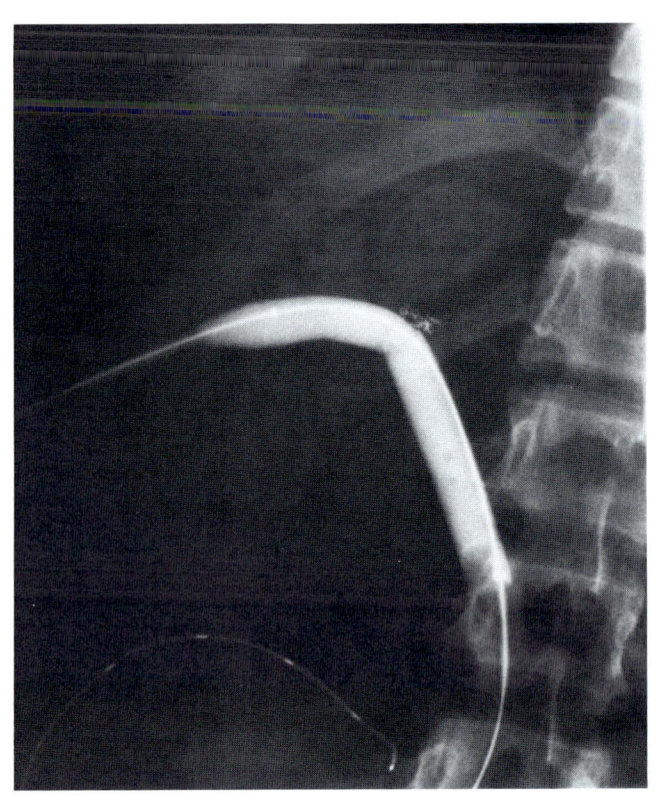

FIGURE 19-7 Transhepatic balloon dilatation of a choledochojejunostomy stricture (Caroli's disease).

BILE DUCT STONES

The diagnosis of common duct or intrahepatic duct stones is suspected by the patient's history and abnormal liver

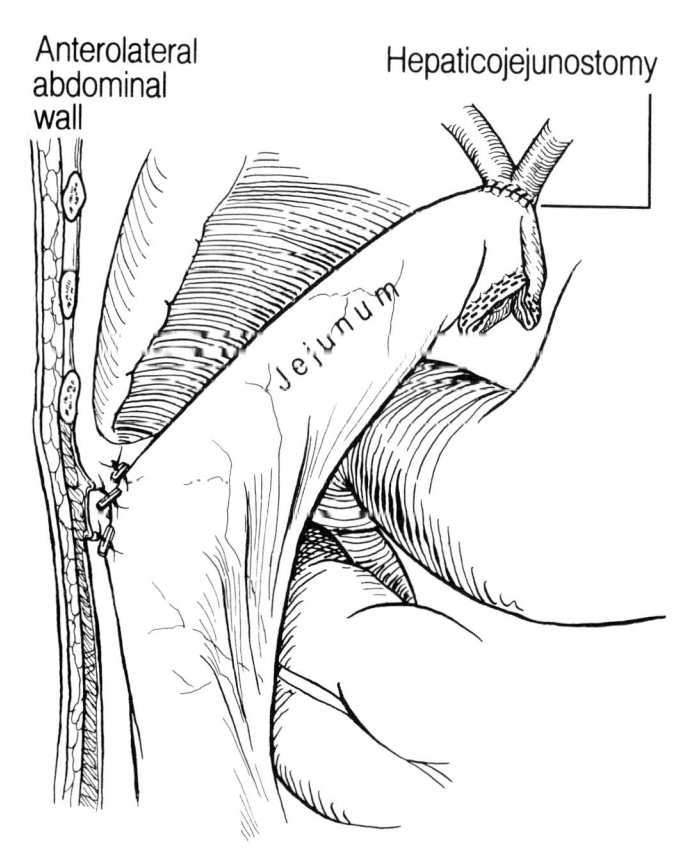

FIGURE 19-8 After hepaticojejunostomy, the Roux limb is sutured (and clipped for x-ray identification) to the lateral abdominal wall, allowing easy percutaneous access to the anastomosis.

function tests. The diagnosis is usually confirmed by endoscopic retrograde cholangiopancreatography and occasionally by thin-needle percutaneous cholangiography. Stone removal is by one of several methods, but endoscopic sphincterotomy is the accepted and usual method. Open surgical or even laparoscopic techniques using general anesthesia are rarely needed to remove bile duct calculi.

For stones up to 3 cm in diameter, endoscopic sphincterotomy is usually successful at removing bile duct stones. When stones are multiple, large, or above a stricture, supplementary techniques such as pulsed-dye laser[21] and electrohydraulic lithotripsy (EHL)[22] may be used to fragment the stone. However, recent basket technology allows the operator either to crush the stone confidently or remove the basket without fear of trapping the instruments within the duct.

ESWL is not widely available in the United States because it is not approved by the Food and Drug Administration. Europeans have successfully used extracorporeal shock wave lithotripsy (ESWL) in more than 400 patients to fragment retained common duct stones. An endoscopic sphincterotomy is performed, and a nasobiliary tube is placed in advance of the ESWL procedure. With fluoroscopic imaging, contrast is injected around the stone for easy shock wave targeting. Calcified and noncalcified stones have been removed using these techniques.[23–25]

For bile duct or intrahepatic stones, percutaneous transhepatic access can be established with a skinny needle and graded dilation if a T-tube tract is unavailable. Small 8- to 10.5-French endoscopes with 1-mm working channels are available to remove calculi. The 11-French sheaths are needed to guide the 10.5-French endoscope. Stones are usually larger than the sheath and can be fragmented with EHL probes.[22] Endoscopy is necessary when using EHL, and the probe must be placed 1 mm from the stone. Failure to visualize the target clearly will result in bile duct injury. Although the pulsed-dye laser is not traumatic to the ducts, the cost is nearly 25 times greater than that of the EHL unit, which is approximately $10,000.

SYMPTOMATIC GALLSTONES: PERCUTANEOUS MANAGEMENT BY ROTATIONAL CONTACT LITHOTRIPSY

This section describes rotational contact lithotripsy in the management of symptomatic gallstones in patients who are not candidates for laparoscopic cholecystectomy or open removal of the gallbladder. The rotational contact lithotripsy device (Kensey-Nash Lithotrite) has undergone animal testing and completed a Phase I human study.[26,27] Other techniques to remove gallstones include pulsed-dye laser, EHL, and methyl-tert-butyl ether injection. Any technique that removes only gallbladder stones plays a minor role currently because of laparoscopic cholecystectomy.

The major advantage of the Lithotrite over other mechanical systems lies in the fact that no targeting is required by the operator. Hospitalization is currently needed for 1 to 2 nights with all fragmenting or dissolution techniques. The Lithotrite device has a stationary six-prong protective cage (Fig. 19-9), which prevents the gallbladder wall from being pulled against the impeller when a vortex is formed. Impeller speeds are up to 30,000 RPM. Animal studies (swine) have revealed excellent fragmentation of surgically implanted human stones with impeller times ranging from 5 to 30 min.[26] Mucosal edema and hemorrhage do result from impact of stone fragments on the wall, but in swine experiments, considerable repair is seen at 5 weeks. At the 3-month follow-up, the mucosa and submucosa show near-normal findings. Our patients have a normal oral cholecystogram at 4 to 6 weeks after the procedure, if the preprocedure study was showed normal gallbladder function.

The patient is informed that the procedure is being used to remove the gallstones and that, since the gallbladder is left in place, 50 percent of patients can expect stones to reform within 5 years.[28]

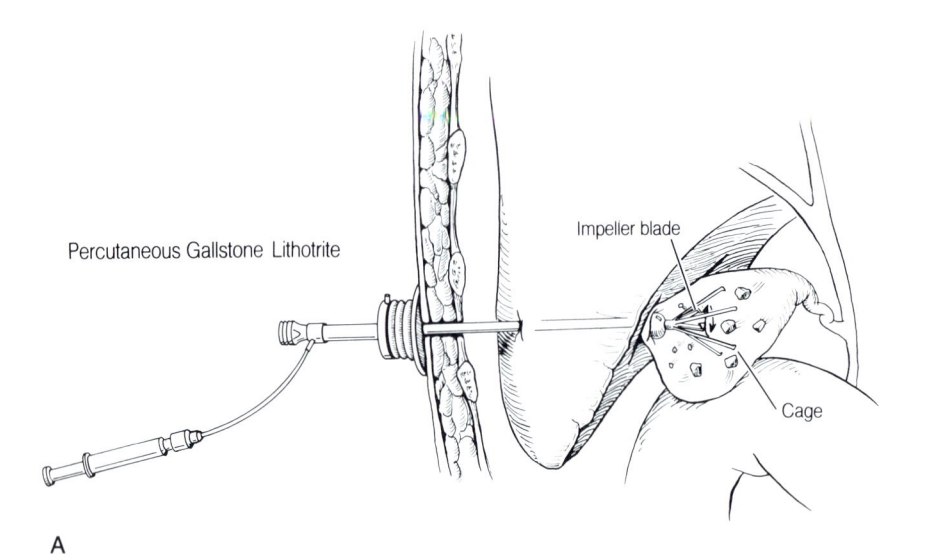

FIGURE 19-9 A. The percutaneous gallstone lithotrite is placed transhepatically and the protective cage opened in the gallbladder to expose the metal impeller. B. The Lithotrite within a patient's gallbladder; the stones were fragmented in less than 2 min.

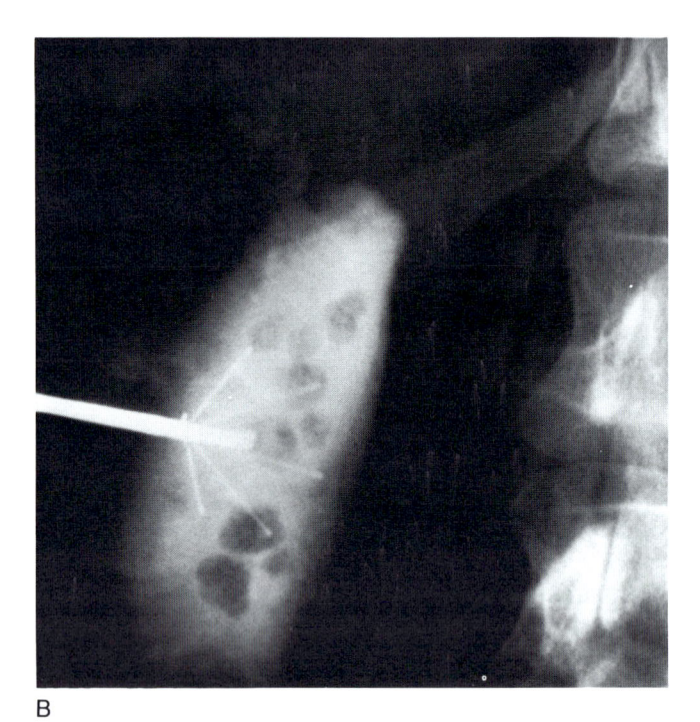

Procedure for Rotational Fragmentation

The patient is placed supine on a radiographic–fluoroscopic table that is then tilted to a 20° to 30° reverse Trendelenburg position, allowing calculi to congregate in the fundus and body instead of the neck of the gallbladder. For anesthesia, we have used epidural blocks in some patients; in others, fentanyl and midazolam are sufficient. We have also performed intercoastal nerve blocks in combination with fentanyl and midazolam and find higher patient acceptance using this latter regimen. Ultrasound guidance with fluoroscopy is the most convenient and expeditious guidance system to puncture the gallbladder and monitor fragmentation. If the patient is obese and preprocedural ultrasound imaging seems less than optimal, CT guidance can be used to target the gallbladder. With the table elevated to 20° to 30°, the puncture is made with a 21-gauge needle, and a 0.038-in Coons or Amplatz wire is advanced and partly coiled within the gallbladder. With the wire coiled inside the gallbladder, the tract is dilated with 8- and 10-French dilators. An 11-French tear-away sheath is then placed over the 0.038-in wire into the gallbladder. A Tuohy-Borst adaptor is attached, and contrast confirms the tip position. Forty-three percent contrast medium is injected to allow slight opacification of the gallbladder. Stones floating toward the neck on injection of contrast medium can be seen, and calculi can transiently enter the cystic duct, resulting in failure of the vortex to pull them into the impeller. Thus, we use the partly upright position and dilute contrast medium to keep stones in the fundus and body of the gallbladder.

The Lithotrite is placed through the 11-French sheath. Constant fluoroscopic imaging of the tip of the sheath must be performed while advancing the impeller shaft.

With the gallbladder distended and opacified, the six prongs are opened by manipulating the proximal end of the impeller shaft. Once open, adequate clearance between the prongs and impeller blade will allow rotation of the blade. Before starting the rotation at 5000 rpm, the shaft is turned manually by one quarter to one half turn clockwise and counterclockwise to ensure that no prongs are engaged in the wall, thereby causing torque on the gallbladder. If torque on the gallbladder wall is detected, slightly inflating the gallbladder with saline is usually sufficient to allow the prongs to become free.

With these safety checks and table tilt at 20° to 30°, over a period of 3 to 5 min, the electrical drive used to power the system is adjusted to bring impeller speeds up to 30,000 rpm. The vortex will automatically pull the stones into the basket and fragment them. The impact of stone material can be palpated while holding the shaft. Rotation of the impeller ranges from 20 to 60 min.

When no visible fragments are seen under fluoroscopy and the impact on the shaft disappears, completion of the procedure is near. The unit is now operated at 30,000 rpm empirically for another 2 min. With completion of rotation, the cage is collapsed and the shaft removed, leaving the sheath in place. A 12-French pigtail catheter is placed in the gallbladder, and all fragmented material is aspirated.

Irrigation with saline is then performed with 40 to 50-mL aliquots four to five times to loosen debris on the wall. A bile bag is attached to the catheter for dependent drainage. We use 10 mL of saline to irrigate the gallbladder during each nursing shift. The drainage catheter is left in place and attached to the leg for another 5 to 6 days to allow a tract to form.

The patients are returned to the ward, and they receive intravenous fluids. Vital signs are taken frequently for 12 h. The patient has nothing by mouth until the following morning, when clear liquids are allowed. If tolerated, a soft low-fat diet is ordered by the evening meal. We find the patients are not ready to eat a regular diet until the second postprocedural day. Patients are discharged by 48 h with the drainage catheter in place.

Because fine debris (usually under 500 μm) can adhere to the gallbladder wall, the patient is instructed to irrigate the catheter with saline twice daily and keep the extension tubing attached to the bile bag. Forty-eight hours before returning to the clinic for removal of the catheter, the patient is instructed to close the stopcock to test the patency of the cystic and extrahepatic ducts.

On follow-up at 7 to 10 days, if ultrasound examination and fluoroscopic spot films are normal, the catheter is removed. The tract is closed with an absorbable gelatin plug to prevent bile leak.

In the United States and Europe, 50 patients have undergone the Lithotrite procedure without mortality. In three centers in the United States, 24 patients have been followed for 5 to 24 months. Ten of 24 are free of stones or debris, 5 have residual debris under 3 mm, and 1 has a 6-mm residual fragment. Eight patients underwent cholecystectomy for various reasons. Two had retained stones, one of which turned out to be a cystic duct carcinoma and in another patient, cholecystectomy was necessary to remove a stone trapped in a phrygian cap.

Three patients had complications resulting in cholecystectomy. One developed an empyema of the gallbladder when the drainage tube dislodged on day 1. A second patient developed a fibrotic mass at the puncture site, and one other developed acute cholecystitis.

A sixth patient had an incidental cholecystectomy (no calculi found) at the time of a gastric stapling procedure 1 year later. Two other patients continued to leak bile after tube removal and underwent cholecystectomy. The latter complication is preventable by closing the tract with a plug of surgical absorbable gelatin.

Two limitations of this technique are that a large burden of stones exceeding 75 percent of gallbladder volume cannot be fragmented (no space for device), and no stone can be larger than 25 mm.

Percutaneous rotational lithotripsy is a reasonable successful nonoperative method to manage symptomatic cholelithiasis. It is indicated for patients who have a prohibitive risk for general anesthesia. Removal of the gallbladder by laparoscopic techniques will continue to be the therapy of choice for cholelithiasis in the vast majority of patients.

ABLATION OF THE GALLBLADDER AND CYSTIC DUCT

Although laparoscopic cholecystectomy has taken the forefront in the treatment of cholelithiasis, the description of another technique using only local anesthetics to remove (ablate) the gallbladder is described here.

Since 1984, Becker and associates[29,30] have developed a three-step procedure to ablate the gallbladder. The technique first requires occlusion of the cystic duct by applying a bipolar coagulation device through a cholecystostomy tube.

Occlusion of the cystic duct is performed by passing a hydrophilic guide wire through the cystic duct and placing a bipolar electrode into the cystic duct. Then 400 W of power is used over a 2-s application. The catheter is pulled back toward the gallbladder after each discharge to apply a current of injury along the entire cystic duct.

A waiting period of 2 weeks is necessary to allow adequate fibrosis to occlude the cystic duct before gallbladder sclerosis is attempted. Ethyl alcohol (95%) and 3% sodium tetradecyl sulfate (STS) are used clinically for vascular sclerosis and have been proved to be safe in humans. The gallbladder is filled with 95% alcohol and 3% STS and left in place for 20 min. Two additional aliquots of alcohol have been used in our laboratory in animals.

In seven of eight animals in Becker's[30] studies, effective ablation resulted. In our animals, 6 of 10 had the gallbladder replaced by fibrosis with 4 of 10 having a small (1 to 2 mL) mucucoele at 6 weeks with residual cells seen at histologic examination.

In the Becker[31] series, eight patients have been treated with the technique and followed with ultrasound, revealing decreasing gallbladder size but small residual lumina. In one patient whose therapy was attempted by us, the cystic duct was too patulous for effective sclerosis by 7-French bipolar, probes and the sclerosis procedure could not be completed.

Although a procedure to remove the gallbladder with local anesthetics would be noteworthy, current sclerosis methods are cumbersome and lengthy. It remains a three-step procedure and requires an indwelling cholecystostomy tube for 6 to 8 weeks, making the technique justifiable in only a few selected high-risk elderly patients. A one-step sclerosing procedure using a local anesthetic continues to be elusive with current agents.

REFERENCES

1. Molnar W, Stockum AE: Relief of obstructive jaundice through percutaneous transhepatic catheter—a new therapeutic method. *Am J Roentgenol* 1974; 122:356.
2. Huibregtse K, Kanton RM, Coene PP, et al: Endoscopic palliative treatment in pancreatic cancer. *Gastrointest Endosc* 1986; 32:334.
3. Marks WM, Feeny PC, Ball TJ, et al: Endoscopic retrograde biliary drainage. *Radiology* 1984; 152:357.
4. Dooley JS, Dick R, George P, et al: Percutaneous transhepatic endoprosthesis for bile duct obstruction: Complications and results. *Gastroenterology* 1984; 86:905.
5. Lammer J, Neumayer K: Biliary drainage endoprostheses: Experience with 201 placements. *Radiology* 1986; 159:625.
6. Gunther RW, Schild H, Thelen M: Percutaneous transhepatic biliary drainage: Experience with 311 procedures. *Cardiovasc Intervent Radiol* 1988; 11:65–71.
7. Klein GE, Lammer J: Primary implantation of expandable Wallstent endoprostheses for relief of obstructive jaundice. *Radiology* 1989; 173P:378.
8. Gillams A, Dick R, Dooley JS, et al: Self-expandable stainless steel braided endoprosthesis for biliary strictures. *Radiology* 1990; 174:137–140.
9. Lossef SV, Druy E, Jelinger E, et al: Use of Hot-Tip laser probes to recanalize occluded expandable metallic biliary endoprostheses. *Am J Roentgenol* 1992; 158:199–201.
10. Hayes JK, Sapozink MD, Miller FJ: Definitive radiation therapy and bile duct cancer. *Int J Radiat Oncol Biol Phys* 1988; 15:735–744.
11. Coons HG, Carey PH: Large-bore, long biliary endoprostheses (biliary stents) for improved drainage. *Radiology* 1983; 148:89.
12. Lameris JS, Stoker J, Nijs HGT, et al: Percutaneous use of self-expandable stents in patients with malignant biliary obstruction. *Radiology* 1991; 179:703–707.
13. Zuidema GD, Cameron JL, Sitzmann JV, et al: Percutaneous transhepatic management of complex biliary problems. *Ann Surg* 1983; 197:584–593.
14. Trambert JJ, Bron KM, Zajiko AB, et al: Percutaneous transhepatic balloon dilatation of benign biliary strictures. *Am J Roentgenol* 1987; 149:945–948.
15. Williams HJ, Bender CE, May GR: Benign postoperative biliary strictures: Dilatation with fluoroscopic guidance. *Radiology* 1987; 163.629–634.
16. Mueller PR, vanSonnenberg E, Ferrucci JT, et al: Biliary stricture dilatation. Multicenter review of clinical management in 73 patients. *Radiology* 1986; 160:17–22.
17. Rossi P, Bezzi M, Salvatori FM, et al: Recurrent benign biliary strictures: Management with self-expanding metallic stents. *Radiology* 1990; 175:661–665.
18. Carrasco CH, Wallace S, Charnsangavej C, et al: Expandable biliary endoprosthesis: An experimental study. *Am J Roentgenol* 1985; 145:1279.
19. Irving JD, Adam A, Dick R, et al: Gianturco expandable metallic biliary stents: Results of a European clinical trial. *Radiology* 1989; 172:321.
20. Russell E, Yrizarry JM, Huber JS, et al: Percutaneous transjejunal biliary dilatation: Alternate management for benign strictures. *Radiology* 1986; 159:209–214.
21. Nishioka NS, Levins PC, Murray SC, et al: Fragmentation of biliary calculi with tunable dye lasers. *Gastroenterology* 1987; 93:250–255.
22. Picus D, Weyman PH, Marx MV: The role of percutaneous intracorporeal electrohydraulic lithotripsy in the treatment of biliary tract calculi. *Radiology* 1989; 170:989–993.
23. Ponchon T, Martin X, Barkun A, et al: Extracorporeal lithotripsy of bile duct stones using ultrasonography for stone localization. *Gastroenterology* 1990; 98:726–732.
24. Sauerbruch T, Stern M, the Study Group for Shock-Wave Lithotripsy of Bile Duct Stones: Fragmentation of bile duct stones by extracorporeal shock waves. A new approach to biliary calculi after failure of routine endoscopic measures. *Gastroenterology* 1989; 96:146–152.
25. Schneider MU, Mattek W, Bauer R, et al: Mechanical lithotripsy of bile duct stones in 209 patients. Effect of technical advances. *Encoscopy* 1988; 20:248–253.
26. Miller FJ, Kensey K, Nash J: Experimental percutaneous gallstone lithotripsy: Results in swine. *Radiology* 1989; 170:985–987.
27. Miller FJ, Rose SC, Buchi KN, et al: Percutaneous rotational contact biliary lithotripsy: Initial clinical results with the Kensey Nash Lithotrite. *Radiology* 1991; 178:781–785.
28. Villanova N, Bazzoli, F, Frabboni R: Gallstone recurrence after successful oral bile acid treatment: A follow-up study and evaluation of post-dissolution treatment. *Gastroenterology* 1987; 92:1789.
29. Becker CD, Quenville NF, Burhenne HJ: Long-term occlusion of the porcine cystic duct by means of endoluminal radiofrequency electrocoagulation. *Radiology* 1988; 167:63.
30. Becker CD, Quenville NF, Burhenne HJ: Gallbladder ablation through radiologic intervention: An experimental alternative to cholecystectomy. *Radiology* 1989; 171:235.
31. Becker CD, Fache JS, Malone DE, et al: Ablation of the cystic duct and gallbladder: Clinical observations. *Radiology* 1990; 176:687.

Chapter 20

Endoluminal Treatment of Tumors and Stones in the Bile Ducts

Jeffrey L. Ponsky

Flexible fiberoptic endoscopy evolved in the 1960s and soon allowed excellent visualization of the upper and lower gastrointestinal tract. Routine cannulation of the ampulla of Vater, allowing contrast imaging of the pancreatic and bile ducts, became possible with the development of the side-viewing duodenoscope.[1] It was only after the description of electrosurgical section of the ampullary sphincter, however, that the era of therapeutic pancreaticobiliary endoscopy began.[2]

Maladies afflicting the bile ducts frequently present with jaundice and may be accompanied by pain, fever, weight loss, or sepsis. Long-standing ductal obstruction may produce biliary cirrhosis. A careful history and physical examination will give clues to the cause of the problem and suggest the required intervention.

The prerequisite to consideration of any biliary therapy is a thorough laboratory evaluation and radiologic imaging of the pancreas and biliary tree. Ultrasound and CT are valuable in assessing the liver and its ductal system. Although only one of these modalities may be needed, each provides slightly different information, and the use of both is often beneficial. Ultrasound clearly demonstrates the substance of the liver, the bile ducts, and the gallbladder. It may fail to image the pancreas because of the presence of intestinal gas. CT provides a more detailed look at the substance of the pancreas and is also useful in demonstrating the liver and bile ducts. It is somewhat less illustrative than ultrasonography in demonstrating the details of ductal size and architecture. Although these examinations provide information regarding ductal size and the presence of mass lesions, they fail to yield outlines of the system detailed enough to provide a "road map" for surgery and offer no therapeutic dimension. Diagnostic endoscopic retrograde cholangiopancreatography (ERCP) and percutaneous transhepatic cholangiography permit direct opacification of the biliary tree and offer a window for minimally invasive therapy. Various articles have been written arguing the value of each of these methods over the other.[3,4] In practice, both are extremely valuable and optimum effectiveness is achieved when they are used selectively and, occasionally, in concert.

ENDOSCOPIC THERAPY FOR BILE DUCT TUMORS

Tumors afflicting the biliary system may be native to the ductal system, as in cholangiocarcinoma, or the result of invasion or compression by neoplasia in adjacent tissue. The latter circumstance is most common, with extrinsic compression of the ductal system caused by pancreatic carcinoma, portal node metastases from visceral cancers, and hepatic tumor deposits. Patients most often present with clinical jaundice, and biliary dilation is confirmed by ultrasound or CT examination. A diagnostic cholangiogram should be obtained before any interventional therapy is employed. Cholangiography can be performed by the percutaneous or endoscopic routes, each offering particular advantages. The percutaneous approach may be particularly valuable when obstruction is believed to be high in the biliary tree. The endoscopic approach offers the opportunity to examine the duodenum and ampulla of Vater and to approach drainage of the system internally, without puncture of the liver capsule or substance.

Careful evaluation of the diagnostic cholangiogram will help to determine which mode of therapy is best pursued. Benign neoplasms of the bile ducts are rare, but do occur, and may be treated endoscopically if accessible. An example of a such a lesion is a papillary adenoma of the common bile duct, which may be excised after endoscopic sphincterotomy (Fig. 20-1). Although most endoscopic therapeutic maneuvers within the biliary tree will require antecedent sphincterotomy, some may be accomplished without spincteric section. When the intention of the endoscopist is to provide biliary drainage by placement of an

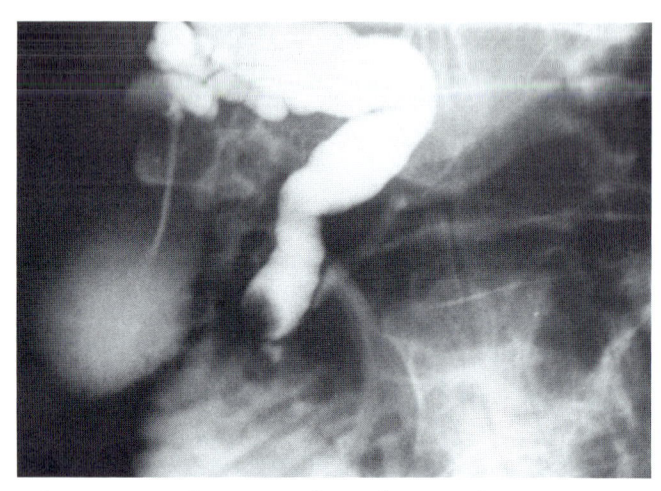

FIGURE 20-1 A benign papillary adenoma of the bile duct is demonstrated by endoscopic retrograde cholangiopancreatography and was excised after endoscopic sphincterotomy.

indwelling biliary stent, sphincterotomy is not always necessary. Indeed, if a cannula and wire can be introduced deeply into the duct and advanced through the narrowed segment, a stent can usually be maneuvered through the intact ampullary orifice and over the wire into the desired position (Fig. 20-2). Pancreatitis is uncommon after this procedure in spite of the relatively tight fit of the stent in the ampulla.

In many cases, it will be necessary, or desirable for the endoscopist to divide the ampulla before further manipulation of the ductal system. This is particularly so if there is a need to obtain cytologic samples from inside the duct. Sphincterotomy is accomplished by selectively cannulating the common bile duct with a sphincterotome cannula. The wire is slightly bowed, and current is applied in short bursts until the tissue in the upper midline of the intramural portion of the ampulla desiccates and divides (Fig. 20-3). The incision should be no longer than necessary for the therapeutic intervention desired and, certainly, should not extend beyond the visible intramural bulge of the bile duct in the duodenal wall. After sphincterotomy, a cytology brush may be inserted into the duct to obtain brushings. On some occasions, it may be useful to use a "mother–daughter" scope combination, the daughter scope being directed up the bile duct to obtain biopsies under direct vision (Fig. 20-4).

After diagnostic maneuvers are accomplished, a stent may be placed to relieve obstruction. Straight plastic stents are most often employed (Fig. 20-5). Generally, stents of 10-French or larger are preferred because clogging is more frequent with smaller stents. Most stents will occlude eventually as a result of deposition of bile and bacterial products. Replacement is usually necessary at intervals of from 4 to 6 months. More recently, expandable mesh metal stents have become available. These stents are less likely to occlude but are expensive and not removable. Although biliary stenting offers little with regard to curative treatment of tumors obstructing the bile ducts, in appropriately selected cases, it provides excellent palliation without the necessity of laparotomy. It is important for the endoscopist to be cognizant of the fact that a number of biliary, ampullary, and perhaps, pancreatic tumors may be curable with radical surgical extirpation. Patients with such lesions should not be deprived of the opportunity for such therapy.

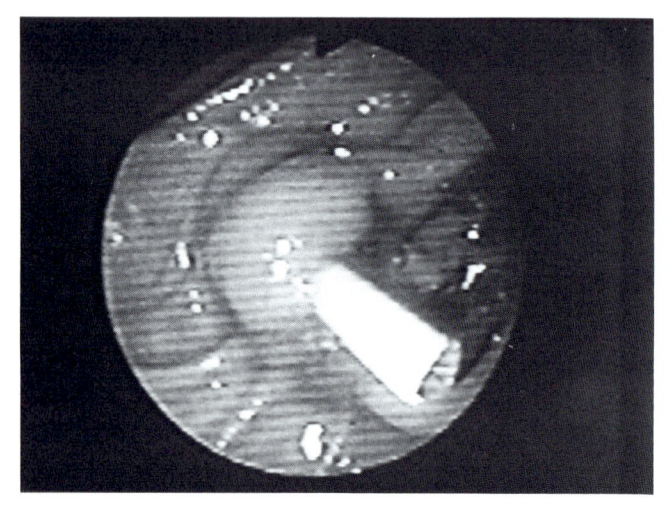

FIGURE 20-2 A 10-French biliary stent placed through the ampulla without sphincterotomy.

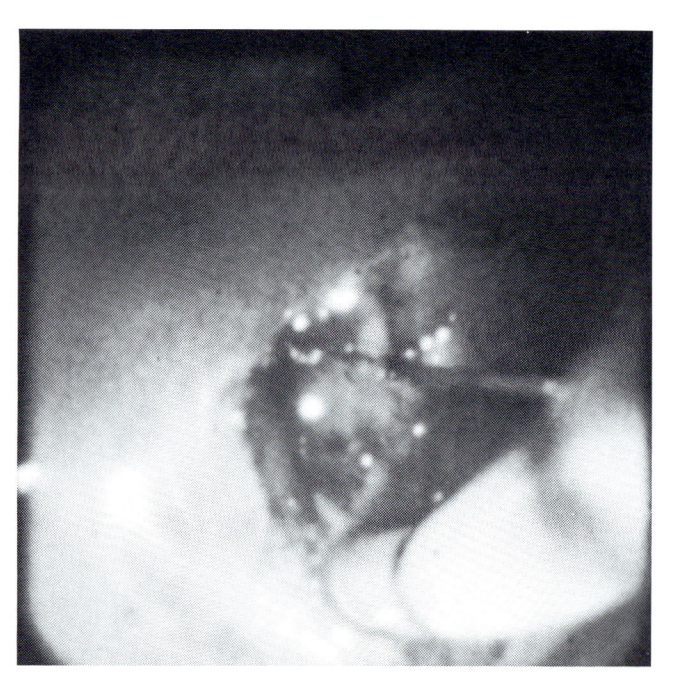

FIGURE 20-3 The sphincterotomy incision is made in a stepwise fashion in the upper midline of the ampullary bulge.

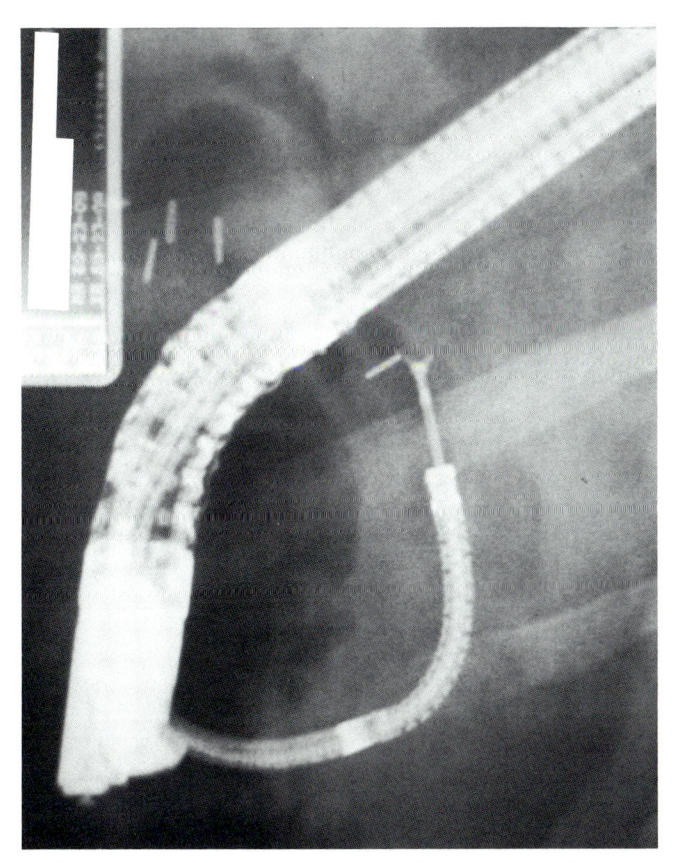

FIGURE 20-4 Using the mother–daughter scope combination, biopsies may be taken from the interior of the bile duct under direct vision.

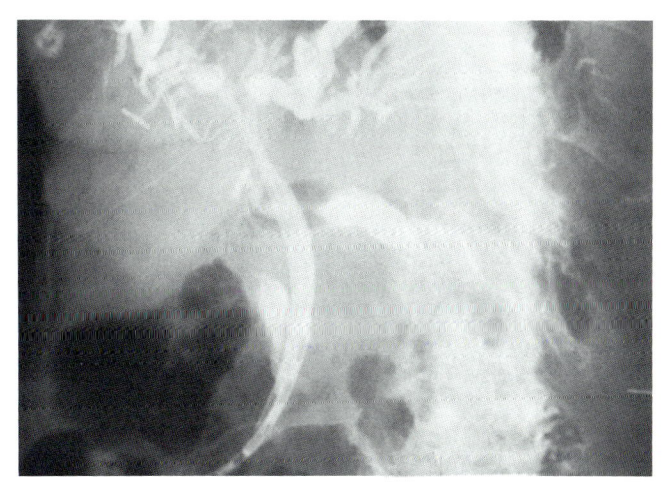

FIGURE 20-5 Two straight stents are positioned into the right and left hepatic ducts through a tumor of the bile duct bifurcation.

ENDOSCOPIC APPROACH TO BILE DUCT STONES

Removal of bile duct stones by means of endoscopic sphincterotomy has become the method of choice for approaching this problem in patients with retained or recurrent stones after cholecystectomy and in selected patients with intact gallbladders deemed unfit for surgery.[5] More recently, this approach has been applied to patients with common bile duct stones before planned laparoscopic cholecystectomy.

When patients who have undergone previous cholecystectomy develop symptoms suggesting biliary colic, jaundice, or abnormal liver function, ultrasonography should be employed to assess the caliber of the biliary tree. Although stones may be suggested at times, the method does not reliably define calculi in the common bile duct. When symptoms, laboratory findings, or ultrasound examination suggest a reasonable probability of choledocholithiasis, an ERCP should be performed. The procedure is not without risk, and particular care should be exercised to avoid overfilling of the pancreatic duct because this may lead to pancreatitis.[6] The demonstration of common duct stones will, in most cases, indicate the performance of an endoscopic sphincterotomy. When gallstone pancreatitis seems likely, in the face of jaundice, pain, and elevation of the serum amylase, the procedure may be performed to relieve biliary and pancreatic obstruction. Emergency decompression of the biliary tract may be indicated in patients with signs of cholangitis. Preparation for the procedure should include assessment of clotting parameters, electrolytes, blood count, and liver function tests. Preoperative antibiotics are indicated when biliary obstruction is present.

The technique of endoscopic sphincterotomy has been well described.[7] An electrosurgical cannula, the sphincterotome, must be selectively introduced into the common bile duct. The position of the cannula may be verified by injection of contrast material under fluoroscopic guidance. Only a short segment of wire should be introduced when cutting because an occasionally precipitous division of the tissue may occur. It is preferable to apply blended cutting and coagulation current in intermittent short bursts to create a gradual desiccation and division of the tissue, inserting more wire as necessary until the desired length of the incision is achieved. Cutting is performed in the upper midline region of the ampulla and should be confined to the visible bulge of the intramural portion of the common bile duct. As the division is continued cephalad, there is increased risk of hemorrhage secondary to division of a transverse artery, which frequently crosses the ampulla. When small stones are present, complete sphincteric section is unnecessary, and an incision just large enough to allow passage or extraction of the stones will suffice. In some cases, selective cannulation may be impossible, and the use of a modified catheter may be necessary to gain access to the duct. One such cannula is the "precut" sphincterotome. The cutting wire exits the tip of the cannula, and the endoscopist incises the ampulla in the position where the common duct orifice is expected.[8] Although this method is effective in expert hands, it clearly carries a greater risk of complication.[9]

After division of the sphincter has been accomplished, some stones will pass spontaneously. Although it was customary a decade ago to allow time for such passage before instrumentation of the duct, it is now the practice of most endoscopists to extract the calculi immediately. The latter may occur spontaneously with sphincteric division or be easily accomplished with ductal irrigation. In most cases, biliary balloon catheters can easily be positioned above the stones and used to drag them through the open sphincter (Fig. 20-6). When multiple stones are present, the most distal stone should be removed first, then the next, and so on. Some stones will require wire baskets to trap or crush them before removal. Stones too large to pass through the sphincteric incision may be captured in a wire basket and crushed by a process of mechanical lithotripsy. The latter method involves the advancement of a metal sheath over the basket wire and sequential tightening of the sheath against the basket until the stone breaks (Fig. 20-7). The fragments are then extracted.

Alternative methods include the introduction of electrohydraulic probes and laser lithotripters into the bile duct. The electrohydraulic probes are extremely effective in fragmenting bile duct calculi. They must be in contact with the stone to work and suffer from their propensity to injure the bile duct wall. Newer methods of more safely delivering the probe may add to the safety and utilization of this method in the future. The pulsed-dye laser has a wavelength of 504 nm and delivers an impulse that is extremely effective in fragmenting stones when the fiber is brought into contact with the stone. The laser produces little damage to the biliary walls and is safer than the electrohydraulic technique. This method suffers, however, from the expense of the laser and difficulty in delivering the fiber to the stone. Mother–daughter scope combinations and special laser baskets, with a central lumen for the laser fiber, have been helpful in performing lithotripsy by this method.

In spite of the increasing array of endoscopic tools for extracting ductal calculi, there are occasionally stones which tax the expertise of the most talented endoscopist. When large or impacted stones appear refractory to extraction by endoscopic techniques, surgery may be the next option (Fig. 20-8). Unfortunately, many of these patients are poor operative candidates and effective biliary decompression may be the best solution. In such cases, a biliary stent can be inserted with its proximal end positioned above the calculi and its distal end exiting the ampulla. Such stents provide excellent palliation in otherwise untenable situations. Another method, which will be of occasional use where available, is the extracorporeal shock wave lithotripter. Although proved unsatisfactory as a routine treatment for cholecystolithiasis, the method may be valuable in fragmenting large or refractory common duct stones after sphincterotomy. In such cases, a nasobiliary drain is first placed endoscopically, and contrast medium is injected so that the stone may be localized fluoroscopically and treated.

SUMMARY

Recent developments in endoscopic technology and technique have permitted minimally invasive access to the bile duct for the diagnosis and treatment of neoplasms and calculus disease. When a patient's history or physical examinations suggests biliary disease, appropriate laboratory studies must be obtained, followed by ultrasound and/or CT examination of the hepatobiliary system. ERCP will offer a detailed image of the bile ducts and suggest the utility and nature of any further intervention. When neoplasm is suspected, biopsy or cytologic sampling may be performed. Decompressive stents can be placed to offer significant palliation of inoperable or advanced disease. Some benign lesions may be excised or destroyed.

The therapeutic impact of retrograde cholangiography

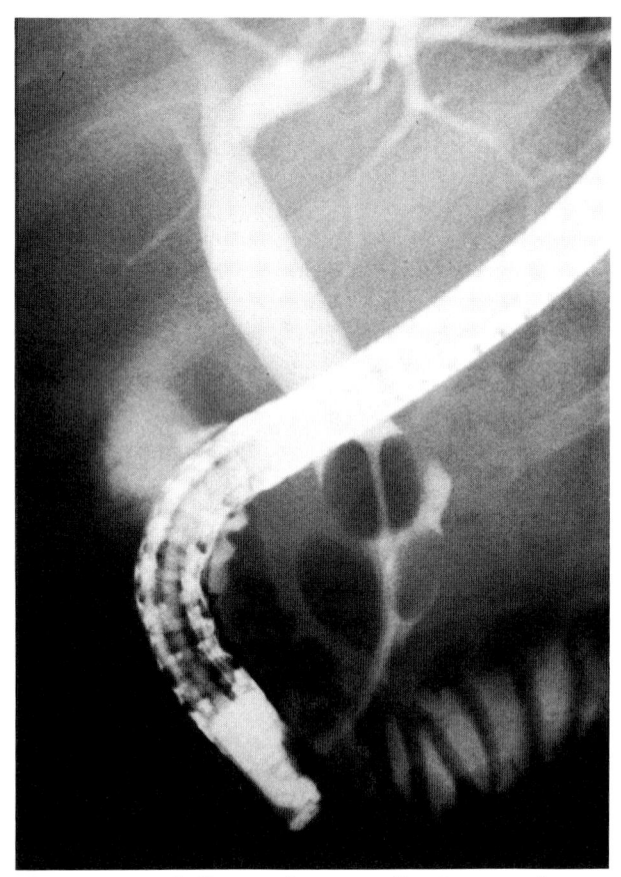

FIGURE 20-6 A balloon catheter is inflated proximal to a bile duct stone and used to deliver it through a sphincterotomy.

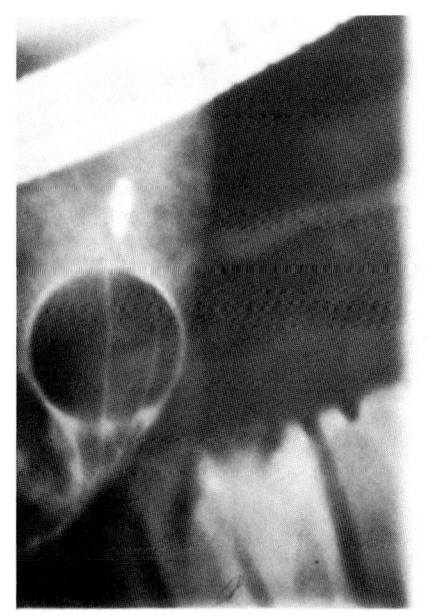

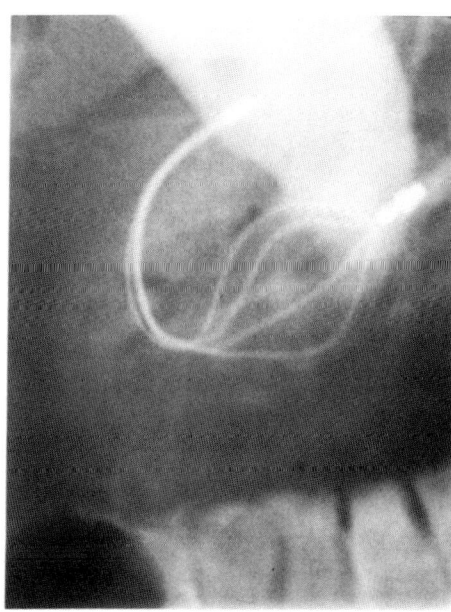

FIGURE 20-7 A large stone is trapped in a lithotripsy basket, and the scope is removed before introduction of a metal sheath used to crush the stone.

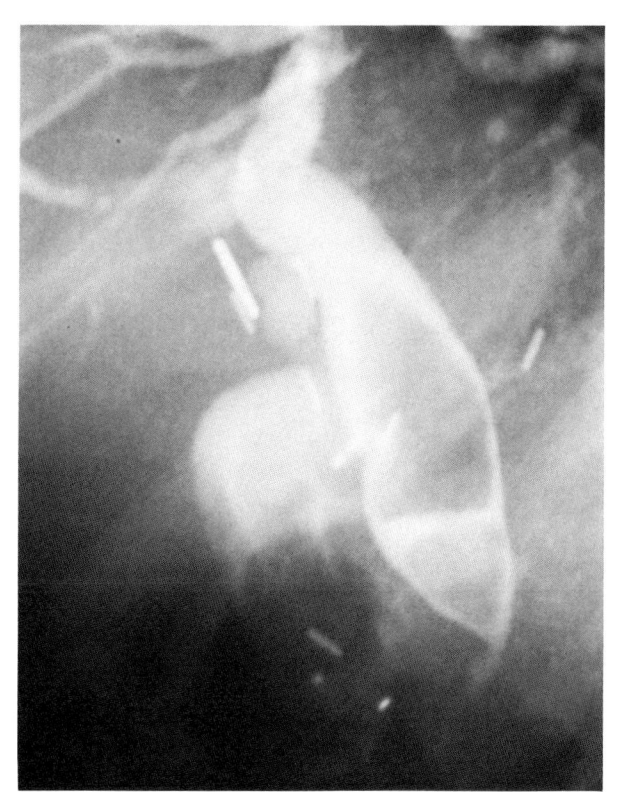

FIGURE 20-8 Extremely large bile duct stones may best be treated by open surgery or, if the patient is unfit for surgery, by placement of a stent to provide biliary decompression.

has been greatest in the management of bile duct stones. The majority of stones retained or recurrent after cholecystectomy can be easily removed by means of endoscopic sphincterotomy. More refractory stones may require complex manipulations, such as mechanical or laser lithotripsy, to assist in their removal. In cases where removal is impossible and surgery is deemed inappropriate, significant palliation may be obtained by stent placement and biliary decompression. The future will undoubtedly present further improvements in access to the bile ducts and expand the therapeutic dimensions of retrograde cholangiography for benign and malignant conditions.

REFERENCES

1. Cotton PB: Progress report: ERCP. *Gut* 1977; 18:316–341.
2. Kawai K, Akasaka Y, Murakami K, et al: Endoscopic sphincterotomy of the ampulla of Vater. *Gastrointest Endosc* 1974; 20:148.
3. Satake K, Cho K, Tatsumi S, et al: Evaluation of cholangiographic procedures in diagnosis of obstructive jaundice. *Am Surg* 1981; 47:387–392.
4. Matzen P, Malchow-Moller A, Lejerstofte J, et al: Endoscopic retrograde cholangiopancreatography and transhepatic cholangiography in patients with suspected obstructive jaundice. A randomized study. *Scand J Gastroenterol* 1982; 17:731–735.
5. Siegel JH, Safrany L, Ben-Zvi JS et al: Duodenoscopic sphincterotomy in patients with gallbladders in situ: Report of a series of 1272 patients. *Am J Gastroenterol* 1988; 83:1255–1258.
6. Hamilton I, Lintott DJ, Rothwell J, et al: Acute pancreatitis following endoscopic retrograde cholangiopancreatography. *Clin Radiol* 1983; 34:543–546.
7. Silvis SE, Vennes JA: Endoscopic retrograde sphincterotomy, in Silvis SE (ed): *Therapeutic Gastrointestinal Endoscopy*. New York, Igaku-Shoin, 1984, pp 198–240.
8. Ponsky JL (ed): *Atlas of Surgical Endoscopy*. Chicago, Mosby Year Book, 1991, pp 114–115.
9. Cotton PB: Precut papillotomy—A risky technique for experts only. *Gastrointest Endosc* 1989; 35:578–579.

Chapter 21

Laparoscopic Cholecystectomy

Jonathan M. Sackler

The first planned cholecystectomy was performed by Langenbuch[1] via a right upper quadrant incision in 1882. This technique was the mainstay of treatment of gallstone disease for the next 105 years.[2] In the late 1980s, a combination of new technologies and aggressive scientific experimentation gave birth to laparoscopic cholecystectomy (LC), which has radically changed the way the medical community and the lay public think about gallstones.

This innovation, as no other in recent years, has single-handedly altered the surgical management of gallstone disease. Internationally, multiple investigators labored independently in a headlong rush to provide the first successful laparoscopic removal of the gallbladder. Phillipe Mouret, a general surgeon and gynecologist in the south of France, usually bears the honor of having been the first to complete this procedure successfully, although Mühe[3] of West Germany claims to have carried out this operation in September 1985. Elsewhere in France, Jacques Perissat and colleagues[4] and Francois Dubois and coworkers[5] also achieved the same goal. In the United States, Reddick and Olsen,[6] McKernan and Saye,[7] Berci and associates,[8] and Airan and Ko[9] all performed cases within a few months of each other. Due credit must be given to the early work of Cuschieri and colleagues[10] in Dundee, who had performed this procedure in a porcine experimental model, and Berci and Cuschieri,[11] who had been proposing laparoscopic cholecystostomy for several years.

It is usual for surgical advances to emanate from detailed laboratory work and carefully controlled prospective clinical trials. This did not happen with the laparoscopic revolution, probably as a result of the pressure to perform this operation because gallbladder disease constitutes about 30 percent of the general surgeon's work load. The publicity attending the introduction of LC led many patients to demand the operation from their surgeons, and before long, any surgeon who was not performing LC was simply not performing cholecystectomies. Additionally, a number of medical equipment companies realized the potential for business expansion by manufacturing laparoscopic instrumentation and accessories, and there was pressure from this group as well for the technique to spread.

Therefore, a large number of training courses were hastily assembled around the world, with widely varying content and quality as manufacturers scrambled to fill orders for instruments that had never been tested. It is important to stress the validity of adequate training because the depth of training has been shown to be related to the number and type of complications.[12–14] Of course, laparoscopy is currently taught within the confines of the residency program along with all other surgical techniques, and this is preferable to the "short-course" format. For those practicing surgeons who had not learned the procedure, course content was suggested and endorsed by, among others, the Society of American Gastrointestinal Endoscopic Surgeons. They proposed that a course should consist of didactic material and experimental animal procedures, including practice on at least two pigs for each position of primary surgeon, assistant, and camera operator.[15] There are several reasons for the unprecedented popularity of LC, including: cosmetic appeal, small incisions, shortened hospital stay, reduced convalescence, lower costs, and less pain.

INDICATIONS

The advent of this new treatment modality has not changed the reasons why gallbladders are removed, and broadly speaking, these include symptomatic cholelithiasis, large gallbladder polyps, and acalculus cholecystitis. Additionally, removal may be indicated in those with asymptomatic gallstones who are at high risk of developing problems, such as diabetic patients or those about to undergo transplantation. There is no reason to remove the gallbladder in a patient with asymptomatic cholelithiasis just because of the existence of the laparoscopic technique. Indeed, these people often have nondilated extrahepatic ductal systems and may be more liable to injury.[16] This complication, which is unpalatable at any time, is made more difficult if the patient did not need cholecystectomy in the first place.

Since LC has been available, many patients have returned to their doctor and requested surgery, having previously refused it when open surgery was the sole technique. Unfortunately, these are often the patients who, as a result of chronic inflammation, may be poor candidates for LC.

CONTRAINDICATIONS

Broadly speaking, the most important factor in identifying contraindications is the surgeon's level of skill at the time of the patient interview, for although a particular case may prove impossible early in one's laparoscopic experience, 1 year or so later, it may be a routine case. A degree of introspection and humility is called for, with the majority of patients undergoing a diagnostic laparoscopy and "trial dissection."[17] If it proves impossible to safely remove the gallbladder laparoscopically, the surgeon can convert to open surgery. Such a judgment call should not be deemed a complication; it merely represents a change in the nature of the incision. Indeed, early conversion to open cholecystectomy may prevent complications, such as injury to the bile duct.

However, there are situations that merit special attention.

Pregnancy

During the first trimester of pregnancy, any surgery that can be avoided should be deferred until later in the pregnancy or after birth. This rationale should not be altered in the era of LC even though a laparoscopic procedure may be technically feasible.[18] During the later stages of gestation, the size of the uterus limits the amount of room available for laparoscopic dissection. There is also concern that the absorption of CO_2 from the pneumoperitoneum may damage the fetus, and early experimental work has suggested this may be true.[19] End-tidal CO_2 monitoring and alteration of ventilation to keep maternal partial CO_2 pressure less than 36 mmHg is vital.

Pacemaker

During open surgery, the use of monopolar electrocautery may cause "detuning" of the pacemaker. While it is being retuned with a magnet, the surgeon may contain bleeding with pressure, but this is difficult under laparoscopic control. Therefore, such patients should either have a temporary external pacemaker positioned, or consideration should be given to using bipolar cautery during the case. Of course, open cholecystectomy is another option.

Coagulopathy

In patients with a bleeding tendency, the laparoscopist should take extreme care in the conduct of the procedure because bleeding from the liver bed, or even the trocar entry site, may be fatal. There are techniques to control hemorrhage, and these will be addressed later.

Obesity

Although it is true that the extremely obese patient may be a difficult operative candidate because of the length of the trocar and instruments required, it is almost certainly easier than an open case, where any incision is often not large enough. It is useful to note in either case that obese women tend to "carry their obesity" in the abdominal pannus, whereas obese men often have a great deal of fat in the peritoneal cavity (e.g., omentum and triangle of Calot).[20,21]

Cirrhosis

These patients often have a caput medusa, which makes abdominal entry difficult, and numerous vessels and adhesions from portal hypertension. Great care should be taken in deciding to perform a cholecystectomy in such a patient.

Previous Surgery

Such patients are more likely to have adhesions between the viscera and the abdominal wall, which may render the creation of a pneumoperitoneum and access to the gallbladder more difficult. During the preoperative gallbladder ultrasound, the radiologist should consider mapping adhesions, using the technique described by Siegel and associates.[22] This consists of comparing how the viscera slide in relation to the abdominal wall; a fair degree of accuracy is available with this method. At the time of surgery, with either the needle or open laparoscopy technique, a suitable entry site may be selected away from the site of the prior surgery.

Acute Cholecystitis

This is usually understood to mean a patient presenting emergently with fever, localized constant pain, and leukocytosis with peritoneal signs. However, very often, we will find a robin's egg blue gallbladder at laparoscopy, which may portend an effortless dissection. Conversely, an elective case may present dense vascular adhesions, with a thickened gallbladder wall, perhaps containing white bile or pus. This confirms the value of performing a diagnostic laparoscopy and trial dissection. The neophyte laparoscopist should heed its warnings and convert to an open procedure early in the procedure.[23,24]

Porcelain Gallbladder

This rare variant, where the gallbladder wall is replaced with calcium, may be almost impossible to remove laparoscopically (Fig. 21-1). Again, a trial dissection is reasonable because the feel of the gallbladder may not be what we would expect based on the preoperative x-ray appearance.[25]

Carcinoma

In cases where malignancy of the gallbladder is suspected, it is probably not appropriate to attempt laparoscopic removal because a liver resection may be required. Obviously, the consent form should reflect the opportunity to make this operative decision. In this era of early discharge of patients, I routinely open the gallbladder after removing it from the abdominal cavity to look for unsuspected polyps. If seen, an early pathologic examination result should be sought so that the patient is not discharged, only to be brought back for the shocking diagnosis of unsuspected carcinoma. Another reason to consider the open route for resection of the malignant gallbladder is that, in drawing it across the abdominal cavity and through the umbilical incision, the gallbladder may rupture, leading to seeding of malignant cells through the exit wound. This would obviously not be as great a concern during open surgery.

PREPARATION

Initially, a thorough history should be taken from the patient to confirm the likely diagnosis of symptomatic gallstones. If there is anything suspicious about the history, despite the presence of gallstones on investigation, other sources for discomfort, such as diverticulosis, hiatal hernia, or peptic ulcer disease, should be considered. Many cases of postcholecystectomy syndrome are "caused" by resection of an asymptomatic gallbladder. Special notice should be taken of symptoms suggestive of cardiorespiratory problems, bleeding disorders, and the nature and site of previous surgery. If the patient has an extremely symptomatic hiatal hernia, this should be addressed during the investigations,[26] and a history of inguinal hernia should likewise be noted.[27] Physical examination should be used to confirm the diagnosis and assess prior abdominal scars, signs of bleeding tendency, or inguinal hernia. Investigations should routinely include chest x-ray and electrocardiography as dictated by hospital policy, blood count, electrolyte panel, and clotting screen as a matter of routine. Liver function tests will help to define the likelihood of common duct stones and may also demonstrate previously unsuspected liver disease. Ultrasound is currently the "gold standard" for diagnosing gallstones and, at this time, comments should be made on the thickness of the gallbladder wall (if greater than 3 mm), the presence of pericholecystic fluid, and the Phrygian cap deformity, which is valuable preoperative knowledge because it helps to avoid misinterpreting the anatomy.[28] Similarly, the ultrasonographer should attempt to note the diameter of the common duct and look for choledocholithiasis. As mentioned previously, at this time, adhesion mapping can be undertaken.[22] If the patient has a symptomatic hiatal hernia, gastroscopy should be performed, and further cardiorespiratory testing will be dictated by the history and physical findings. Full and informed consent is vital for this, as in any procedure, and should include permission to explore the common bile duct and convert to open cholecystectomy. The issue as to whether to tell patients in great detail about the possible complications must be addressed by each surgeon individually. There is a fine line between "full and frank discussion" and terrifying the general public with what are, after all, rare complications.

At time of surgery, the patient should be shaved and prepared with povidone iodine (or chlorhexidine if there is an allergy to iodine). The bladder should be decompressed with a Foley catheter and an orogastric tube passed to deflate the stomach.[27] Because of the raised intraabdominal pressure and reverse Trendelenburg position used during LC, it is possible that deep venous thrombosis is more likely. Therefore, prophylaxis should be utilized. I prefer sequential compression stockings for this purpose.[29] If the patient does have an inguinal hernia, it may be worthwhile applying a truss preoperatively to prevent the embarrassing and painful condition of scrotal emphysema.

The patient should be placed supine on the operating table with preferably the left arm extended if the anesthesiologist so desires. A footboard should be positioned to prevent the patient slipping off, and straps should be applied also. The earthing plate for monopolar electrocautery should ideally be placed on the anterior surface of the

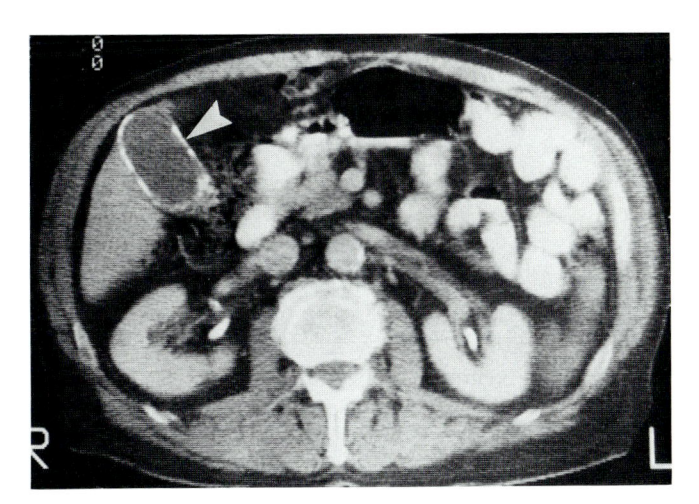

FIGURE 21-1 CT scan of abdomen showing porcelain gallbladder (arrow).

thigh to prevent disconnection and the danger of pooling of fluid that is more likely when it is placed on the buttock.

EQUIPMENT

In laparoscopic surgery, we rely totally on effective, well-maintained instrumentation, and it is vital that the surgeon be conversant with the construction of each piece of equipment and knowledgeable in problem solving. First, we must survey the operating room setup, which consists of monitors for both the surgeon and assistant and also possibly one for observers (see Chap. 33). Surgeons should be able to see the insufflator because readings from this device may inform them of impending or future problems, such as an empty gas tank. On the surgeon's side of the operating room should be the energy source for dissection, the irrigation, suction, and documentation cart. Each piece of equipment will now be considered in turn.

Insufflator

It is vital to have a machine capable of delivering up to 10 L/min of gas because, with multiple ports, gas loss is greater and reinsufflation is vital. The machine should have a preset limit, and after this pressure is reached, insufflation should automatically cease. The display should include the volume of gas in the tank, the current pressure, the preset pressure, the current flow rate, and the preset flow rate. The usual insufflating agent is carbon dioxide, which may cause a decrease in pH, a rise in the partial pressure of CO_2, and a depression in the partial pressure of oxygen. It is therefore important for the anesthesiologist to monitor the patient carefully.[30] The gas line from the cylinder to the insufflator should have a wrench and spare gaskets attached, and the surgeon should be familiar with techniques of changing the cylinder. A spare gas cylinder with a regulator should be kept in the room.

There is some concern that particulate matter may be carried in the gas, especially because many cylinders are very old and are refilled repeatedly. It may be worthwhile placing a microfilter in line between the insufflator and the patient (Hunter JG. Personal communication, 1991).

With long procedures, concern about the physiologic effects of CO_2 has been expressed, and this has led to a new technique. After an initial pneumoperitoneum has been created, a curved needle is inserted to the left of the falciform ligament and brought out to the right. This is followed with a wider metal tube, which may be attached to an overhead gantry and thereby act as an abdominal retractor. This tube has perforations to allow for the evacuation of smoke, and no further insufflation is required.[31,32] Further work needs to be done to evaluate whether this is a true advance or whether it causes extensive abdominal wall bruising.

Light Source

Magnification and distance viewing are required. It is necessary to use a 300-W xenon light source. These are inappropriately called "cold" light sources—they are anything but cold, and great care must be taken when the telescope is withdrawn from the abdomen because contact with paper drapes may lead to an operating room fire. In addition, the light is so bright that it will damage the vision of the operating room team for the duration of the procedure, and light feedback may also damage the camera. Therefore, when withdrawing the telescope from the abdomen, the light should be turned down. The cable to attach the telescope to the light source must be securely attached at both ends, and it is preferable to use a fluid-filled cable because this conducts up to 30 percent more light. Before commencing the operation, the light cable should be checked for broken fibers or damaged quartz plugs.

Television Screens

High-definition monitors are required (in the United States, 480 and, in the United Kingdom, 625 lines). Newer television screens will double the number of lines and thereby improve definition considerably. The monitor should be large enough to allow the surgeon to see the operative field clearly without straining.

Camera

The details of camera technology have been covered in Chapter 2. Currently, the single-chip camera is ideal and should be white balanced and focused. The focal length should be reduced to the minimum at the commencement of the operation. Currently, the camera and laparoscope may be purchased as a single unit, and it is likely that digitized laparoscopes will soon be available. In addition, the quality of the captured image may be improved by digitalization techniques.

Some surgeons still like to use the beam splitter, which allows a monocular view through the telescope and the television image to be captured.

Energy Source

A great deal of attention has been paid to the different techniques of removing the gallbladder from the liver bed. It is likely that the skill of the surgeon and familiarity with the chosen source is more important than the inherent characteristics of any of the modalities. Each has its advantages and disadvantages and these will be listed in turn.

MONOPOLAR ELECTROCAUTERY

This is the most familiar type to most surgeons. The machinery is inexpensive, and if it becomes dysfunctional, another unit is always available. Research has demonstrated that this is the easiest for surgeons to utilize and leads to the fastest laparoscopic cholecystectomy.[33,34] However, there are concerns that if the insulation fails, leakage may occur with consequent damage (see Chap. 5). In addition, the phenomenon of coupled capacitive discharge may occur (see Chap. 5). Surgeons may avoid these problems by using the lowest current setting available, activating the machine in short bursts, and if a tissue effect is not seen, instead of turning up the power, checking the circuit. By varying the pressure of the hook, spatula, or other electrocautery tool on the tissue, a different effect may be achieved, either slow coagulation or fast dessication.

BIPOLAR ELECTROCAUTERY

This system avoids the risk of extraneous current alluded to previously, but it is much slower, the instruments are somewhat bulky, they need to be cleaned frequently, and the generators are more expensive. Work has demonstrated that it is safe but slow.[35]

FREE BEAM LASER

The KTP device is expensive and requires precautions such as safety goggles, notices on doors, and the presence of a laser safety officer. Although the technique is elegant,[36] there are dangers of *past pointing* injuries, and concern has been expressed that the wavelength of this laser may have adverse genetic effects (Cuschieri A. Personal communication, 1990).

CONTACT LASER

This has the same drawbacks as the preceding technique, and, although elegant, is slower and associated with more gallbladder perforations.[37]

HYDRODISSECTION

This enables tissue planes to be separated by a water jet.[38] The most commonly used system is that devised by Nezhat-Dorsey. It is an interesting idea but is rather slow for cholecystectomy. It may have some role to play in other laparoscopic operations, but it is unlikely to achieve widespread use.

CUSA

The cavitronic ultrasound aspirator (CUSA) plays a role in neurosurgery and mucosal proctectomy. It is an expensive alternative to monopolar electrocautery.[39]

HARMONIC SCAPEL

This is another variant using sound waves to separate tissue planes, which is said to be hemostatic. Further work needs to be done to elucidate whether this indeed has any advantages, although it is very costly (Amaral JF. Personal communication, 1991).

Irrigation

Just as in open surgery, it is necessary to have a clear field. Irrigation is vital in this regard because even the smallest drop of blood will occlude the surgeon's view. Most surgeons use a single instrument for suction, irrigation, and coagulation because it limits the time necessary for instrument changes. One may simply attach the instrument to a liter of saline held in a pressurized bag, similar to that found in every emergency room. Alternatively, a rotary pump activated by a foot switch may be used or a nitrogen-driven system. A novel approach is to utilize a laparoscope with an additional channel through which the irrigant may be delivered to either clean the lens or wash blood away from an oozing area.

Suction

The "workhorse" of laparoscopic cholecystectomy must be connected to the wall suction by clear plastic tubing. It is imperative that the surgeon check that this works before the operation commences because it is frustrating to have to try to initiate suction in urgent circumstances.

Documentation

It is important to keep a record of cases for teaching, research, and medicolegal purposes. It has yet to be defined as to whether a video tape constitutes part of the patient's record and if the surgeon is bound to keep a recording after it is made. It is likely that our legal colleagues will define these issues for us. The use of ¾-in U-matic tapes provides the best quality and allows for later editing. The machine is large and expensive, and the tapes are bulky to store. Alternatively, ½-in VHS tapes are simpler to store, and the machines are cheaper and more accessible, although not as suitable for editing. Eight-millimeter tapes are the smallest of all and are ideal for storage.[40] We should remember that, when making a video tape, always to record the patient's name on the tape and on the box for ease of identification. Occasionally, it is useful to show these tapes to the referring physician, and patients may occasionally even want to see a portion of their operations.

The easiest way to secure prints or slides of a phase of the operation is to attach a 35-mm single-lens-reflex camera to the laparoscope, but this is time consuming and runs the risk of breaching the sterile field, although the quality of the images are superb. Alternatively, different devices for image capture are available, and a number of copies of each image may be produced and kept in the surgeon's office, the patient's chart, and even given to the referring physician. A digital image may be captured and later processed, but the hardware for this system is expensive, and each individual slide is similarly costly.

Mixing Desk

This device is extremely useful when common duct stones are encountered because the image from the choledochoscope and the laparoscope may be mixed and presented as a "picture-in-picture" format (see Chap. 7).

Veress Needle

The needle, or closed technique, of creating a pneumoperitoneum is the most commonly used. This needle was devised by Janos Veress[41] in the 1930s. It consists of a sharp outer trocar containing a sprung, blunt, hollow obturator. When passing through the abdominal wall, the blunt inner tube is recessed and then springs out after the peritoneal cavity has been entered. They are available in both reusable and disposable forms, and it is necessary for safe entry to see the top move up and down, to feel this, and to hear an audible click from the spring. Some maintain that the tap should be kept closed on entering the abdomen in case a large vessel is entered to prevent air embolus. Others maintain that by keeping the tap open, air enters and allows the intestines to fall away from the approaching needle.

Trocars

A wide variety of trocars exist with sizes from 4 to 35 mm in disposable and reusable forms. The reusable trocars have the advantage of reduced cost and elegance. Some have a hollow sharp trocar that allows the whistle of an escaping pneumoperitoneum to be heard as the cavity is entered. The drawbacks to these instruments are that they require constant maintenance and sharpening. Some surgeons have concerns about their sterility. The main advantage of the disposable trocars is that they are sharp, thereby requiring less force to achieve entry,[42] and are guaranteed to be sterile. Many have a safety-shield mechanism that should limit the number of visceral or vascular injuries. One new approach to trocar introduction is to use an electrically heated stylette that will cut through the abdominal wall, much like a diathermy probe in open surgery. Without doubt, the most important issue in trocar introduction is not the design, but the method by which it is placed in the abdomen by the surgeon, that is, with thought and care.

Telescope

Routinely, surgeons use a Hopkins rod–lens system, which, with its unique design, allows for optimal light conduction and image generation. Most would advocate the use of the 10-mm scope for operative laparoscopy (the 4 mm is suitable for diagnostic procedures). The scope comes in a variety of viewing angles from 0° to 45°. The 30° angle seems ideal, because it allows several different perspectives on any given structure.

Laparoscope Cleaner

It is necessary to clean and antifog the scope before introducing it into the peritoneal cavity. There are a number of approaches that include commercial antifogging agents and to wet and heat the laparoscope above body temperature. One way to achieve this is to have a blood warmer at the side of the operating table with a sterile plastic bottle of saline that may be easily accessed by the surgeon. Another approach is to use a thermos flask on the Mayo stand, which will keep water hot for the duration of the operation and antifogs and cleans the telescope at the same time at minimal cost.

Clip Applier

These are available in reusable single-shot and disposable multishot forms. Most clips currently are made of titanium to minimize problems with later CT or MRI scans. Again, the most important issue is surgeon choice, although cost is an important concern.

Pretied Catgut Loops

The techniques of suturing are dealt with in Chapter 14. It is useful for the surgeon to have these available to secure the cystic duct stump and to close perforations in the gallbladder.

Sutures and Needle Holders

Again, this has been dealt with in Chapter 14. The surgeon should know how to use this equipment, especially if the common duct is to be approached. It is occasionally necessary to fashion an intra- or extracorporeal knot around an enlarged cystic duct.[43]

Cholangiography

Whether the surgeon is a proponent of routine, selective, or no cholangiography for open cholecystectomy, the situation is radically different for the laparoscopic technique.[44–46] In open surgery, the surgeon is able to palpate the duct for stones and visualize its diameter, thereby deciding whether a cholangiogram is necessary to detect unsuspected stones. In the difficult case, retrograde or *fundus-first* cholecystectomy may be performed. However, in laparoscopic surgery, the common duct is not so easily assessed, and cholangiography is the most sensitive method for detecting unsuspected common duct stones. In addition, with cholangiography, the anatomy will be clearly defined, helping the surgeon to avoid such potential pitfalls as the short cystic duct, the cystic duct draining into the right hepatic, or an accessory duct draining into the cystic duct or into the gallbladder (duct of Luschka). If the surgeon has inadvertently catheterized the common bile duct, a cholangiogram also will allow this error to be detected before any duct is divided. Without cholangiography, a simple incision would become a disastrous resection of the extrahepatic ductal system (Fig. 21-2).

The best way to perform cholangiography is with fluoroscopy, and either a ceiling-suspended or mobile unit is ideal.[47,48] It is useful to have a coaxial cable linking the operating room with the radiology suite so that an audiovisual link exists between the surgeon and radiologist, allowing them to discuss the films. There are a number of techniques of performing cholangiography, and these will be covered in the next section.

Hand Instruments

The basic laparoscopic cholecystectomy set consists of the following: forceps with medium serration to grasp the gallbladder, locking grasping forceps with fine serrations, two pairs of nonlocking grasping forceps for grasping and teasing adhesions, large scissors for cutting sutures and micro-

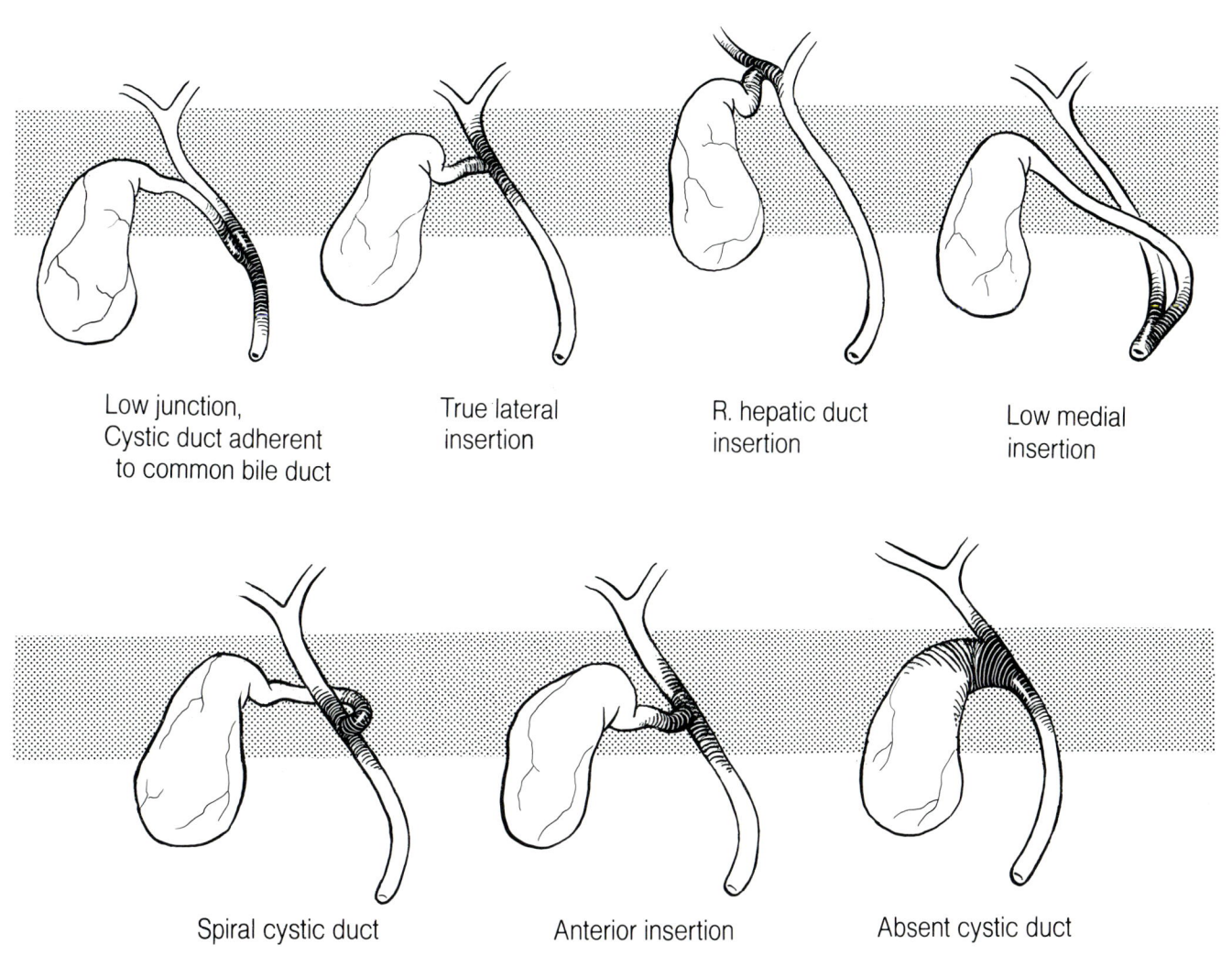

Low junction, Cystic duct adherent to common bile duct

True lateral insertion

R. hepatic duct insertion

Low medial insertion

Spiral cystic duct

Anterior insertion

Absent cystic duct

FIGURE 21-2 Operative cholangiography will delineate the wide variations in biliary anatomy. The cystic duct may insert into the extrahepatic biliary system anywhere from the high right hepatic duct to the ampulla of Vater. It may course anterior to or posterior to and insert on any aspect of the common hepatic duct. In one percent of cases, the cystic duct is so patulous it is essentially nonexistent. These latter cases present the greatest difficulty for the inexperienced surgeon.

scissors for incising the duct, a cholangiograsper, a suction–coagulation–irrigation probe with a variety of tips, and a variety of dissecting probes, reducers, and other specialized instruments, such as stone-retrieval forceps, which will be dealt with later. All of these instruments are available in disposable forms, and the choice of which to use will be predicated on the surgeon's preference and the availability of instruments.

ANESTHETIC CONSIDERATIONS

Because of the physiologic effects of gaseous exchange and abdominal distention from the pneumoperitoneum, a careful anesthetic input is mandatory. Ideally, the anesthesiologist will not use nitrous oxide because this may lead to intestinal distention. Narcotic analgesics should be avoided and antiemetics administered to reduce postoperative nausea. Additional drugs which the anesthesiologist may consider giving are: morphine and fentanyl if there is free flow into the duodenum during cholangiography (to cause sphincter spasm). Likewise, if there is no flow into the duodenum and there is concern about either spasm at the sphincter or a small calculus, the anesthesiologist may administer intravenous glucagon.

A careful watch should be kept on the blood pressure, pulse, electrocardiogram tracing, and pulse oximetry. Measurement of end-tidal carbon dioxide is also useful. If the partial pressure of CO_2 is rising, then the tidal volume and respiratory rate may be increased until a more normal situation is achieved.[49] It is also vital that the anesthesiologist keep the patient well relaxed because a semirigid abdominal wall will minimize the space the surgeon has to work in, just as with open surgery.

TECHNIQUE

It is possible for laparoscopic cholecystectomy to be carried out by one surgeon working with a scrub nurse and instrument holders. However, most work with an assistant surgeon and a camera operator who may be a trained technician, resident, or medical student. The techniques of single-surgeon cholecystectomy are covered in Chapter 7.

Having prepared and draped the abdomen, the pneumoperitoneum will be instituted. For the closed technique, the Veress needle, whose function has been previously checked by the scrub nurse, is inserted at 90° to the abdominal wall, which is held up by the surgeon and assistant. Usually this will be at the lower border of the umbilicus through a small incision, but previous surgery may dictate another insertion point (Fig. 21-3). A 10-mL syringe filled with saline is attached to the needle, followed by aspiration, to determine whether proper entry has been achieved into the abdominal cavity. If blood is aspirated, the needle should be repositioned. If blood is seen to spurt into the needle, laparotomy should be undertaken because this indicates penetration of a major vessel. If bowel contents are retrieved, the laparoscopy should be continued, and the damage assessed after the needle has been repositioned. Saline should be irrigated, and then the whole procedure repeated. If the saline is retrieved at the second aspiration, this means the needle is in the preperitoneal space.

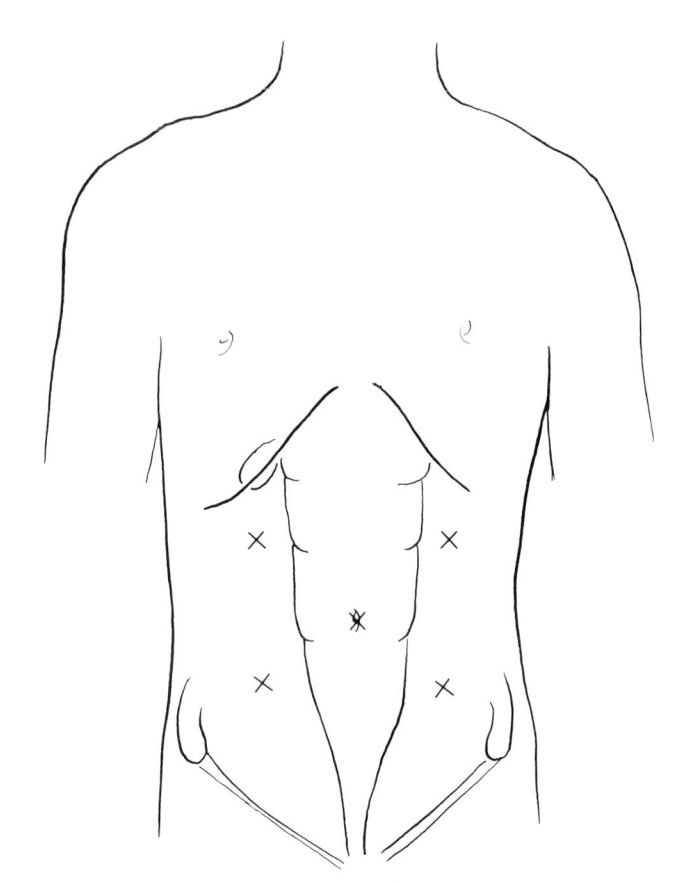

FIGURE 21-3 The usual position for Veress needle insertion is the lower border of the umbilicus. Alternative positions, based on prior surgery, are indicated.

Tubing from the CO_2 insufflator is attached, and insufflation commences, initially at no more than 1.5 L/min. This ensures that, if the needle is in a vessel, the anesthesiologist will have an opportunity to detect a problem before fatal air embolus occurs. Also, rupture of the diaphragm[50] or disturbance of cardiorespiratory function is less likely at these low flow rates. If a good flow rate is maintained, but low pressure continues despite the infusion of several liters of gas, this means that the needle is probably in the lumen of the bowel, there is a large inguinal or hiatal hernia, or there is a leak from the system. If low pressure and high flow rates are indicated, this implies the needle is in the correct place. After an intraabdominal pressure of 14 to 15 mm Hg is achieved, the needle is removed, and the incision is enlarged to accommodate the

11-mm trocar, which is introduced. One should be certain not to enlarge the incision too much because otherwise there will be a troublesome gas leak around the cannula sheath. If there has been concern about adhesions, one may attach a syringe with saline to the Veress needle and try to instill saline, which should be effortless, and then aspirate, at which time gas should be retrieved. By doing this in a circumferential fashion, an area free of adhesions may be "mapped" out.[51]

Some surgeons routinely prefer the Hasson trocar technique,[52] especially if the patient has an umbilical hernia that will require repair, there is concern about adhesions, or Veress needle insertion has failed. Here a circumumbilical incision is made, the median raphé is grasped between two Kocher clamps, and two stay sutures are inserted. A bold incision is then made with Mayo scissors into the peritoneal cavity, and the Hasson trocar is positioned and secured in place with sutures (Fig. 21-4).

The prewarmed laparoscope is introduced into the abdomen, and the area of the needle and trocar incision is checked for damage. It is then vital to perform a full diagnostic laparoscopy.[53] After the diagnosis has been confirmed and no other problems are evident, steps are taken to commence cholecystectomy.

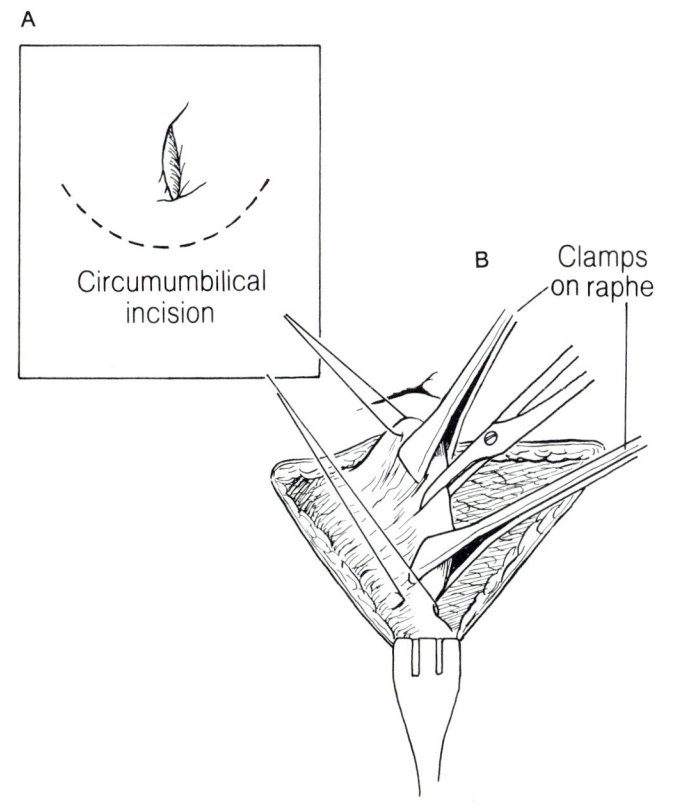

FIGURE 21-4 To insert the Hasson cannula, (A) an incision is made around the lower border of the umbilicus (B), the midline raphé is grasped, and two stay sutures are inserted. An incision is made with Mayo scissors into the peritoneal cavity.

The patient is placed in the reverse Trendelenburg position with the right side tilted up. A vertical incision is made in the midline below the xiphisternum, and a 10-mm trocar is introduced through the midline but just to the right of the falciform fat pad to avoid damage and bleeding. With the reducer in place, the fundus of the gallbladder is grasped and elevated.

The appropriate positions of the trocars are then determined based on a number of parameters. First, it is vital that the instruments not be coaxial with the telescope, or one will be unable to see the tip of the instrument. Likewise it is disadvantageous to have instruments moving toward the telescope because the field will be diminished. There are, in fact, only small angles, close to 90°, suitable for instrument introduction. Also to be taken into account is that trocar insertion sites must not traumatize abdominal wall vessels and underlying structures and must not be so far away that the instruments will not reach the target tissue (Fig. 21-5).

By holding the fundus, the site of the next two trocars may be decided. Broadly speaking, the third trocar, a 5-mm instrument, is introduced in the anterior axillary line above the anterior superior iliac spine. Through this trocar, a locking grasping forceps is used to hold the fundus of the gallbladder up and over the liver. After an ideal position has been obtained, it is fixed with a towel clip to the drape. An additional gas line may be taken from a Y connector and joined to this trocar so that any lost gas lost will be sooner replaced. The fourth trocar is introduced, generally, in the midclavicular line below the right costal margin, and it is this that will provide medial and lateral retraction of Hartmann's pouch (Fig. 21-6). It is vital that all these trocars be placed under direct vision; it is unacceptable to cause injury at this stage. There may be adhesions to the gallbladder, which should be teased down toward, never up away from, the common bile duct to avoid avulsing the cystic duct from the common bile duct (Fig. 21-7).

Attention should be turned to the area of Hartmann's pouch. Careful maneuvers with limited electrocautery and blunt and sharp dissection should free up the attachments, both lateral and medial, to the gallbladder. Use of the 30° scope allows one to create a window behind the gallbladder, which will then help the surgeon define the junction of the gallbladder and cystic duct and prevent damage to the common bile duct.[54] This is then secured via a clip applier placed through the subxiphisternal trocar (Fig. 21-8).

In preparation for cholangiography, an incision is made with a microscissors introduced through the midclavicular portal. There are several ways to perform the cholangiogram.

First, a 4-French catheter placed through a cholangiograsper is introduced through the midclavicular line portal, passed into the duct, and grasped in place. If there are difficulties introducing the catheter because of the valves of Heister, a hydrophilic floppy-tipped guide wire may be

222 PART II Old Diseases

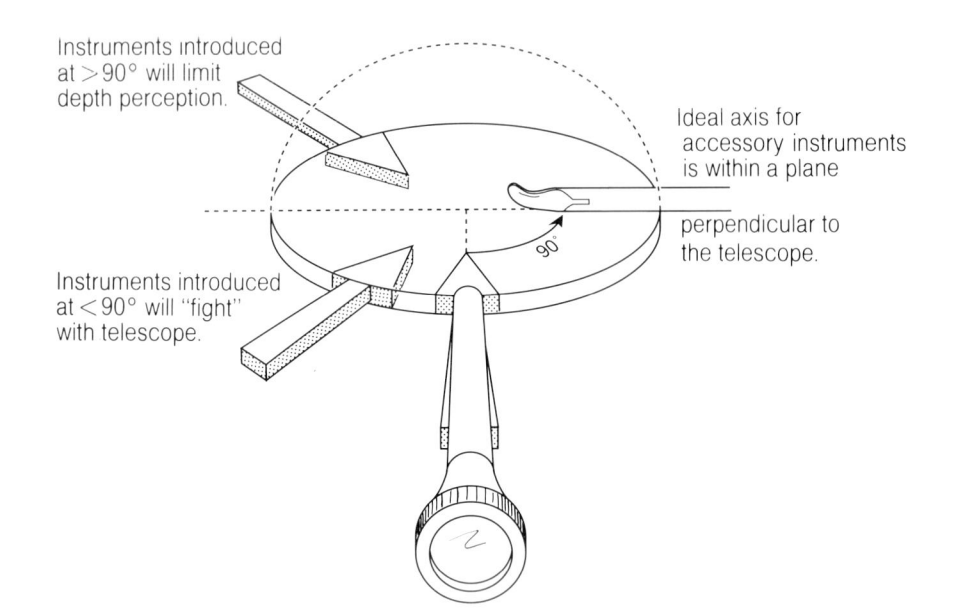

FIGURE 21-5 This diagram shows that trocars should not be introduced toward or coaxial with the laparoscope. The ideal position is at 90° to the line of vision.

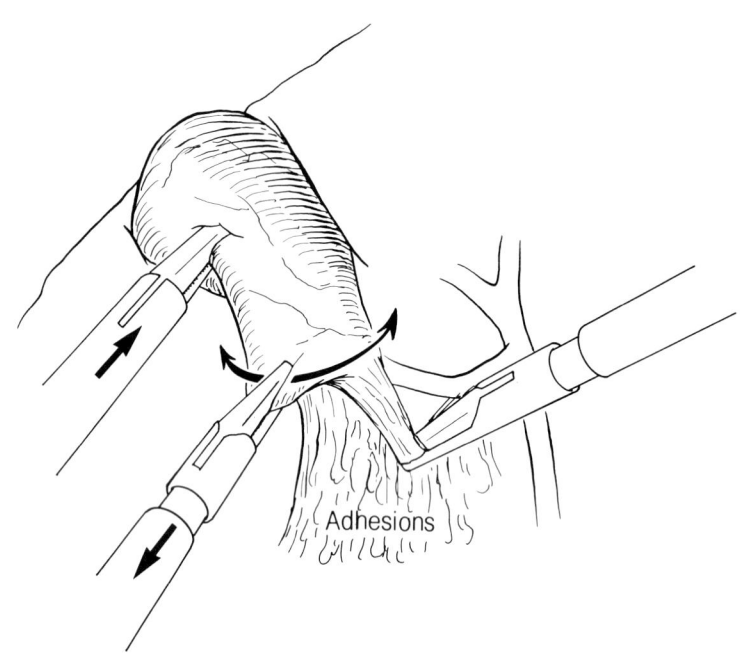

FIGURE 21-7 The fundus of the gallbladder is retracted in a cephalic direction and Hartmann's pouch is moved side to side. A grasper is used to tease adhesions down.

introduced through the catheter, although this may lead to air bubbles on the films (Fig. 21-9).[55]

The second method is an intravenous catheter passed percutaneously directly over the duct. Through this, an umbilical feeding catheter can be positioned in the cystic duct (Fig. 21-10).[56] This is useful when no cholangiograsper is available. A guide wire may also be used in this method.

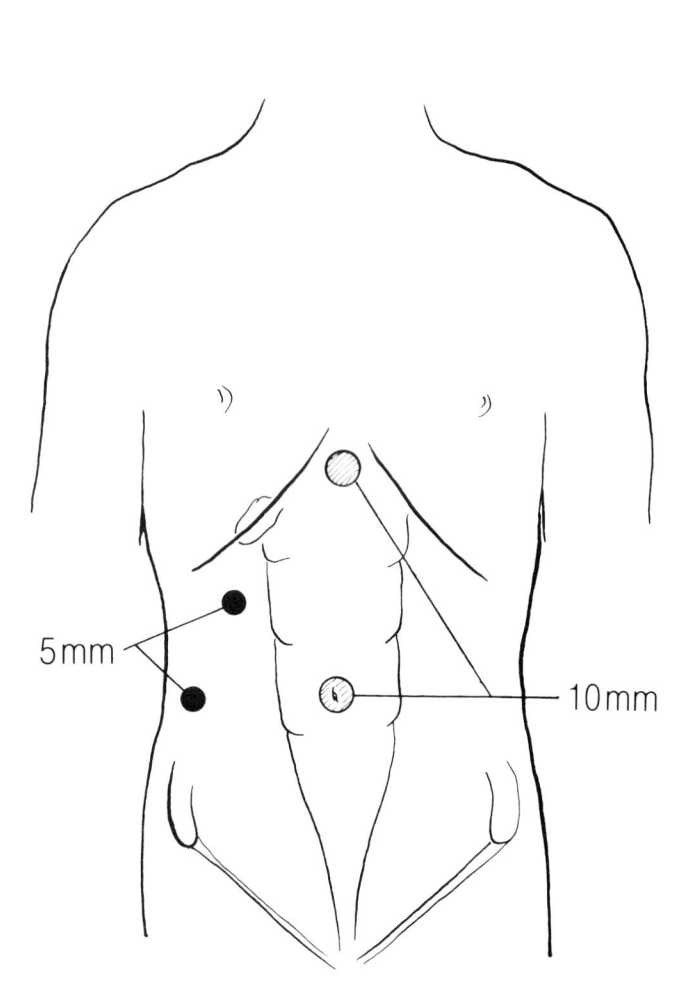

FIGURE 21-6 The standard positions of the trocars for laparoscopic cholecystectomy.

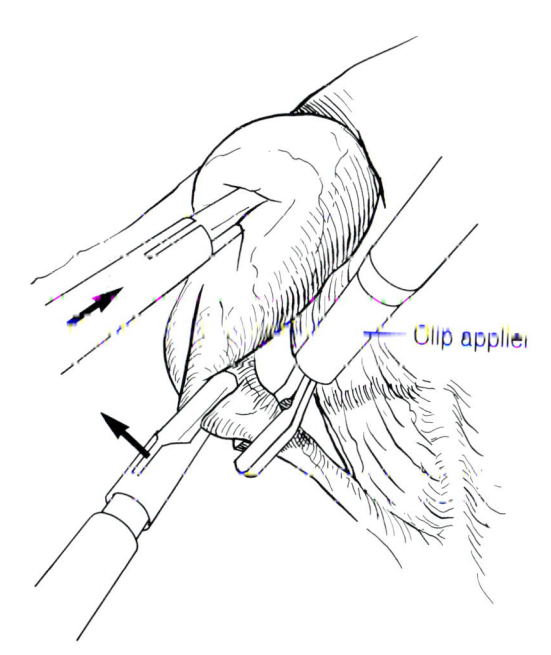

FIGURE 21-8 The peritoneal attachments of the gallblader to the liver are incised to create a window behind Hartmann's pouch, which may be viewed with the 30° laparoscope and allow for safe placement of a clip.

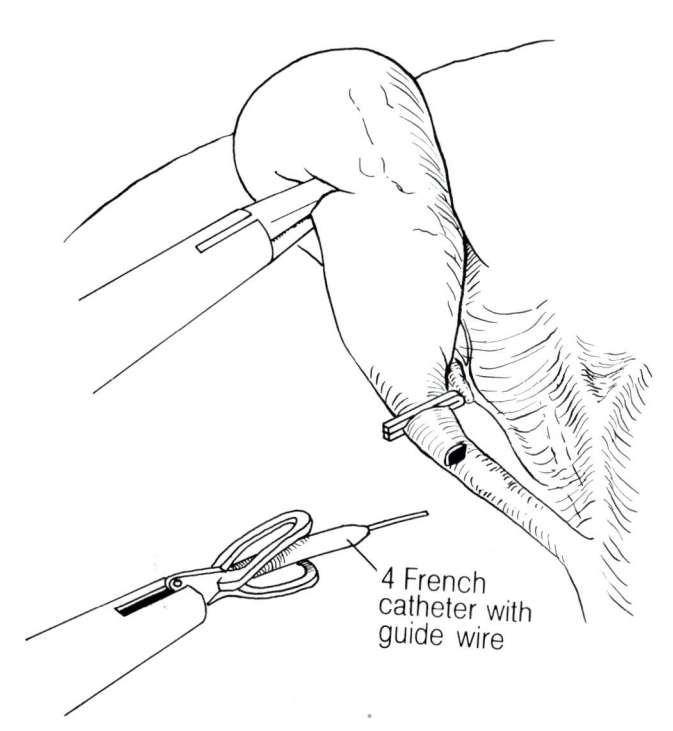

FIGURE 21-9 The cystic duct–gallbladder junction has been clipped and the cystic duct incised. A cholangio-grasper is introduced, which contains a 4-French ureteral catheter and guide wire to aid insertion.

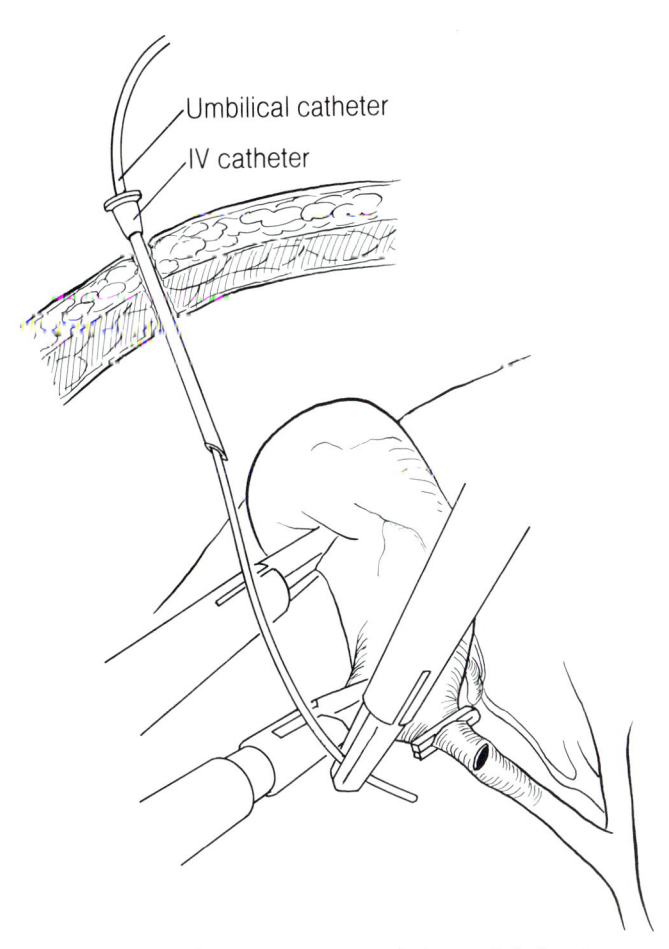

FIGURE 21-10 The percutaneous technique of cholangiography using an intravenous needle and umbilical catheter, which will be held in place by a clip.

There is a diverse range of cholangiocatheters available, some retaining by means of balloons, others by Malecot-type devices. If a metal trocar has been used in the subxiphisternal position, it may be replaced over a radiolucent trocar to prevent a shadow impeding interpretation of the cholangiogram.[57] The laparoscope should be withdrawn and the patient placed supine with the left side up to move the common duct away from the spine during the x-rays.

After satisfactory cholangiograms have been obtained (Fig. 21-11), the telescope is reintroduced and the trocar, repositioned. The cholangiocatheter is withdrawn, and the assistant surgeon again holds Hartmann's pouch. The cystic duct should be secured with either clips or pretied Roeder catgut loops. The latter are preferable because the migration of metal clips into the common bile duct from the cystic duct has been reported, with subsequent common duct stone formation (Fig. 21-12).[58] Even absorbable clips have been known to find their way into the common duct and cause symptoms.[59] If the cystic duct is extremely short, it may be tied in continuity before division.

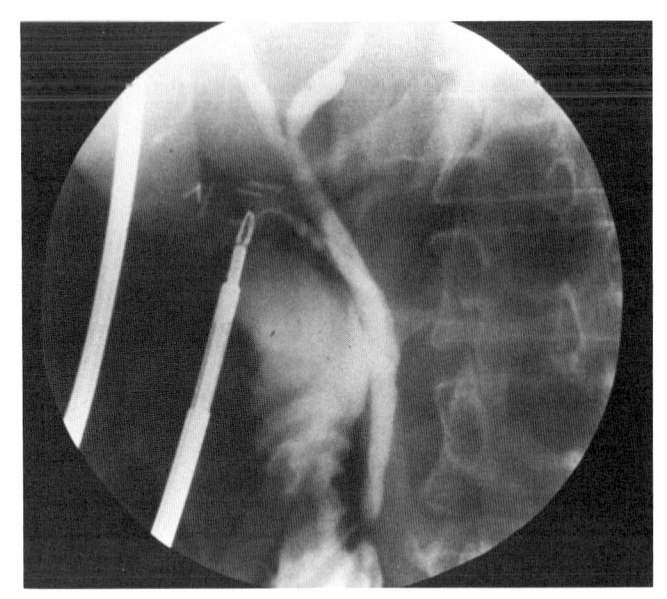

FIGURE 21-11 A normal intraoperative cholangiogram showing the entire extrahepatic ductal system, free flow into the duodenum, no filling defects or accessory ducts, and a long cystic duct segment, which may be safely secured.

One must then address the cystic artery. It is preferable to refrain from dividing this until the cystic duct has been dealt with because it helps to hold up structures toward the gallbladder. Obviously, if the cystic artery crosses the cystic duct, it may be necessary to clip and divide it first. Three clips are positioned, two below and one above, via the subxiphisternal portal, and the artery is then divided (Fig. 21-13).

The gallbladder is then dissected free of the liver by alternately retracting it laterally and dissecting the medial side and then bringing it medially and attacking the lateral aspect (Fig. 21-14A). Care must be taken to look for a posterior cystic artery lying in the liver bed or duct of Luschka, which may have been suggested during gallbladder filling on the cholangiogram. Just before the gallbladder has been totally removed from the liver bed, thorough irrigation and inspection should be carried out because, as a result of the retraction afforded by the gallbladder, this will be the surgeon's last opportunity to review the duct and artery thoroughly for secure closure (Fig. 21-14B).

After the gallbladder has been removed, the abdomen should be lavaged and aspirated. Because the parietal peritoneum is pain sensitive, it can be anesthetized by injecting 1% lidocaine with epinephrine 1:200,000, raising a wheal, and then injecting the skin incision of the xiphisternal and two lateral trocar sites (Fig. 21-15). The telescope should then be moved from the umbilical to the subxiphisternal

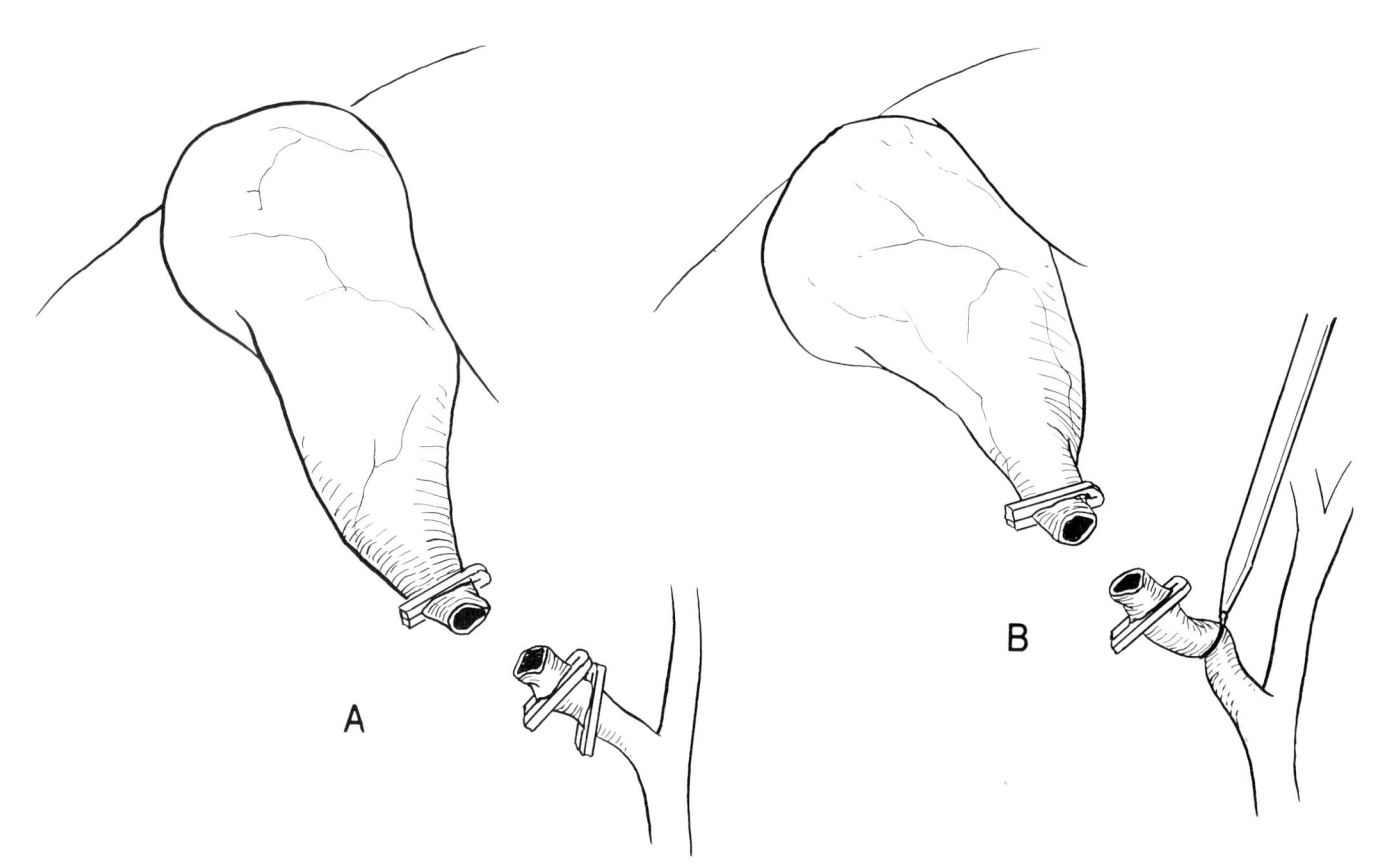

FIGURE 21-12 The cystic duct stump may be closed with (A) two clips, (B) a clip and a pretied Roeder loop, or if large, tied in continuity.

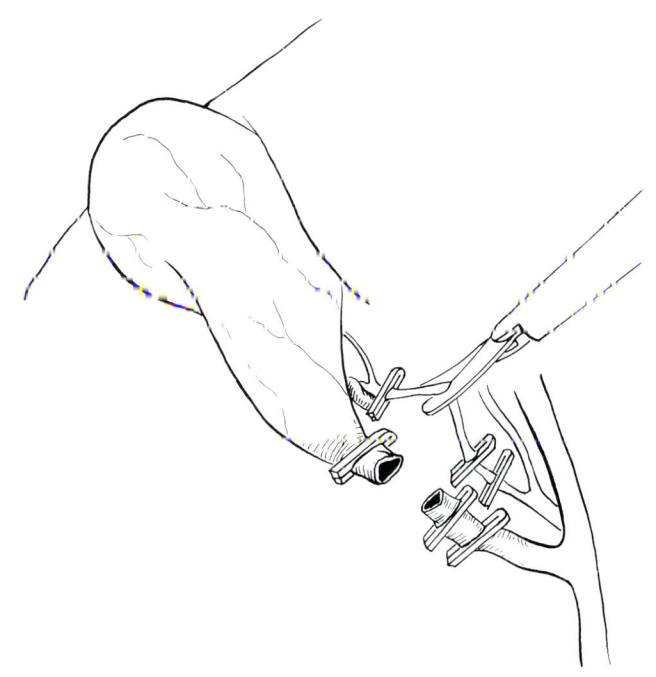

FIGURE 21-13 The cystic duct has been secured with two clips and the artery has been clipped. Both structures are divided.

position. This allows the surgeon to access the lower reaches of the abdomen adequately and permits removal of the gallbladder from the umbilicus, which is the thinnest part of the abdominal wall, the most easily extended incision, and the area most likely to become infected.

After the neck of the gallbladder has been grasped through the umbilical incision and brought out, the bile may be aspirated and the stone load reduced, allowing removal (Fig. 21-16). With a finger obstructing the umbilical incision, the scope should be used for a final review of the trocar insertion sites, and anesthesia may be introduced as before, raising a wheal on the peritoneum and in the skin before releasing the pneumoperitoneum and removing the instruments. When releasing the pneumoperitoneum, this should be done into damp gauze swabs or using a suction device to prevent the surgical team from inhaling this potentially virus-laden gas. The fascia at the umbilical incision should be closed with a strong absorbable suture and subcuticular sutures applied to all the incisions, which are then closed with adhesive strips. The patient should have the oro- or nasogastric tube and Foley catheter removed before transfer to the recovery area.

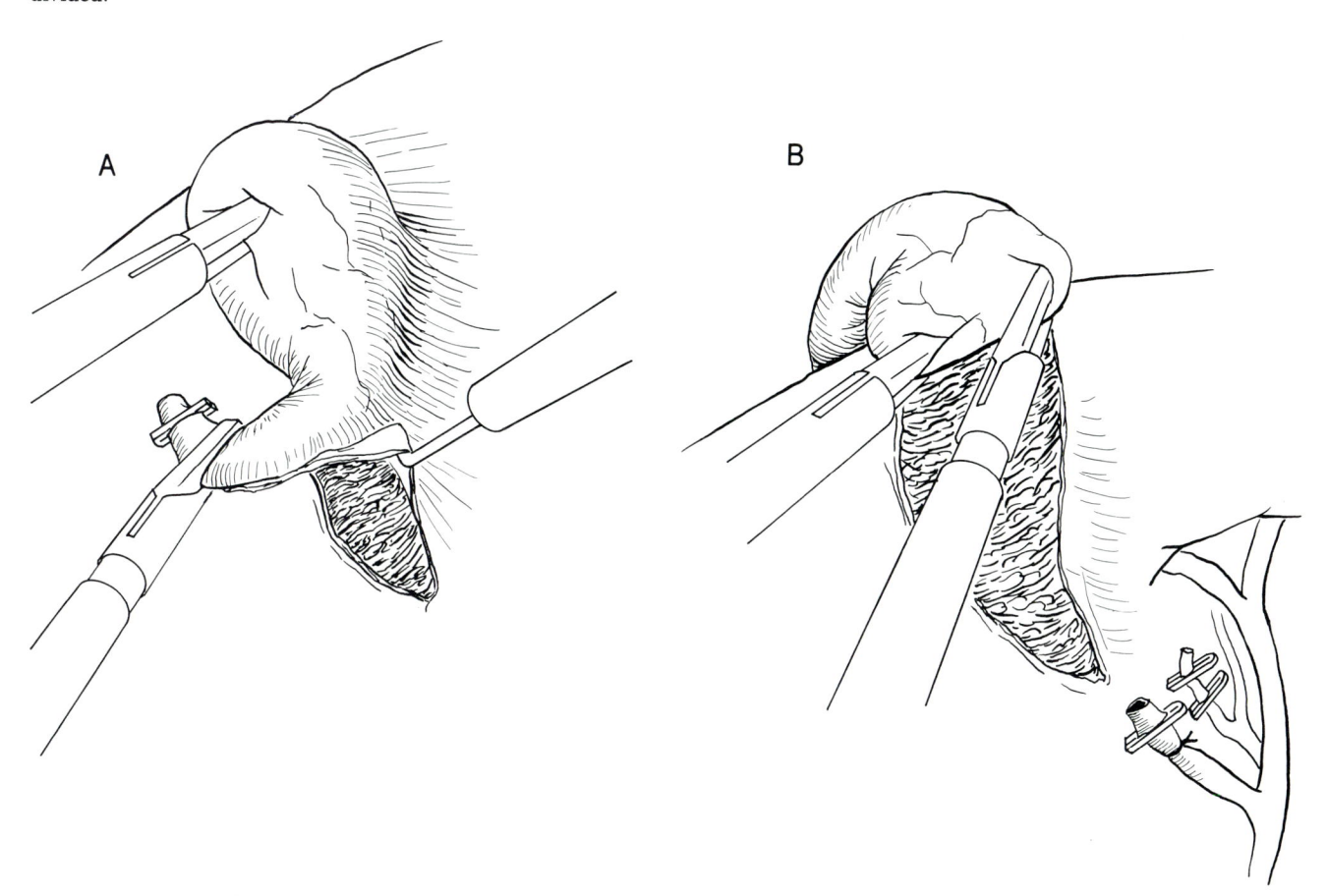

FIGURE 21-14 A. The gallbladder is dissected free of the liver by moving from medial to lateral and elevating the gallbladder to place the interposing tissue under tension, thus facilitating division. B. Before final removal, the elevated gallbladder allows the surgeon to review the liver bed, duct, and artery.

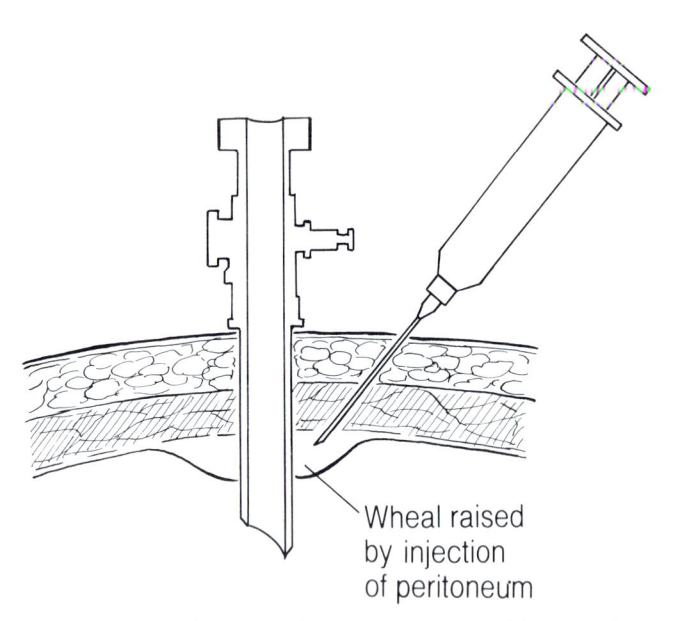

FIGURE 21-15 The parietal peritoneum is sensitive to pain and may be anesthetized with 1% lidocaine with epinephrine.

COMPLICATIONS AND RESULTS

Acute Cholecystitis

There are special problems attending this situation that should discourage surgeons from performing such procedures early in their experience. First, it may be difficult to grasp the gallbladder because of its thickened wall. It is useful to introduce a needle probe into the midclavicular portal, through which the gallbladder can be decompressed with a suction trap to obtain some fluid for culture (Fig. 21-17). If "white bile" is retrieved, this indicates to the surgeon that the cystic duct is blocked, and great care must be taken in dissection because there will often be a short cystic duct. If bile has been retrieved and the anatomy is not at all clear, cholecystocholangiography may be performed. If the patient is extremely ill and unlikely to tolerate a lengthy LC, discretion may be the better part of valor, and the surgeon should merely insert a cholecystostomy tube and terminate the procedure.[11,60]

To help define the anatomy, a Doppler probe to locate the cystic artery is useful. If the gallbladder is in continuity with the common bile duct, pressure on the gallbladder will cause a surge of bile through the cystic duct, which can be detected with the probe.

After the gallbladder has been decompressed, the hole can be closed with a pretied Roeder catgut loop, and this provides a "ledge," which can then be grasped. When removing an inflamed and possibly gangrenous gallbladder, a drain should be left in situ. There are many ways of inserting these, but the largest may be positioned by placing a grasper through the midclavicular portal and bringing it out through the subxiphisternal skin incision, using the trocar as a guide. The portion of the drain that will lay outside the abdomen is then grasped, brought across the abdominal wall, and then withdrawn from the midclavicular portal. The subxiphisternal trocar is then reinserted, and the drain is positioned.

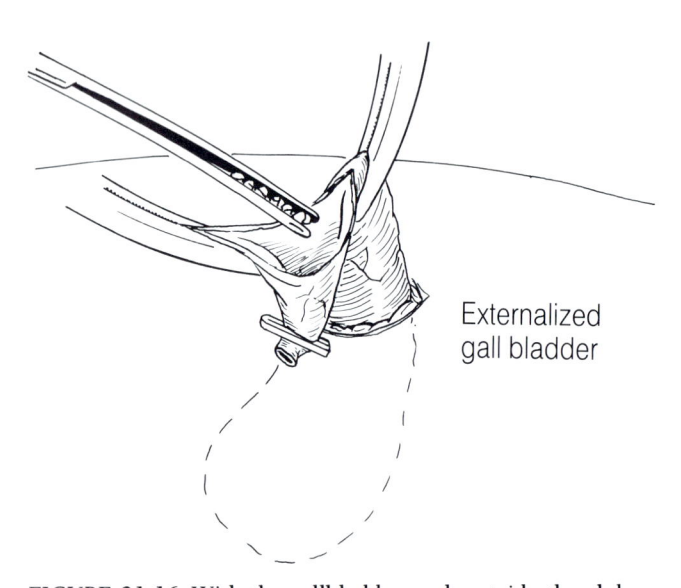

FIGURE 21-16 With the gallbladder neck outside the abdomen and swabs protecting the umbilical incision, bile is aspirated and stones removed with Randalls or Desjardins forceps.

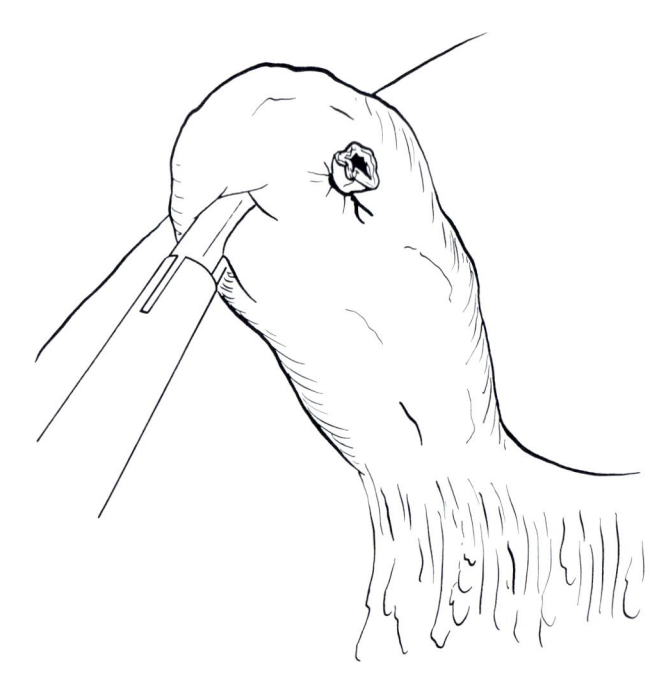

FIGURE 21-17 In acute cholecystitis, aspiration of bile and application of a Roeder loop allows the surgeon to grasp a "ledge" of tissue.

Bleeding

If a trocar site is seen to be oozing during the procedure, monopolar electrocautery can be used to control hemorrhage. During the case, a Foley catheter can be used, with the balloon inside the trocar wound to provide effective tamponade. If this is unsuccessful, especially in a patient with cirrhosis, a Keith needle can be inserted on one side of the trocar, retrieved within the abdominal cavity, and then passed in and out several more times to create a purse-string ligature around the trocar site that can be tied externally over a bolster for a couple of days. If bleeding is encountered during laparoscopic cholecystectomy, the first sign is usually loss of vision as a result of blood on the telescope. It should be withdrawn, irrigation and aspiration commenced, and, if necessary, an additional trocar positioned. If the bleeding seems to come from the area of the porta, the surgeon should not hesitate to open the patient because cautery or clip application here may make a minor injury fatal or may lead to a clip being inadvertently placed on the common bile duct.

When bleeding emanates from the liver bed, one may tamponade this by pressing the gallbladder into the liver bed, switching the fundal grasper to Hartmann's pouch, and using this latter grasper as a means of pressing against the bleeding area, a move described by Airan and Ko.[9] However, local hemostatic agents and cautery will usually suffice.

Spilled Stones

It is not uncommon, especially in acute cholecystitis or early in a surgeon's experience, to rupture the gallbladder and lose stones. When this happens, the surgeon should attempt to close the hole with a pretied Roeder catgut loop and aspirate the stones. Occasionally, many will be lost, and the use of bags to hold the spilled stones and the gallbladder is helpful (see Chap. 7). Alternatively, the 10-mm scoop forceps may be utilized to pick up stones. Initial literature reports suggested that these stones were of no consequence,[61] but there are sporadic reports currently of subphrenic and subhepatic abscesses as a result (Berci G. Personal communication, 1991). Therefore, it is probably judicious to administer additional antibiotics at this point in the procedure, thoroughly irrigate and aspirate the abdomen, and place a drain.

Occasionally, there will be too many stones within the gallbladder to allow easy removal from the abdominal wall. A number of possibilities exist. The first of these is to extend the umbilical incision, which appears not to increase pain medication requirements[63] and does little to negate the cosmetic advantage of laparoscopic surgery if the incision is made at the base of the umbilicus. Secondly, we may lift the stones out of the open gallbladder neck one at a time, but this is tiresome and frustrating.[61] Additionally, one runs the risk of perforating the gallbladder with Randall stone forceps. A third alternative is to fragment the gallstones with a rotary gallstone lithotrite, which has been shown experimentally to be efficacious and is useful in a number of circumstances.[65] It is important that the gallbladder be free of perforations because it may not achieve distention with saline, a necessary prerequisite of this technique of lithotripsy.

When to Convert to Open Cholecystectomy

It is much better for a surgeon to recognize that a procedure is progressing unsatisfactorily and convert by choice rather than be driven by necessity to open the patient. The well-prepared surgical team should have a large knife and a number of laparotomy pads present on the Mayo stand during every LC so that, if conversion is necessary, it can be undertaken rapidly, and an urgent situation, such as profuse hemorrhage, can be controlled while the laparotomy set is opened. As a rule of thumb, if the operation is not progressing after 1 h and no clear anatomy has been obtained, then conversion is a wise move. Obligatory conversion will occur if a visceral, vascular, or bile duct injury is detected and found to be laparoscopically nonrepairable. Detection of another pathologic condition and irretrievable loss of the gallbladder after its complete dissection (if fluoroscopy has failed to locate it) are other reasons to consider conversion.

Postoperative Management

After 2 h in the recovery room, the patient should be returned to the floor and commence a clear liquid diet upon awakening. Pain relief will be dictated by the patient's procedure and personality, but most require only oral, nonsteroidal anti-inflammatory drugs and, perhaps, one dose of a parenteral narcotic. An antiemetic should be administered, as required, and the patient encouraged to mobilize. Blood pressure, pulse, temperature, and respiration should, as usual, be followed regularly after surgery and then every 4 h thereafter. Most patients are freely mobile and using the toilet and eating by the same evening of surgery. The decision to allow patients to be discharged on the same day will depend on their personal circumstances, the procedure they have undergone, and the surgeon's comfort level.[66] It has already been such a major advance to send patients home after 1 day compared with the 5 or 6 days after conventional surgery that we are perhaps a little premature to consider same-day surgery in this setting. If, on the day after surgery, patients have fever, a change in hemodynamic parameters, vague symptoms or signs, they should be kept in the hospital and investigated because these may be the first indicators of bowel damage or ductal injury.

Initially, leukocyte count and liver function tests should

be taken and an ultrasound, performed, as required. If a bile duct injury is suspected, biliary scintigraphy is useful, and if this fails to show excretion of dye into the gastrointestinal tract, percutaneous drainage under CT scan guidance, followed by nasobiliary drainage instituted after endoscopic retrograde cholangiopancreatography, is valuable. If there is any postoperative concern about a patient's stability or if an injury to vascular, visceral, or ductal structures is thought to have occurred, laparotomy should be instituted forthwith.

REFERENCES

1. Langenbuch C: Ein Fall von Exterpation der Gallenblase wegen chronischer Cholelithiasis: Heilung. *Klin Wochenschr* 1882; 19:725–727.
2. McSherry C: The gold standard. *Am J Surg* 1989: 158:174–178.
3. Mühe E: The first cholecystectomy through the laparoscope. *Langenbecks Arch Chir* 1986; 369:804.
4. Perissat J, Collet D, Belliard R: Gallstones: Laparoscopic treatment—Cholecystectomy and lithotripsy. Our own technique. *Surg Endosc* 1990; 4:15–17.
5. Dubois F, Berthelot G, Levard H: Cholecystectomie par coelioscopie. *Presse Med* 1989; 18:980–982.
6. Reddick EJ, Olsen DO: Laparoscopic laser cholecystectomy. *Surg Endosc* 1989; 3:131–133.
7. McKernan JB, Saye WB: Laparoscopic general surgery. *J Med Assoc Ga* 1990; 79:157–159.
8. Berci G, Sackier JM, Paz-Partlow M: Laparoscopic cholecystectomy: Mini-access surgery—Reality or utopia? *Postgrad Gen Surg* 1990; 2:50–54.
9. Ko ST, Airan MC: Review of 300 consecutive laparoscopic cholecystectomies. Development, evolution and results. *Surg Endosc* 1991; 5:103–108.
10. Cuschieri A, Berci G, Sackier JM, et al: Clinical aspects of laparoscopic cholecystectomy, in Cuschieri A, Berci G (eds): *Laparoscopic Biliary Surgery.* London, Blackwell, 1990, pp 82–88.
11. Berci G, Cuschieri A: *Practical Laparoscopy.* London, Baillière Tindal, 1986.
12. Bailey RW, Imbembo AL, Zucker KA: Establishment of a laparoscopic cholecystectomy training program. *Am Surg* 1991; 57:231–236.
13. Sackier JM: Training and education in laparoscopic surgery, in Cuschieri A, Berci G (eds): *Laparoscopic Biliary Surgery.* London, Blackwell, 1990, pp 1–8.
14. Chamberlain GVP, Carron Brown JA: *Report of the Working Party of the Confidential Inquiry into Gynaecological Laparoscopy.* London, Royal College of Obstetricians and Gynaecologists, 1978.
15. Society of American Gastrointestinal Endoscopic Surgeons: Guidelines on privileging and credentialling: Standards of practice and continuing medical education of laparoscopic cholecystectomy. *Am J Surg* 1991; 161:324–325.
16. Moossa AR, Easter DW, van Sonnenberg E, et al: Laparoscopic injuries to the bile duct: A cause for concern. *Ann Surg* 1992; 215:203–208.
17. Nathanson LK, Shimi S, Cuschieri A: Laparoscopic cholecystectomy: The Dundee technique. *Br J Surg* 1991; 78:155–159.
18. Arvidsson D, Gerdin E: Laparoscopic cholecystectomy during pregnancy. *Surg Laparosc Endosc* 1991; 1:193–194.
19. Hunter JG: Laparoscopy in the pregnant patient. *Surg Endosc* 1992; 6:52–53.
20. Sackier JM: The complicated laparoscopic cholecystectomy. *Gastrointest Endosc Clin North Am,* in press.
21. Reddick EJ, Olsen DO, Spaw A, et al. Safe performance of difficult laparoscopic cholecystectomies. *Am J Surg* 1991; 161:377–381.
22. Siegel B, Golub RM, Loiacano L, et al: Technique of ultrasonic detection and mapping of abdominal wall adhesions. *Surg Endosc* 1991; 5:161–163.
23. Cooperman AM: Laparoscopic cholecystectomy for severe, acute, gangrenous cholecystitis. *J Laparoendosc Surg* 1990; 1:37–40.
24. Flowers JL, Bailey RW, Scovill WA, et al: The Baltimore experience with laparoscopic management of acute cholecystitis. *Am J Surg* 1991; 161:388–392.
25. Welch NT, Fitzgibbons RJ, Hinder RA: Beware of the porcelain gallbladder during laparoscopic cholecystectomy. *Surg Laparosc Endosc* 1991; 1:202–205.
26. Gomel V: Laparoscopy. *Can Med Assoc J* 1974; 111:167–169.
27. Sackier JM, Berci G, Paz-Partlow M: Elective diagnostic laparoscopy. *Am J Surg* 1991; 161:326–331.
28. Sarti DA: *Diagnostic Ultrasound: Text and Cases.* Chicago, Year Book Medical, 1987, pp 142–213.
29. Berci G, Sackier JM, Paz-Partlow M: A new endoscopic treatment for symptomatic gallbladder disease—Laparoscopic cholecystectomy. *Gastrointest Endosc Clin North Am* 1991; 1:191–203.
30. Shantha TR, Harden J: Laparoscopic cholecystectomy: Anesthesia related complications and guidelines. *Surg Laparosc Endosc* 1991; 1:173–178.
31. Nagai H, Kondo Y, Yasuda T, et al: A new method of laparoscopic cholecystectomy and other abdominal surgery: An abdominal wall-life technique not utilizing peritoneal insufflation. *Surg Endosc* 1992; 6:87.
32. Kitano S, Moriyama M, Sugimachi K: A newly designed U-shaped retractor for laparoscopic cholecystectomy. *Surg Endosc* 1992; 6:101.
33. Voyles CR, Meena AL, Petro AB, et al: Electrocautery is superior to laser for laparoscopic cholecystectomy (editorial). *Am J Surg* 1990; 160:457.
34. Easter DW, Moossa AR: Laser and laparoscopic cholecystectomy: A hazardous union. *Arch Surg* 1991; 126:423–424.
35. Olsen DO, Corbitt JD, Edelman DS, et al: Clinical experience using a bipolar electrosurgical device for laparoscopic cholecystectomy. *Surg Endosc* 1992; 6:104.
36. Reddick EJ, Olsen DO: Laparoscopic laser cholecystectomy: A comparison with mini-lap cholecystectomy. *Surg Endosc* 1989; 3:131–133.
37. Bordelon BM, Hobday KA, Hunter JG: Laser versus electrosurgery in laparoscopic cholecystectomy: A prospective, randomized trial. *Arch Surg,* in press.
38. Nezhat C, Nezhat FR: Safe laser endoscopic excision or vaporization of peritoneal endometriosis. *Fertil Steril* 1989; 52:149–151.
39. Wetter LA, Payne J, Kirschenbaum G, et al: The ultrasonic dissector (CUSA) facilitates laparoscopic cholecystectomy. *Arch Surg,* in press.
40. Paz-Partlow M: Documentation for laparoscopy, in Berci G, Cuschieri A (eds): *Practical Laparoscopy.* London, Baillière Tindal, 1986, pp 19–32.
41. Veress J: Neues Instrument zue Ausfuhrung von Brust Oder Bauchpunktionen. *Dtsch Med Wochenschr* 1938; 41:1480–1481.
42. Corson SL, Batzer FR, Gocial B, et al: Measurement of the force necessary for laparoscopic trocar entry. *J Reprod Med* 1989; 44:282–284.
43. Ko ST, Airan MC: Therapeutic laparoscopic suturing techniques. *Surg Endosc* 1992; 6:41–46.
44. Sackier JM, Berci G, Phillips E, et al: The role of cholangiography in laparoscopic cholecystectomy. *Arch Surg* 1991; 126:1021–1026.

45. Flowers JL, Zucker KA, Graham SM, et al: Laparoscopic cholangiography: Results and indications. *Ann Surg* 1992; 215:209–216.
46. Berci G: Cholangiography and choledochoscopy during laparoscopic cholecystectomy, its place and value. *Dig Surg* 1991; 8:92–96.
47. Berci G, Hamlin JA: *Operative Biliary Radiology*. Baltimore, Williams and Wilkins, 1981, pp 63–109.
48. Hardy JE, Rose SC, Nieves AS, et al: Intraoperative cholangiography: Use of portable fluroscopy and transmitted images. *Radiology* 1991; 181:205–207.
49. Wittgen CM, Andrus CH, Fitzgerald SD, et al: Analysis of the hemodynamic and ventilatory effects of laparoscopic cholecystectomy. *Arch Surg* 1991; 126:997–1001.
50. Doctor HN, Hussain Z: Bilateral pneumothorax associated with laparoscopy: A case report of a rare hazard and review of the literature. *Anesthesiology* 1973; 28:75–81.
51. Palmer R: Security in laparoscopy, in, Phillips JM, Keith L (eds): *Gynecological Laparoscopy: Principles and Techniques*. New York, Symposia Specialists Medical Books, 1974, pp 17–26.
52. Hasson HM: Open laparoscopy vs. closed laparoscopy. A comparison of complication rates. *Adv Planned Parenthood* 1978; 13:41–43.
53. Hennington MH, Croom RD, Koruda MJ, et al. The importance of intra-abdominal laparoscopic examination during laparoscopic cholecystectomy. *N C Med J* 1991; 52:545–546.
54. Hunter JG: Avoidance of bile duct injury during laparoscopic cholecystectomy. *Am J Surg* 1991; 162:71–76.
55. Phillips EH, Berci G, Carroll B, et al: The importance of intraoperative cholangiography during laparoscopic cholecystectomy. *Am Surg* 1990; 56:789–795.
56. Petelin J: Laparoscopic approach to common duct pathology. *Surg Laparosc Endosc* 1991; 1:33–41.
57. Berci G, Sackier JM, Paz-Partlow M: New ideas and improved instrumentation for laparoscopic cholecystectomy. *Surg Endosc* 1991; 5:1–3.
58. Janson JA, Cotton PB: Endoscopic treatment of bile duct stone containing a surgical staple. *HPB Surg* 1990; 3:67–71.
59. Onghena T, Vereecken L, Vanden Dwey K, et al: Common bile duct foreign body: an unusual case. *Surg Laparosc Endosc* 1992; 2:8–10.
60. Perissat J, Collet DR, Belliard R: Gallstones: Laparoscopic treatment, intracorporeal lithotripsy followed by cholecystostomy or cholecystectomy—A personal technique. *Endoscopy* 1989; 21:373–374.
61. Soper NJ, Dunnegan DL: Does intraoperative gallbladder perforation influence the early outcome of laparoscopic cholecystectomy? *Surg Laparosc Endosc* 1991; 1:156–161.
62. Ponsky JL: Complications of laparoscopic cholecystectomy. *Am J Surg* 1991; 161:393–395.
63. Bordelon B, Hobday K, Hunter JG: Incision extension is the optimal method to remove the large gallbladder in laparoscopic cholecystectomy. *Surg Endosc* 1992; 6:225–227.
64. Donohue JH, Grant CS, Farnell MB, et al: Laparoscopic cholecystectomy: Operative technique. *Mayo Clin Proc* 1992; 67:441–448.
65. Sackier JM, Hunter JG, Paz-Partlow M, et al: The rotary gallstone Lithotrite to aid gallbladder extraction in laparoscopic cholecystectomy. *Surg Endosc* 1992; 6:235–238.
66. Reddick EJ, Olsen DO: Outpatient laparoscopic laser cholecystectomy. *Am J Surg* 1990; 160:485–489.

Common Bile Duct Exploration

Lee L. Swanstrom

The need for addressing the necessity and preferred methods of common bile duct exploration (CBDE) in the current climate of minimally invasive surgery is imperative. The technique of laparoscopic cholecystectomy has taken the surgical community by storm to the point that it has become apparent that the majority of cholecystectomies done in the United States during the 1990s will be performed with this technique. Lagging behind our knowledge of current options for gallbladder removal is our understanding of the indications for cholangiography and how to deal with abnormal findings, whether encountered preoperatively or postoperatively. An 8 to 14 percent incidence of common duct calculi during cholecystectomy has been well documented.[1,2] Less described, but certainly present, is the occurrence of common duct pathologic conditions other than bile duct stones. Berci and Shore[3] have noted an 11 percent incidence of noncalculus pathologic findings encountered during CBDE. Considering the large number of cholecystectomies done worldwide every year, the amount of common duct disease to be dealt with is not insignificant.

During the initial learning phase of laparoscopic cholecystectomy, the preoperative suspicion of choledocholithiasis represented a relative contraindication for the laparascopic approach.[4] This conservative approach soon fell victim to the generalized collapse of most of the contraindications to the procedure and to the futility of trying to determine preoperatively the presence of common duct disease. Abandonment of the avoidance technique of dealing with common duct pathologic conditions was hastened by the development of techniques and equipment to perform CBDE laparoscopically.

There also seems to be a widespread feeling that the majority of common duct stones found incidentally will pass without complication. Unfortunately, complications, when they do occur, can be catastrophic, and there are no reliable criteria to differentiate safe stones from dangerous ones. At the end of the 1980s, it was readily apparent that minimally invasive approaches to common duct disease were needed. Three philosophic approaches were advocated: preemptive treatment, intraoperative surgical techniques, or postoperative damage control.

Preoperative detection of all stones requires a high index of suspicion and liberal indications for preoperative cholangiography. When stones stones are present, treatment can consist of preoperative endoscopic retrograde cholangiopancreatography (ERCP)/sphincterotomy,[5] extracorporeal shock-wave lithotripsy,[6] transhepatic retrieval,[7] or dissolution therapy.[8] The problem with the preoperative approach is obvious; up to 85 percent of patients with no common duct abnormalities may be suspected to harbor stones based on current methods of preoperative assessment[9] and will, therefore, receive unneeded intervention at great expense and great potential for complication.

A much more acceptable approach has been taken by a large number of surgeons, that is, to deal with abnormal cholangiograms or postoperative symptoms after the patient has recovered from the laparoscopic operation. The rationale is, of course, to avoid unnecessary preoperative studies, false-positive intraoperative cholangiograms, and clinically irrelevant findings. This approach relies primarily on the use of postoperative ERCP for retrograde stone removal. This approach is not without its costs, failures (11 to 30 percent), and complications (8 to 12 percent).[10–12] In spite of these drawbacks, postoperative ERCP has been a popular alternative to converting to open CBDE even though the latter is probably preferable on the basis of efficacy, patient safety, and cost effectiveness.[13]

Our own preference has been to perform routine cholangiography and laparoscopic CBDE (LCBDE) for positive findings. This avoids unnecessary procedures related to false-positive preoperative assessment and, by dealing with them all, skirts the issue of whether some stones could be left alone. It also obviates a second postoperative procedure, with its risks, costs, and patient discomfort.

TECHNIQUE OF LCBDE

There are three basic approaches to LCBDE, each with varying demands for equipment, technical proficiency, and potential for success. The ultimate goal should be for surgeons who perform laparoscopic cholecystectomy to become proficient in all three methods because each is probably useful in at least some cases.

The technique LCBDE is based on several precepts that run counter to prevailing practices of open CBDE. One of these is the preferability of transcystic duct exploration, the main benefit of which is the avoidance of having to open the common duct. Although exploration is easy through a choledochotomy, the opening must then be closed, and T-tube placement and/or suture repair of the choledochotomy probably represents the most technically delicate laparoscopic procedure currently performed. Certainly, the consequences of an error are disastrous. Bile leaks are annoying, and common duct strictures are disabling or even life threatening. Transcyst duct exploration has been advocated for open cases in the past.[14] However, in spite of persuasive arguments and good results, this technique has failed to gain wide acceptance over more traditional approaches. Today, with the majority of LCBDEs being successfully performed through the cystic duct, the logic of this approach is being vindicated.

A second concept, which had been advocated and defended but never widely accepted until the advent of LCBDE, is that of selective common bile duct drainage after exploration. A classic paper on this approach was published in the 1960s by Sawyers and associates,[15] which presented excellent results after exploration and primary repair of the choledochotomy. Common duct drainage was reserved for cases that did not drain after exploration, usually because of sphincter spasm. Although it is easy laparoscopically to place a single limb common duct drain via the cystic duct and possible to place a T-tube, not having to do either significantly simplifies both the procedure and postoperative care.

Two other technical concepts, although less explicitly stated and more generally accepted, have had an impact on the development and acceptance of LCBDE: direct visualization as the "gold standard" for exploration and the benefit of minimizing ductal and ampullary trauma by using refined technique and instrumentation. Many of the same instruments and techniques used to achieve the latter goal are also used in LCBDE, and choledochoscopy or fluoroscopic visualization is necessitated by the lack of tactile input so heavily relied on in techniques of the past.

Fluoroscopically Directed Stone Removal

Fluoroscopically guided common duct stone retrieval (FGSR) is a technique lifted directly from the urologic armamentarium, as have been most of the laparoscopic common duct techniques. It has been called both the *blind technique* and the *low-tech approach,* although these descriptions are true in only a relative sense. Attempts to perform this technique without radiologic visualization or with inadequate instrumentation will only create frustration for the surgeon and offer potential harm to the patient.

EQUIPMENT

The equipment needed is simpler than that required for other exploration methods but no less critical. It includes the following:

1. A cholangiography setup; we use a 4-French ureteral catheter and a cholangiogram (Olsen) clamp (model no. 28378CH, Karl Storz, Culver City, CA).
2. A high-resolution imaging system, preferably a digital fluoroscopy unit.
3. 4- and 5-French six-wire helical stone retrieval baskets with soft filiform leaders (e.g., model no. GU6354, Baxter, Deerfield, IL).
4. A long (22-cm) introducer sheath with an airtight gasket (Karl Storz) for wires and baskets.
5. 4-French vascular embolectomy catheter.
6. An extra 5-mm trocar.
7. Glucagon for ampullary relaxation.
8. Pretied suture ligatures (endoloops) and 5-mm round closed suction drains are sometimes needed.

The instruments required and initial trocar placement are unchanged from that in routine laparoscopic cholecystectomy, which is not surprising considering the frequency of abnormal cholangiograms that were unsuspected preoperatively. Using FGSR, it is frequently possible to perform the stone retrieval using the midclavicular 5-mm port. Unless the cystic duct is very broad and short, however, this can sometimes be difficult because of the acute angles involved, and we currently routinely place a fifth 5-mm port immediately below the costal margin in the midclavicular line for all methods of LCBDE (Fig. 22-1). An alternative to this for FGSR is to use a 14- or 16-French angiocatheter instead of a trocar, a method previously described for cholangiography.[16]

We inject 1 mg of glucagon, an effective smooth muscle relaxant, intravenously when a common duct pathologic condition is found by cholangiography. This relaxes the sphincter of Oddi, easing the passage of instruments into the duodenum, and minimizing trauma to the distal duct.

Another area where frustration can be avoided is in the use of imaging equipment. Although this procedure can be done using standard radiographs, the need constantly to confirm the presence of the basket is awkward and time consuming. Most operating rooms have high-resolution real-time fluoroscopy equipment for vascular, urologic, and orthopedic applications, which lends itself nicely to this technique and should be used, if at all possible. Digitally enhanced units can deliver images that equal or surpass those of still films.[17] Leaving a free passage for the C-arm to

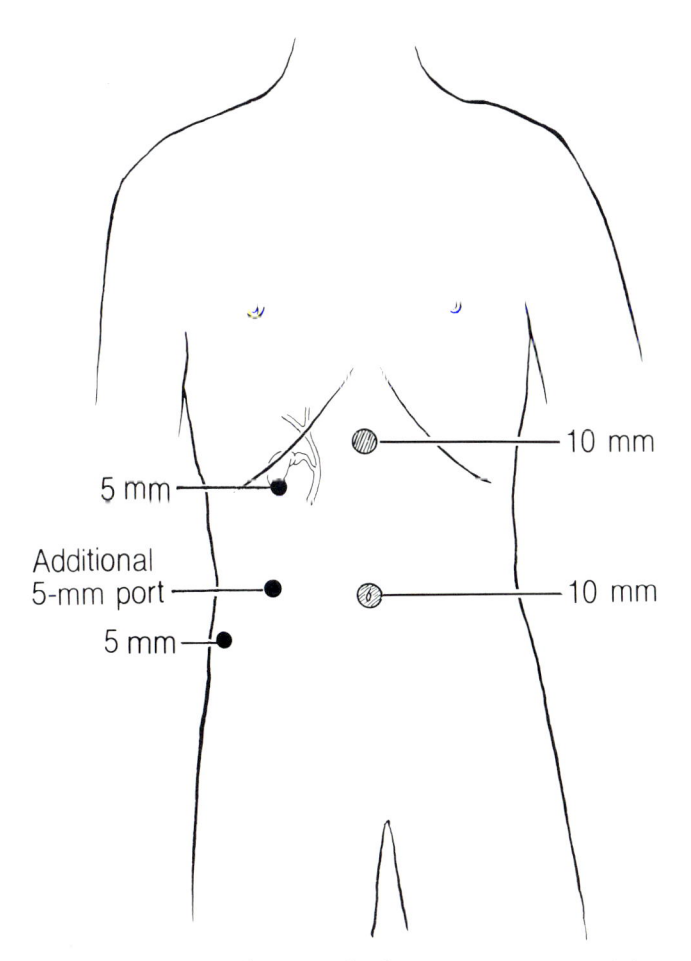

FIGURE 22-1 Port placement for laparoscopic common bile duct exploration (LCBDE). Standard port placement is enhanced by the addition of a 5-mm port to access the proximal common bile duct with the choledochoscope.

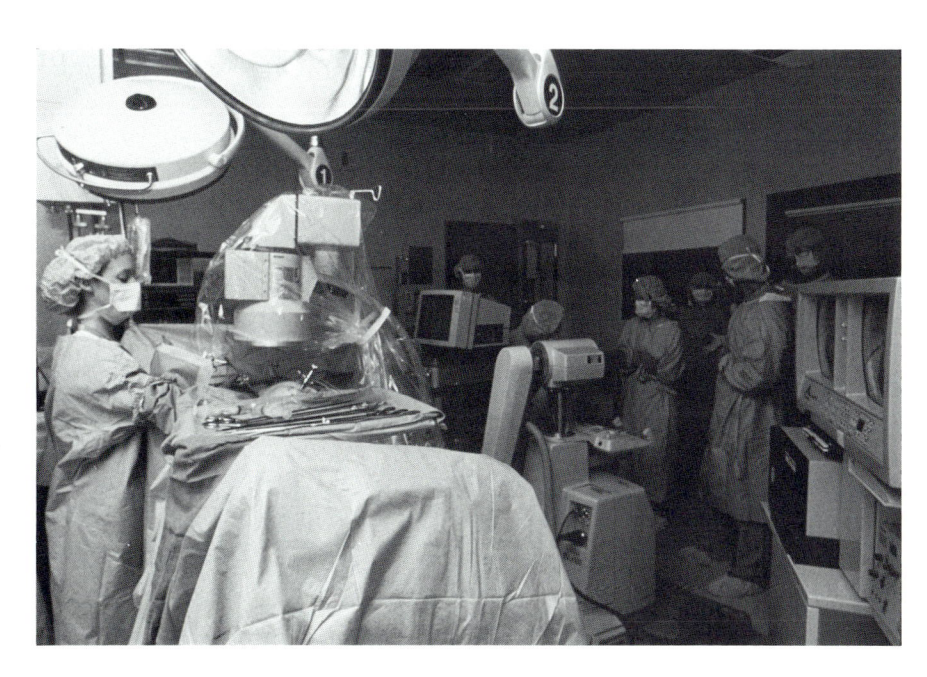

FIGURE 22-2 Operating room setup for fluoroscopic cholangiography and LCBDE. the C-arm enters from the patient's left, the x-ray monitors are placed off the left foot of the table, and the surgeon stands behind a sterile draped lead shield on the right of the patient.

enter from the patient's left, free from all table supports, is the first step toward successful FGSR (Fig. 22-2).

The baskets used are of key importance. Baskets less than 4 French tend to be too soft to pass on their own and are also very fragile; those greater than 5 French are much too stiff to thread into the common duct safely. There also are many basket wire configurations, and for this application, a helical basket is an absolute necessity (Fig. 22-3). While withdrawing the basket back through the common duct, the surgeon twists the catheter in a clockwise manner; this both opens the basket wires and tunnels the stone into the tightly woven apex of the basket, where it will remain until the surgeon closes the basket for removal (Fig. 22-4). This is in contrast to the straight wire Sugura-type basket (Fig. 22-5), which must be placed precisely around the stone and carefully tightened to hold the stone for removal, a procedure obviously requiring direct visualization.

The number of wires comprising the basket also is important. Between three and eight wires are available, but a four- or six-wire basket is most often used for common duct work; the choice depends on the size of the stones. The smaller the stone is, the more wires are needed to trap and hold it. Conversely, large stones will not be able to work their way between closely spaced wires; therefore, a three- or four-wire basket would be more effective.

Vascular embolectomy catheters can sometimes be helpful in dislodging impacted stones and repositioning a stone for engagement by the basket. Similar catheters designed for open biliary duct work are too short, and depending on the duct size, 2- to 5-French Fogarty-type embolectomy catheters are usually what is needed. The smaller-sized catheters come with an optional stiffening stylet, which is necessary to pass the catheter past stones or other instruments.

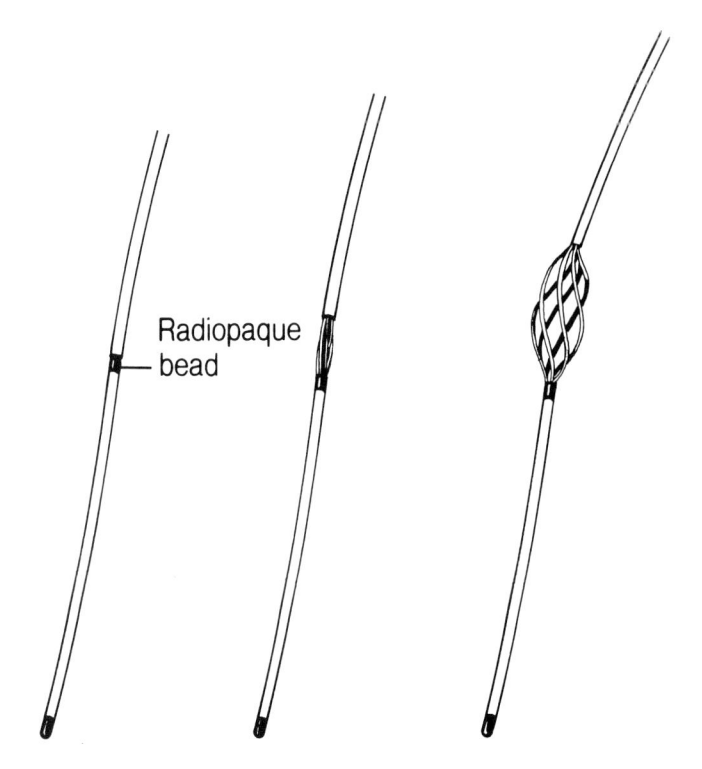

FIGURE 22-3 A six-wire helical stone basket is used for fluoroscopic transcystic bile duct exploration. This basket is preceded by a soft filiform tip, which prevents injury to the bile duct or duodenum. A radiopaque bead marks the position of the basket, and as the sheath is slowly withdrawn, the basket opens.

Endoloops are used to secure any cystic ducts that require dilatation, are especially large, or look abused at the completion of stone removal. Not dividing the cystic artery before duct closure helps in the application of the endoloop by preventing the transsected duct from retracting into the porta hepatis. A closed suction drain is occasionally necessary for similar indications, namely, tenuous closure of the cystic duct stump or the possibility of small guidewire or closed-basket perforations. The 5-mm round drains are easily inserted and directed via one of the lateral 5-mm ports and are easily removed before the patient goes home if they have drained no bile.

PROCEDURE NOTES

Our current method of performing FGSR is as follows. When a true-positive cholangiogram is obtained (false-positive ones are aggressively ruled out by various maneuvers, including saline flushes, repeated films, real-time contrast injections, and tilting the patient to spot air bubbles), the anesthesiologist is instructed to administer intravenously 1 mg of glucagon. The cholangiocatheter is left in position, and an additional 5-mm port is placed as shown in Figure 22-1.

An appropriately sized helical stone basket is loaded into a 5 mm guide, using either a second cholangiogram clamp or a catheter guide with an airtight reducing nipple. While counter traction is applied on the distal gallbladder via the subxiphoid port, the closed stone basket is inserted into the cystic duct alongside the cholangiocatheter from the first assistant's side of the table (the patient's right). The basket is gently advanced until it meets resistance, usually representing the stone or the ampulla. At this time, the C-arm is prepared and brought into position, usually from the left side of the table.

Dilute contrast medium is injected under real-time fluoroscopy to ascertain the position of the basket relative to the stone. While watching the x-ray monitor, the closed basket is gently pushed past the stone and through the ampulla. Under visualization, the basket is opened after it is in the proper position between the stone and the ampulla. It is extremely important not to open the basket while it is still in the duodenum and then try to pull it back through the ampulla because there have been instances of the basket capturing a slightly prolapsed papilla and becoming trapped or causing a serious laceration. It is equally important not to open the basket while advancing the catheter because the basket can capture the stone while advancing and carry it through the ampulla into the duodenum. Because of the one-way valve-like nature of the ampullary sphincter, the basket with stone often will not reenter the common duct, and by design, stones are difficult to dislodge from a helical basket. Opening the patient or an upper endoscopy soon follows.

After the basket is in a satisfactory position, it is opened and, using clockwise twisting, pulled past the stone. Capture of the stone is confirmed by watching it move with the basket on the fluoroscope. The basket is then slowly closed and withdrawn from the cystic duct. This process is repeated as many times as needed as indicated by repeated cholangiograms. If ampullary spasm occurs with repeated instrumentation, additional glucagon can be given, or gentle dilatation of the sphincter with a 4-French Fogarty balloon catheter can be performed. Caution should be used to avoid overaggressive dilatation because reports have implicated such maneuvers in severe postprocedural pancreatitis.[18]

Basket retrieval works best if the stone is free in the duct so the basket wires can fully expand. Impacted distal stones can sometimes be dislodged by slipping an embolectomy catheter past the stone, inflating the balloon, and slowly pulling back. Care must be taken not to withdraw stones too far back, or they will end up in the relatively inaccessible proximal bile ducts. Other tricks that occasionally work include vigorously irrigating the stone with a catheter placed in the distal duct and opening and closing the basket when it directly overlies the stone, as indicated by fluoroscopy. Obviously, all tricks occasionally fail, and a decision must be made whether to progress to another method of LCBDE or convert to an open procedure.

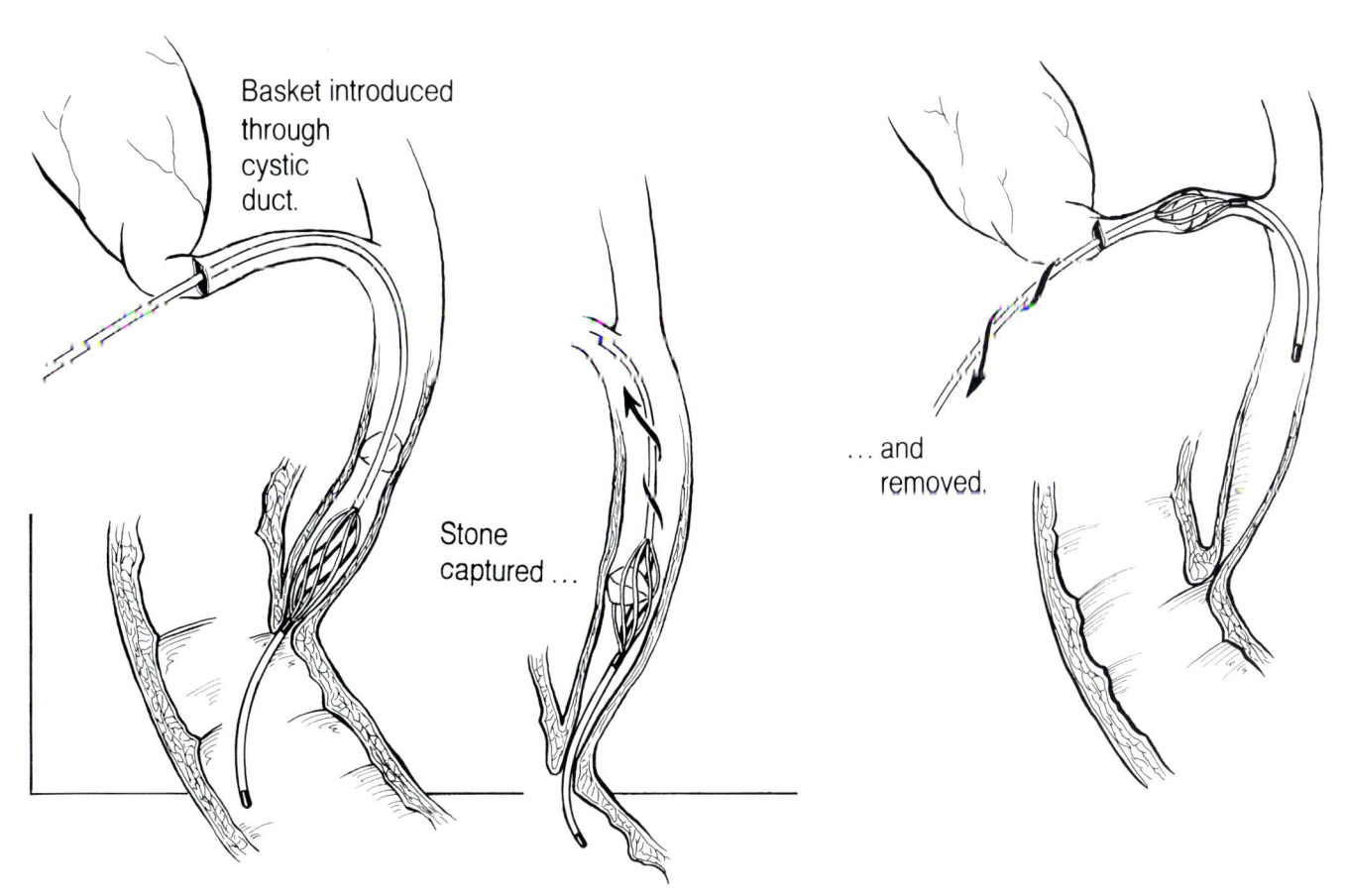

FIGURE 22-4 After fluoroscopic confirmation of basket position has been obtained, the basket is rotated clockwise as it is withdrawn. This entraps the stone within the helical cage. When the cystic duct orifice is reached, the basket is closed and, with continued clockwise rotation, pulled from the cystic dochotomy.

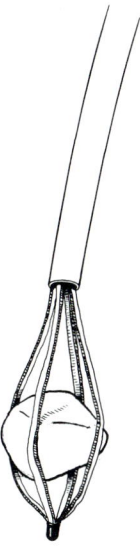

FIGURE 22-5 For choledochoscopic stone extraction, a three- or 4-flat wire stone basket is used. Here a stone is seen captured within the basket.

Rarely, the common duct stone will be larger than the cystic duct diameter. This is unusual considering where the stone came from and, unfortunately, is usually only discovered after the stone has been captured. Almost always, slow progressive pressure while closing the stone basket will crush the stone. If not, a balloon dilator can be advanced into the cystic duct alongside the basket and the duct dilated enough to permit removal of the stone. Any stone larger and harder than these tricks will handle is best treated by some other procedure.

Stones in the proximal common duct present a problem for FGSR. Current stone baskets are not steerable and, unless the ductal anatomy happens to lend itself to it, usually are not able to be maneuvered into the proximal ducts. Irrigation or patient repositioning may bring the stone into the distal duct. If not, an alternative procedure is again necessary.

One difficulty in performing FGSR is the inability to pass the stone basket through the cystic duct. This can often be handled by adjusting the angle of attack, improving countertraction, or switching to a smaller-sized catheter. Occasionally, a closed basket will be seen on the fluoro-monitor to perforate the cystic or common duct. It is extremely important not to open the basket if it has violated the common duct wall because this could turn a clinically insignificant perforation into a 1-cm rent. The message here is to use imaging at all times to confirm basket placement.

Engaging the stone can be a problem at times. Aside from previously discussed techniques of stone dislodgement and rotating the basket to the correct position, we should consider changing to a basket with more or less wires (depending on the stone size) or trying to pull the stone into a wider portion of the duct with an embolectomy catheter. Finally, if a basket with a stone should become stuck, try to crush or release the stone, but do not hesitate to perform an esophagogastroduodenoscopy or open procedure. It is much better in the end to do a minor second procedure than to deal with a torn or avulsed common duct or duodenum.

The rate of successful explorations by FGSR is good in some hands,[19] although not as high as with other methods. Also, the reported risk of complication is fairly high. In our rather limited experience with this technique, we have had three failed attempts, one common duct perforation, one ampullary laceration with bleeding, and only two successful retrievals. None of these complications required intervention or had adverse clinical sequelae, but we have been asked to consult on an incident of a stone and basket becoming trapped in the duodenum, which required an open procedure with duodenotomy.

Choledochoscopy

Distress with the limitations of the basket retrieval method, our understanding of the current state of the art for open CBDE, and our own prelaparoscopy clinical approach to common duct stones have made choledochoscopy the mainstay of our approach to LCBDE. Although technically more involved than FGSR, it is both safer and more effective, while preserving the advantages of a transcystic-duct minimally invasive procedure.

Choledochoscopy was first described by Bakes[20] in 1923, and it has subsequently undergone a slow evolution from a cumbersome experimental technique with crude rigid instruments to a fast and simple procedure, which, in the last decade, has become the new gold standard for CBDE.[21-23] The primary factor in the replacement of the so-called Bakes dilator and Randall forceps school of exploration with choledochoscopic techniques was the fiberoptic revolution of the late 1970s and '80s. The availability of small flexible easy-to-use endoscopes, with excellent optics and useful working channels, combined with a newly demonstrated need to decrease ductal trauma, dramatically increased the acceptance of the technique. Indeed, the incidence of retained stones and complications of explorations decreased markedly with the employment of choledochoscopy in open CBDE and provided excellent results; thus, we saw no reason to change when we began performing laparoscopic explorations.

Equipment

The equipment needed for choledochoscopic exploration is more technologically advanced, expensive, and generally less available than that used for other techniques. On the other hand, most, if not all, of the needed equipment is used by urologists for nephroureteral procedures, and purchasing these instruments for dual departmental use is often a possibility. The equipment needed is as follows:

1. Routine cholangiography equipment (see previous description under FGSR section).
2. Two complete camera setups or, alternatively, a dual-head split-screen device (e.g., model no. GS9400-S, Solos Medusacam, Norcross, GA).
3. An assortment of soft-tip guide wires, 0.018 to 0.038 cm in diameter and 145 cm in length.
4. Coaxial balloon dilators e.g., a 5-French catheter with a 15-French by 4-cm balloon (e.g., model no. 72401260 Baxter).
5. Flexible choledochoscope, primarily a 9- to 10-French steerable scope with a 1.2-mm working channel, e.g., model no. 511276, Storz; model no. AUR 9, American ACMI, (Stamford, CT); or model no. URF-P2, Olympus, (Lake Success, NY); but on occasion, a 4-French scope is useful (e.g., model no. AF14, Olympus).
6. Stone baskets (e.g., 3-French, three- or four-wire Segura-type baskets (model no. 319-103, Microvasive, Watertown, MA).
7. Lithotripter units, either a pulsed-dye laser or a electrohydraulic lithotriptor, are extremely useful if available.
8. Glucagon, 1 mg, for sphincter relaxation.
9. Pretied endoloops to ligate the cystic duct securely usually stretched and thinned out, after the exploration.
10. A 5-mm round closed suction drain.

It is possible to perform laparoscopic choledochoscopy with a single camera setup, but this is awkward at best. It is necessary to switch the camera head constantly between laparoscope and choledochoscope, leaving a critical blind spot either intraabdominally or inside the duct. Current split-screen setups or, alternatively, a second complete camera setup wired to one of the monitors greatly streamlines the procedure, both technically and with regard to time, and is probably worth the extra cost.

An array of guide wires is useful with this technique. They aid in insertion by stiffening and guiding scopes and other instruments, or they can be used as probes to palpate, manipulate, and dislodge stones. Hydrophilic-coated wires (e.g., model no. 630-100, Microvasive) have proved especially useful in difficult cases, passing through tortuous cystic ducts or past tightly wedged stones when nothing else could. The size of the wires varies and ranges from 0.018-in wires for small 3-French endoscopes to 0.038-in for larger scopes or for passing alone. The most common wires that we use are 0.035-in soft, straight, or angled-tipped noncoated varieties, but a full selection is always available on the choledochoscopy cart.

The single most critical element in performing laparoscopic choledochoscopy is the choledochoscope itself. Flexible endoscopes have undergone tremendous evolution since their introduction and continue to improve yearly, especially in the criteria important for effective choledochoscopy: size, optical clarity, good light transmission, steerability, and functional working channel. Relatively few companies are manufacturing scopes specifically for LCBDE, and the majority of endoscopes being used were actually designed for vascular or ureteral work. This will undoubtedly change as LCBDE gains wider acceptance. Compared with arteries and ureters, the common duct is short, dark, and cavernous. Other differences include the acute angulations of the ductal anatomy and the size differences between the cystic and common ducts. Considering these factors, the perfect choledochoscope should be only long enough to pass through the trocar, intraabdominal space, and cystic and common ducts. It should be as small as possible and have a tapered or beveled tip to ease introduction into the cystic duct. It should transmit sufficient light to illuminate the interior of large dilated ducts and be extremely steerable to negotiate acute changes in direction. Finally, it should have a large working channel (ideally, 4 French) to allow passage of a wide array of instruments. Although this ideal scope is not yet in existence, it undoubtedly will be.

The scope that we use most often is a 9.5-French ureteronephroscope with a beveled tip, bidirectional flexion, and a 1.2-mm working channel. If unable to insert this scope, we use a 4.2-French angioscope, which only has unidirectional flexion and a 2.4-French working channel, making it less useful but still functional. A final consideration is that of cost; flexible endoscopes require a large financial commitment. Several manufacturers have developed disposable or semidisposable flexible endoscopes in an attempt to mitigate this cost element. Unfortunately, these scopes fall far short in the optics and flexibility categories, rendering them poor bargains. The only other option would be joint purchasing with other departments with whom the endoscopes and cost could be shared.

Dilatation of the cystic duct is frequently necessary to allow easy passage of the choledochoscope. There are currently two options for duct dilatation: semirigid tapered dilators or coaxial balloon dilators. Although some have effectively used the guide wire tapered dilators,[16] we find that they almost always avulse the partially divided cystic duct because of the high frictional shearing forces created. Coaxial balloon dilatation averts this problem and has routinely allowed safe dilatation of even small ducts to 15 French or more. Such balloons come in a wide variety of sizes and designs. We find the most useful to be a 5-French soft filiform-tipped over-guide-wire catheter with a 4-cm 15-French balloon. This usually permits easy insertion of a standard 9.5 French endoscope and minimizes the danger of over dilatation and rupture of the cystic duct.

A different size and type of stone basket from that used in FGSR is required for explorations via the choledochoscope. The size of catheter is restricted by the size of the working channel of the scope, usually between 2 and 3-French. Also, three- or four-wire straight-wire (Segura type) baskets are needed for precise placement and closure around visualized stones. Helical-type baskets are not able to be rotated to capture the stone because of the fineness of the catheters and their tight fit within the endoscope. One problem with these baskets is their small size, which makes them fragile and easily bent out of shape. Once misshapen, they are all but useless and need to be replaced. This delicateness also makes it impossible to crush any but the softest common duct stones. These baskets are, however, stiffer than guide wires and can perforate the duct wall. For this reason, they should only be advanced and opened under direct vision.

Intraductal lithotripsy has proved extremely useful in LCBDE. This is particularly true for large impacted stones, which can be especially difficult to surround and remove with stone baskets. There are two basic technologies currently being used for intracorporeal lithotripsy: pulsed-dye laser and spark gap-generated shock waves. Laser lithotripsy utilizes energy generated by a coumarin dye laser, which is trasmitted by flexible quartz fibers of either 320 or 550 μm. The stone-breaking force comes from a strong plasma field exerted against solid objects at the tip of the fiber. This force is very effective at fracturing stones but, with normal use, has the important benefit of minimally affecting soft tissues. This is obviously important in common bile duct work.

There are, however, drawbacks to using the laser lithotripter. One is its high initial cost and the cost of added operative personnel needed to run and maintain it, costs which are usually passed on to the patient. The other concern is in regard to the quartz fibers. These are rather stiff, very brittle, and quite sharp. Care must be taken not to perforate the duct or break the fiber by using it as a probe.

Electrohydraulic lithotriptors, on the other hand, are comparatively inexpensive, portable, easy to set up, and do not require extra operating room personnel to run them. The 3-French electrode wires are flexible, fairly durable, and can be resterilized, reducing the cost to the patient.

The drawbacks to electrohydraulic devices are a result of the technology itself. The force used to fracture the stone comes from a strong hydraulic wave induced by an electric discharge at the tip of the probe. Like all waves, the generated force falls off fairly sharply but still propagates beyond the immediate area. This opens the possibility of inadvertent injury to tissues remote from the intended target, a possibility increasing as the energy used increases. This danger is compounded by the fact that, unlike the plasma field of the pulsed-dye laser, a hydraulic wave does not differentiate between soft tissue and calculus. The Food and Drug Administration has recently approved newer low-energy units for use in the common duct (e.g., model no. AEH-2, American ACMI; or Storz Calcutrip 27080), but care must be taken even with these units to prevent injury to the ductal mucosa or ductal perforations. The lowest energy and pulse rate settings should be used and the device never fired unless it is fully visible and directed only at the center of the stone.

PROCEDURE NOTES

We have found that keeping together all the necessary equipment for performing LCBDE in a cabinet that can be wheeled into the operating room is a tremendous time-saving device. When an abnormal cholangiogram is encountered, the extra equipment, including a second camera system, can be rapidly set up, while attempts are made to rule out a false-positive finding. Once again, the anesthetist intravenously administers 1 mg of glucagon for sphincter relaxation.

A 0.035-in guide wire is then passed down the cholangiocatheter and into the duodenum, when possible. The cholangiocatheter is removed, and a 5-French coaxial balloon dilator is advanced over the guide wire and positioned in the cystic duct. The balloon is slowly inflated to the recommended pressure, usually about 3 atm and maintained for 3 to 5 min. Dilating for a shorter length of time often will fail to stretch the spiral valves adequately and make it more difficult to insert the endoscope. The balloon is then deflated, and balloon and guide wire are removed.

A fifth 5-mm trocar is then inserted directly over the opened cystic duct (see Fig. 22-1), and an extra long (22-cm) 3.5-mm reducing sheath is inserted through it. A 9.5-French choledochoscope is advanced through the reducer, and the tip is placed immediately above the opening in the cystic duct. The guide wire is next reinserted into the common duct via the operating port of the scope, and the scope is advanced over the wire into the ducts. Insertion is facilitated by gently twisting the scope around the guide wire, which is epicentrically placed at the end of the scope. If the scope still hangs up on the cystic duct opening (frequently with a nonbevel-tipped scope), the anterior lip of the opening can be grasped and retracted with a fine dissecting instrument inserted through the lower midclavicular port. This and firm countertraction via the subxiphoid port will almost always allow insertion of the scopes. The second camera, or a split-viewing-system camera, is then attached to the scope so that both the intraabdominal view and the intraductal image are visible. It is important to watch the insertion trocar and intraabdominal portion of the scope to prevent a loop from occurring and pulling the scope out of the duct. Once in the common duct, a high-pressure irrigation supply, either a roller-pump device or a simple pressure bag, is connected to the endoscope. If using a pressure bag, it must be checked frequently for pressure maintenance (maximum, 150 cmH$_2$O) to keep the duct distended and irrigated freely of debris.

The scope is then advanced until the stone is seen. If the stone is free within the duct, the guide wire is exchanged for the 3-French stone basket, which is advanced up to the stone, opened, carefully manipulated around the stone, and closed (Fig. 22-6). The endoscope and trapped stones are then removed from the duct, and the process is repeated, as needed. Trapped stones that are too large for removal via the cystic duct should be crushed by closing the basket down tightly. If this fails, lithotripsy is another choice for impacted distal stones, although, with time and persistence, such stones can usually be mobilized sufficiently for basket removal by careful probing with a guide wire. If a pulsed-dye laser is used to break a stone, an initial power setting of 60 mW, with a 10-Hz pulse rate, is used. The fiber tip is placed at the center of the stone, and short bursts of power are applied until cracks are seen. A guide wire or closed stone basket can then be used to probe the fracture line and

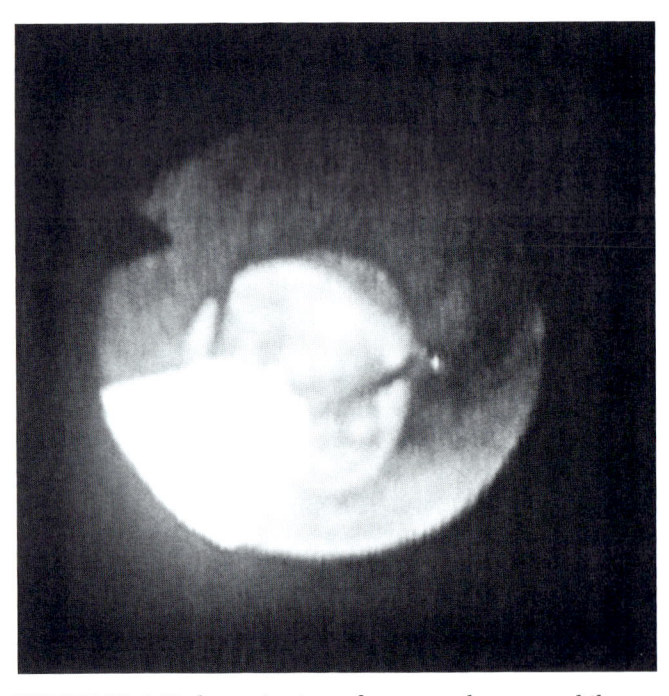

FIGURE 22-6 Endoscopic view of entrapped common bile duct stone.

dislodge the fragments, which are then retrieved. If an electrohydraulic unit is used, the electrode tip needs to be positioned 1 mm or less from the center of the stone and short pulses of low energy, starting with the lowest settings, usually 3600 V as a single pulse, are used until the stone breaks. Once the stone has fracture lines, lithotripsy should be stopped because further breakage will only create more fragments to retrieve and a fine debris, which compromises visibility.

When all visible stones have been removed, a guide wire is inserted through the choledochoscope and into the duodenum. The scope is then gently manipulated through the ampulla to ensure distal duct patency. If the scope does not easily pass through the ampulla, it should be withdrawn into the cystic duct, and a cholangiogram should be taken by injecting dye through the irrigating port. This should show flow into the duodenum and a stone-free distal duct. If no flow is seen, even after a repeat dose of glucagon, a single limb common duct drain can be inserted through the cystic duct and secured with an endoloop.

After the duct is cleared and distal patency established, the attenuated cystic duct is divided and endo-looped, and the gallbladder is removed. A 5-mm round closed suction drain is left close to the cystic duct stump as a prophylactic measure against missed bile leaks.

Some difficulties and questions remain with regard to this procedure. Failure to negotiate the cystic duct with the scope after a reasonable effort is best solved by trying one of the other methods of duct exploration. The presence of large numbers of common duct stones is, perhaps, a relative contraindication to transcystic duct removal, although, given time and patience, multiple stones can be removed. Multiple scope reintroductions can sometimes be facilitated by placing an introducer sheath into the common duct after cystic duct dilatation. Use of a large Swan-Ganz introducer sheath has been described,[24–25] or we have used a flexible ureteral introducer sheath (model no. 11276BS, Storz). Whichever is used, it must be placed far down the cystic duct to prevent it from dislodging with abdominal wall motion or during stone extraction.

Stones in the proximal biliary tree present a true challenge for the choledochoscopist and, fortunately, are unusual. Proximal choledochoscopy is sometimes possible via the cystic duct and requires a highly flexible scope and dissection of the cystic duct down to the common duct junction. As shown in Figure 22-7, medial traction of the cystic duct will sometimes permit the scope to be directed into the common hepatic duct. If the scope will not go proximally, we can try to draw the stones into the distal duct by alternating forceful irrigation with aspiration or other such maneuvers. Alternatively, we could insert the scope through a choledochotomy, as is discussed in the next section. If a complete choledochoscopy, proximal and distal, is performed, a completion cholangiogram is not needed; otherwise, one should be carried out to make certain that a stone was not washed proximally during choledochoscopy.

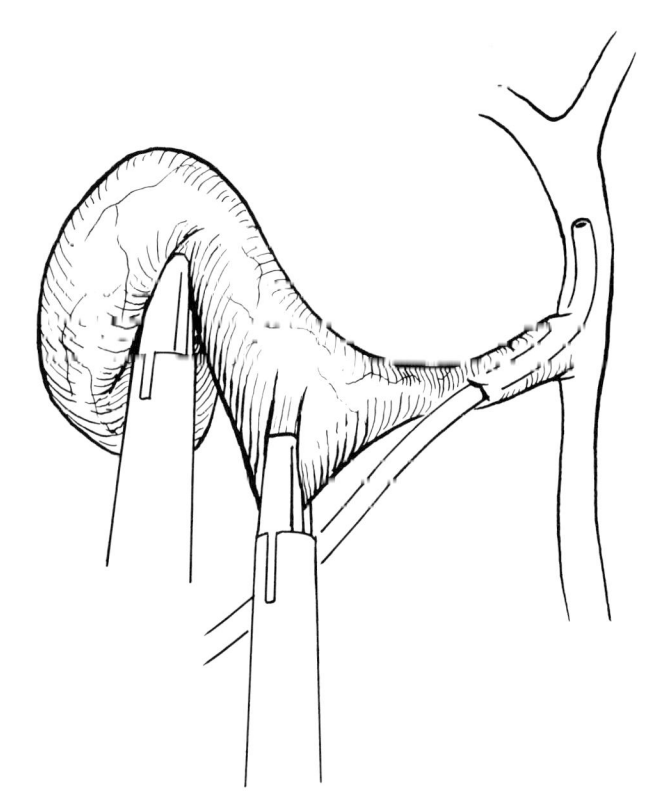

FIGURE 22-7 Proximal choledochoscopy. The infundibulum of the gallbladder is retracted inferiorly to bring the cystic duct to an angle where the scope may be passed superiorly. The success of this maneuver is clearly dependent upon cystic duct anatomy.

Occasionally, CBDE is indicated for reasons other than stones. If a bile duct tumor is encountered, it is possible to obtain biopsies using small cytologic brushes or a 3-French biopsy grasper. It may even be possible to perform more aggressive resections using a contact tip laser, such as the YAG or potassium titanyl phosphate, although the risks would be substantial and, for suspected malignancies, probably not the procedure of choice.

Distal common duct stricture is another occasional finding during laparoscopic cholecystectomy. Unfortunately, other than obtaining cytologic examination to rule out a ductal malignancy, there is not much to be done laparoscopically if this is the case. Retrograde stricture dilatation has not been very successful, and an antegrade sphincterotomy using a hot-wire sphincterotome, as is used with ERCP sphincterotomies, would likely perforate the duct because the most of the cut would be in the relatively thin-walled common duct. In cases of strictured ducts, we would probably just leave a decompressing drain in and refer the patient for postoperative ERCP, or convert to an open procedure for a choledochoenterotomy.

Laparoscopic Choledochotomy

Exploration of the common duct via a choledochotomy is, of course, the manner in which the majority of CBDEs were performed before laparoscopic cholecystectomy. This well-established method also is feasible for laparoscopic techniques, although it demands fairly advanced laparoscopic skills.[26] We currently use laparoscopic choledochotomy as a backup method should transcystic methods fail.

EQUIPMENT

The equipment needed to perform LC includes the following:

1. A 10-mm 30° (forward-oblique) Hopkins rod lens laparoscope (Storz).
2. A laparoscopic needle driver.
3. A 5-mm suture knot pusher (e.g., model no. MP782, Marlow, Willoughby, OH).
4. Suture material. We use a 4–0 monofilament absorbable suture on either a ski-shaped needle (e.g., model no. D7836, Ethicon, Somerville, NJ) or a small tapered straight needle (e.g., model no. 2639-31, Davis and Geck, Wayne, NJ).
5. A 12- or 14-French T-tube.
6. Choledochoscope, guide wires, stone baskets, and Fogarty embolectomy catheters, as previously described in the choledoscopic exploration section.
7. Glucagon, 5-mm closed suction drains, and setups for cholangiography are used as previously described.

The necessity of suturing the common duct closed around the T-tube is what makes this procedure a technically difficult one. Suturing is usually performed through the subxiphoid port, and the "forceps" (usually a second needle holder) are placed through the midclavicular port. There are several types of laparoscopic needle holders available, none of which is perfect. According to individual preference, we can choose between guillotine or standard jaw, diamond or striated jaw, and single or double action holders. There are pros and cons to each, and one should try them all to find the one that is most user friendly.

There are several ways to tie laparoscopically placed sutures. Extracorporeal knot tying is probably the easiest way to approach endoscopic suturing first, although the technique involves several instrument changes and an annoying loss of pneumoperitoneum. Monofilament suture is preferred because it slides better and frays less. The long suture is brought out through the trocar, where each throw can then be placed and, using a knot pusher device, slid back down the trochar to approximate the tissue edges. Alternatively, a Roeder slip knot can be tied outside the abdomen and pushed down in one step.[27]

Knots can also be placed within the abdomen by using the familiar technique of instrument tying. Intracorporeal knot tying allows the surgeon to keep attention focused on the video screen and minimizes instrument changes, thereby saving time and pneumoperitoneum. Unfortunately, this technique requires much more practice and video coordination to master and, until mastered, can easily turn the most mild-mannered and accomplished surgeons into surly raving idiots. As in open cases, a running suture can be a time-saving method of placing multiple stitches. Such a suture line is usually started by passing the needle back through a pretied loop at the end of the stitch after the first bite. At the end of the suture line, an intracorporeal knot can be tied, or alternatively, ligating clips can be applied to anchor the stitch.

The type of suture material used to close the choledochotomy depends on the surgeon's preference and the technique of knot tying used. Typically, a fine monofilament absorbable suture is used for extracorporeal knots and an absorbable woven suture, for intraabdominal ties. Almost any needle can be used, but because of the limitations of current needle drivers, either a short, straight, tapered, or a ski-shaped needle works best.

The remainder of the equipment and instruments used for laparoscopic choledochotomy is similar to that needed for choledochoscopy and T-tube placement during the corresponding open procedure.

PROCEDURE NOTES

The procedure itself is familiar and, therefore, an easy one for surgeons to conceptualize. The gallbladder is left in situ to provide a handle to lift the liver away from the common duct. Clips are placed on the distal cystic duct, but it is not divided to maintain tension on the common duct. The anterior wall of the common duct can then be carefully cleared at the most distal level possible. Care should be taken to use the gentlest techniques and a minimum of low-wattage coagulation to prevent damage to the duct and the possibility of delayed strictures. Placing the usual stay sutures has not been helpful and incurs the risk of their tearing out and damaging the common duct. A very small longitudinal duchotomy, approximately the same size as the circumference of the suspected stone, is made using a microscissors or arthroscopy scalpel (Fig. 22-8A). The choledochoscope can then be inserted directly into the duct and stone removal accomplished as described in the section on transcystic choledochoscopy (Fig. 22-8B).

Complete stone removal is confirmed by proximal and distal choledochoscopy, ideally including passage of the scope into the duodenum. A 12- or 14-French T-tube is passed completely into the peritoneal cavity through the 10-mm port. Proximal and distal limbs are then manipulated into the common duct, a task that is guaranteed to be easier said than done (Fig. 22-8C). Next, fine suture repair of the choledochotomy is performed; we like 4–0 in-

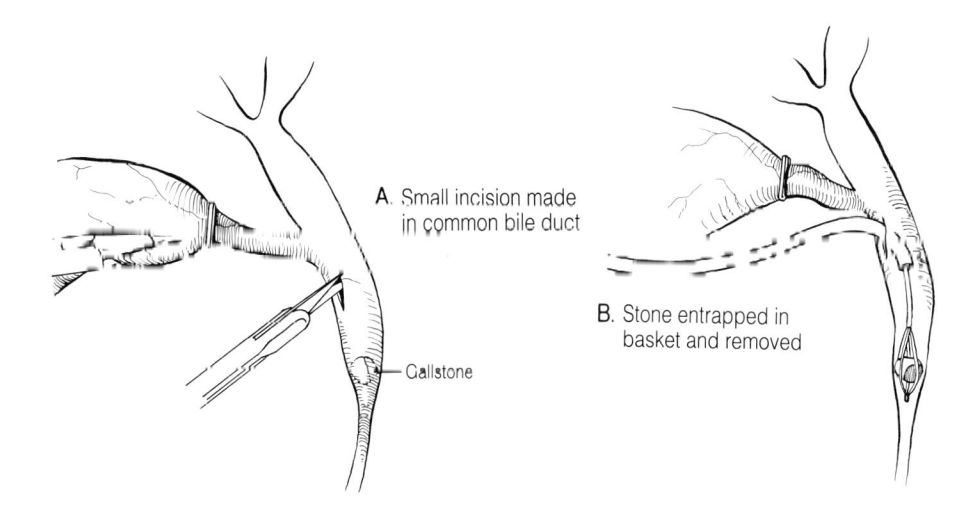

FIGURE 22-8 Laparoscopic choledochotomy and bile duct exploration. A. With the microscissors, a vertical choledochotomy is made. Note that the cystic duct has not been divided. The gallbladder makes an excellent retractor and avoids the requirement for stay sutures. The choledochotomy is as long as the gallstone is wide. B. The choledochoscope is introduced through the choledochotomy and the stone is entrapped with a basket. C. A short-armed T-tube is placed through the choledochotomy. D. The T-tube is secured in place with two interrupted absorbable sutures. The T-tube is then brought out through the right subcostal trocar site.

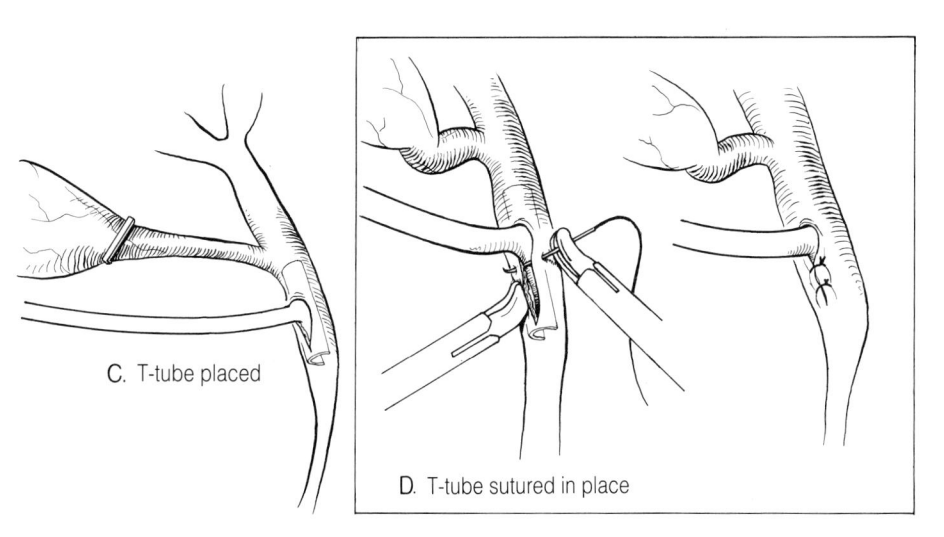

terrupted sutures tied intracorporeally for a secure closure of the choledochotomy (Fig. 22-8D). If desired, a T-tube cholangiogram can be performed, although, after a good choledochoscopic examination, this is probably redundant. The cystic duct and artery can then be divided and the gallbladder removed in the standard fashion. A closed suction drain should be placed near the repair to complete the procedure.

The technical demands of endoscopic repair of the common duct cannot be understated. Although placing the T-tube can be agonizing, suturing the common duct can be equally frustrating and dangerous. It takes much practice with endoscopic suturing techniques to gain the ability to place the precise atraumatic stitches needed, and mistakes can result in lacerated common ducts, bile leaks, sewn-in T-tubes, or bile duct strictures.

There has long been discussion regarding the true need of postexploration common duct drainage and the function of the T-tube as a stent.[28] Although primary duct repair without drainage may be the ideal, it seems prudent currently to go ahead and struggle with laparoscopic T-tube placement until a consensus is achieved.

RESULTS

Currently, we treat positive cholangiograms under a protocol that applies the algorithm in Figure 22-9. It should be noted that, although, transcystic choledochoscopy is our preferred approach, both fluoroscopic-guided stone retrieval and choledochotomy are important backup methods. Our results have been good to date. Cholangiograms were obtained in 378 of 400 laparoscopic cholecystectomies (97 percent). Of these, 40 (10.5 percent) were abnormal. One

Positive Cholangiogram

```
Positive Cholangiogram
        |
Cystic duct dilation
        |
Transcystic choledochoscopy
    /          \
Succeeds      Fails
  /    \         |
Free   Impacted  Fluoroscopic basket retrieval
stone  stone           |
  |       |          Fails
Basket ← Lithotripsy   |
retrieval          Lap choledochotomy
  |                    |
Completion           Fails
cholangiogram          |
                  Open exploration
```

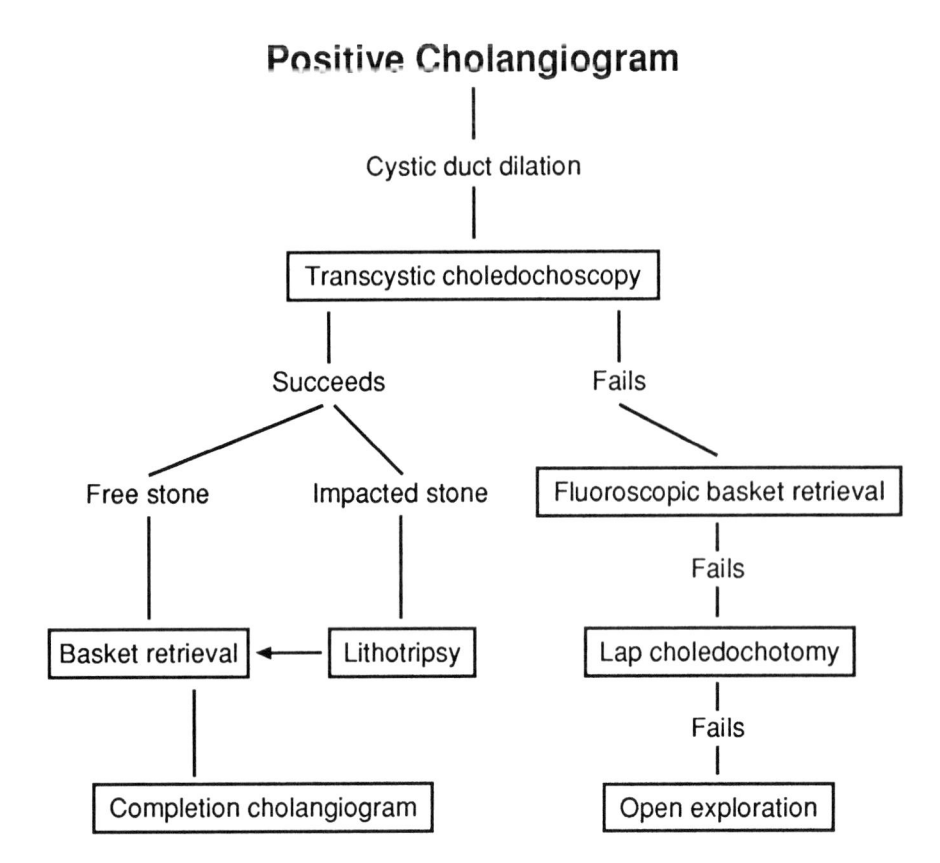

FIGURE 22-9 Procedure algorithm for laparoscopic common bile duct exploration.

case was encountered before the development of laparoscopic exploration techniques and was treated successfully with postoperative ERCP. Under our current treatment protocol, we have been able successfully to perform transcystic duct choledochoscopic explorations in 33 cases, with 12 cases employing stone retrieval by fluoroscopic-guided baskets when the scope was unable to be passed. One last case entailed choledochoscopy, stone retrieval, and T-tube placement via a choledochotomy.

The total success rate for LCBDE was 36 of 39 attempts, or 92 percent. The three failed attempts were encountered early in our experience and before laparoscopic choledochotomy was added to our algorithm. Two of these patients underwent open explorations, and one, by preoperative request, had postoperative ERCP. There have been no failures using the laparoscopic approach in the last 25 attempts.

Complications have included one retained stone after both choledochoscopy and a normal completion cholangiogram, which became clinically significant 72 h postoperatively and which required ERCP for removal. None of the other complications required intervention, including one postoperative ileus lasting 4 days, two ampullary lacerations with bleeding, and two common duct perforations with closed stone baskets.

The ileus showed no cause by CT scan or ERCP and resolved with conservative therapy. The ampullary lacerations were caused by open stone baskets, one during FGSR and one under direct visualization. Saline duct irrigation was initiated in both cases until bleeding stopped, and a cholangiogram was performed to rule out perforation. The two instances of perforation, one with a 5-French basket during FGSR and the other with a 3-French basket during choledochoscopy, required no treatment other than placement of a closed suction drain in the gallbladder fossa. There was no bile leakage in either case postoperatively. The patient who had a choledochotomy was readmitted on postoperative day 5 for 24 h after an episode of apparent transient cholangitis. The T-tube cholangiogram was normal, and the symptoms rapidly resolved with antibiotics. No incidents of postoperative wound infection, pancreatitis, or bile leaks have been encountered.

The complication rates have been similar to those in other larger series (Hunter J. Personal communication, March 1992),[28,29] with serious complications (abscesses, bile leaks, or clinical pancreatitis) being rare, 0 to 9 percent, and minor complications (postoperative ileus, nonleaking wire perforations, or transient fevers) in about 10 percent of cases.

Length of stay for LCBDE patients was only slightly increased over that of a regular laparoscopic cholecystectomy, an average of 29 h in the hospital versus 23 h. There seems to be a slight tendency for more postoperative nausea, but pain medication usage is the same for both, as

TABLE 22-1 Reported laparoscopic common bile duct exploration series

			Successful LCBDE			
Author	No. positive cholangiogram (%)	No. attempted LCBDE (%)	FGRS	Transcystic choledochoscopy	Laparoscopic choledochotomy (No.)	Total success rate
Current series	40 (10.5%)	39 (97%)	5%	85%	3% (1)	92%
Petelin J[28]	71 (9.0%)	54 (76%)	31%	61%	8% (4)	94%
Carroll et al.[29]	57 (10.1%)	11 (72%)	0%	90%	2% (1)	98%
Hunter J	25 (8.0%)	24 (96%)	62%	33%	5% (1)	88%

LCBDE = laparoscopic common bile duct explorations; FGRS = fluoroscopic-guided stone retrieval.

is the length of time to resumption of normal activity. As in regular laparoscopic cholecystectomy, drains are removed before hospital discharge unless there is apparent bile.

Data from other reported series, presented in Table 22-1, further confirm the possibility, effectiveness, and safety of LCBDE.

CONCLUSION

Considering the current prevalence of laparoscopic cholecystectomy, a major task of the 1990s is to find equally high-tech solutions for common duct disease. Several interesting methods have been attempted, but unfortunately, most of these fail to address underlying conditions or lack the cost effectiveness found in traditional methods. For now, only LCBDE seems to provide an acceptable answer to the problem of choledocholithiasis.

Data from several series indicate that LCBDE is safe and cost effective. An argument has also been advanced that, because choledochoscopy is the current gold standard for open CBDE, use of the endoscope also should be the first choice during LCBDE. New high-resolution digital fluoroscopic units may advance completion cholangiography close to the resolution of choledochoscopy but will probably always be slightly inferior to direct visualization.

Also LCBDE has succeeded in pushing the envelope of current practice forward, with the majority of explorations being performed via the cystic duct, disimpacting stones with special guide wires or lithotripters, and retrieving fragments with miniature baskets. Most of these minimally invasive explorations can be completed without T-tube drainage of the bile duct.

This is certainly not to say that this technique has reached full maturity. Refinements still need to be made, for example, the optics are imperfect, equipment costs are high, proximal choledochoscopy is difficult, and retrieval instruments are very fragile. As interest grows and technologic advances occur, however, these problems will be solved. For other, more philosophic questions, it will take longer to achieve a consensus. These questions include such issues as whether all common duct stones need to be addressed, exactly when it is necessary to visualize the proximal common ducts, who should have sphincterotomies, and whether there are safe antegrade methods of doing so. Of course, after these issues have been solved and instruments invented to perform them, new questions demanding new answers will take their place as part of the continued evolution of CBDE.

REFERENCES

1. Way LW, Admirand WJ, Dunphy JE: Management of choledocholithiasis. *Ann Surg* 1972; 176:347–359.
2. DenBesten L, Doty JE: Choledocholithiasis. *Surg Clin North Am* 1981; 61:893–907.
3. Shore M, Berci G: Choledochoscopy, in Wright R, Alberti K, Karren S (eds): *Liver & Biliary Disease*. London, WB Sanders, 1979, pp. 529–542.
4. Phillips E, Daykhovsky L, Carroll B, et al: Laparoscopic cholecystectomy: Instrumentation and technique. *J Laparoendosc Surg* 1990; 1:13–15.
5. Arregui M, Davis C, Arkush A, et al: Laparoscopic cholecystectomy combined with endoscopic sphincterotomy and stone extraction or laparoscopic choledochoscopy and electrohydraulic lithotripsy for management of cholelithiasis with choledocholithiasis. *Surg Endosc* 1992; 6:10–15.
6. Fried LA, LeBrun GP, Norman RW, et al: Extracorporeal shockwave lithotripsy in the management of bile duct stones. *Am J Radiol* 1988; 151:923–926.
7. Shimada H, Nihmoto S, Matsuda A, et al: Experience with percutaneous transhepatic fiberoptic choledochoscopy for retained stones in the biliary tract. Report on 15 patients. *Surg Endosc* 1987; 1:189–194.
8. Palmer KR, Hofmann AF: Intraductal mono-octanoin for the direct dissolution of bile duct stones: Experience in 343 patients. *Gut* 1986; 27:196–202.
9. Swanstrom L, Sangster W: Laparoscopic management of common bile duct stones. Presented at the British Columbia Surgical Society, Vancouver, BC, May 10, 1991.
10. Stain S, Cohen H, Tsuishoysha M, et al: Choledocholithiasis. *Ann Surg* 1991; 6:627–632.

11. Cotton PB, Lehman G, Vennes J, et al: Endoscopic sphincterotomy complication and their management: An attempt at consensus. *Gastrointest Endosc* 1991; 37:383–393.
12. Miller BM, Kozarek RA, Ryan JA, et al: Surgical versus endoscopic management of common bile duct stones. *Ann Surg* 1988; 207:135–141.
13. Neoptolemos JP, Carr-Locke DL, Fossard DP: Prospective randomized study of preoperative endoscopic sphincterotomy versus surgery alone for common bile duct stones. *BMJ* 1987; 294:470–474.
14. Reid DA: Choledochoscopy of the cystic duct as a new approach to the biliary tree. *Surg Gynecol Obstet* 1989; 169:68–70.
15. Sawyers J, Herington J, Edwards W: Primary closure of the common bile duct. *Am J Surg* 1965; 109:107–112.
16. Petelin JB: Laparoscopic approach to common duct pathology. *Surg Laparosc Endosc* 1991; 1:33–41.
17. Berci G, Sackier J, Paz-Partlow M: Routine of selected intraoperative cholangiography during laparoscopic cholecystectomy? *Am J Surg* 1991; 161:355–360.
18. Phillips E, Carroll B, Fallas M: Laparoscopic antegrade balloon dilatation of the sphincter of Oddi. *Surg Endosc*, in press.
19. Hunter J: Laparoscopic transcystic CBDE. *Am J Surg* 1992; 103:53–58.
20. Bakes J: Die Choledoscopapilloskopie nebst Bemerkungen uber Hepaticusdrainage und Dilatation der Papille. *Arch Klin Chir* 1923; 126:473–476.
21. Escat J, Fourtanier G, Maigne C, et al: Choledochoscopy in common bile duct surgery for choledocholithiasis: A must. *Am Surg* 1985; 51:166–167.
22. Motson R, Wetter L: Operative choledochoscopy: Common bile duct exploration is incomplete without it. *Br J Surg* 1990; 77:975–982.
23. Kappes S, Adams M, Wilson S: Intraoperative biliary endoscopy. *Arch Surg* 1982; 117:603–607.
24. Graber J: Laparoscopic CBD access. *Surg Alert* 1992; 8:730–732.
25. Stokar M, Leveillee R, McCann A, et al: Laparoscopic CBDE. *J Laparoendosc Surg* 1991; 1:5287–5293.
26. Ko S, Airan M: Therapeutic laparoscopic suturing techniques. *Surg Endosc* 1992; 6:41–46.
27. Chande S, Devitt J: T-tubes, the surgical amulet after choledochotomy. 1973; *Surg Gynecol Obstet* 136:100–102.
28. Petelin J: Laparoscopic CBDE. Presented to American College of Surgeons Post-Graduate Course, Chicago, IL, October 23, 1991.
29. Carroll B, Phillips E, Daykhovsky L, et al: Laparoscopic choledochoscopy: An effective approach to the common duct. *J Laparoendosc Surg* 1992; 2:115–121.

Chapter 23

Endoscopic Intervention for Pancreatic Disorders

Aaron S. Fink

Endoscopic retrograde cholangiopancreatography (ERCP) and its therapeutic extensions constitute a means to treat, and frequently cure, biliary tract pathologic disorders. Indeed, in many circumstances (e.g., retained common bile duct stones or biliary fistulae after cholecystectomy, or palliation of unresectable malignant biliary obstruction), endoscopic intervention is considered the optimal mode of treatment. With the technologic advances of the last two decades, these therapeutic endoscopic techniques are being applied increasingly to primary pancreatic disorders. Although experience is often limited and anecdotal, the benefits of endoscopic intervention for pancreatic disorders will undoubtedly generate increased interest. Most of these endoscopic interventions have focused on pancreatitis and its sequelae. The various indications for endoscopic intervention in pancreatic disease will be discussed relative to the timing of clinical presentation.

ENDOSCOPIC INTERVENTION DURING ACUTE PANCREATITIS

Acute pancreatitis frequently follows gallstone impaction at the ampulla. In most cases, these impacted stones pass spontaneously, and the patient rapidly improves after limited supportive treatment. Occasionally, however, the patient fails to respond to conservative management.

Gallstone Pancreatitis

Early common duct exploration in severe gallstone pancreatitis usually reveals stones,[1,2] and several authors have recommended urgent biliary surgery in such patients in an effort to obtain prompt clinical improvement after disimpaction of residual common duct stones.[1–7] In general, these surgical series have failed to document beneficial results from this aggressive surgical approach.[1,5–7]

During an attack of pancreatitis, the technique of ERCP can be used to predict severity and identify patients who are likely to benefit from urgent intervention. Acute pancreatitis is generally considered to be a contraindication to ERCP; however, this mandate is under reconsideration. Cremer[8] analyzed the results of ERCP in 355 patients with acute pancreatitis. Although the diagnostic information was less helpful than anticipated (normal study in most patients), this study clearly demonstrated that, in patients with acute pancreatitis, ERCP is safe and does not adversely affect ultimate clinical outcome. Although reservations regarding the use of ERCP during acute pancreatitis are based on assumed risks, it must be acknowledged, however, that data supporting the apparent safety of retrograde injection of contrast into the acutely inflamed pancreas remain limited. Thus, endoscopic intervention during acute pancreatitis requires careful attention to technique and should only be undertaken by those with considerable expertise in therapeutic ERCP. Furthermore, such endoscopic intervention must be applied only under the strictest of indications, as discussed subsequently.

Endoscopic sphincterotomy in the treatment of gallstone pancreatitis seems to be an ideal alternative to early surgical intervention involving laparotomy and duodenotomy. Several uncontrolled reports[9–15] have demonstrated the relative safety and potential benefit of urgent endoscopic sphincterotomy for selected cases (usually severe) of acute gallstone pancreatitis. The compiled results from these retrospective series are found in Table 23-1.

Randomized prospective data regarding this critical issue are also available. In a recent study, Neoptolemos and coworkers[16] compared early (< 72 h) ERCP and endoscopic sphincterotomy with conservative management in patients with acute gallstone pancreatitis. All patients underwent ultrasound and biochemical testing within 24 h of admission and severity prediction (modified Glasgow scale[17]) within 48 h. Exclusion criteria included acute or

245

TABLE 23-1 Endoscopic sphincterotomy for gallstone pancreatitis in 393 patients*

Successful procedure	93%
Morbidity	6%
Mortality	2.8%

*Data compiled from uncontrolled series.[9-15]

chronic ethanol abuse or an identified nonbiliary cause of pancreatitis. After screening, if gallstones were suspected, patients were randomized to receive early ERCP and sphincterotomy (59 patients) or conservative management (62 patients). Local and systemic complications and mortality were compared in each group. Overall complications were significantly decreased in patients treated endoscopically (17 versus 34 percent). As illustrated in Table 23-2, the results were particularly striking in those patients suspected of having a severe attack of pancreatitis.

Consideration of these data suggests that, on admission, the severity of pancreatitis should be assessed using one of the objective prognostic factor systems.[17-22] Gallstones should then be sought via ultrasonographic examination. If expert endoscopic support is available, urgent ERCP and sphincterotomy should be considered in patients with severe disease and gallstones, especially if clinical deterioration continues or rapid resolution fails to occur. Urgent ERCP should also be considered in those patients with unremitting disease and equivocal ultrasonographic examinations if there is a high risk of a biliary cause, as judged by clinical and biochemical criteria.[23-25] If choledocholithiasis is demonstrated, endoscopic sphincterotomy should then be performed.

Traumatic Pancreatitis

Acute traumatic pancreatitis represents another potential indication for endoscopic intervention. Although emergency laparotomy should not be deferred in the unstable patient, ERCP is generally underutilized in the evaluation of the stable trauma victim with hyperamylasemia. Fourteen such cases were reported by Barkin and associates.[26] Computerized tomographic scans, obtained in 12 of the 14 patients, demonstrated pancreatic abnormalities in 9 patients. In all 14 patients, these authors were able to obtain endoscopic pancreatograms without complication. These studies revealed major ductal abnormalities (extravasation) in four patients, minimal abnormality in one patient (mild ductal irregularity in the midbody of the pancreas), and no abnormalities in nine patients. At laparotomy, lacerated ducts were found in all four patients with contrast extravasation on pancreatogram. The patient with mild abnormality and five of the nine patients with normal pancreatograms recovered without surgical exploration. Three of the remaining patients were explored and found to have either a normal pancreas (one patient) or mild pancreatitis (two patients); all recovered without further pancreatic intervention. Thus, endoscopic intervention can delineate the need for surgical exploration in stable trauma patients with hyperamylasemia. Indeed, although not reported, it is conceivable that an isolated pancreatic ductal injury might be managed endoscopically, utilizing pancreatic duct decompressive techniques. Taxier and colleagues[27] have also reported benefits of ERCP in patients with pancreatic trauma.

ENDOSCOPIC INTERVENTION AFTER ACUTE PANCREATITIS

As noted, acute pancreatitis usually resolves with conservative treatment in the majority (80 percent) of cases. Depending on the clinical population served, however, the cause of the pancreatitis may remain obscure in 15 to 40 percent of cases, even after multiple diagnostic tests.[28] Cotton and Beales[29] successfully obtained endoscopic pancreatograms in 25 of 31 such patients with unexplained recurrent pancreatitis. Surgically correctable lesions (e.g., strictures, obstructions, or pseudocysts) were identified in 12 of the 25 patients. Guided by the results of pancreatography, successful surgical exploration was accomplished in most patients. It is notable that periampullary pancreatic duct obstruction was discovered in three of the six patients in whom endoscopic pancreatography failed.

Idiopathic Pancreatitis

Others have found ERCP to be beneficial after recovery from idiopathic pancreatitis. Thus, in 38 to 46 percent of patients, previously unappreciated lesions amenable to surgical or endoscopic therapy were identified using ERCP.[30-32] These lesions included undiagnosed gallstones, choledochocele (Fig. 23-1), ampullary disorders (e.g., stenosis, tumors, or sphincter of Oddi dysfunction), pancreat-

TABLE 23-2 Endoscopic versus conservative treatment of severe acute gallstone pancreatitis*

Results	Endoscopic treatment	Conservative treatment
Complications	6/25 (24%)†	17/28 (61%)
Hospital stay (days)	9.5†	17.0
Mortality	1/25 (2%)	5/28 (18%)

*Adapted from Ref. 16.

†$P < 0.05$ versus conservative therapy.

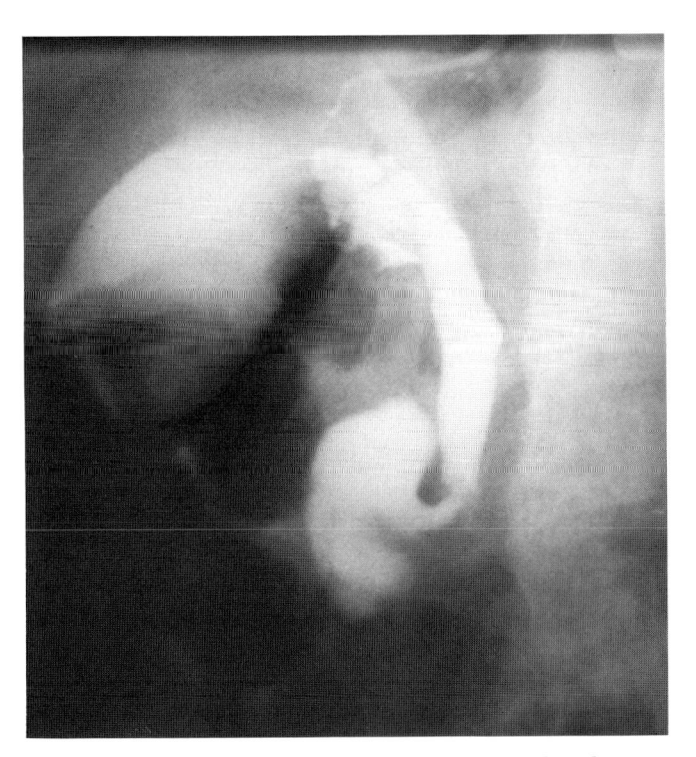

FIGURE 23-1 In this elderly gentleman who developed unexplained pancreatitis while recovering from multiple orthopedic injuries, endoscopic retrograde cholangiopancreatography (ERCP) revealed this choledochocele.

ic ductal abnormalities (e.g., pancreas divisum [Fig. 23-2] or strictures),[33] congenital duodenal wall cysts,[34,35] and unrecognized chronic pancreatitis.

Preoperative "Road Map"

Endoscopic identification of previously unappreciated chronic pancreatitis may lead to a recommendation for surgical intervention. During surgery for chronic pancreatitis, the value of the road map provided by ERCP is well known. Similar value may accrue if ERCP is used preoperatively in patients with pancreatic pseudocysts (Fig. 23-3).

Nealon and associates[36] prospectively evaluated the role of routine preoperative ERCP in patients with pancreatic pseudocysts who were referred for operative intervention. Over a 36-month period, ERCP was performed in 41 consecutive patients with pseudocysts. Twenty-four of the 41 patients were believed to be recovering from acute pancreatitis. Successful ERCP was obtained in 39 of the 41 patients and revealed unsuspected chronic pancreatitis in 9 of the patients originally believed to have acute disease. Dilated pancreatic and common bile ducts were observed in 23 and 12 patients, respectively; these abnormalities were only seen in patients with chronic pancreatitis. Most importantly, ERCP findings led to alteration of the operative plan in 24 of the 41 patients, 22 of whom had chronic pancreatitis. Sugawa and Walt[37] and O'Connor and associates,[38] in earlier retrospective studies, documented sim-

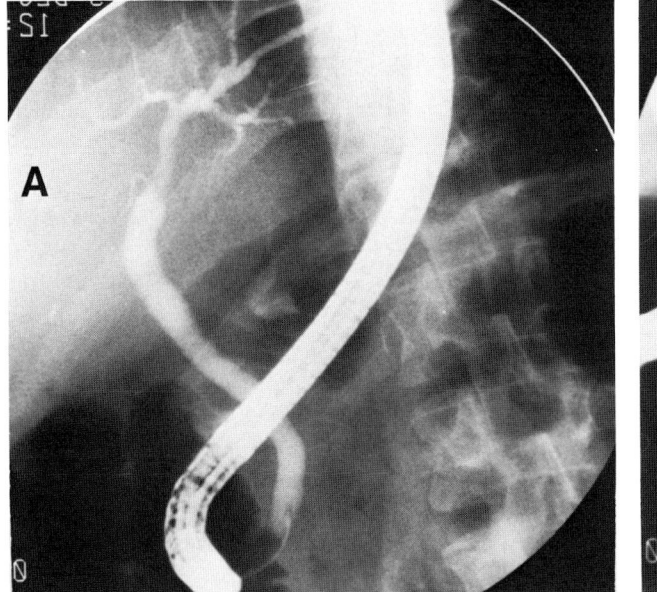

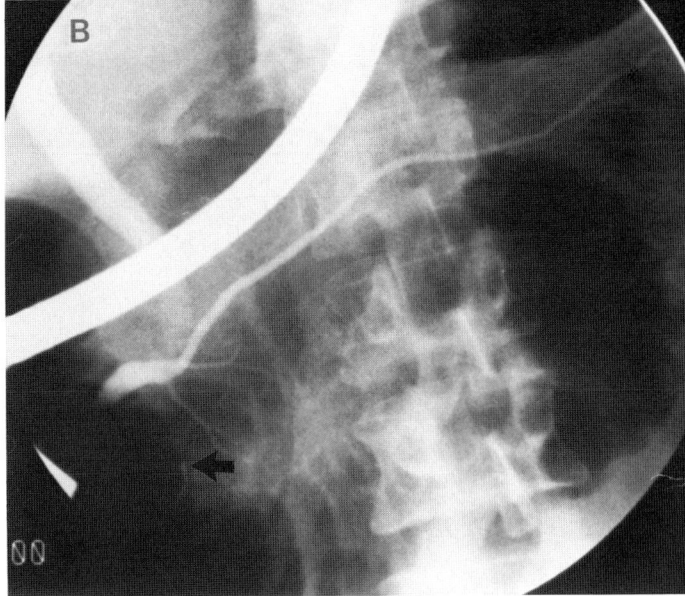

FIGURE 23-2 This 45-year-old renal transplant patient developed persistent idiopathic pancreatitis. A. Initial injection of the main papilla failed to fill the pancreatic duct. B. Cannulation of the minor papilla allowed opacification of a complete pancreas divisum. Note the catheter (arrow) placed at the main papillary orifice.

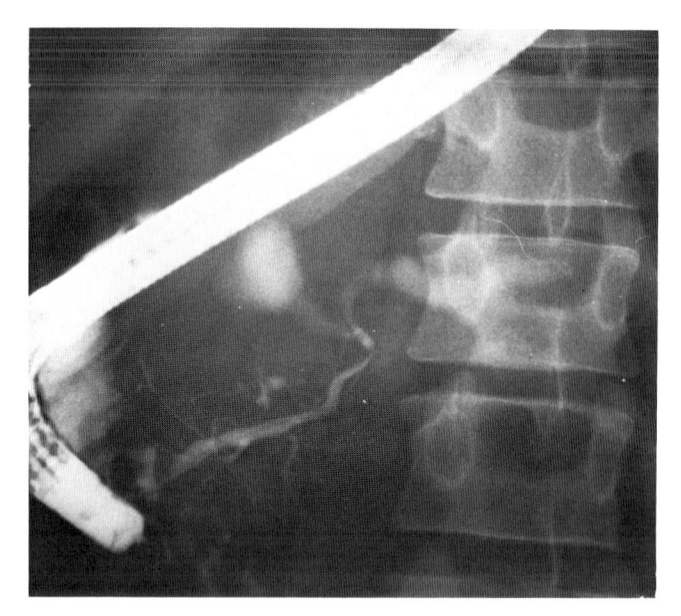

FIGURE 23-3 Preoperative ERCP in this 30-year-old patient with a pancreatic pseudocyst revealed a communicating pseudocyst and dilated pancreatic duct proximal to a mid-duct stricture. These findings altered the planned operative therapy.

ilar beneficial results of preoperative ERCP in patients with pseudocysts.

Ahearne and coworkers[39] have further suggested that preoperative ERCP can be used as the basis of an algorithm to select appropriate therapeutic modalities for patients with pancreatic pseudocysts. In their algorithm (Fig. 23-4), it is assumed that pseudocysts associated with pancreatic duct obstruction or pancreatic ductal communication require surgical intervention. Thus, in elective cases, if preoperative ERCP reveals either pancreatic duct obstruction or pseudocyst communication, surgery is indicated; a lack of both findings permits percutaneous drainage.

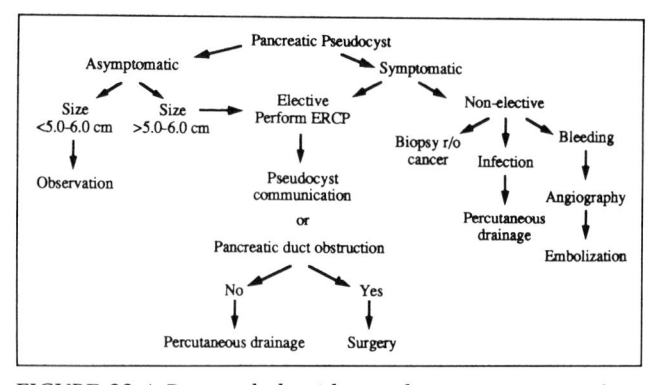

FIGURE 23-4 Proposed algorithm outlining appropriate therapy for pancreatic pseudocysts based on preoperative ERCP findings. (Adapted from Ref. 39.)

Among 102 patients with pseudocysts seen over a 6-year period,[39] adequate preoperative ERCP had been obtained in 40 of 69 electively treated patients. Retrospective application of the algorithm to these 40 patients revealed that, in 26 patients, the treatment course followed the algorithm. In 14 patients, the selected therapy differed from the algorithm. Although there was no significant difference in clinical criteria (e.g., age, length of hospitalization, APACHE II score, Ranson criteria, or pseudocyst size) between the two patient groups, the treatment outcome did differ. In the group that followed the algorithm, there was one treatment failure and two complications (3 of 26, 12 percent). In the group that did not follow the algorithm, 6 of 14 (43 percent) experienced either treatment failure or complication. The authors propose prospective testing of their algorithm (see Fig. 23-3) to prove its validity.

Massive Pancreatic Necrosis

ERCP may be beneficial in evaluating ductal anatomy in patients recovering from massive pancreatic necrosis and be useful, therefore, in delineating internal fistulae that have developed.[40] Howard and Wagner[41] reported ERCP results in 12 survivors of severe acute pancreatitis; all patients had required extensive debridement and external drainage of massive pancreatic necrosis. Surprisingly, the main pancreatic duct maintained its normal length and configuration in 8 of the 12 patients. Necrosis or stricture of the pancreatic duct, although rare, was seen primarily in patients who developed diabetes.

Endoscopic sphincterotomy may be indicated for patients who recover from acute gallstone pancreatitis but are unacceptable candidates for cholecystectomy. Davidson and associates[42] described 19 such patients who underwent endoscopic sphincterotomy with the gallbladder left in situ after recovery from pancreatitis. All 19 patients remained free from recurrent pancreatitis during a mean follow-up of 39 months.

ENDOSCOPIC INTERVENTION IN CHRONIC PANCREATITIS

Diagnostic Considerations

Endoscopic intervention has greatly enhanced the diagnosis and management of chronic pancreatitis. ERCP can be particularly useful in identifying noncalcific chronic pancreatitis, often a difficult diagnosis. Conventions for establishing this diagnosis, outlined in Table 23-3, were refined at the International Workshop on Pancreatitis held in Cambridge in 1983.[43] Although these definitions have facilitated interpretation of endoscopic pancreatograms, the protocol is still plagued by a lack of correlation between structural and functional abnormalities.[44–46] Furthermore, ERCP is not always needed for diagnosis. The pathog-

TABLE 23-3 Cambridge classification of endoscopic pancreatographic changes in chronic pancreatitis*

Terminology	Main pancreatic duct	Abnormal main pancreatic duct branches	Additional features
Normal	Normal	None	None
Equivocal	Normal	<3	None
Mild	Normal	≥3	None
Moderate	Abnormal	≥3	None
Severe	Abnormal	≥3	One or more: large cavity, obstruction, filling defects, severe dilation, or irregularity

*Adapted from Ref. 43.

nomy of chronic pancreatitis can be demonstrated by pancreatic calcification on plain abdominal films. Indeed, the pattern of radiologic calcification can predict the findings of endoscopic pancreatography.[47]

Before elective exploration, however, ERCP provides a vital road map, which offers critical morphologic information. This information may not only determine potential surgical options (e.g., pancreaticojejunostomy versus resection), but it may also reveal other pathologic conditions (e.g., ampullary tumor, stricture, fistula, or cyst), which will influence the ultimate surgical procedure performed. Therefore, in chronic calcific pancreatitis, diagnostic ERCP is indicated preoperatively to provide a precise anatomic road map.

Occasionally, it may be difficult to distinguish the endoscopic findings of chronic pancreatitis from those of pancreatic carcinoma. This distinction may be particularly difficult in the presence of pancreatic duct obstruction. The diagnosis is facilitated by accurate evaluation of the ductal and extraductal characteristics, especially at the point of obstruction.[48] Unfortunately, preliminary experience with endoscopic ultrasonography has failed to identify findings pathognomonic for either entity.[49]

Recurrent Postoperative Symptoms

Endoscopy is also helpful in evaluating the patient with persistent or recurrent symptoms after pancreatic surgery. Possible findings include stenosed sphincteroplasty, undrained duct segments after pancreaticojejunostomy,[50] or progressive pancreatic changes. Some of these findings may warrant further therapeutic intervention.

Endoscopic Therapy

Various techniques utilized in endoscopic biliary therapy are currently being applied to primary pancreatic disorders.

The ongoing interest in the development of surgical alternatives guarantees continued progress in this area. However, because of limited experience, many of these procedures are considered to be investigational. The modalities that have been applied to pancreatic disorders are listed in Table 23-4.

SPHINCTER OF ODDI DYSFUNCTION

As discussed earlier, endoscopic sphincterotomy may be useful in biliary pancreatitis, either rarely during the severe acute attack or more commonly after recovery in patients unsuitable for subsequent cholecystectomy. Sphincterotomy has also been used to treat recurrent acute pancreatitis secondary to sphincter of Oddi dysfunction. The latter entity refers to a group of variably defined clinical syndromes attributable to abnormal sphincter of Oddi motility.

The diagnosis of sphincter of Oddi dysfunction remains somewhat problematic. Two broad clinical syndromes have been identified: (1) biliary-type pain with or without abnormal liver function tests (especially aspartate transaminase and alkaline phosphatase[51]) and (2) idiopathic acute pancreatitis[52] after exclusion of other unusual causes. In view of the lack of specificity of these clinical and laboratory criteria, a multitude of other tests have been developed to identify biliary abnormalities caused by sphincter dysfunction (Table 23-5).

The recent development of endoscopic manometric techniques has allowed direct measurement of sphincter of Oddi pressures and contractility. Although the diagnostic criteria remain controversial, several groups have identified distinct manometric abnormalities in patients with idiopathic pancreatitis. Toouli and coworkers[52] reported findings that, in a group of 28 patients with idiopathic pancreatitis, 25 had abnormal sphincter of Oddi motility. The abnormalities included increased basal pressure (n = 16), increased frequency of phasic contractions (n = 9), increased frequency of retrograde contractions (9 of 20), absence of phasic contractions (n = 3), and paradoxic response to cholecystokinin (n = 2).

TABLE 23-4 Endoscopic therapeutic techniques utilized for pancreatic disorders

Sphincterotomy: biliary, pancreatic
Nasopancreatic drainage
Balloon dilatation
Endoprosthesis insertion (± ESWL)
Pancreatic stone fragmentation and removal
Pancreatic cystenterostomy
Pancreatic ductal occlusion

ESWL = extracorporeal shock-wave lithotripsy.

TABLE 23-5 Criteria for nonmanometric assessment of sphincter of Oddi dysfunction

ERCP abnormalities:
  Common bile duct dilation ≥ 12 mm
  Delayed common bile duct emptying ≥ 45 min in supine position
Hepatobiliary scintigraphy
  Biliary clearance of radiopharmaceutical
  Time to maximal biliary uptake (T_{max}) of radiopharmaceutical
Calibration of the sphincter
Morphine neostigmine test
Fatty-meal sonography

Adapted with permission from Keith RG, Hadjis NS: Pancreas divisum and sphincter of Oddi dysfunction. *Pancreas* 1991; 6(suppl 1):S60.

Geenen and associates[53] used other diagnostic criteria to denote sphincter of Oddi dysfunction: elevated basal sphincter of Oddi pressure (40 mmHg above duodenal pressure), delayed biliary or pancreatic ductal drainage (> 45 min or > 10 min, respectively), and duct dilation. Using these criteria over a 10-year period, the authors diagnosed 36 cases of sphincter of Oddi dysfunction in 555 patients with acute recurrent pancreatitis. Thirty of these 36 patients ultimately underwent sphincterotomy (22 initially and 8 at a later date). In patients treated with sphincterotomy, 70 percent remained free of pain and pancreatitis. In those patients treated medically, only 7 percent remained asymptomatic.

On retrospective review of the data, the only diagnostic criterion resulting in good outcome after sphincterotomy was elevated basal sphincter of Oddi pressure.[53] If verified, these data suggest that sphincterotomy may be indicated in patients with acute recurrent pancreatitis and elevated basal sphincter of Oddi pressure. Although balloon dilatation of the main papilla has been utilized as an alternative to endoscopic or surgical sphincterotomy, it appears to offer only temporary symptomatic improvement at the cost of frequent postdilatation pancreatitis.[54]

PANCREATIC SPHINCTEROTOMY

Several authors have noted that sphincter of Oddi hypertension can be limited to the pancreatic duct sphincter and can lead to recurrent acute pancreatitis.[52,55,56] In this situation, biliary sphincterotomy alone is generally effective because it leaves a short hypotensive pancreatic sphincter segment.[57] However, endoscopic manometry has demonstrated persistent pancreatic sphincter hypertension after endoscopic or surgical sphincterotomy.[58] Thus, if symptoms persist after biliary sphincterotomy and residual pancreatic hypertension is demonstrated, consideration should be given to opening the pancreatic duct orifice. Although this is usually achieved with surgical septectomy, endoscopic pancreatic sphincterotomy has been described and is gaining interest as a primary therapy.[58–66]

Assessment of complications and results of endoscopic pancreatic sphincterotomy is difficult because it is usually combined with other therapeutic modalities (e.g., stone removal or endoprosthesis insertion). In chronic pancreatitis, the procedure appears to be relatively safe, especially when combined with pancreatic duct decompression. However, this procedure imposes great risk of severe pancreatitis in patients with an otherwise normal pancreas.[65] Thus, until ancillary technical or pharmacologic measures are shown to afford greater safety, pancreatic sphincterotomy should not be performed in patients with pancreatic sphincter stenosis or dysfunction and minimal pancreatic disease.

NASOPANCREATIC DECOMPRESSION AFTER DIFFICULT CANNULATION

A potentially beneficial ancillary technical procedure is nasopancreatic drainage, which provides temporary pancreatic duct decompression. Geenen[53] utilized this decompressive technique in attempting to reduce post-ERCP pancreatitis after difficult endoscopic intervention. Patients at high risk for post-ERCP pancreatitis were randomized to receive either 24 or 48 h of nasopancreatic drainage or no drainage. As noted in Table 23-6, nasopancreatic drainage significantly decreased the incidence of post-ERCP hyperamylasemia and clinical pancreatitis.

PANCREATIC ENDOPROSTHESIS WITH OR WITHOUT LITHOTRIPSY

In view of the success of biliary endoprosthesis insertion, several groups have extended this technology to pancreatic disorders.[59,61,62,64,66,67] Pancreatic duct decompression has been utilized as either a temporary or permanent therapeutic intervention (Fig. 23-5).

Endoscopic pancreatic stents are inserted in a fashion similar to biliary endoprostheses. Initially, a 0.025-in or 0.035-in guide wire is passed into the main pancreatic duct and advanced toward the tail. A 5- or 7-French stent is then passed over the guide wire and positioned through the

TABLE 23-6 Prevention of postendoscopic retrograde cholangiopancreatography induced pancreatitis with nasopancreatic drainage*

Condition	No drainage	Nasopancreatic drainage
Number	12	11
Elevated amylase (5 × normal)	12	3[†]
Pancreatitis	5	1[†]

*Adapted from Ref. 53.
[†]$P < 0.05$ versus no drainage.

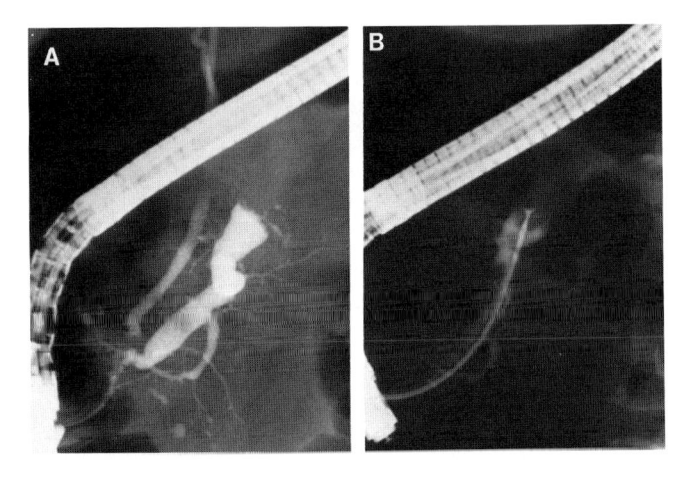

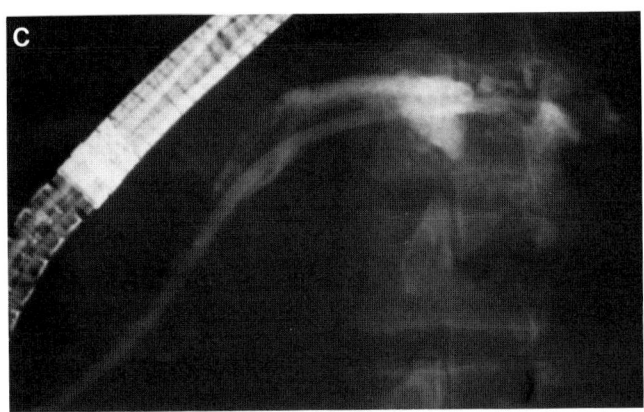

FIGURE 23-5 A. ERCP in this patient revealed an obstructing pancreatic ductal lesion in the neck of the gland. B. Biopsy was obtained after deeply cannulating the pancreatic duct with a biopsy forceps. The lesion proved to be a benign mucus-secreting tumor. C. A long pancreatic duct endoprosthesis was inserted for decompression. (Courtesy of Dr. Peter B. Cotton, Duke University Medical Center, Durham, NC.)

major papilla. Rarely, 10-French stents can be inserted into patients with significantly dilated pancreatic ducts. As would be expected, given the small caliber of pancreatic stents and the nature of pancreatic secretion, it is not surprising that pancreatic endoprostheses are prone to occlusion. In addition, there is evidence to suggest that the endoprosthesis itself may induce ductal changes that resemble chronic pancreatitis.

Temporary decompression has been used to decompress acutely the pancreatic ductal system after potentially traumatic endoscopic intervention, following extracorporeal lithotripsy of pancreaticolithiasis, or as a means of selecting patients best suited for more permanent drainage procedures. An example of the latter was published by Pullano and coworkers.[68] These authors proposed that patients with pancreas divisum might be best selected for surgical intervention on the basis of their response to temporary endoscopic stenting of the minor papilla (Fig. 23-6).

Reports suggesting that permanent endoscopic pancreatic drainage (achieved by combining sphincterotomy, stone extraction, stricture dilatation, and stenting) might offer long-term benefits in patients with chronic pancreatitis have generated much interest.[61,62,64,66,67] Thirty such patients were treated by Huibregste and associates[61] with a combination of pancreatic sphincterotomy and endoprosthesis insertion. Seventeen of their 21 patients with chronic relapsing pancreatitis improved. Furthermore, 7 of 10 patients with chronic pain improved, 6 of whom became pain-free over a 10- to 34-month follow-up period. These promising results were not obtained without complications. Pancreatic abscess developed in two patients; pancreatic ductal disruption occurred in one patient, who subsequently died. The authors indicated that patients with a dominant main duct stricture were most likely to respond favorably to endoscopic therapy.

Similar results were documented in 14 patients by McCarthy and colleagues,[66] who also noted the favorable prognosis for patients with dominant main duct stricture. These authors reported successful placement of pancreatic endoprostheses across the minor papilla in 26 patients with pancreas divisum, 18 of whom experienced symptomatic improvement.

Grimm and coworkers[62] reported a more extensive experience with endoscopic therapy for chronic pancreatitis. Seventy patients suffering from intractable pain associated with chronic pancreatitis were treated with a combination of pancreatic sphincterotomy, stone extraction, and stenting. Endoscopic intervention was successful in 61 patients (87 percent). One third of the patients developed mild pancreatitis, which resolved with supportive therapy. Two patients died after endoscopic intervention (3 percent procedure-related mortality): one from hemorrhagic pancreatic infarction and one from pulmonary embolism after surgery for septic complications (two infected pseudocysts and one hepatic abscess). Fifty of the 61 (82 percent) successfully treated patients experienced initial pain relief. On follow-up, however, only 35 (57 percent) remained pain-free.

As mentioned previously, removal of pancreatic duct stones is a frequent component of endoscopic therapeutic intervention. Symptomatic improvement generally follows removal of these stones, especially when they are confined to the main pancreatic duct.[59–62,64,69] Recently, extracorporeal shock-wave lithotripsy (ESWL) has been used in the management of pancreaticolithiasis.[62,70–72]

The most extensive experience has been in Brussels,[72] where 123 patients were treated with a combination of ESWL and endoscopic intervention. With endoscopic pancreatic sphincterotomy and other ancillary procedures (e.g., nasopancreatic drainage, Fogarty or balloon extraction, and stenting), ERCP was undertaken several hours after ESWL. Pancreatic stones were successfully fragmented in all but one patient. Although the main pancreatic duct was completely cleared in only 59 percent of patients,

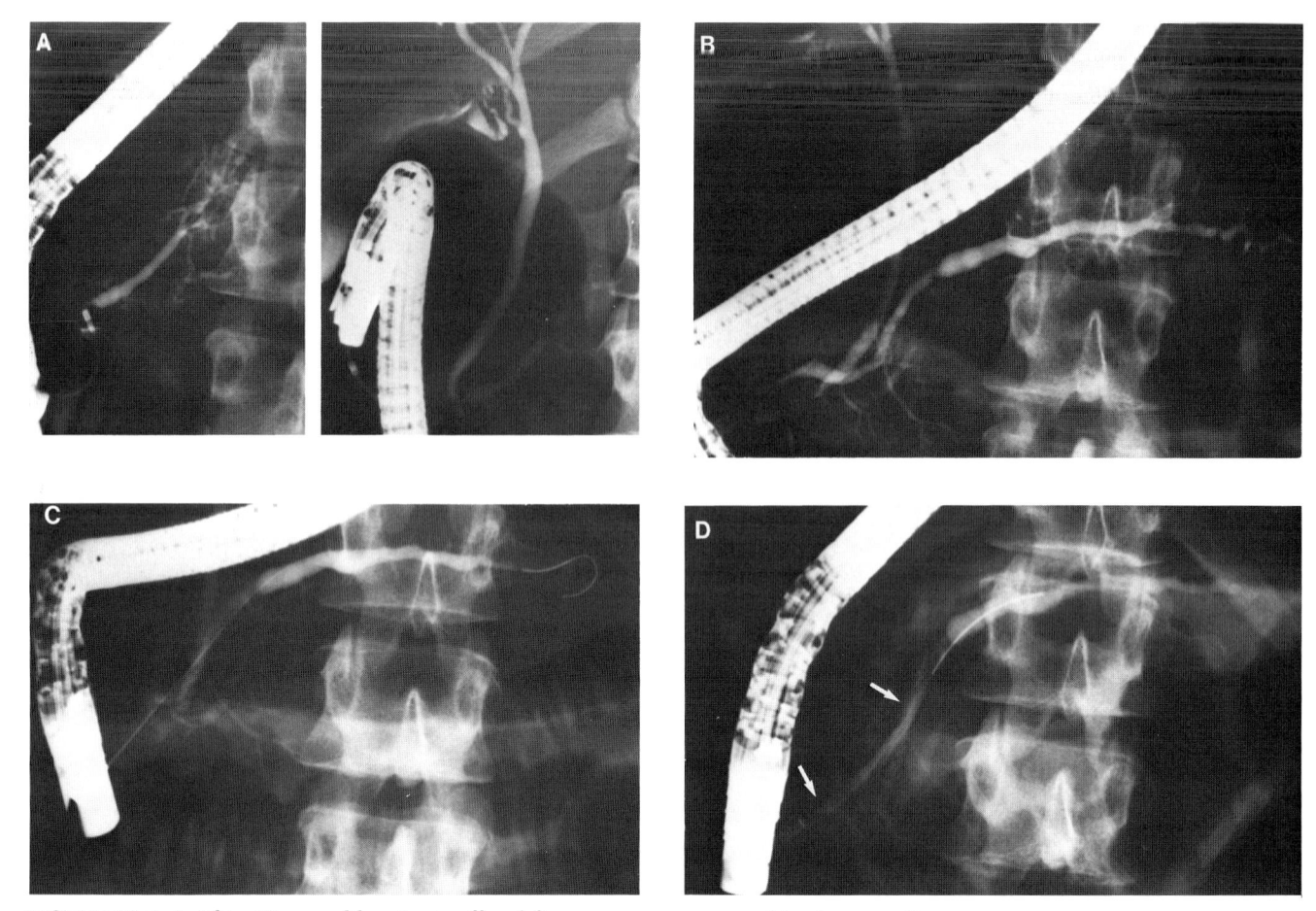

FIGURE 23-6 A. This 18-year-old patient suffered from recurrent pancreatitis since age 2 years. Endoscopic pancreatogram initially filled only the ventral pancreas. B. Pancreas divisum was confirmed after cannulation of the minor papilla. C. A long guide wire was passed to the pancreatic tail. D. An endoprosthesis (arrow) was inserted into the dorsal pancreatic duct. (Courtesy of Dr. Peter B. Cotton, Duke University Medical Center, Durham, NC.)

most patients (90 percent) experienced some decrease in ductal diameter. Although there were no reports of procedure-related mortality, 34 percent of patients developed "sepsis of pancreatic origin." The authors claim that complications were "relatively minor and not life-threatening." Many patients developed complete or partial pain relief; recurrent pain was most common in patients in whom nasopancreatic drains could not be inserted or in whom pancreatic duct diameter failed to decrease after therapy. Frequency of pain relief also decreased with length of follow-up.

PSEUDOCYSTS

Pancreatic pseudocysts have been approached endoscopically in several centers with pancreatic expertise.[61,67,72-74] Nasopancreatic drains[67] or endoprostheses[61] have been used to drain these cysts when they communicate with the main pancreatic duct. If a mature cyst impinges on the stomach or duodenum, endoscopically created cystoenterostomy has been utilized for drainage.[73,74] Cremer and associates[74] reported 22 endoscopic cystoduodenostomies; these were successful in 96 percent of patients, with only a 9 percent recurrence rate. Pain relief was obtained in 20 of the 22 patients. This group also reported 11 endoscopic cystogastrostomies, resulting in a 100 percent success rate, 19 percent relapse rate, and pain relief in 9 of 11 patients. Although these results are promising, complication rates, especially bleeding, have been high. Thus, the role of endoscopically created cystoenterostomy remains to be established.

SUMMARY

This review demonstrates the impact of endoscopy on diagnosis and management of pancreatic disorders. Although experience is limited, the reports of endoscopic therapeutic intervention for chronic pancreatitis offer great promise. Their ultimate role awaits clarification of appropriate indications, safety, efficacy, and long-term follow-up.

REFERENCES

1. Kelly TR: Gallstone pancreatitis: The timing of surgery. Surgery 1980; 88:345.
2. Stone HH, Fabian TC, Dunlop WE: Gallstone pancreatitis: Biliary tract pathology in relation to time of surgery. Ann Surg 1981; 194:305.
3. Acosta JM, Rossi R, Galli OMR, et al: Early surgery for acute gallstone pancreatitis: Evaluation of a systematic approach. Surgery 1978; 83:367.
4. Mercer LC, Saltzstein ED, Peacock JB, et al: Early surgery for biliary pancreatitis. Am J Surg 1984; 148:749.
5. Tondelli P, Stutz K, Harder F, et al: Acute gallstone pancreatitis: Best timing for biliary surgery. Br J Surg 1982; 69:709.
6. Osborne DH, Imrie C, Carter DC: Biliary surgery in the same admission for gallstone-associated acute pancreatitis. Br J Surg 1981; 68:758.
7. Kelly TR, Wagner DS: Gallstone pancreatitis: A prospective randomized trial of the timing of surgery. Surgery 1988; 104:600.
8. Cremer M: Personal communication to Geenen JE. Cited in Geenen JE: A/S/G/E distinguished lecture—Endoscopic therapy of pancreatic disease: A new horizon. Gastrointest Endosc 1988; 34:386.
9. Safrany L, Cotton PB: A preliminary report: Urgent duodenoscopic sphincterotomy for acute gallstone pancreatitis. Surgery 1981; 89:424.
10. van der Spuy S: Endoscopic sphincterotomy in the management of gallstone pancreatitis. Endoscopy 1981; 13:25.
11. Rosseland AR, Solhaug JH: Early or delayed endoscopic papillotomy (EPT) in gallstone pancreatitis. Ann Surg 1984; 199:165.
12. Ligoury CI, Meduri B, DiGiulio E, et al: Endoscopic treatment of acute pancreatitis, in Banks PA, Bianchi Porro G (eds): Acute Pancreatitis: Advances in Pathogenesis, Diagnosis, and Treatment. Milan, Masson Italia Editori, 1984, pp 151–160.
13. Tulassay Z, Farkas IE: Endoscopic sphincterotomy in acute gallstone pancreatitis. Lancet 1988; 2:1314.
14. Neoptolemos JP, London N, Slater ND, et al: A prospective study of ERCP and endoscopic sphincterotomy in the diagnosis and treatment of acute gallstone pancreatitis. Arch Surg 1986; 121:697.
15. Delmotte JS, Pommelet P, Houcke P, et al: Initial duodenoscopic sphincterotomy in patients with acute cholangitis or pancreatitis complicating biliary stones. Gastroenterology 1982; 82:1042.
16. Neoptolemos JP, Carr-Locke DL, London NJ, et al: Controlled trial of urgent endoscopic retrograde cholangiopancreatography and endoscopic sphincterotomy versus conservative treatment for acute pancreatitis due to gallstones. Lancet 1988; 2:979.
17. Blamey SL, Imrie CW, O'Neill J, et al: Prognostic factors in acute pancreatitis. Gut 1984; 25:1340.
18. Ranson JHC, Rifkind KM, Roses DF, et al: Prognostic signs and the role of operative management in acute pancreatitis. Surg Gynecol Obstet 1974; 139:69.
19. Dammann HG, Dreyer M, Walter TA, et al: Prognostic indicators in acute pancreatitis: clinical experience and limitations, in Beger HG, Buchler M (eds): Acute Pancreatitis. Berlin; Springer-Verlag, 1987; pp 181–197.
20. Mayer AD, McMahon MJ: The diagnostic and prognostic value of peritoneal lavage in patients with acute pancreatitis. Surg Gynecol Obstet 1985; 160:507.
21. Bank S, Wise L, Gersten M: Risk factors in acute pancreatitis. Am J Gastroenterol 1983; 78:637.
22. Agarwal N, Pitchumoni CS: Simplified prognostic criteria in acute pancreatitis. Pancreas 1986; 1:69.
23. Blamey SL, Osborne DH, Gilmour WH, et al: The early identification of patients with gallstone associated pancreatitis using clinical and biochemical factors only. Ann Surg 1983; 198:574.
24. Davidson BR, Neoptolemos JP, Leese T, et al: Biochemical prediction of gallstones in acute pancreatitis. A prospective study of three systems. Br J Surg 1988; 75:213.
25. Mayer AD, McMahon MJ: Biochemical identification of patients with gallstones associated with acute pancreatitis on the day of admission to hospital. Ann Surg 1985; 201:68.
26. Barkin JS, Ferstenberg RM, Panullo W, et al: Endoscopic retrograde cholangiopancreatography in pancreatic trauma. Gastrointest Endosc 1988; 34:102.
27. Taxier M, Sivak MV Jr, Cooperman AM, et al: Endoscopic retrograde pancreatography in the evaluation of trauma to the pancreas. Surg Gynecol Obstet 1980; 150:65.
28. Ranson JHC: Etiological and prognostic factors in human acute pancreatitis: A review. Am J Gastroenterol 1983; 77:633.
29. Cotton PB, Beales JSM: Endoscopic pancreatography in management of relapsing acute pancreatitis. BMJ 1974; 1:608.
30. Cooperman M, Ferrara JJ, Carey LC, et al: Idiopathic acute pancreatitis: The value of endoscopic retrograde cholangiopancreatography. Surgery 1981; 90:666.
31. Hamilton I, Bradley P, Lintott DJ, et al: Endoscopic retrograde cholangio-pancreatography in the investigation and management of patients after acute pancreatitis. Br J Surg 1982; 69:504.
32. Venu R, Geenen JE, Hogan WE, et al: Idiopathic recurrent pancreatitis. An approach to diagnosis and treatment. Dig Dis Sci 1989; 34:56.
33. Leese T, Chiche L, Bismuth H: Pancreatitis caused by congenital anomalies of the pancreatic ducts. Surgery 1989; 105:125.
34. Kalvaria I, Bornman PC, Girdwood AH, et al: Periampullary cyst: A surgically remedial cause of pancreatitis. Gut 1987; 28:358.
35. Holstege A, Barner S, Brambs HJ, et al: Relapsing pancreatitis associated with duodenal wall cysts: Diagnostic approach and treatment. Gastroenterology 1985; 88:814.
36. Nealon WH, Townsend CM, Thompson JC: Preoperative endoscopic retrograde cholangiopancreatography (ERCP) in patients with pancreatic pseudocyst associated with resolving acute and chronic pancreatitis. Ann Surg 1989; 209:532.
37. Sugawa C, Walt AJ: Endoscopic retrograde cholangiopancreatography in the surgery of pancreatic pseudocysts. Surgery 1979; 86:639.
38. O'Connor M, Kolars J, Ansel H, et al: Preoperative endoscopic retrograde cholangiopancreatography in the surgical management of pancreatic pseudocysts. Am J Surg 1986; 151:18.
39. Ahearne PM, Baillie JM, Cotton PB, et al: An endoscopic retrograde cholangio-pancreatography (ERCP)-based algorithm for the management of pancreatic pseudocysts. Am J Surg 1992; 163:111.
40. McLatchie GR, Meek D, Irmie CW: The use of endoscopic retrograde choledochopancreatography (ERCP) in the diagnosis of internal fistulae complicating severe acute pancreatitis. Br J Radiol 1985; 58:395.
41. Howard JM, Wagner SM: Pancreatography after recovery from massive pancreatic necrosis. Ann Surg 1989; 209:31.
42. Davidson BR, Neoptolemos JP, Carr-Locke DL: Endoscopic sphincterotomy for common bile duct calculi in patients with gall bladder in situ considered unfit for surgery. Gut 1988; 29:114.

43. Axon ATR, Classen M, Cotton PB, et al: Pancreatography in chronic pancreatitis: International definitions. *Gut* 1984; 25:1107.
44. Nakano S, Horiguchi Y, Takeda T, et al: Comparative diagnostic value of endoscopic pancreatography and pancreatic function tests. *Scand J Gastroenterol* 1974; 9:383.
45. Braganza JM, Hunt LP, Warwick F: Relationship between pancreatic exocrine function and ductal morphology in chronic pancreatitis. *Gastroenterology* 1982; 82:1341.
46. Caletti G, Brocchi E, Agostini D, et al: Sensitivity of endoscopic retrograde pancreatography in chronic pancreatitis. *Br J Surg* 1982; 69:507.
47. Gilinsky NH, Leung JWC, Heron C, et al: Calcific pancreatitis: Calcification patterns and pancreatogram correlations. *Clin Radiol* 1984; 35:401.
48. Rohrmann CA, Silvis SE, Vennes JA: The significance of pancreatic ductal obstruction in differential diagnosis of the abnormal endoscopic retrograde pancreatogram. *Radiology* 1976; 121:311.
49. Kaufman AR, Sivak MV Jr: Endoscopic ultrasonography in the differential diagnosis of pancreatic disease. *Gastrointest Endosc* 1989; 35:214.
50. Prinz RA, Aranha GV, Greenlee HB: Redrainage of the pancreatic duct in chronic pancreatitis. *Am J Surg* 1986; 151:150.
51. Hogan WJ, Geenen JE, Dodds WJ: Dysmotility disturbances of the biliary tract: Classification, diagnosis, and treatment. *Semin Liver Dis* 1987; 7:302.
52. Toouli J, Roberts-Thomson IC, Dent J, et al: Sphincter of Oddi motility disorders in patients with idiopathic recurrent pancreatitis. *Br J Surg* 1985; 72:859.
53. Geenen JE: A/S/G/E distinguished lecture—Endoscopic therapy of pancreatic disease: A new horizon. *Gastrointest Endosc* 1988; 34:386.
54. Kozarek RA: Balloon dilatation of the sphincter of Oddi. *Endoscopy* 1988; 20:207.
55. Guelrud M, Siegel JH: Hypertensive pancreatic duct sphincters as a cause of pancreatitis. *Dig Dis Sci* 1984; 29:225.
56. Raddawi HM, Geenen JE, Hogan WJ, et al: Pressure measurements from biliary and pancreatic segments of sphincter of Oddi. *Dig Dis Sci* 1991; 36:71.
57. Delmont J, Harris AG: Advantages and limitations of endoscopic manometry of the sphincter of Oddi, in Siegel JH (ed): *Endoscopic Retrograde Cholangiopancreatography: Technique, Diagnosis, and Therapy*. New York; Raven, 1992, pp 113–122.
58. Hogan WJ, Geenen JE, Kruidenier J: Ineffectiveness of conventional sphincteroplasty in relieving pancreatic duct sphincter pressure in patients with idiopathic recurrent pancreatitis. *Gastroenterology* 1983; 84:1189.
59. Fugi T, Amano H, Harima K, et al: Pancreatic sphincterotomy and pancreatic endoprosthesis. *Endoscopy* 1985; 17:69.
60. Schneider MU, Lux G: Floating pancreatic duct concrements in chronic pancreatitis. *Endoscopy* 1985; 17:8.
61. Huibregtse MD, Schneider B, Vrij AA, et al: Endoscopic drainage in chronic pancreatitis. *Gastrointest Endosc* 1988; 34:9.
62. Grimm H, Meyer W-H, Ch Nam V, et al: New modalities for treating chronic pancreatitis. *Endoscopy* 1989; 21:70.
63. Fuji T, Amano H, Ohmura R, et al: Endoscopic pancreatic sphincterotomy technique and evaluation. *Endoscopy* 1989; 21:27.
64. Sherman S, Lehman GA, Hawes RH, et al: Pancreatic ductal stones: Frequency of successful endoscopic removal and improvement in symptoms. *Gastrointest Endosc* 1991; 37:511.
65. Sherman S, Lehman GA: Endoscopy and pancreatic disease, in Cotton PB, Tytgat GNJ, Williams CB (eds): *1990 Annual of Gastrointestinal Endoscopy*. London; Current Science, 1990, pp 69–77.
66. McCarthy J, Geenen JE, Hogan WJ: Preliminary experience with endoscopic stent placement in benign pancreatic diseases. *Gastrointest Endosc* 1988; 34:16.
67. Kozarek RA, Patterson DJ, Ball TJ, et al: Endoscopic placement of pancreatic stents and drains in the management of pancreatitis. *Ann Surg* 1989; 209:261.
68. Pullano WE, Siegel JH, Ramsey WH, et al: Pancreas divisum: The camps are divided—To decompress preoperatively is the answer. *Gastrointest Endosc* 1986; 32:153.
69. Ponsky JL, Duppler DW: Endoscopic sphincterotomy and removal of pancreatic duct stones. *Am Surg* 1987; 53:613.
70. Kerzel W, Ell C, Schneider HT, et al: Extracorporeal piezoelectric shockwave lithotripsy of multiple pancreatic duct stones under ultrasonographic control. *Endoscopy* 1989; 21:229.
71. Sauerbruch T, Holl J, Sackmann M, et al: Extracorporeal shock wave lithotripsy of pancreatic stones. *Gut* 1989; 30:1406.
72. Delhaye M, Vandermeeren A, Baize M, et al: Extracorporeal shock-wave lithotripsy of pancreatic calculi. *Gastroenterology* 1992; 102:610.
73. Sahel J, Bastid C, Pellat B, et al: Endoscopic cystoduodenostomy of cysts of chronic calcifying pancreatitis: A report of 20 cases. *Pancreas* 1987; 2:447.
74. Cremer M, Deviere J, Engelholm L: Endoscopic management of cysts and pseudocysts in chronic pancreatitis: Long-term follow-up after 7 years of experience. *Gastrointest Endosc* 1989; 35:1.

Chapter 24

Percutaneous Approaches to Liver Neoplasms

Philip D. Schneider / John P. McGahan

Some patients with intrahepatic malignancies are not candidates for potentially curative liver resection. Generally, systemic metastatic disease or intraabdominal disease outside the liver form the bulk of the contraindications to surgical resection. Although it appears that resection of up to three or four lesions in the liver may be associated with longevity in the setting of metastatic colorectal cancer,[1] it is possible that the location of one or two lesions within the liver may be such that standard resection is not possible. In addition, patients may have major medical illnesses, including liver diseases with substantial reduction of liver function, which make them unsuitable for liver resection. In recent years, it has also become apparent that patients with metastatic neuroendocrine tumors, such as carcinoid and gastrinoma, may achieve substantial symptomatic benefit by ablation of hepatic metastases, even when the primary or every metastatic site is not controlled. Generally, the value of resecting multiple intrahepatic foci of malignancy is still somewhat uncertain, and although technically feasible, the risk of surgery may outweigh the benefit. As an alternative to surgery, ablation of these foci minimizes surgical morbidity and mortality and provides curative or palliative benefit for those unable or unwilling to undergo hepatic resection.

Investigators have searched for alternative means to treat liver lesions in situ to control the disease and avoid complications associated with surgery. Impetus has been given to the possible role of in situ tumor treatment by accumulated evidence indicating that the beneficial results of resection include patients who have had surgical margins as close as 1 cm around the metastatic lesion.[1,2] Specific information about margins is not available for small primary hepatocellular carcinomas. However, there is extensive evidence of palliative benefit from localized resection of small hepatomas in those patients who are not candidates for major liver resection because of extensive coincidental cirrhosis. Thus, the goal of effective in situ treatment, with margins that might allow a cure, has been a reasonable pursuit. Techniques used for the interstitial treatment of hepatic tumors include cryosurgery, alcohol injection, interstitial radiation implantation, laser hyperthermia, and radiofrequency electrodesiccation.

The use of interstitial therapies has been driven by the fact that, even with careful selection, the majority of patients who undergo liver resection for metastatic disease or hepatocellular carcinoma will ultimately succumb to their disease. If a relatively safe means could be employed to ablate and cure the few patients who are curable and, at the same time, reduce the morbidity and mortality of the therapy, most patients with liver cancer would be better served. There is early promise that interstitial ablation may provide the means to achieve reasonable cure rates, with reduced risk compared with standard liver resections.

TECHNIQUE FOR PERCUTANEOUS APPROACHES TO INTERSTITIAL ABLATION OF HEPATIC MALIGNANCIES

Materials and Protocol

Imaging studies are reviewed, and an appropriate interstitial ablation technique is selected. An intravenous crystalloid solution is started, and attention is directed toward adequate sedation and pain control during the procedure. The steps taken are as follows:

1. Real-time ultrasound is used to locate the lesion to be ablated, or if necessary, CT guidance can be used.

2. Utilizing real-time ultrasound, a Chiba needle is placed in the desired position within or near the tumor. Aspiration biopsy confirms the nature of the lesion.

3. For alcohol ablation techniques, alcohol can be in-

jected at this point, and its tracking through the interstitium followed by ultrasound.

4. For the placement of laser fibers for percutaneous interstitial hyperthermia, a 14-gauge needle and trocar are placed percutaneously into the lesion by ultrasound. For Nd:YAG laser treatment, the trocar is withdrawn, and the bare fiberoptic cable is placed into the lesion in the appropriate position.

5. If a percutaneous cryoprobe is to be used after the Chiba needle is in place, a guide wire is placed into the tumor, and a dilator is passed over the wire, sequentially dilating the tract to a size appropriate to accept the percutaneously introduced probe.

6. If interstitial radiation therapy is the chosen modality, large-bore needles, 14 gauge or larger, are percutaneously placed into the lesion, and iridium seeds are placed directly into the lesion. Alternatively, large afterloading catheters are left in place, and the introducing needles are withdrawn. The patient is subsequently placed in a shielded room or removed to the radiation oncology suite for afterloading of the interstitial catheters previously placed.

7. A specially sheathed, long, 18- or 20-gauge needle can be placed into the tumor when radiofrequency electrodesiccation is to be used. Radiofrequency can be applied and ultrasound used to monitor tumor destruction.

Procedure Notes

With the techniques indicated, real-time ultrasound monitors tissue destruction when laser hyperthermia or radiofrequency electrodesiccation is used. With alcohol injection, however, the distribution of the alcohol can be tracked with ultrasound, but this does not necessarily correlate with the extent of tumor destruction. Therefore, with alcohol ablation and interstitial radiation therapy techniques, the extent of tissue necrosis can only be judged with imaging studies performed days to weeks after treatment.

After completion of the therapy and confirmation of adequate tissue distribution of the destructive agent, the patient is monitored for complications. Broad-spectrum antibiotics are continued, and the patient is discharged. Combination therapies with either systemic or regional chemotherapy and/or radiation therapy can be considered at this point. Serum or urine biochemical markers are periodically used with CT or magnetic resonance imaging (MRI) to assess treatment results.

It is useful for surgeons and interventional radiologists to understand more than the anatomy of the major perihepatic vessels, including the hepatic artery, portal vein, hepatic veins, and vena cava. Understanding intrahepatic segmental anatomy is also useful.[3,4] The hepatic artery divides in the hilum to form two branches, 3 to 5 mm in diameter. Segmental hepatic artery branches are 1 to 2 mm in size. Arterioles within the periphery of the liver parenchyma are generally 25 μm in diameter. The right and left portal veins range from 5 to 15 mm in diameter. Large distributing branches of the portal vein up to 280 μm in diameter are found at the level of the hepatic segments and successively branch to become portal venules, averaging 35 μm in size in the periphery of the hepatic lobule. The artery, vein, and bile ducts traverse the parenchyma as the portal vein triads. The hepatic sinusoids are approximately 7 to 15 μm in width. Centrally in the hepatic lobule, terminal hepatic venules are close to 45 μm in size and, as tributaries coalesce, rapidly increase in size as the vessels approach the 8- to 20-mm diameter hepatic veins proper in the posterior aspect of the liver. Therefore, the majority of the liver has vessels of small diameter and low flow that are amenable to coagulation by a variety of means, including heat, freezing, or desiccation.

The bile ducts can be more easily injured by these modalities than surrounding vessels. Although large vessels, such as the portal and hepatic veins, rapidly dissipate heat and cold, bile ducts are unable to dissipate thermal energy. Photothermal, electrothermal, and cryosurgical physical effects are dissipated via large-vessel convection, enabling percutaneous treatment of lesions close to major vessels without vessel injury. However, because bile is static within the ducts, the potential for biliary stricture and occlusion must be considered, whether treating near the hilum and the major bile ducts or peripherally near the major segmental biliary tributaries.

As with liver resection, physiologic parameters, which are as yet difficult to quantify but have been termed *hepatic reserve*, will have a profound influence on the likelihood of interventional complications. Thus, transcatheter embolization may result in substantial impairment of hepatic reserve and occasional hepatic failure, even with careful selective embolization. In situ ablation can alleviate this problem and enable tumor destruction without the danger of initiating fatal liver failure.

Improved hepatic imaging, in particular the development of percutaneous real-time ultrasound, has facilitated percutaneous visualization of liver lesions in the size range of 2 cm in diameter. Ultrasound is useful both for identifying the site of a metastasis and directing an interstitial treatment modality to the tumor site. Ultrasound is helpful in defining the margins of the tumor and can be used to monitor the ongoing effects of tissue damage occurring as a result of thermal injury. The tracking of the alcohol into the liver interstitium after ethanol injection can also be monitored with ultrasound by visualizing the sonographic features of alcohol dispersion. Follow-up analysis by CT or MRI can then be employed as an anatomic indication of treatment effectiveness. Tumor markers, such as carcinoembryonic antigen, α-fetoprotein, or neuroendocrine secretory products, can also be used as indirect means of assessing the efficacy of treatment, although radiologic imaging is the preferred method of assessing the response to therapy and evaluating a possible recurrence within and outside the liver.

RESULTS OF PERCUTANEOUS INTERSTITIAL ABLATION

Cryotherapy

In 1987, Ravikumar and associates[5] reported their surgical experience with hepatic cryosurgery for metastatic colon cancer to the liver. The development of 8- to 12-mm liquid-nitrogen-cooled probes suitable for surgical placement within the liver marked the advent of interstitial therapy. Verification of the effectiveness of therapy was determined anatomically by the use of real-time ultrasound to measure the size of the increasing ice ball caused by freezing. Freezing and thawing for three cycles was an effective means of ensuring tumor necrosis.[6,7] The average size of lesions treated in this series was under 3 cm.

Zhou and colleagues,[8] in the following year, published results of their use of cryosurgery for hepatocellular carcinomas. Sixty patients were treated using surface freezing, with hemispheric areas of necrosis of 9 cm in diameter via a 6-cm probe or 6 cm via a 3-cm probe accomplished by placing the freezing plate onto the surface of the liver. Survival appeared to be improved in 27 cases treated with cryosurgery alone, with a 2-year survival rate of 23 percent and a 5-year survival rate of 4 percent, although this represents a select group of patients. Three papers report a total of 35 patients who underwent cryotherapy for metastatic disease.[5-7] Smaller lesions (< 4 cm) appear to respond well, and uncontrolled survival data appear promising. Newer smaller probes are being produced for percutaneous placement via a successively dilated tract. Clinical experimentation with these 3- to 5-mm probes is underway.

The disadvantage of cryotherapy appears to be that it requires an operation to place the large (8 and 12 mm) probes near the lesions. Thus, the surgical risks must be factored into the analysis of morbidity and mortality. The new smaller percutaneous probes will have risks that differ from those of surgical cryotherapy.

The surgical placement of cryoprobes appears to be safe, with no frequent treatment-associated complications recorded. Air embolus can occur with the technique of interstitial treatment via the tract of the dilator used to place the cryoprobes, and an unusual nitrogen embolus has been described.[6,9] Bleeding after freeze–thaw "cracking" of the liver and myoglobinuria have been reported in isolated instances.[7,9] Vessels tolerate cooling well, but bile duct stricture or occlusion occurs readily. By contrast, although avoiding surgery, percutaneous probe placement carries other risks. Rigid dilators and large tracts for percutaneous-

ly placed cryoprobes will result in greater risks of bleeding and liver laceration. Air embolus and hemobilia are potential complications. Combining laparoscopy with ultrasound and cryotherapy might reduce the risks of percutaneous treatment, but again, it reintroduces surgical risks.

Percutaneous Ethanol Injection

There is a recent tide of enthusiasm for percutaneous injection of absolute alcohol directly into hepatic tumors. Most research is directed toward treatment of hepatocellular carcinomas (HCC), with ultrasound used for guidance of needle placement. Livraghi and coworkers[10-12] have published several articles about this technique in the treatment of small HCC. Their most recent report describes 51 patients with 72 lesions, in whom 745 separate alcohol treatments were performed, an average of 10 treatments per lesion. There was no significant complications. In 40 of the 51 patients, there was complete remission of the lesions. In 11 of 51 patients, there was partial remission. The 1-, 2-, and 3-year survival rates for these patients were 100, 89, and 58 percent, respectively. In patients with single HCC, the 1-, 2-, and 3-year survival rates were 100, 94, and 71 percent, respectively. These authors think that percutaneous ethanol injection into HCC is a better treatment than surgical resection for lesions less than 3 cm in size and, in addition, should be used in those patients who are poor operative risks for lesions less than 5 cm.[11]

Their data were confirmed by other reports. Ebara and colleagues[13] reviewed their experience with this technique in the treatment of 120 lesions in 95 patients with HCC smaller than 3 cm. Their 1-, 2-, 3-, 4-, and 5-year survival rates, based on the Kaplan-Meier method, were 93, 81, 65, 52, and 28 percent, respectively. There have been a number of other series that substantiate the effectiveness of absolute alcohol treatment for small HCC.[14,15]

In most series, the technique for percutaneous ethanol injection of HCC is similar. Generally, 2 to 8 mL of 99.5% absolute alcohol is injected into the lesion at each treatment session.[16] There is variation as to the number of treatment sessions and the amount of alcohol injected. For instance, Livraghi and associates[11] performed 745 treatments on 72 lesions, or 10 treatments per lesion. Borghetti and colleagues[14] performed 78 treatments on 14 HCC, or 5.6 treatments per lesion. Shiina and coworkers[16] proposed the total amount of ethanol injected in separate sessions to be based on the total tumor volume plus a margin of safety. Their volume calculation is as follows:

$$V = 4/3 \, \pi \, (r + 0.5)^3$$

where V is the volume in milliliters, r is the radius in centimeters, and 0.5 is the margin of safety. This margin is provided to ensure that a certain amount of surrounding tissue is treated to accomplish complete tumor kill. Shiina and colleagues[17] proposed simultaneous use of multiple injection needles to increase delivery of alcohol and, thus, decrease number of treatment sessions. We have found that, in small lesions, the needle may be repositioned for reinjection, thus providing a more even delivery of alcohol into the entire tumor in one session. In lesions greater than 3 cm, we have repositioned the same needle in a number of different portions of the tumor for multiple treatments at one session.

The most commonly used guide for needle placement during percutaneous ethanol injection is ultrasound under real-time control. Dispersion of ethanol, which is visualized by ultrasound as an echogenic focus, marks the area of treatment (Fig. 24-1). If a lesion is encapsulated, ethanol is delivered precisely to the lesion. However, in poorly encapsulated lesions, there is a lack of geometric dispersion of the ethanol.

Percutaneous ethanol injection of these lesions may be followed by: (1) imaging procedures, such as ultrasound, CT, or MRI, which demonstrate necrosis or disappearance of the tumor; (2) use of fine-needle aspiration techniques, demonstrating lack of retrieval of tumor cells; or (3) a decrease in serologic markers.[11,14,16] Injection of alcohol into laboratory animal livers has shown no significant systemic side effects. Percutaneous ethanol injection into the liver produces an area of coagulation necrosis whose size is determined by the amount of injection. Remote necrosis occurs with increased doses of alcohol, which produce unpredictable diffusion.[18]

Some authors have advocated combined arterial chemoembolization and alcohol injection. Tanaka and associates[19] believe that, in lesions greater than 3 cm, diffusion of ethanol through the entire tumor was not always possible because of tumor size, or heterogeneity

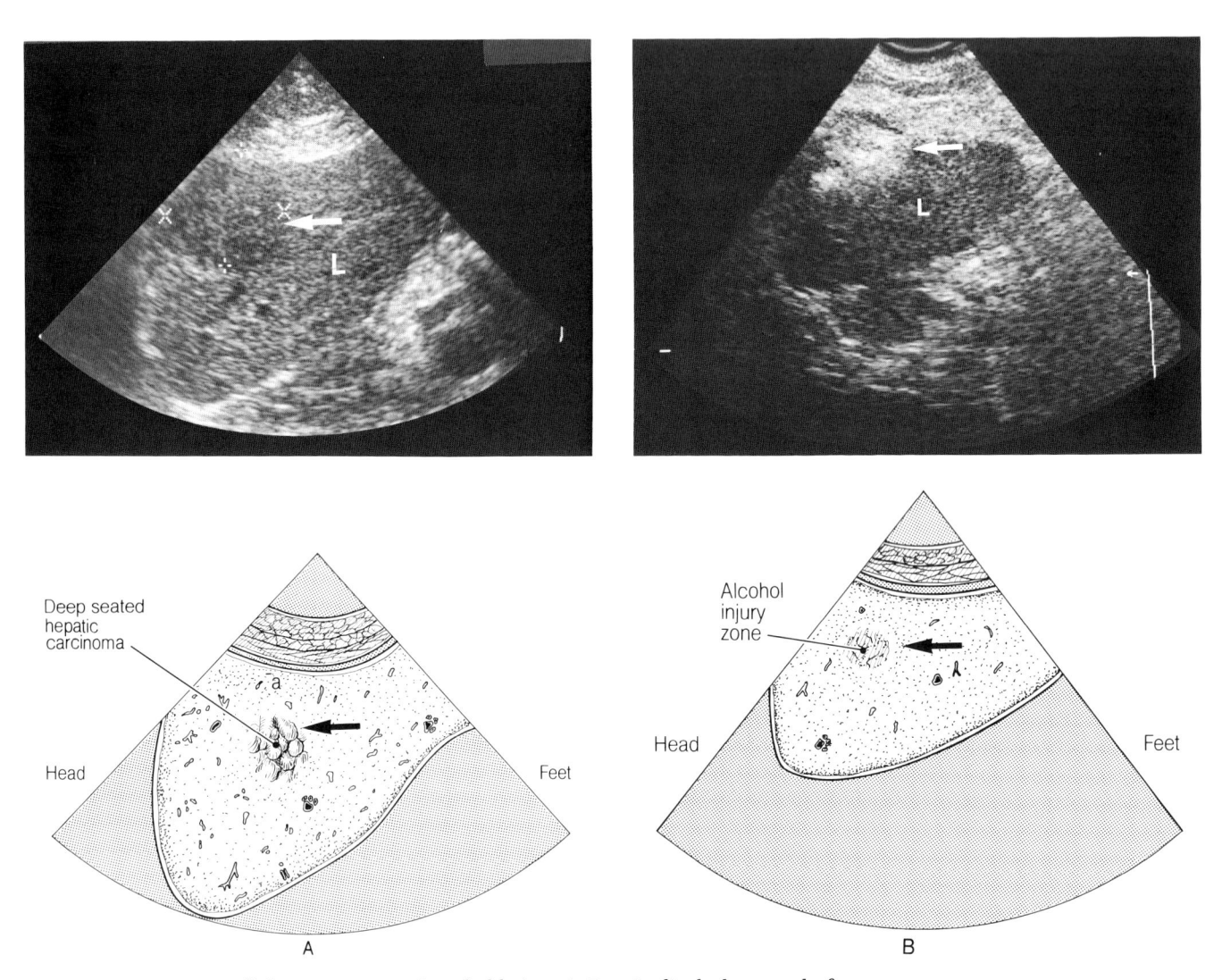

FIGURE 24-1 Hepatocellular carcinoma: ethanol ablation. A. Longitudinal ultrasound of a well-marginated hepatocellular carcinoma (arrow). The diagnosis was made by fine-needle aspiration biopsy (L = liver). B. Longitudinal ultrasound after treatment demonstrates the mass is now diffusely echogenic (arrow) after alcohol treatment (L = liver).

(e.g., cystic or solid components). Likewise, it has been shown that with transarterial embolization (TAE) of HCC necrosis is incomplete, with tumor cells remaining at portions of the lesions.[20] Therefore, Tanaka and associates[19] thought that initial utilization of TAE would alter the texture of HCC, causing tumor necrosis and easy diffusion and infiltration of the entire tumor with injection of absolute alcohol. In their protocol for TAE, they used (1) iodized oil; (2) an anticancer agent (doxorubicin hydrochloride), followed by (3) an injection of gelatin sponge, thus effecting chemoembolization. This is performed before percutaneous ethanol injection. In four patients, with HCC ranging from 3 to 9 cm in diameter, who later underwent surgical resection, there was complete tumor necrosis in all tumors with this combined therapy.[21]

Shiina and coworkers[16] reported long-term follow-up results of patients receiving alcohol injection alone (n = 23) or with TAE (n = 54), with combined 1-, 2-, 3-, and 4-year survival rates of 89, 74, 68, and 60 percent, respectively. These results, like those of Livraghi[10-12] and Ebara,[13] are comparable to surgical series employing limited resection for small HCC. Nakamura and associates[21] concurred that combined chemoembolization and percutaneous ethanol injection provide a safe and effective means of treating HCC.

Although there is extensive experience in percutaneous ethanol ablation of HCC, the experience of percutaneous techniques and treatment for metastatic disease is limited. Giovannini and coworkers[22] published a report on a series of eight patients, of whom six with metastatic disease were treated with alcohol injection. There were 59 injections involving 11 lesions. There was complete necrosis in four lesions, partial necrosis in three, and no change in four. Livraghi and colleagues[23] treated 14 patients with 21 hepatic metastases ranging from 1 to 3.8 cm in diameter. They performed 171 treatments on 21 lesions, or 8.1 treatments per lesion. There was complete response in 11 of 21 lesions. However, these authors were less enthusiastic about alcohol injection for liver metastases compared with HCC. They believe that the natural course of metastatic disease may preclude the widespread use of this type of treatment of liver metastases.

Interstitial Radiotherapy

Little information exists about interstitial or brachytherapy of intrahepatic malignancies despite the known utility of the technique for tumors close to the body surfaces or when employed at laparotomy or thoracotomy for adjuvant or palliative management of difficult tumors. The two methods, implantation of the tumor with radioactive iridium seeds or employment of afterloading catheters (which can be used to guide radiation source placement), have benefited from technical advances in computer planning, stereotactic guidance of catheter placement, and high-speed computerized source distributon via afterloading catheters, such as is provided by the Gamma Med II irradiator.[24] However, treatment of liver tumors with ultrasound-guided placement of catheters or radioactive sources has, thus far, been utilized in only a few patients.[25] The only means of following up on the effects of therapy is subsequent imaging over several weeks or months.

Interstitial Laser Hyperthermia

In 1985, Hashimoto and associates[26] were the first to apply the concept of interstitial thermal injury clinically by utilizing laser light. They recognized that light administered by the Nd:YAG laser could deliver light energy at the tip of an interstitially placed transmission fiber. Previous experimental work by others had established that the nature of such an injury was a spheric lesion at the tip of the fiber, which, as with the other modalities discussed previously, could be followed using real-time ultrasound. Since their report, others, including Hahl and coworkers,[27] established that the technique was safe and, as with alcohol injection, the laser fibers could be inserted via percutaneously placed needles introduced under ultrasonic guidance. However, the size of the fiber necessitates a 14-gauge needle with stylet for placement.

The extent of thermal injury is determined, as with all laser techniques, by the power in watts, exposure time, characteristics of light wavelength intensity, and absorption characteristics of the tissue. Using the Nd:YAG laser, applied power has ranged from 0 to 6 W, and exposure times have ranged from 500 to 1000 s. An advantage within the liver (especially with tumors located near major vascular structures that we wish to preserve) is the thermal conduction and protection afforded by blood flow, which will save major vessels from injury. Thus, the technique has potential application for lesions that are near structures that make them surgically unresectable.[9] Heat, however, has the potential of causing bile duct injury, resulting in obstruction or narrowing, as previously mentioned.

An additional danger is related to the power setting, as has been reported by Schröder and colleagues.[28] With the Nd:YAG laser at low power settings, in the range of 0.5 to 1.5 W, no cooling is needed. However, if 4 to 6 W of power are applied to decrease the exposure time, most investigators have used coaxial gas flow in the range of 1 L/min to provide cooling and avoid the vaporization that causes tissue disruption or vapor emboli. The application of heat and gas under pressure in a closed space has led to an instance of fatal air embolism.[28] It appears that the lower power settings will at least have the advantage of diminishing the risk of embolus because gas cooling is not required, although the time required for creating therapeutic heat injury will be longer.

A physical danger is introduced by the large, rigid, 14-gauge introducing needles. Liver laceration, bleeding, and

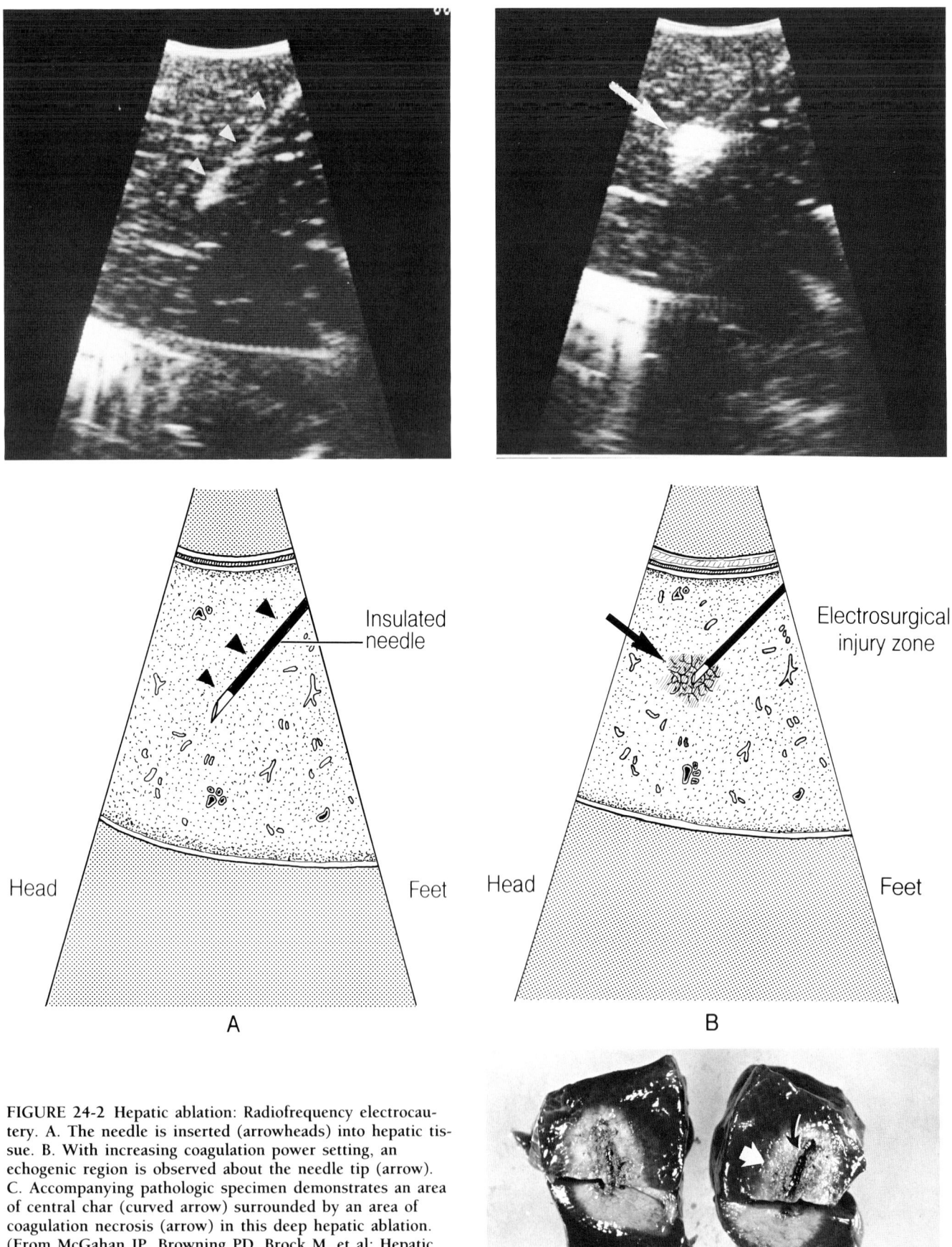

FIGURE 24-2 Hepatic ablation: Radiofrequency electrocautery. A. The needle is inserted (arrowheads) into hepatic tissue. B. With increasing coagulation power setting, an echogenic region is observed about the needle tip (arrow). C. Accompanying pathologic specimen demonstrates an area of central char (curved arrow) surrounded by an area of coagulation necrosis (arrow) in this deep hepatic ablation. (From McGahan JP, Browning PD, Brock M, et al: Hepatic ablation using radiofrequency electrocautery. *Invest Radiol* 1990; 25:267–270.)

hemobilia are much more likely to occur than with the smaller-gauge needles required for alcohol injection.[29,30]

To treat larger lesions, we must carefully place a pattern of fibers such that the entire tumor is encompassed to ensure total ablation. A spread or pattern of laser fibers can achieve this effect. The major advantage of this technique is that the extent of necrosis can be monitored using real-time ultrasound and can be adjusted at the time of treatment. The injury is predictably spheric, unlike the irregular lesions resulting from alcohol injection.[31]

Radiofrequency Desiccation

In 1990, McGahan and colleagues[32] published a report on percutaneous ablation of liver tissue with radiofrequency electrocautery. This concept was novel because it proposed the use of focal application of radiofrequency electrocautery in the animal liver via ultrasound guidance. A monopolar electrocautery with an 18- to 20-gauge needle was placed deep in the liver parenchyma. The distal 1 cm of the needle tip was uninsulated and placed in the area of treatment. With gradual application of current, an elliptic echogenic focus was observed sonographically (Fig. 24-2).

Pathologically, the echogenic lesion corresponded to an area of coagulation necrosis surrounded by a rim of partially destroyed tissue. The lesion size increased with added current. A larger volume of the liver could be destroyed by placement of multiple needles for treatment (Fig. 24-3). The authors believed that this percutaneous technique had great potential because (1) the lesion was well controlled, (2) the technique allowed for retreatment, (3) there seemed to be a few complications, (4) it could be performed without hospitalization, and (5) the technique could be combined with other therapeutic methods.[32]

The authors have treated three patients with this technique, and an additional 14 patients have been treated by authors reporting this technique based on similar animal experimentation.[33] Follow-up is too short to determine efficacy.

CONCLUSION

The introduction of ablative probes into the liver interstitium, with large areas of resulting necrosis, may predispose to infection. As with a variety of transcatheter embolization techniques, larger tumors that become necrotic have increased rates of infection. Thus, antibiotic prophylaxis and monitoring for infection are required in patients undergoing interstitial therapies. Although complications appear to be few in the short term and the discomforts of the procedures are well tolerated by most patients, the potential for bile duct injury from heat, cold, radiation, or alcohol must be considered. In addition, although it is established that healing of the ablated areas occurs eventually by contraction and fibrosis, we must be alert with all these techniques to the possibility and long-term risk of hemobilia, especially when using 14-gauge introducers or afterloading catheters.[29]

Table 24-1 provides a comparison of these interstitial and in situ techniques, assessing several parameters. Obviously, existing resources, both human and material, influence the qualitative value of techniques at a given institution. The rapid advancement of technology and cross fertilization between groups using different interstitial techniques will lead to an understanding of the benefits and limitations of each technique. However, there is essentially no information at this time to suggest that these techniques should be used in lieu of hepatic resection in an attempt to cure patients who are good operative risks. There is insufficient data to determine that survival is comparable between patients undergoing hepatic resection and those treated with interstitial techniques. The majority of patients treated have had HCC and results are promising. Metastatic disease poses special problems and few such patients have been treated with any of these techniques.

Nevertheless, it is clear that these interstitial treatments cause reproducible tissue destruction and are well tolerated, with low risk to the patients. It is conceivable that interstitial techniques may replace hepatic resection in some instances in the future, particularly for lesions less than 3 cm in size. Combining therapies, such as transcatheter regional chemotherapy or systemic chemotherapy with percutaneous ablative techniques, may be worthwhile. Patients who are candidates for curative resection, but for

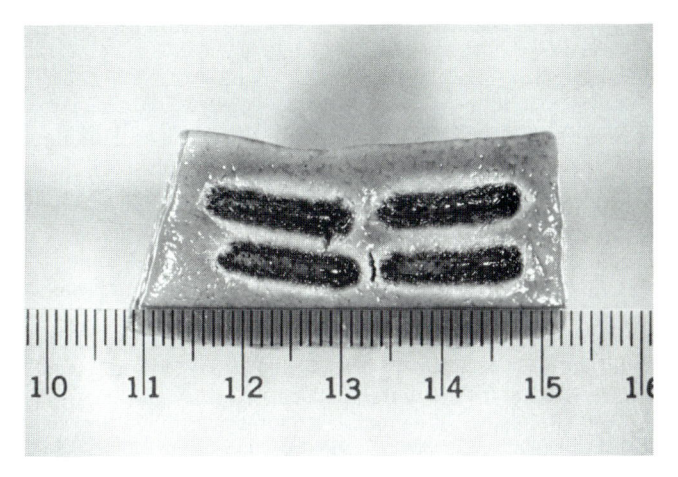

FIGURE 24-3 Radiofrequency hepatic ablation: contiguous treatment. Four separate treatments are performed, demonstrating the possibility of increasing the volume of tissue necrosis by contiguous placement of needles for hepatic treatment. [From McGahan JP: Interventional US: Aspiration/drainage techniques, in Rifkin JW, Charboneau JW, Laing FC (eds): *Syllabus: Special Course in Ultrasound 1992.* Oak Brook, IL, Radiological Society of North America, 1991, pp 73–80.]

TABLE 24-1 Qualitative assessment of techniques for interstitial in situ hepatic tumor ablation

Criteria	Percutaneous cryotherapy	Percutaneous alcohol injection	Percutaneous laser hyperthermia	Percutaneous interstitial radiotherapy	Percutaneous radiofrequency electrodesiccation
Ease of application	Fair	Excellent	Good	Poor	Good
Precision and predictability	Fair	Fair	Good	Fair	Excellent
Ease of real-time monitoring	Good	Poor	Good	Not possible	Good
Accessibility to all liver	Fair	Good	Fair	Fair	Good
Treatment frequency	Good	Poor	Good	Good	Good
Ease of retreatment	Fair	Excellent	Good	Fair	Excellent
Equipment expense	Fair	Excellent	Poor	Poor	Good
Hospitalization time	Good	Excellent	Good	Fair	Good
Staff required	Radiologist, possibly anesthesiologist	Interventional radiologist	Interventional radiologist, technician	Interventional radiologist, physicist, radiation therapist	Interventional radiologist, possibly anesthesiologist

whom surgical resection is not an option, should be offered participation in carefully conducted clinical trials utilizing any of these interstitial techniques. This is an evolving technology-based clinical treatment, with too little data regarding long-term results. We must proceed carefully and document our results meticulously.

REFERENCES

1. Hughes KS, Rosenstein RB, Songhorabodi S, et al: Resection of the liver for colorectal carcinoma metastases: A multi-institutional study of long-term survivors. *Dis Colon Rectum* 1988; 31:1-4.
2. Hughes KS, Simon R, Songhorabodi S, et al: Resection of the liver for colorectal carcinoma metastases: A multi-institutional study of patterns of recurrence. *Surgery* 1986; 100:278–284.
3. Campra JL, Reynolds TB: The hepatic circulation in the liver: Biology and pathobiology, in Arias I, Popper H, Schacter D, et al (eds): *The Liver: Biology and Pathobiology*. New York, Raven Press, 1982, pp 627–645.
4. Rappaport AM: Physioanatomic considerations, in Schiff L, Schiff ER (eds): *Diseases of the Liver*. Philadelphia, JB Lippincott, 1982, pp 1–57.
5. Ravikumar TS, Kane R, Cady B, et al: Hepatic cryosurgery with intraoperative ultrasound monitoring for metastatic colon carcinoma. *Arch Surg* 1987; 122:403–409.
6. Onik G, Rubinsky B, Zemel R, et al: Ultrasound-guided hepatic cryosurgery in the treatment of metastatic colon carcinoma, preliminary results. *Cancer* 1991; 67:901–907.
7. Ravikumar TS, Steele GD: Hepatic cryosurgery. *Surg Clin North Am* 1989; 69:433–440.
8. Zhou XD, Tang ZY, Yu YQ, et al: Clinical evaluation of cryosurgery in the treatment of primary liver cancer. *Cancer* 1988; 61:1889–1892.
9. Masters A, Steger AC, Bown SG: Role of interstitial therapy in the treatment of liver cancer. *Br J Surg* 1991; 78:5189–5523.
10. Livraghi T, Salmi A, Bolondi L, et al: Small hepatocellular carcinoma: Percutaneous alcohol injection—Results in 23 patients. *Radiology* 1988; 168:313–317.
11. Livraghi T, Torzilli G: Percutaneous alcoholization of the small hepatocarcinoma. *Ann Ital Chir* 1991; 62:19–23.
12. Livraghi T, Vettori C: Percutaneous ethanol injection therapy of hepatoma. *Cardiovasc Intervent Radiol* 1990; 13:146–152.
13. Ebara M, Ohto M, Sugiura N, et al: Percutaneous ethanol injection for the treatment of small hepatocellular carcinoma: Study of 95 patients. *J Gastroenterol Hepatol* 1990; 5:616–626.
14. Borghetti M, Benelli G, Bonardi R: Treatment of small hepatocarcinomas by percutaneous ultrasound-guided alcohol injection: Personal experience in 14 lesions. *Radiol Med* 1991; 81:502–509.
15. Seki T, Nonaka T, Kubota Y, et al: Ultrasonically guided percutaneous ethanol injection therapy for hepatocellular carcinoma. *Am J Gastroenterol* 1989; 84:1400–1407.
16. Shiina S, Tagawa K, Unuma T, et al: Percutaneous ethanol injection therapy of hepatocellular carcinoma: Analysis of 77 patients. *AJR Am J Roentgenol* 1990; 155:1221–1226.
17. Shiina S, Hata Y, Niwa Y, et al: Multiple-needle insertion method in percutaneous ethanol injection therapy for liver neoplasms. *Gastroenterol Jpn* 1991; 26:47–50.
18. Festi D, Monti F, Casanova S, et al: Morphological and biochemical effects of intrahepatic alcohol injection in the rabbit. *J Gastroenterol Hepatol* 1990; 5:402–406.
19. Tanaka K, Okazaki H, Nakamura S, et al: Hepatocellular carcinoma: Treatment with a combination therapy of transcatheter arterial embolization and percutaneous ethanol injection. *Radiology* 1991; 179:713–717.
20. Nakamura H, Tanaka T, Hori S, et al: Transcatheter embolization of hepatocellular carcinoma: Assessment of efficacy in cases of resection following embolization. *Radiology* 1983; 147:401–405.
21. Nakamura H, Hashimoto T, Suyama Y, et al: Combined therapy

with transcatheter chemo-embolization and percutaneous ethanol injection. *Jpn J Cancer Chemother* 1990; 17:1740–1743.
22. Giovannini M, Seitz JF, Rosello R, et al: Treatment of minor hepatic tumors with ultrasonically guided percutaneous injection of absolute alcohol: Results in 8 patients. *Gastroenterol Clin Biol* 1989; 13:974–977
23. Livraghi T, Vettor C, Lazzaroni S: Liver metastases: Results of percutaneous ethanol injection in 14 patients. *Radiology* 1991; 179:709–712.
24. Dritschild A, Grant EG, Harter KW, et al: Interstitial radiation therapy for hepatic metastases: Sonographic guidance for applicator placement. *AJR Am J Roentgenol* 1986; 146:275–278.
25. Holt RW, Nauta RJ, Lee TC, et al: Intraoperative interstitial radiation therapy for hepatic metastases from colorectal carcinomas. *Am Surg* 1988; 54:231–233.
26. Hashimoto D, Takami M, Idezuki M: In depth radiation therapy by Nd:YAG laser for malignant tumors of the liver under ultrasonic imaging. *Gastroenterology* 1985; 88:A1663.
27. Hahl J, Haapiainen R, Ovaska J, et al: Laser-induced hyperthermia in the treatment of liver tumors. *Lasers Surg Med* 1990; 10:319–321.
28. Schröder TM, Puolakkainen PA, Hahl J, et al: Fatal air embolism as a complication of laser-induced hyperthermia. *Lasers Surg Med* 1989; 9:1983–1985.
29. Merrell S, Schneider PD: Hemobilia: Evolution of current diagnosis and treatment. *West J Med* 1991; 155:621–625.
30. Okuda K, Musha H, Nakajima Y, et al: Frequency of intrahepatic arteriovenous fistula as a sequela to percutaneous needle puncture of the liver. *Gastroenterology* 1978; 74:1204–1207.
31. Bosman S, Phoa SSK, Bosma A, et al: Effect of percutaneous interstitial thermal laser on normal liver of pigs: Sonographic and histopathologic correlations. *Br J Surg* 1991; 78:572–575.
32. McGahan JP, Browning PD, Brock JM, et al: Hepatic ablation using radiofrequency electrocautery. *Invest Radiol* 1990; 25:267–270.
33. Rossi S, Fornari F, Pathies C, et al: Thermal lesions induced by 108 KHz localized current field in guinea pig and pig liver. *Tumori* 1990; 76:54–57.

Chapter 25

Laparoscopic Approaches to Diseases of the Liver

Jonathan M. Sackier / John G. Hunter

Although there is little doubt that formal anatomic resections of the liver can and will be performed using laparoscopic techniques, the problems associated with removing a large volume of tissue and controlling bleeding have limited laparoscopic surgery of the liver to several distinct indications. In this chapter, we will address laparoscopic liver biopsy, treatment of hepatic cysts, and wedge resection of peripheral lesions.

LIVER BIOPSY

Diseases of the liver often require directed biopsy for definitive diagnosis. There are a variety of ways in which tissue may be retrieved from the liver for pathologic examination, including blind percutaneous, CT-directed, and ultrasound-directed biopsy. These techniques are limited by their ability to detect and sample small lesions and by the risk of hemorrhage in patients with coagulopathy.

Laparoscopic liver biopsy has none of these drawbacks, allows the surgeon to dictate the timing of the biopsy, and provides the opportunity to biopsy areas not otherwise accessible, such as the domes of the liver. The ability to detect and sample small lesions is especially valuable in oncologic surgery, where direct inspection of the liver allows detection of liver metastases too small to be seen with computerized axial tomographic scan, ultrasound, or magnetic resonance imaging. Because 43 percent of patients with pancreatic cancer who are thought to be metastasis-free after CT and angiography, indeed, have metastases detectable with laparoscopy, this diagnostic procedure should be a part of the preoperative evaluation of any patient being considered for pancreaticoduodenectomy.[1]

Techniques

The preoperative evaluation of patients referred for laparoscopic liver biopsy includes inspection for scars from previous abdominal incisions, correction of coagulopathy, examination for ascites, and assessment of risk for general anesthesia should it become necessary to complete an uncomfortable procedure or correct a complication of laparoscopic biopsy.

If biopsy is to be part of a more major laparoscopic procedure or if the patient is uncooperative, general anesthesia will be required. Otherwise, laparoscopic biopsy may be performed under local anesthesia with intravenous sedation. If laparoscopy is to be performed with the patient awake, N_2O should be used to create the pneumoperitoneum because it is less irritating than CO_2.[2] Under local anesthesia, the insufflation pressures also should be kept below 10 mmHg.

With laparoscopic guidance, the following types of tissue may be retrieved.

1. Fine-needle aspiration of solid organs.
2. Peritoneal washings.
3. Aspiration of fluid (e.g., gallbladder contents or cyst contents).
4. Trucut needle biopsy.
5. Pinch or punch biopsy.
6. Excisional biopsy (e.g., small liver lesions or lymph nodes).

Procedure Notes

As usual, the laparoscope is introduced through the umbilicus. For diagnostic procedures, a 5-mm telescope will suffice. An additional 5-mm trocar is placed in the right midclavicular line at about the level of the anterior superior iliac spine. This trocar accommodates a "workhorse" probe that can deliver electrosurgery, suction, and irrigation (Fig. 25-1).

If an area on the liver has been identified on a previous abdominal CT scan or ultrasound, it is palpated with the probe to ensure that it is solid and not a hemangioma. If a core biopsy is required, a third 1- to 2-mm puncture is made over the lesion from which the biopsy will be obtained to introduce the biopsy needle. If a cirrhotic liver is to be sampled, the lateral segment of the left lobe is a convenient target. The biopsy needle is brought into the peritoneal cavity under direct vision, and the surgeon checks to ascertain that the coagulation probe can reach the site. The surgeon should then raise the liver edge to gain an impression of its thickness so that deeper structures, such as the stomach, are not accidentally sampled.

The patient is asked to suspend breathing, or respiration is stopped if controlled ventilation is being employed. Omitting this step, carries the risk of tearing the liver capsule, with subsequent hemorrhage. The sample is retrieved, and immediate pressure is brought to bear on the biopsy site with the suction–coagulation probe. After maintaining pressure for several minutes, short bursts of coagulation (about 25 to 40 W) are applied as the probe is withdrawn. The liver is then elevated to ascertain that there is no exit-site bleeding resulting from full-thickness penetration of the needle.

If an exophytic lesion of the liver is to be sampled, then a pinch forceps is used. The punch forceps and biopsy needle are more effective in cases of intrahepatic lesions that are visible through the capsule or have been located with the aid of ultrasound.

Ascites

Although laparoscopy is often useful for evaluation of the patient with ascites of unknown origin, there are several important considerations in these severely ill patients. First, an evaluation of clotting ability, including prothrombin time, partial thromboplastin time, and platelet count, is imperative. The referring doctor should be discouraged from performing a preoperative ascitic tap because this may predispose to a chronic leak of ascitic fluid. Before the procedure, the surgeon should mark the position of the liver and spleen because these may be enlarged. One should then carefully search for collateral vessels around the umbilicus. If a caput medusae is detected, it is wise to perform the initial puncture and trocar insertion to the left of the umbilicus.

Initially, the patient should be placed in reverse Trendelenburg position so that the gas-filled viscera float up on the pool of ascites, thus avoiding the introduced needle. Although these patients may have a distended abdomen, a pneumoperitoneum is, nevertheless, mandatory. To prevent frothing of the proteinaceous ascitic fluid during insufflation, it is helpful to aspirate as much fluid as possible through the Veress needle and then drop the hub of the needle so that the needle tip is above the surface of the ascitic pool. After the accessory trocar has been introduced, the remainder of the ascites may be slowly withdrawn (saving some for analysis) and replaced in a stepwise fashion with gas.

Many of these patients tend to have a bleeding diathesis; thus, careful attention must be paid to any biopsy needle and trocar insertion sites. If troublesome bleeding occurs on the peritoneal surface, it can be controlled using electrocautery or a Foley catheter with the balloon blown up inside the abdomen to tamponade the bleeding. If neither of these steps is effective, a full-thickness suture may be placed percutaneously and tied over a bolster for a few days. At the end of the procedure, it is mandatory to close the incision in layers to prevent a chronic ascitic leak.

Postoperatively, the patient is kept at bed rest for several hours and observed for signs of bleeding. Same-day discharge is generally appropriate. The most frequent complication of laparoscopic liver biopsy is an ascitic leak. Bleeding is exceedingly rare.

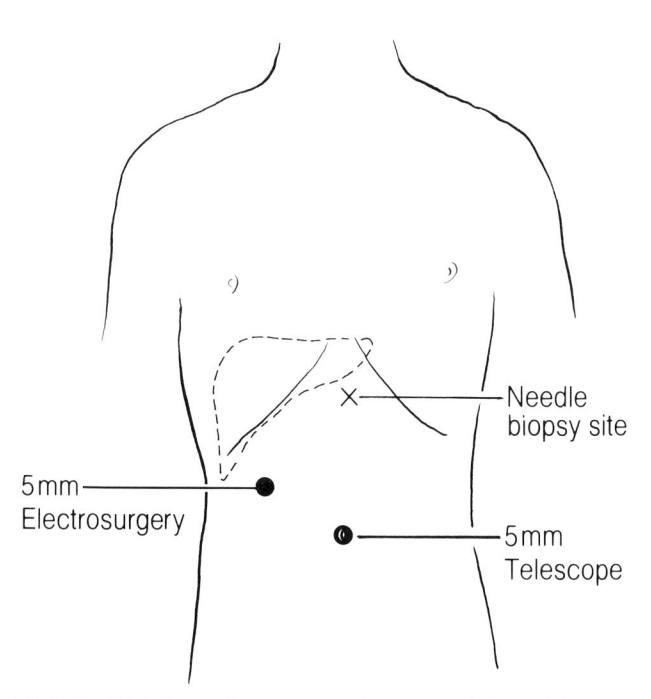

FIGURE 25-1 Port placement for laparoscopic liver biopsy. The stab wound necessary for the core biopsy may be made anywhere beneath the costal margin that allows the best access to the liver lesion requiring biopsy. In a diffusely cirrhotic liver, biopsy of the lateral segment of the left lobe can be made through a stab wound, high in the midline.

BENIGN HEPATIC CYSTS

Fenestration and packing of hepatic cysts is an ideal procedure for laparoscopic surgery. Hepatic cysts are most commonly congenital and benign. They may be filled with clear fluid or, occasionally, with biliary fluid if a connection with a bile duct is present. Hepatic cysts require treatment only if symptomatic, and the most common symptom is upper abdominal fullness. Although older surgical texts recommend excision of the cyst,[3] more recent data have shown that unroofing and omental packing is adequate therapy.[1] If one is tempted to simplify the management and only unroof the cyst, the edges of resection may fall together, leading to cyst recurrence. Although it has frequently been stated that the finding of bile in a cyst requires closure of the communication with the biliary tree or Roux-en-Y cyst jejunostomy, recent experience suggests that external drainage will control any bile extravasation while the connections of the cyst to the biliary tract seal (Way L. Personal communication, June 1992). If spontaneous closure does not occur and a persistent bile fistula develops from the base of a cyst, placement of a nasobiliary tube or endoscopic stent will eliminate elevated biliary pressure from an intact sphincter of Oddi, and allow closure of the fistula.

Another technique for management of hepatic cysts involves unroofing and sclerosis of the cyst lining with electrocautery or chemical agents. It appears that, if these cysts are kept adequately fenestrated by omental packing, sclerotherapy of the cyst lining is unnecessary. The biggest drawback to laparotomy for carrying out cyst fenestration is that it is too much incision for too few symptoms, often leaving the patient with incisional pain that is worse than the symptoms of the cyst.

It is against this background that CT-guided percutaneous drainage and sclerotherapy with alcohol has arisen, but recurrence is common despite aggressive cyst sclerosis.[5] Laparoscopy provides adequate access the first time, without incurring the pain and morbidity of an incision.

TECHNIQUE OF LAPAROSCOPIC CYSTOTOMY

Laparoscopic cystotomy requires two or three trocars in addition to the viewing telescope. The trocar positions will depend on the location of the cyst, but a slight modification of laparoscopic cholecystectomy positioning seems ideal (Fig. 25-2). If the surgeon uses a two-handed technique, the majority of the operation can be performed unassisted. A surgical assistant, using an expandable retractor or a blunt rod to expose the surface of the cyst, may be a welcome addition to the operating team. Using a grasper in the left hand and an electrosurgical hook with suction and irrigation in the right hand, the surgeon, standing on the

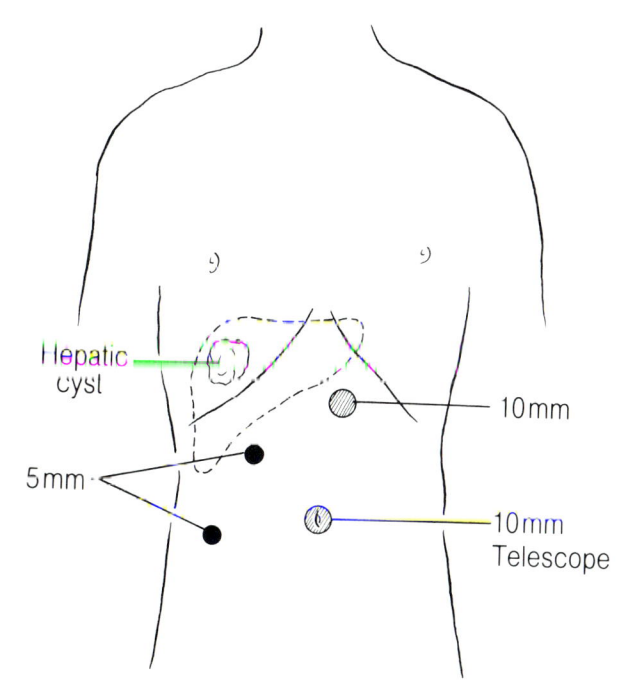

FIGURE 25-2 Port placement for hepatic cystotomy. The trocar positions are dependent on cyst location. If the cyst is located centrally, slight modifications of laparoscopic cholecystectomy trocar placement will usually suffice. Through the 10-mm midepigastric port, the dissection is performed by the surgeon standing on the patient's left. A larger port is necessary to tack omentum into the defect after wide unroofing has occurred. The surgeon uses the midclavicular port for the left hand, and the first assistant uses the most lateral port for retraction, irrigation, and aspiration. A 30° telescope is a must for this procedure.

left side of the patient, cauterizes a hole into the cyst and aspirates its contents for cytologic examination, culture, and chemical analysis, if desired. The cyst can then be entirely unroofed using the electrosurgical hook.

The dissection begins at the most dependent point of the cyst surface to prevent blood run down from obscuring the field during subsequent unroofing. When the cyst has been entirely unroofed, a piece of the cyst wall is taken out for the pathologist, and the inner surface of the cyst is examined to ensure that the preoperative diagnosis has been correct.

The surgeon then uses two graspers to mobilize a portion of the omentum, rotating it up to the right upper quadrant. While the first assistant holds the omentum in place, the surgeon anchors the omentum in this position with either staples or interrupted sutures.

RESULTS OF HEPATIC CYSTOTOMY

Although a very limited number of hepatic cystotomies have been performed, it appears that the procedure is quite successful when properly performed (Way L. Personal communication, June 1992).[6] The most frequent adverse outcome is that of cyst recurrence, which occurs in cases of deep-seated cysts, especially if inadequate omentum was available for thorough packing within the cyst cavity. A second cause of recurrence is inadequate unroofing of the cyst or inadequate fixation of omentum in the cyst cavity. Certainly, bleeding and persistent bile fistula can occasionally be expected with this technique, but currently, this complication has not been reported.

The postoperative care of these patients is the same as that for patients after laparoscopic cholecystectomy. They are observed for hemodynamic stability and the absence of an ileus. The patient may be discharged the morning after surgery.

LAPAROSCOPIC LIVER RESECTION

Fewer than 10 cases of laparoscopic liver resection have been reported, and thus, it is difficult to say much about this procedure. Intuitively, it makes a great deal of sense that small superficial lesions could be adequately saucerized and removed in a tissue specimen bag (see Chaps. 7 and 21). The scenario in which such an approach might be reasonable is that of the patient with colonic cancer who has CT evidence of one to four small peripheral nodules, consistent with recurrent metastasis. In this patient, intraoperative laparoscopic ultrasonography would be helpful to ensure that the lesions seen on CT scan represented all that were present. The technique would then involve removing a 1-cm margin of normal tissue around the metastasis and slowly deepening the resection.

Desirable instrumentation would include an electrosurgical hook dissector for the liver capsule and a CUSA (Cavitational Ultrasonic Surgical Aspirator, Valleylab, Inc., Boulder, CO) for deeper dissection. High-frequency ultrasonic waves from the CUSA mechanically disrupt tissue with a very high water content, leaving fibrous and elastic tissue, such as vessel walls, unaffected. When moved rapidly side to side, the CUSA does an excellent job of removing hepatocytes with very little bleeding. Exposed vessels are controlled with clips. Oozing may be arrested with an argon beam coagulator (Birtcher Medical, Irvine, CA).

Another disease process for which laparoscopic hepatic resection has been utilized is echinococcal (hydatid) cyst.[7] In the treatment described, the cyst is aspirated and filled with a scolicidal agent, such as cetrimide, to kill the viable scolices and minimize the risk of intraperitoneal spillage of cyst contents (which may cause anaphylactic shock). As reported, the resection technique requires that the surgeon, using an Nd:YAG laser (although CUSA and electrosurgery might be more hemostatic), come through the liver at the edge of the cyst. Large-volume bleeding was not encountered in the few cases that were reported, but this certainly remains one of our concerns. After cyst resection is complete, a number of closed suction drains are placed near the raw surface of the liver and left until drainage becomes minimal.

CONCLUSION

Diseases requiring biopsy of the liver or hepatotomy are ideal for application of minimally invasive approaches. When resection involves removing a large volume of hepatic tissue or a centrally located lesion, minimally invasive procedures carry the risk of large-scale bleeding and problematic removal of tissue from the abdomen. Despite these drawbacks, the inventive courageous laparoscopic surgeon will discover ways to circumvent these difficulties and eventually perform formal anatomic hepatic resections. Until then, the techniques we have described will obviate laparotomy in many patients with simple problems requiring liver surgery.

REFERENCES

1. Warshaw AL, Tepper JE, Shipley WU: Laparoscopy in the staging and planning of therapy for pancreatic cancer. *Am J Surg* 1986; 151:76–80.
2. Minoli G, Terruzzi V, Spinzi GC, et al: The influence of carbon dioxide and nitrous oxide on pain during laparoscopy: A double-blind, controlled trial. *Gastrointest Endosc* 1982; 28:173.
3. Jones RS: Liver cysts, in Cameron JL (ed): *Current Surgical Therapy*—2. St. Louis, CV Mosby, 1986, pp 157–160.
4. Schwartz SI: Liver cysts, in Cameron JL (ed): *Current Surgical Therapy*—3. Philadelphia, Decker, 1989, pp 209–212.
5. Bean WJ, Rodan BA: Hepatic cysts: Treatment with alcohol. *AJR* 1985; 144:237–241.
6. Fabiani P, Katkhouda N, Iovine L, et al: Laparoscopic fenestration of biliary cysts. *Surg Laparosc Endosc* 1991; 1:162–165.
7. Katkhouda N, Fabiani P, Benizri E, et al: Laser resection of a liver hydatid cyst under video laparoscopy. *Br J Surg* 1992; 79:560–561.

Chapter 26

Transjugular Intrahepatic Portosystemic Shunts

Robert E. Barton / Josef Rösch / Frederick S. Keller / Barry Uchida

The treatment of hemorrhage from gastroesphageal varices caused by portal hypertension is a challenging clinical problem. Although several therapeutic modalities are available, none are ideal. Most patients with bleeding esophageal varices are treated initially by endoscopic sclerotherapy. This does nothing to relieve the underlying portal hypertension, however, so the incidence of rebleeding and retreatment are relatively high. Patients who fail sclerotherapy usually undergo creation of a surgical portosystemic shunt. Although shunts are highly effective in preventing further bleeding, they are associated with significant morbidity and mortality when performed in patients with poor hepatic function, particularly when performed on an emergency basis. Liver transplantation is the ultimate treatment for variceal hemorrhage because it addresses the underlying liver disease leading to the development of portal hypertension and varices. Transplantation, however, is costly and may not be warranted in many patients. It is also not feasible as an emergency procedure.

The shortcomings of these currently accepted therapies have led to a search for additional treatment options. The transjugular intrahepatic portosystemic shunt (TIPS) represents a new alternative in the management of portal hypertension. Early results suggest that the application of this technique may improve outcomes in high-risk patients with variceal bleeding.

HISTORY

The idea of TIPS was conceived by Rösch and associates[1] in 1969. They created a tract between the portal and hepatic veins in dogs using long coaxial dilators and stented it with plastic tubing to create a shunt; however, occlusion of these small-diameter shunts invariably occurred after a short period of time. These investigators continued their work using a variety of larger-diameter tubing, including coil spring stents, but they were unable to achieve long-term patency of portosystemic shunts in animals.[2] They also successfully created TIPS in cadavers, but the technology available at the time precluded clinical application of this technique.

Interest in TIPS was renewed with the development of the angioplasty balloon catheter. Colapinto and associates[3] reported the first TIPS in a human in 1982. They embolized gastroesophageal varices in a patient with severe cirrhosis and variceal hemorrhage through a transjugular approach. After embolization, a portosystemic shunt was created by inflating an angioplasty balloon in the tract between the hepatic and portal veins. No stent was used. This technique was eventually used to treat 15 patients and resulted in an average decrease of portal venous pressure of only 5.9 mmHg.[4] Although hemorrhage was controlled for a short period of time, recurrent variceal hemorrhage occurred in more than half of the patients. All but two patients died within 6 months of the procedure. Clearly, this technique did not provide adequate portal decompression.

The introduction of expandable stents was the final technologic development that brought TIPS to its current state. Palmaz and associates[5] first reported using Palmaz balloon-expandable stents in the creation of TIPS between the inferior vena cava and portal bifurcation in dogs in 1985. They later performed TIPS in dogs with portal hypertension, and the shunts remained patent during the 48-week duration of the study with the stents showing early endothelialization.[6] Rösch and colleagues[7] used the modified Gianturco-Rösch Z-stent for TIPS creation in young swine in 1987. This successful animal work set the stage for clinical trials.

Richter and coworkers[8] performed the first TIPS using metallic stents in a human in Freiberg, Germany in January 1988. They have continued their work and have performed this procedure in more than 75 patients currently. In the United States, the first clinical experience was reported by Zemel and associates[9] at the Miami Vascular Institute and

LaBerge and coworkers[10] at the University of California, San Francisco. At the Charles Dotter Institute of Interventional Therapy, we have performed TIPS in 40 patients. Interest in TIPS is growing rapidly, and the number of procedures being performed worldwide will increase dramatically in the near future.

INDICATION FOR TIPS

The indications for TIPS are evolving as more is learned about this new procedure. Initially, TIPS was performed only on an emergency basis in patients with massive bleeding and severe liver disease who had failed sclerotherapy and were not considered candidates for emergency surgical portosystemic shunts. Indications for the procedure were expanded after early results showed TIPS to be effective in the control of variceal hemorrhage. Currently, TIPS is performed often in patients who are candidates for liver transplantation that develop bleeding refractory to sclerotherapy before a donor liver becomes available. Here, TIPS is preferable to shunt surgery, which increases the difficulty of subsequent liver transplantation.[11] It can effectively control variceal hemorrhage without complicating subsequent transplantation because the entire shunt is intrahepatic and no laparotomy is required.[12] We and other investigators are also performing TIPS electively as an alternative to shunt surgery in higher-risk patients who rebleed after sclerotherapy or who have varices inaccessible to sclerotherapy, particularly gastric and duodenal varices or varices around an ileostomy or colostomy.

Indications for TIPS may ultimately be expanded even further. The ultimate role of this procedure will depend upon the results of prospective randomized trials comparing TIPS with other treatment modalities.

TECHNIQUE

Before the TIPS procedure, it is essential to confirm the patency of the portal vein and to evaluate portal venous anatomy. In early patients, this was accomplished by performing transhepatic portography with placement of a Dormia basket at the portal bifurcation through a transhepatic tract to act as a target for portal vein puncture.[8] This technique has been abandoned because it unnecessarily increases the risk of the procedure and led to two of the described procedure-related deaths.[13] Ultrasound is currently used by some to document portal vein patency and to guide the puncture.[13] We routinely use arterial portography to demonstrate portal venous anatomy. Injection of both the splenic and superior mesenteric arteries can provide a complete view of the portal venous system and may reveal unsuspected causes of variceal hemorrhage, such as splenic vein occlusion. Arterial portography may fail to demonstrate the portal vein in patients with very advanced liver disease and hepatofugal portal venous flow. In this case, wedged hepatic venography should be performed at the time of the TIPS procedure to visualize the portal vein. We prefer to perform the angiographic study on the day before TIPS, but in emergencies, it is combined with the TIPS procedure.

Little specific patient preparation is required. We routinely prescribe broad-spectrum antibiotics before the TIPS procedure. In patients with massive ascites, we have found it helpful to drain the ascites before TIPS when feasible. This aids in the hepatic vein catheterization and the portal venous puncture by decreasing the angle between the hepatic veins and the inferior vena cava. In addition, a higher-quality fluoroscopic image can also be obtained if ascites is decreased. Most investigators have not attempted to correct coagulopathy before TIPS. The procedure has been performed in a number of patients with markedly prolonged prothrombin times and/or profound thrombocytopenia without complications. We prefer, however, to correct bleeding disorders if possible to permit safe pre-TIPS arteriography and to minimize the risk of serious bleeding should the liver capsule be inadvertently punctured during creation of the shunt.

The TIPS procedure itself is performed under intravenous sedation. It is important that the patient be alert enough to cooperate, particularly with breath holding. The right internal jugular vein is entered high in the neck, and a large vascular sheath is placed. If the right internal jugular vein cannot be used, the procedure can be performed through the left internal jugular vein with minimal discomfort to the patient. Most investigators use the Colapinto transjugular liver biopsy needle (Cook, Bloomington, IN) for the liver puncture. We prefer a recently developed coaxial catheter needle system.[14] This system has the advantages of being rigid, allowing precise needle orientation for liver puncture, and having a very sharp small needle, making it less traumatic. It also allows placement of a large vascular sheath into the portal vein, which is required for use of the modified Gianturco-Rösch Z-stent and the Palmaz stent.

The coaxial catheter system is placed selectively in the right hepatic vein (Fig. 26-1A). A test injection of contrast medium is performed to confirm the suitability of the hepatic vein for creation of the TIPS. In patients in whom the portal vein could not be visualized as a result of hepatofugal flow, a wedged hepatic venogram is performed to demonstrate portal venous anatomy.

A puncture site is then selected in the hepatic vein above the portal bifurcation. The catheter with a needle inside is rotated anteriorly in the proximal hepatic vein and wedged against the wall of the vein. The needle is then advanced with a forceful thrust to puncture the liver and portal vein (Fig. 26-1B). Ideally, the right portal vein should be entered about 2 cm from its bifurcation. A more central puncture

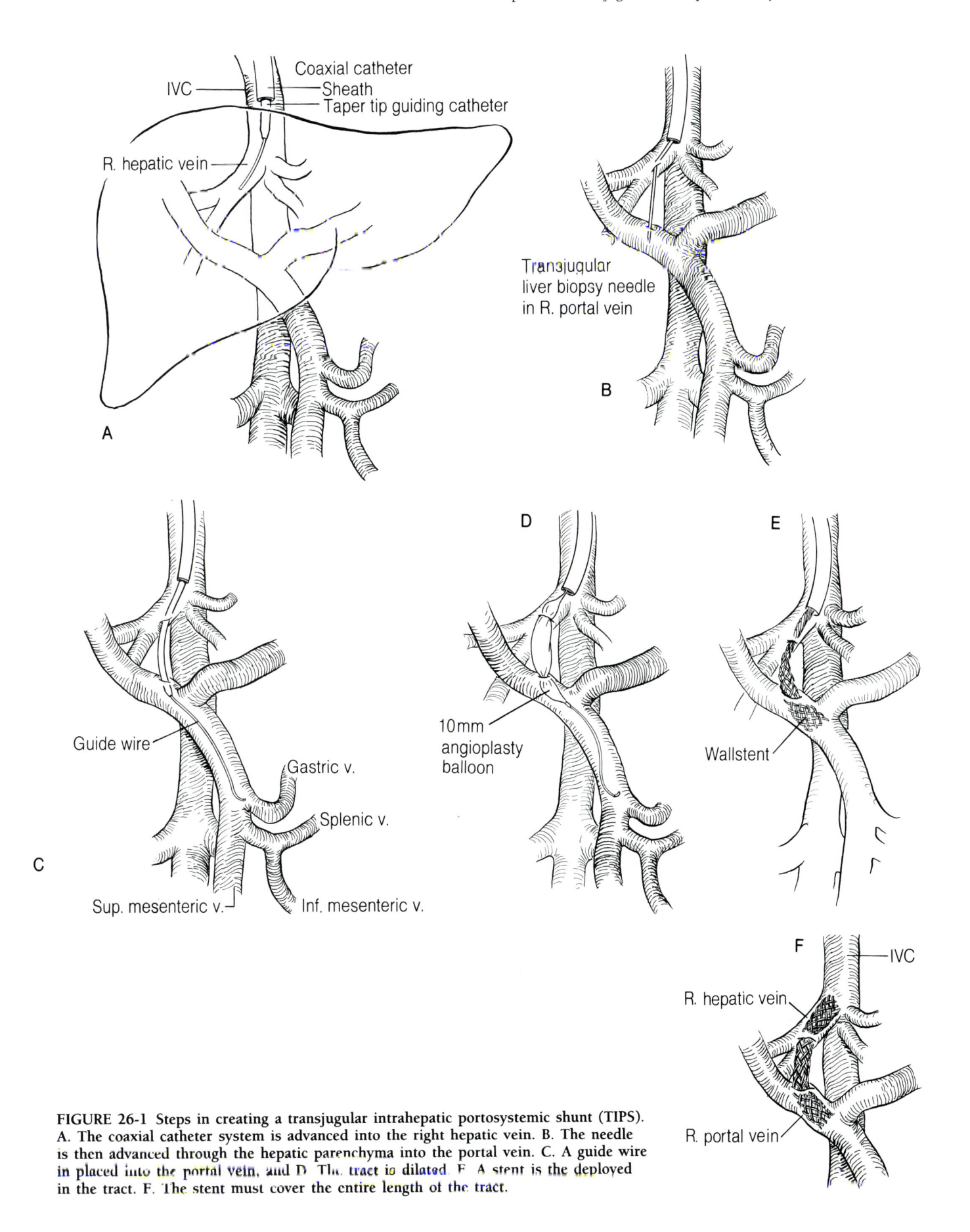

FIGURE 26-1 Steps in creating a transjugular intrahepatic portosystemic shunt (TIPS). A. The coaxial catheter system is advanced into the right hepatic vein. B. The needle is then advanced through the hepatic parenchyma into the portal vein. C. A guide wire is placed into the portal vein, and D. The tract is dilated. E. A stent is then deployed in the tract. F. The stent must cover the entire length of the tract.

carries additional risk because the portal vein bifurcation might be entered outside the liver and creation of the TIPS could cause massive intraperitoneal hemorrhage.[12] A more peripheral puncture is safe but may make catheterization of the portal vein more difficult and may result in a curved tract, which requires use of a more flexible stent. Portal vein puncture is usually the most difficult part of the procedure, with success being closely related to the operator's experience.

After the puncture, suction is applied to the needle as it is slowly withdrawn. When blood is freely aspirated, contrast material is injected through the needle to confirm that a suitable portal vein branch has been entered. A floppy-tipped guide wire is then advanced through the needle and down the portal vein (Fig. 26-1C). A multisidehole catheter is then introduced into the portal vein for pressure measurement and direct portal venography. Placement of the catheter relatively far out the splenic vein provides optimal visualization of gastroesophageal varices. The diagnostic catheter is then removed over a stiff guide wire, and an angioplasty balloon catheter with a 10-mm diameter and a 4- to 6-cm-long high-pressure balloon is introduced. The balloon is positioned within the intrahepatic tract and inflated (Fig. 26-1D). A long waist seen along the balloon when it is partially inflated marks the parenchymal tract and aids in subsequent stent placement. The hepatic parenchyma usually dilates easily; however, the hepatic vein wall and, particularly, the portal vein wall resist dilatation. The patient usually experiences significant discomfort during dilatation of the tract, requiring additional analgesia.

The tract is now ready for stent placement (Figs. 26-1E and F). The specific steps for stent deployment depend on the type of stent being used. Three types of stents developed for biliary stenting are currently being used for creation of TIPS: the Wallstent (Schneider, Minneapolis, MN), the Palmaz stent (Johnson & Johnson Interventional Systems, Warren, NJ), and the Gianturco-Rösch Z-stent (Cook, Inc., Bloomington, IN). The stents are shown in Figure 26-2. Each has its own advantages and disadvantages.

The Wallstent is a self-expanding device consisting of 24 stainless-steel monofilaments, which have been woven to form a cylinder (Figs. 26-2 and 26-3). The stent most frequently used has a diameter of 10 mm and a length of either 4.2 or 6.8 cm when fully expanded. It comes premounted on a flexible 7-French catheter. The stent is compressed and covered by a thin membrane, which is rolled back to release the stent (see Fig. 26-1D). Its main advantages are its ease of deployment and its extreme flexibility, which allow it to be placed even around extreme curves. This stent, however, is not very radiopaque, making it difficult to see with fluoroscopy. It also shortens significantly when it is deployed, making precise positioning difficult. The maximum diameter of the stent is only 10 mm, which may provide inadequate portal decompression in some patients.[10]

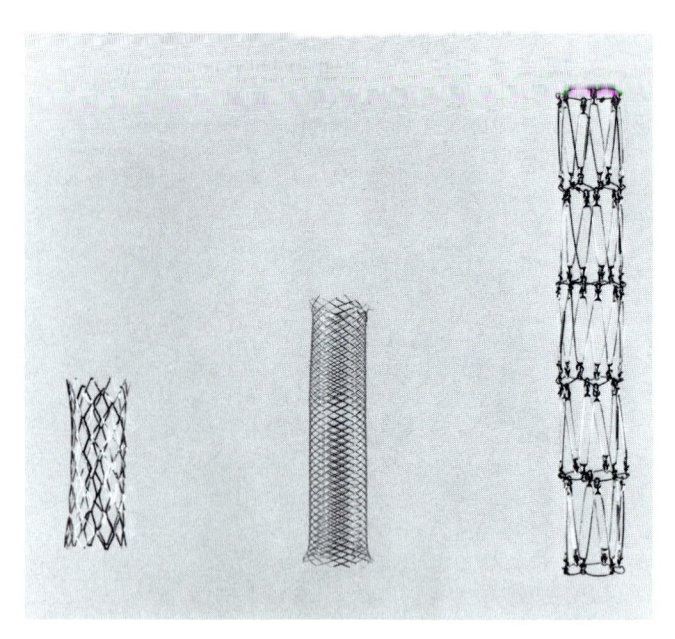

FIGURE 26-2 Stents currently used for TIPS (from left to right): Palmaz stent, Wallstent, and Gianturco-Rösch Z-stent.

The Palmaz stent is a balloon-expandable stent consisting of a tube of electropolished medical-grade stainless steel with staggered parallel slots etched through the wall. It is crimped onto an angioplasty balloon, which is then positioned at the desired site. The stent is expanded by inflating the angioplasty balloon to the desired diameter. The primary advantage to the use of this stent is that its size can be precisely controlled through selection of the balloon used to deploy it. Initially, the stent is dilated to 8 mm. If adequate pressure reduction is not achieved, the stent can then be expanded to 10 mm and, ultimately, to 12 mm if necessary. The primary disadvantages to this stent are its short length (2.5 cm deployed) and its rigidity. The stent is completely inflexible, making it impossible to employ around curves. Frequently, multiple stents are required to cover the length of the tract.[16]

The Gianturco-Rösch Z-stent is a self-expanding stent consisting of multiple stent bodies, which are connected together (Figs. 26-2 and 26-4). Each body is made of a single stainless-steel wire, which has been folded in a zigzag fashion to create a short tube. Individual bodies are connected together with monofilament suture to form a longer stent. The stent that we routinely use has a diameter of 12 mm and a length of 7.5 cm (five bodies). This stent is quite radiopaque and is easy to position because it does not shorten when deployed. It demonstrates moderate flexibility but can kink if curved too much. The stent is positioned by advancing a 10-French sheath through the intrahepatic tract and pushing the stent through the sheath to its end. It is then deployed by withdrawing the outer sheath while the pusher is held in place. The 12-mm-diameter Z-stent ex-

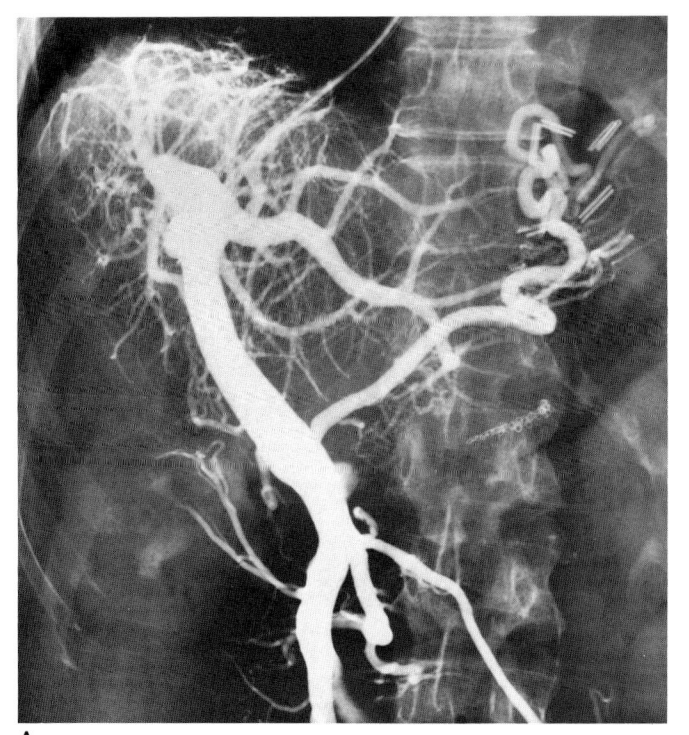

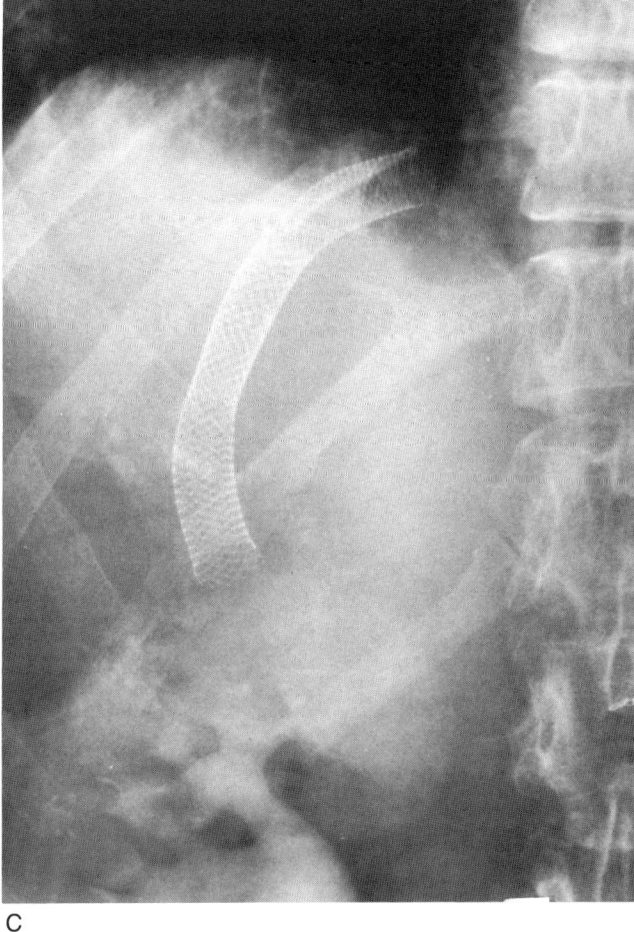

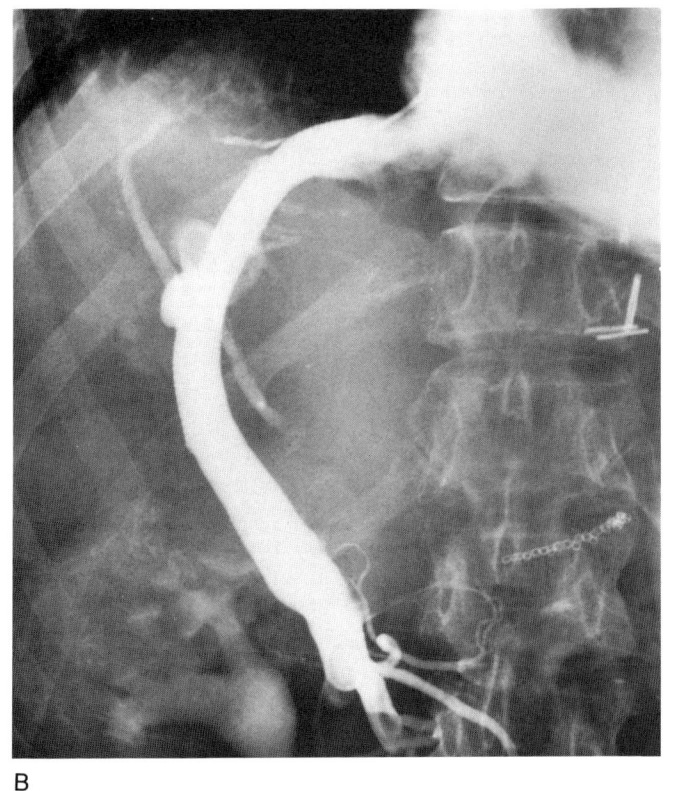

FIGURE 26-3 TIPS created with Wallstent. A. The initial direct portal venogram shows a patent portal vein with filling of intrahepatic portal vein branches and gastroesophageal varices. B. After TIPS creation there is excellent flow through the shunt with no filling of varices and minimal filling of intrahepatic portal vein branches. C. A plain film shows the final position of two overlapping Wallstents used to create the shunt.

pands on its own to 10 mm after being pushed through the sheath. However, it can be fully expanded to its maximum diameter using a 12-mm angioplasty balloon.

The entire length of the parenchymal tract must be covered with stents. If the first stent does not completely cover the tract, an additional stent must be placed to achieve adequate portal decompression. Placement of additional stents is required most often with the Palmaz stent.

After stent placement, a multisidehole catheter is again advanced into the portal venous system, preferably into the splenic vein, and follow-up portal venography is performed along with portal venous pressure measurements. If filling of varices persists on the portogram and reduction in portal venous pressure is not adequate, the stents can be dilated to their maximum diameter with a balloon catheter. Most

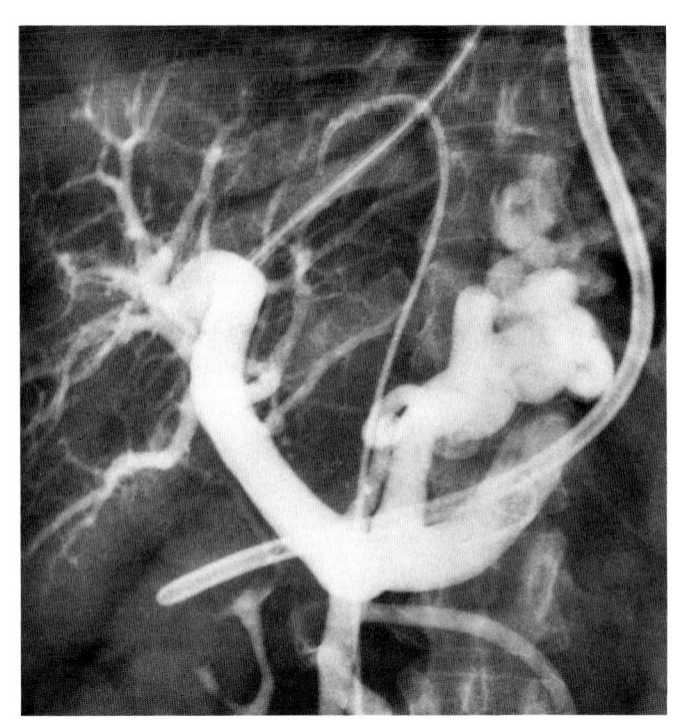

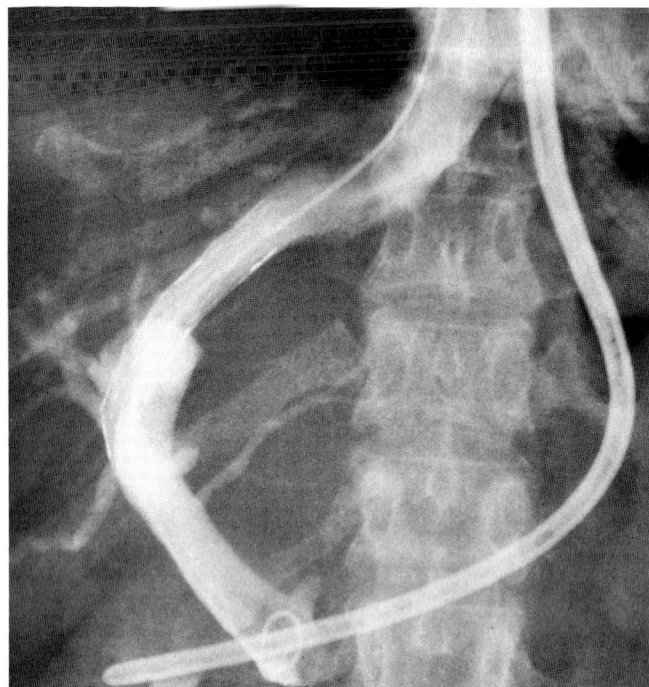

FIGURE 26-4 TIPS created with Gianturco-Rösch Z-stent. A. Initial portal venogram demonstrates huge gastroesophageal varices. B. The final portal venogram shows excellent flow through the shunt with no filling of varices. There is only minimal filling of intrahepatic portal vein branches.

investigators advocate reducing the portosystemic gradient to 10 mmHg. Should filling of varices persist after maximum expansion of the stents, transcatheter embolization of varices can be performed.

After the procedure, the patients are observed for evidence of additional variceal bleeding, intraperitoneal hemorrhage, or encephalopathy. The length of the subsequent hospitalization is determined by the patient's overall clinical condition. About one half of our patients were discharged within 3 days after the TIPS procedure. Should a patient develop recurrent variceal bleeding, the shunt should be recatheterized from the jugular or femoral approach for diagnostic portal venography and pressure measurements. Any stenosis in the shunt can be dilated at that time, additional stents can be placed, and any persistent varices can be embolized.

RESULTS AND DISCUSSION

Because TIPS has been performed clinically for a very short time, little data have yet been published regarding this procedure. The groups of Richter,[8,13,16] LaBerge,[10] and Zemel[9] have all reported small series of patients. A number of papers on TIPS were presented at the meeting of the Society of Cardiovascular and Interventional Radiology in April 1992, which together represent the most complete collection of data on this new technique. The data from that meeting are summarized in Table 26-1 and are the basis for the following discussion.

These early results show clearly that TIPS can be successfully performed in nearly all patients. Most investigators report 100 percent success rates. We have also been successful in all 40 patients in which we have attempted this procedure. LaBerge and associates[17] reported being unable to complete the procedure in only 4 of 100 patients. Three of these failures occurred in patients with chronic portal vein occlusion. The 90 percent success rate of Noeldge and coworkers[21] is the worst reported, with most of their failures occurring early in their experience.

The success of any shunt procedure depends on its ability to reduce portal pressure adequately. Most investigators performing TIPS have sought to reduce the portosystemic gradient to about 10 mmHg. This has been

TABLE 26-1 Results of transjugular intrahepatic portosystemic shunts presented at 17th Annual Meeting of the Society of Cardiovascular and Interventional Radiology

Reference	No. of patients	Child class and no. of patients	Technical success	Gradients (mmHg) Pre-TIPS	Gradients (mmHg) Post-TIPS	30-day mortality	Rebleeding Varices	Rebleeding Other	New encephalopthy
LaBerge et al.[17]	100	10A, 35B, 55C	96%		10.2	14.0%	10%	7%	10%
Zemel et al.[18]	42	5A, 22B, 14C	100%	34	10.0	2.4%	7%		10%
Darcy et al.[19]	21		100%	23	11.5		10%	14%	43%
Maynar et al.[20]	18	13A, 7B, 11C	100%	27	13.0	5.5%	0%	0%	0%
Noelge et al.[21]	75	30A, 30B, 15C	99%			5.3%	10%	4%	5%
Rösch et al. (Unpublished data, 1992).	40		100%			5.0%	8%	5%	5%

TIPS = transjugular intrahepatic portosystemic shunts

accomplished with nearly uniform success. Reported pressure gradients of 23 to 34 mmHg have been reduced to 10 to 13 mmHg after TIPS creation. The ability to adjust portal pressure during the procedure is one of the potential advantages of TIPS. Controlling the portosystemic gradient is particularly simple with the Palmaz balloon-expandable stent. An 8-mm shunt is created initially. The shunt is then progressively enlarged by dilating it with angioplasty balloons of increasing size until the desired portal pressure is achieved. Portal pressure can also be controlled using the 12-mm Z-stent, which initially expands to 10 mm on its own, but which can be further expanded to its maximum diameter with an angioplasty balloon if required for adequate portal decompression. Regulation of portal pressure is more difficult with the Wallstent if its 10-mm maximum diameter results in inadequate portal decompression. LaBerge and associates[17] report having created a second intrahepatic shunt in 10 patients with persistently elevated portal pressures after creation of the initial shunt.

The TIPS procedure appears to be effective in controlling acute variceal hemorrhage. LaBerge and coworkers[17] successfully created TIPS in 30 of 32 patients who were actively bleeding at the time of the procedure. Of these, 28 patients stopped bleeding immediately, and one of the two who did not respond was found to be bleeding from an ulcer at follow-up endoscopy. Hemorrhage has ceased immediately in all patients that we have treated who were actively bleeding.

Rebleeding from varices after TIPS creation is infrequent and is usually related to problems with the intrahepatic shunt. Zemel and associates[18] report rebleeding in 3 of 41 patients. Two of these patients were treated by dilating existing 10-mm shunts to a diameter of 12 mm with no further bleeding. Most of the nine patients reported by LaBerge and coworkers[17] who rebled were found to have stenotic or occluded shunts. All these shunts were successfully recanalized using angiographic techniques.

Two of 40 patients we have treated rebled from varices 2 and 4 months, respectively, after the procedure. In both cases, the shunt had become stenotic, and portal pressure was again elevated. The stenoses were treated by placing additional stents inside the shunts, which resulted in good portal decompression and no further bleeding. Others report frequencies of rebleeding of about 10 percent but do not indicate causes.

The low incidence of rebleeding is due in large part to the relatively high patency rates that have been achieved. LaBerge and coworkers[17] report an overall shunt patency rate of 98 percent. All their surviving patients have patent shunts, and all patients undergoing transplantation had patent shunts at the time of transplantation. Two of 20 patients in their series who died had occluded shunts. Eleven patients in their series, however, required some intervention to maintain or restore shunt patency, resulting in a primary patency of 86 percent. Others report primary patency rates of about 90 percent.

In addition, TIPS can be of particular benefit to prospective liver transplant patients with variceal bleeding uncontrolled by sclerotherapy because it requires no laparotomy or alteration of extrahepatic portal venous anatomy. Iwatsuki and colleagues[11] have shown a trend toward an adverse outcome when liver transplantation is preceded by surgical portosystemic shunting. Surgical shunt procedures result in intraabdominal adhesions, which can make subsequent liver transplantation more difficult. In addition, the surgical shunt must be taken down at the time of transplantation, which further extends the operation. A properly performed TIPS procedure avoids both of these problems. It is important, however, that the stents placed during TIPS not extend into the extrahepatic portal vein or the suprahepatic inferior vena cava where they could complicate a subsequent transplant operation. Early results using TIPS in pretransplant patients have been encouraging.[17]

Besides control of variceal hemorrhage, a couple of additional benefits of TIPS have been noted. Zemel and associates[18] report complete resolution of ascites after TIPS in 29 of 31 patients with ascites in their series. LaBerge's group[17] also reported doubling of platelet counts in one half of their patients with severe thrombocytopenia.

Few serious complications attributable to the procedure have been described. Intraperitoneal hemorrhage is the most feared complication, but it has occurred rarely. Noeldge and associates[21] reported two deaths attributed to intraperitoneal bleeding from transhepatic tracts early in their experience. In these cases, initial portal vein catheterization was performed through a percutaneous transhepatic approach to aid in creating the TIPS. The tracts, however, could not be embolized at the end of the procedures, resulting in fatal hemorrhage. Because of this, the practice of placing transhepatic catheters to assist TIPS creation has been completely abandoned. Perarnau and associates[15] have reported one case of fatal intraperitoneal hemorrhage resulting from the creation of the TIPS. In that case, the portal vein was entered too centrally so that the created shunt was partially extrahepatic, resulting in massive intraperitoneal bleeding. Several other cases of less severe bleeding have also been reported. The groups of LaBerge[17] and Noeldge[21] have both reported single cases of intraperitoneal bleeding, which required transfusion but no other therapy. Zemel and associates[18] described one case where frank extravasation of contrast medium into the peritoneal space was demonstrated on the initial portal venogram after entry into the portal vein. After a stent was deployed to create the shunt, portal pressure decreased, and no extravasation was seen on follow-up venography. The patient did well.

Assorted other complications related directly to the procedure have also been described. Zemel and coworkers[18] report one case of migration of a Palmaz stent to the pulmonary artery. The stent was retrieved and deployed in the infrarenal inferior vena cava without harm to the patient. One case of hemobilia[17] and one case of segmental hepatic infarction[19] have also been reported.

Procedure-related mortality has been remarkably low considering the patient populations treated. Thirty-day mortality rates are as low as 2.4 percent. The 14 percent mortality reported by LaBerge and associates[17] was the highest figure and reflects the severity of disease in patients they treated. Fifty-five percent of their patients were Child Class C and 32 percent were actively bleeding at the time of the procedure. The two patients who died early in our series were moribund when the procedure was performed and received shunts in a last ditch effort to stop variceal hemorrhage. Both patients stopped bleeding after the TIPS procedure only to succumb to adult respiratory distress syndrome and liver failure.

Hepatic encephalopathy and liver failure have been major problems in patients after nonselective surgical portosystemic shunts.[22,23] Total diversion of portal venous flow has been blamed for these complications.[24] It has recently been suggested that partial portal decompression may decrease the incidence of encephalopathy and liver failure. Sarfeh and Rypins[25] created progressive smaller portocaval H-grafts in patients over several years. Their patients with small (8- to 10-mm) grafts had an incidence of encephalopathy of 16 percent compared with 39 percent in those with large-caliber grafts. The small grafts resulted in residual portosystemic gradients of 17 cmH_2O and 12 cmH_2O for 8- and 10-mm grafts, respectively, whereas the large grafts caused complete portal decompression. Johansen[26] reported encephalopathy in 6 percent and liver failure in 6 percent of patients receiving small caliber H-grafts with resultant portosystemic gradients of 10.4 mmHg. Transjugular intrahepatic portosystemic shunts are similar to these small-caliber shunts in their hemodynamic effects and should therefore result in similar rates of encephalopathy and liver failure.

The incidence of encephalopathy in patients undergoing TIPS appears relatively low. LaBerge group[17] reported encephalopathy in 24 of their 96 patients who underwent TIPS; however, only 9 of these patients did not have encephalopathy before the procedure. Among the other series reported, only Darcy and associates[19] reported a rate of encephalopathy greater than 10 percent. Patients in this one series underwent detailed psychometric testing to search for encephalopathy, whereas patients in other series were assessed on more subjective clinical grounds. Differences in criteria used to determine if a patient was encephalopathic account for some of the difference between their results and those of others. In addition to encephalopathy, there have been a few reports of liver failure after TIPS, but the incidence of this complication is uncertain at this time.

CONCLUSIONS

Although the data concerning TIPS are preliminary they support conclusions drawn by LaBerge and associates[10] after their first 25 cases. First, intraheptic portosystemic shunts can be created reliably and safely through a percutaneous approach. Second, TIPS is effective in controlling variceal hemorrhage by lowering portal pressure. Third, the incidence of encephalopathy and liver failure is relatively low. Fourth, TIPS does not hinder subsequent liver transplantation. Conclusions regarding the long-term efficacy of this treatment require further study.

The potential advantage of TIPS over surgical shunts is that TIPS creation is essentially an angiographic procedure that does not require general anesthesia or laparotomy, and in experienced hands it can be completed in less than 2 h. This may result in improved survival when performed in critically ill patients and certainly shortens the duration of hospitalization. The TIPS procedure is technically challenging, however. Considerable expertise in angiographic techniques and transjugular liver biopsy are required for its successful completion.

Despite encouraging early results, it must be remembered that TIPS is still an experimental procedure. Many questions regarding this procedure remain unanswered and require further study. For example, it is unknown which stent will perform best and what long-term patency rates will be achieved. The best end point for the procedure remains to be established. Is partial portal decompression adequate therapy or should varices be embolized concomitantly? Finally, how will rates of hepatic encephalopathy, liver failure, and survival in patients undergoing TIPS compare with those in similar patients treated by sclerotherapy or surgery? The ultimate role of tranjugular intrahepatic portosystemic shunts in the management of portal hypertension and its complications rests on the answers to these questions.

REFERENCES

1. Rösch J, Hanafee WN, Snow H: Transjugular portal venography and radiologic portacaval shunt: An experimental study. *Radiology* 1969, 92:1112–1114.
2. Rösch J, Hanafee W, Snow H, et al: Transjugular intrahepatic portacaval shunt. *Am J Surg* 1971; 121:588–592.
3. Colapinto RF, Stronell TD, Birch SJ, et al: Creation of an intrahepatic portosystemic shunt with a Gruntzig balloon catheter. *Can Med Assoc J* 1982; 126:267–268.
4. Gordon JD, Colapinto RF, Abecassis M, et al: Transjugular intrahepatic portosystemic shunt: A nonoperative approach to life-threatening variceal bleeding. *Can J Surg* 1987; 30:45–49.
5. Palmaz JC, Sibbitt RR, Reuter SR, et al: Expandable intrahepatic portacaval shunt stents: Early experience in the dog. *Am J Roentgenol* 1985; 145:821–825.
6. Palmaz JC, Garcia F, Sibbitt RR, et al: Expandable intrahepatic shunt stents in dogs with chronic portal hypertension. *Am J Roentgenol* 1986; 147:1251–1254.
7. Rösch J, Uchida BT, Putnam JS: Experimental intrahepatic portacaval anastomosis: Use of expandable Gianturco stents. *Radiology* 1987; 162:481–485.
8. Richter GM, Noeldge G, Palmaz JC, et al: Transjugular intrahepatic portacaval stent shunt: Preliminary clinical results. *Radiology* 1990; 174:1027–1030.
9. Zemel G, Katzen BT, Becker GJ, et al: Percutaneous transjugular portosystemic shunt. *JAMA* 1991; 266:390–393.
10. LaBerge JM, Ring EJ, Lake JR, et al: Transjugular intrahepatic portosystemic shunts (TIPS): Preliminary results in 25 patients. *J Vasc Surg* 1992; 16:258–267.
11. Iwatsuki S, Starzl TE, Todo S, et al: Liver transplantation in the treatment of bleeding esophageal varices. *Surgery* 1988; 104:697–705.
12. Ring EJ, Lake JR, Roberts JP, et al: Percutaneous intrahepatic portosystemic shunts to control variceal bleeding prior to transplantation. *Ann Intern Med* 1992; 116:304–309.
13. Richter GM, Noeldge G, Palmaz JC, et al: The transjugular intrahepatic portosystemic stent-shunt (TIPSS): Results of a pilot study. *Cardiovasc Intervent Radiol* 1990; 13:200–207.
14. Uchida BT, Putnam JS, Rösch JR: "Atraumatic" transjugular needle for portal vein puncture in swine. *Radiology* 1987; 163:580.
15. Perarnau JM, Rössle M, Noeldge G, et al: Transjugular intrahepatic shunts: An improved technique. Presented at the Third International Meeting of the Society of Minimally Invasive Therapy, Boston, MA, November 1991.
16. Richter GM, Noeldge G, Roessle M, et al: Evolution and clinical introduction of TIPSS, the transjugular intrahepatic portosystemic shunt. *Semin Intervent Radiol* 1991; 8:331–340.
17. LaBerge JM, Gordon RL, Ring EJ: Transjugular intrahepatic portosystemic shunts with use of the Wallstent endoprosthesis: Midterm results. Presented at the 17th Annual Meeting of the Society of Cardiovascular and Interventional Radiology, Washington, DC, April 1992.
18. Zemel G, Becker GJ, Benenati JF, et al: Transjugular intrahepatic shunts. Presented at the 17th Annual Meeting of the Society of Cardiovascular and Interventional Radiology, Washington, DC, April 1992.
19. Darcy MD, Picus D, Hicks ME, et al: Transjugular intrahepatic portosystemic shunts with use of the Wallstent. Presented at the 17th Annual Meeting of the Society of Cardiovascular and Interventional Radiology, Washington, DC, April 1992.
20. Maynar M, Cabrera J, Pulido-Duque JM, et al: Transjugular intrahepatic stunts. Presented at the 17th Annual Meeting of the Society of Cardiovascular and Interventional Radiology, Washington, DC, April 1992.
21. Noeldge G, Rössle M, Perarneau JM, et al: Transjugular intrahepatic shunt. Presented at the 17th Annual Meeting of the Society of Cardiovascular and Interventional Radiology, Washington, DC, April 1992.
22. Warren WD, Millikan WJ, Henderson JM, et al: Ten years portal hypertensive surgery at Emory. *Ann Surg* 1982; 195:530–542.
23. Villeneuve JP, Pomier-Layrargues G, Duguay L, et al: Emergency portacaval shunt for variceal hemorrhage. *Am J Surg* 1987; 206:48–51.
24. Warren WD: Control of variceal bleeding: Reassessment of rationale. *Am J Surg* 1983; 145:8–16.
25. Sarfeh IJ, Rypins EB, Mason GR: A systematic appraisal of portacaval H-graft diameters. *Ann Surg* 1986; 204:356–363.
26. Johansen K: Partial portal decompression for variceal hemorrhage. *Am J Surg* 1989; 157:479–482.

Chapter 27

Laparoscopic Pelvic Lymphadenectomy

Ralph V. Clayman / Elspeth M. McDougall / Louis R. Kavoussi

Despite reports as early as 1976 of laparoscopic exploration for the cryptorchid testicle, it was not until 1989 that the potential application of laparoscoic surgery to adult urology became evident.[1,2] Dr. William Schuessler,[3] a urologist, teamed with Dr. Thierry Vancaillie, a gynecologist, to perform the first laparoscopic pelvic lymphadenectomy in October of 1989. Subsequently, they have performed over 100 of these procedures and have spent countless hours teaching their technique to other urologists, including these authors. Currently, laparoscopic lymphadenectomy is practiced in many medical centers throughout the country, and the urologist's skill with the laparoscope is rapidly increasing. As a direct result of this experience, other laparoscopic urologic procedures have been and are being perfected: varicocelectomy, ureterolysis, lymphocelectomy, bladder neck suspension, and most recently, nephrectomy. The refinement of laparoscopic equipment and the enhanced laparoscopic capabilities of the urologist will likely lead to the use of this technology in other areas of urology that only a few years ago seemed unlikely if not impossible: nephroureterectomy, ureteral reimplantation, partial and total cystectomy, urinary conduits, and radical prostatectomy.

INDICATIONS

The indications for laparoscopic pelvic lymphadenectomy vary with the urologist's philosophy for treating clinically localized prostatic cancer. If the primary therapeutic modality is a radiotherapeutic approach (external beam or implantation of radioactive seeds), then laparoscopic lymphadenectomy is reasonable in all patients with clinically localized prostatic cancer. Parenthetically, among patients who are destined to receive external beam therapy, the radiation therapist needs to be notified that the node dissection was performed laparoscopically (i.e., transperitoneally) so that the usual pelvic nodal ports are eliminated. If this is not done, there is a potential risk of radiation enteritis developing in bowel loops that may have become adherent at the lymphadenectomy sites.

When the primary therapeutic modality is a surgical approach, then the indications for a laparoscopic lymphadenectomy are dependent on the type of prostatectomy planned. In the case of a planned perineal prostatectomy, all patients are again candidates for a laparoscopic lymphadenectomy.

However, when the surgical approach to radical prostatectomy is via a retropubic route, then the indications for laparoscopic pelvic lymphadenectomy become more limited. First of all, laparoscopic lymphadenectomy should only be done when documentation of nodal metastases (i.e., Stage D1) would preclude the prostatectomy. Next, the morbidity of the laparoscopic procedure must be weighed against the possibility of positive nodal disease. To labor for 2 to 3 h to perform a laparoscopic lymph node dissection and then to proceed to open the patient to remove the prostate retropubically makes little sense if the chances for node-positive disease were extremely low from the outset. The chief benefit of laparoscopic lymph node dissection to the potential patient who will undergo retropubic radical prostatectomy is only when nodal metastases are discovered, thereby sparing the patient an open procedure.

Patients with localized carcinoma of the prostate and metastases to pelvic lymph nodes can expect to develop more distant metastases within 2 to 3 years.[4] Therefore, it is imperative that the preoperative assessment determine whether or not the disease is confined to the prostate. Patients with a Gleason grade of 8 or more have a 20 to 93 percent chance of having pelvic lymph node disease involvement.[5,6] Among patients with an elevated acid phosphatase level (stage D0 disease), upwards of 70 percent will have positive lymph nodes. Indeed, for patients in the high normal range, upward of one half will have metastatic lymphadenopathy.[5]

By contrast, prostate specific antigen is not specific for detecting nodal metastatic prostatic cancer. Among patients with prostatic cancer, the prostate-specific antigen is elevated in approximately 10 percent of patients with clinical Stage A disease, 24 percent with Stage B, 53 percent with Stage C, and 92 percent with Stage D disease.[7,8]

In a series of 72 patients with Stage D prostatic cancer, the prostate-specific antigen level ranged from 68 to 169 ng/mL, whereas 21 patients with Stage B and 15 with Stage C disease had a range of levels from 1 to 34 ng/mL and 3 to 107 ng/mL, respectively.[8] Similarly in a series of 17 patients with proven stage D1 disease, the positive predictive value of a prostate-specific antigen level greater than 15 ng/mL was only 41 percent.[9]

Clinical staging of prostatic cancer is likewise a poor predictor of nodal status. Among patients with clinical stage A1, A2, B1, and B2 disease, the incidence of nodal involvement in a recent report was only 0, 3.3, 5.3, and 9.7 percent, respectively.[10] This is in marked contrast to earlier studies in which 52 percent of patients with clinical Stage B2 disease had positive nodal metastases. This discrepancy between the recent and older study is unexplained. Clinical Stage C disease is associated with nodal metastases in 59 percent; however, data more recent than 1980 are not available.[11]

In summary, laparoscopic pelvic lymph node dissection offers the patient the least invasive definitive evaluation for nodal metastases. Those patients who are candidates for a retropubic prostatectomy and have a high Gleason grade (≥ 8), bulky (clinical Stage C) disease, Stage D0 disease (i.e., isolated elevation of the prostatic acid phosphatase level), or pelvic lymphadenopathy on a CT scan (with a negative CT-guided biopsy) deserve a laparoscopic analysis of the pelvic lymph nodes. In our medical center, more than 250 radical retropubic prostatectomies are performed annually; overall, by adhering to the aforementioned criteria, less than 15 percent of these patients would benefit from a laparoscopic lymphadenectomy.

TECHNIQUE

Patient Informed Consent

The major impetus for patients to elect to undergo a laparoscopic lymphadenectomy is to avoid the morbidity associated with an open lymphadenectomy. Although the laparoscopic procedure is more lengthy than its surgical counterpart, the morbidity appears to be less, and the hospital stay is brief. Indeed, the laparoscopic patient is usually eating the same day as the procedure and is discharged from the hospital on the first postoperative day. Convalescence occurs in less than 2 weeks.

Despite these sanguine results, it is important when obtaining informed consent that the patient be made aware that an open procedure may be necessary, either as a result of anatomic conditions precluding a safe laparoscopic approach (i.e., dense scar tissue from either previous pelvic surgery or from intraabdominal disease, such as a ruptured appendix or diverticulitis) or complications occurring during the laparoscopic procedure (i.e., vascular, bowel, or bladder injury). As such, each patient must consent to possible laparotomy, and this should be clearly stated on the operative permission. In addition, there are certain complications unique to laparoscopy, for example, CO_2 embolus, subcutaneous emphysema, pneumoscrotum, pneumopenis, possible damage to the spermatic cord, hemorrhage from the trocar insertion sites, and intraabdominal injury to bowel, bladder, aorta, inferior vena cava, and/or common iliac vessels. The other risks of the procedure are identical to those resulting from an open lymphadenectomy: wound/trocar site infection, wound herniation, vascular injury, thromboembolism, bladder injury, lymphocele formation, and damage to the obturator nerve. Also, it must be stressed to the patient that this is a relatively new procedure, and the incidence and type of late complications have not yet been reported. Lastly, surgeons need to be very straightforward with their patients regarding their experience with this technique. If the surgeon is still in the stage of being proctored, then this should also be explained to the patient. Such attention to detail and forthrightness should help preclude the adverse legal aspects that inevitably accompany the advent of any new procedure.

Patient Preparation

Before the procedure, we instruct the patient to undergo a complete mechanical and antibiotic bowel preparation on an outpatient basis. This consists of the following regimen: a clear liquid diet for 2 days before the procedure, 2 g of neomycin orally at 7 P.M. and 11 P.M. before the day of surgery, 2 g of metronidazole orally at 7 P.M. and 11 P.M. before the day of surgery, and 4 to 6 L of a colonic lavage solution over 5 h beginning at 1 P.M. on the day before surgery. This regimen results in marked decompression of the bowels, thereby facilitating laparoscopy. Also, after this type of bowel preparation, should a small bowel injury occur, it can be oversewn rather than converting to a laparotomy. The total cost of this outpatient bowel preparation is small ($30) compared with the potential benefits.

Immediately before the procedure, the patient is given a dose of an intravenous antibiotic (usually a cephalosporin). Currently, we have not given minidose heparin before this procedure; however, antiembolism pneumatic compression stockings are routinely used in the operating room.

Instrumentation

To perform a laparoscopic lymphadenectomy, a variety of instruments are required. To initiate the procedure a 14-

gauge Veress needle is required and a high-flow (up to 6 L/min) CO$_2$ insufflator. For gaining access to the abdomen, two 11-mm and two 5-mm laparoscopic trocars are used. Visualization of the abdomen is achieved with a 0° lens 10-mm endoscope attached to a high-power xenon light source. The endoscope is coupled to an endoscopic camera; therefore, all images are viewed on a video monitor. Two atraumatic (i.e., dolphin or duckbill type) and one traumatic (i.e., alligator or rattooth type) 5-mm grasping forceps are used during the procedure. In addition, a 10-mm spoon biopsy or 10-mm rat tooth forceps is needed to retrieve the nodal packet. The dissection is performed with an electrocautery spatula or, more recently, a curved electrocautery scissors (Endoshears, US Surgical, Inc, Norwalk, CT). At times, a hook electrode may also be helpful for incising tissue closely adherent to the pubic bone or external iliac vein. Lastly, it is important to have a functional irrigation–aspiration apparatus. The best of these has a pool suction-type tip, which limits clogging from aspirated tissue. The irrigation solution consists of 1000 mL of normal saline with 5000 units of heparin and 1 g of cefazolin. The pressure in the irrigation bag is raised to 250 mmHg with the aid of a pressure bag (Biomedical Dynamics, Minneapolis, MN). The aspiration port of the instrument is connected to wall suction. This instrument is extremely valuable if bleeding is encountered because it allows the surgeon to clear the field rapidly. Also, the heparin in the solution prevents the formation of blood clots, which might obscure the operative field. Lastly, it is helpful to have titanium clips and a laparoscopic clip applier (single or multiple load) available. This can be helpful in case of bleeding or in the event that an aberrant obturator vein needs to be secured.

Procedure

In the operating room, the patient is placed in a supine position; the legs are separated and placed on spreader bars. A cart, containing the monitor and insufflator is positioned at the foot of the table. Next, a general or regional anesthetic is given. After this, pneumatic compression stockings are applied to both legs, and a nasogastric tube and Foley catheter are placed.

The procedure is performed by the surgeon and one assistant. The former operates via two ports and uses a dissecting instrument and a grasping instrument simultaneously. The assistant operates the camera attached to the endoscope and a second grasping instrument (Fig. 27-1).

The entire abdomen, scrotum, and penis are prepared and draped. A gauze wrap is applied as a turban dressing to the scrotum, trapping both testicles within the scrotum. Likewise, a separate gauze wrap is placed around the phallus. This will preclude the development of a pneumoscrotum or pneumopenis.

For all laparoscopic procedures, there are four basic phases: obtaining the pneumoperitoneum, trocar placement, the lymphadenectomy itself, and trocar removal. Each of these phases will be discussed in order.

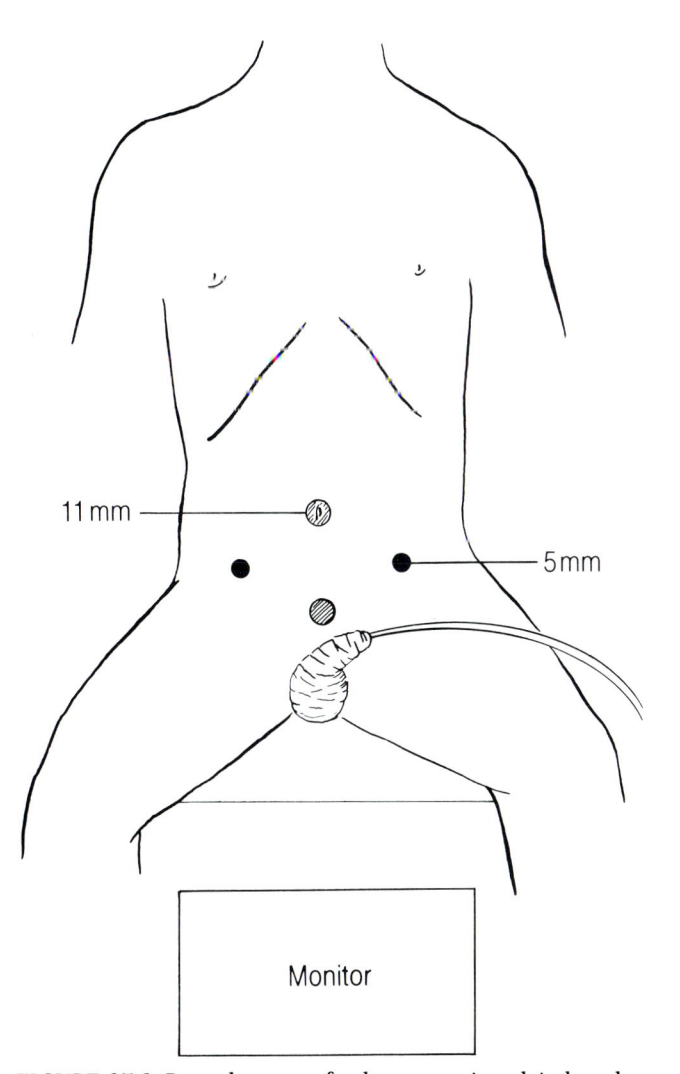

FIGURE 27-1 Port placement for laparoscopic pelvic lymphadenectomy. Note the video screen and insufflator are placed on the same cart (labeled "monitor") that is positioned at the foot of the table. This arrangement affords the surgeon and assistant an excellent view of the laparoscopic television monitor and of the intraabdominal pressure being generated by the insufflator.

PHASE I: THE PNEUMOPERITONEUM

This is obtained in routine fashion with a Veress needle or the technique of open trocar placement (i.e., Hasson cannula) is used selectively.

PHASE II: PLACEMENT OF LAPAROSCOPIC TROCARS

Each trocar site is determined and marked with a sterile marking pen: an 11-mm trocar at the umbilicus, an 11-mm trocar midway between the umbilicus and the symphysis pubis, and two 5-mm trocars, one on the right and one on the left midway between the umbilicus and the iliac crest (see Fig. 27-1).

Just before passage of the 11-mm trocar, the patient is placed in a 30 to 40° head-down position. The intraabdominal pressure is allowed to momentarily increase to 20 to 25 mmHg. The Veress needle is then withdrawn, and the skin incision at the umbilicus is widened (not lengthened) to accommodate the 11-mm trocar. It is often helpful to use a Kelly clamp to spread the incision open a bit; this maneuver rounds out the incision, thereby facilitating trocar placement without making an overly larger incision. If too large an incision is made, the operator will be plagued with leakage of CO_2 around the trocar throughout the case.

Before passage, the trocar is checked to make sure that the safety shield, if present, is operational and to be certain that the flap valve mechanism is working smoothly. The trocar is then introduced into the peritoneal cavity, and the gas line is attached.

A 10.5-mm reducer is applied to the top of the trocar and the 10-mm 0° lens, endoscope is introduced. The abdominal contents are carefully inspected for any evidence of bleeding or bowel injury. With the abdomen still inflated to 20 to 25 mmHg, the two 5-mm ports and the additional 11-mm port are introduced under endoscopic control to prevent accidental injury. Again, the skin incisions should be no larger than the trocar that is going to be introduced. Also, for cosmetic reasons, each skin incision should be made in the direction of the natural abdominal skin folds (i.e., transversely). In addition, just before making the skin incision, it is advisable to transilluminate the planned site of entry with the laparoscope, thereby avoiding injuring any vessels coursing beneath the skin.

It is important to realize that each trocar site has a "memory" for the direction in which the trocar was introduced. As such it is important to direct the second 11-mm trocar directly perpendicular and to direct each of the 5-mm trocars such that they are pointing at a 45° angle downward and toward the symphysis pubis. After introduction of the trocars, the pneumoperitoneum is decreased to 15 mmHg or less.

If, at this point, there is a hissing sound, then CO_2 is likely leaking around a trocar. Several steps can be taken to remedy this problem. First, a purse-string suture of no. 2 polypropylene can be placed and secured around the trocar. Next, white petroleum gauze can be wrapped around the trocar and pushed down against the skin. Last, in some cases, bone wax may help provide a better seal. None of these options is ideal. Quite simply, the best way to deal with leakage around the trocar is not to cause it at all. In this regard, a properly-sized skin incision for each port is essential.

PHASE III: THE PROCEDURE

The next decision is whether to begin the node dissection on the left or right side. In general, it is preferable to start with the side on which the surgeon believes a nodal metastasis is more likely. As such, the dissection should begin on the same side as the palpated prostatic nodule, the side which demonstrates lymphadenopathy on a computed tomogram, or for clinically occult carcinoma, on the side yielding a positive biopsy. If both sides of the prostate are involved, then the side with the higher-grade lesion should be chosen. This practice should enhance the chances of discovering nodal involvement early in the procedure, thereby precluding an unnecessary bilateral node dissection.

The problem of trocar dislodgement can be prevented from occurring or recurring by placing a no. 2 polypropylene suture in the skin and securing it to the sidearm of the port. This is the simplest way to secure the port. Although ports can be purchased with self-retaining features, many of these, as they currently exist, result in a larger skin wound. In our experience, suture fixation remains an inexpensive and effective solution.

Conceptually, there are five steps to performing a laparoscopic lymphadenectomy. In order of their performance they are: identification of the medial umbilical ligament (the remnant of the ipsilateral umbilical artery that is often still patent at the level of bladder where it may provide arterial branches to the bladder), identification and incision of the vas deferens, identification of the pubic bone, identification and dissection of the external iliac vein, and identification and dissection of the obturator nerve.

At the outset of the procedure, the table is rotated so that the side on which the node dissection is to be started, is elevated 30°. The patient is also maintained in a 30 to 40° head-down (Trendelenburg) position. The insufflator is set at 15 mmHg and high flow (i.e., 6 L/min). The surgeon stands on the side of the table opposite to where the node dissection is to be performed (see Fig. 27-1). The surgeon works through the 11-mm midline infraumbilical port with a grasping forceps and uses a cutting instrument through the contralateral 5-mm port. The laparoscope attached to a camera is placed through the midline umbilical 11-mm port; this port and the 5-mm port on the side of the planned node dissection (i.e., ipsilateral side) are controlled by the assistant. Two video monitors are helpful; they should be placed just below each of the operators on either side of the table. Alternatively, if only one monitor is available, it should be placed directly at the foot of the table in between the patient's legs (see Fig. 27-1).

Fogging of the endoscope is particularly noisome; this problem can be limited in several ways. First, it is helpful to have a warming plate on the back table, which can keep a tall container of water heated. If the endoscope fogs, it can be withdrawn and completely bathed in the warm water, wiped, and then reinserted. Alternatively, two endoscopes can be used for each case, with one of them being left on a warming tray to exchange should the endoscope being used become fogged. In addition, there are several antifogging solutions available. In the authors' experience, these have worked extremely well. Lastly, the coupling between the lens and the camera should be checked to be certain it is as tight as possible, in order to preclude the build-up of moisture on the lens itself.

Before the dissection, the laparoscope is momentarily inserted in the lower midline 11-mm port. The point of entry of the umbilical 11-mm port is checked to be certain that, during the blind insertion of the first trocar, neither bowel nor omentum was transversed. The laparoscope is then returned to the 11-mm umbilical port.

Conceptually, the dissection proceeds through the use of traction and countertraction provided by the grasping forceps passed through the ipsilateral 5-mm port and the lower midline 11-mm port. Electrosurgery works best when the tissue to be incised is stretched taut. In this regard, the assistant, working through the ipsilateral 5-mm port, will always be retracting tissue laterally or posteriorly, while the surgeon, working through the 11-mm midline port, will be retracting tissue medially or anteriorly. For dissection purposes, we prefer to use a dolphin or duckbill grasper because these hold the tissue tightly, yet are atraumatic. The contralateral 5-mm port is used by the surgeon for passage of the cutting instrument because instruments introduced through this port will naturally pass between the other two ports.

At the outset, the urachus and medial umbilical ligaments on either side are identified (Fig. 27-2). The former lies directly in the midline and anterior; the medial umbilical ligaments attach to the anterolateral border of the bladder. Each medial umbilical ligament appears as a fatty extension of the abdominal wall. The spermatic cord on either side may be readily identified by gently pulling on the respective testicle (secured within the turban dressing) and looking along the lateral abdominal wall for movement of the spermatic cord. Any visible adhesions near the pelvic inlet should be carefully incised close to the abdominal wall so the colon can be retracted cephalad. These adhesions are more common on the left side.

The steps of laparoscopic pelvic lymphadenectomy are demonstrated in Figure 27-3. The peritoneal reflection immediately lateral to the medial umbilical ligament is incised. To do this, the tissue on either side of the ligament is grasped and pulled taut; the incision may then be made with a scissors, potassium titanyl phosphate laser, electrosurgery probe, or scissors. We prefer the last and have recently been quite pleased using an electrosurgery curved scissors. This is discussed in the list of equipment on pages 280–281. Upon incising the peritoneal reflection, the retroperitoneal fat is immediately seen. The incision in the peritoneum is carried inferiorly along the medial umbilical ligament and to a level approximately 3 to 4 cm below the level of the internal ring. It is important to stay directly along the lateral border of the medial umbilical ligament and medial to the spermatic cord to avoid carrying the dissection too far laterally. Likewise, if the incision

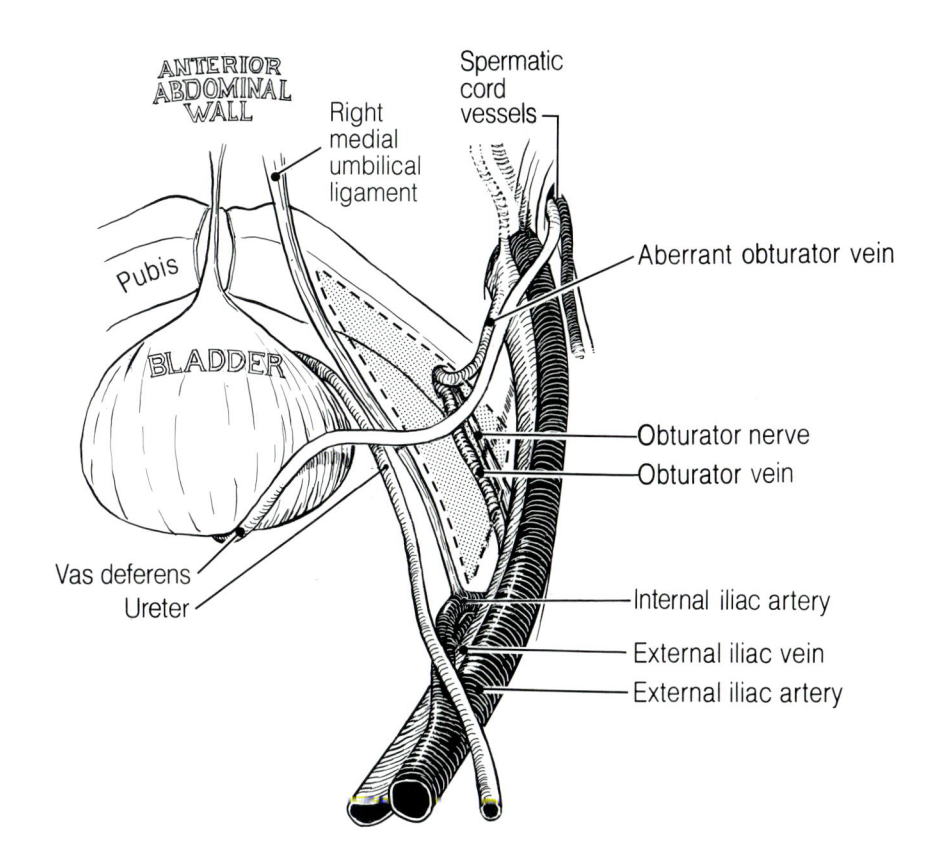

FIGURE 27-2 Laparoscopic pelvic anatomy (right side). The shaded area represents the triangle of pelvic lymphadenectomy for prostatic cancer.

284 PART II Old Diseases

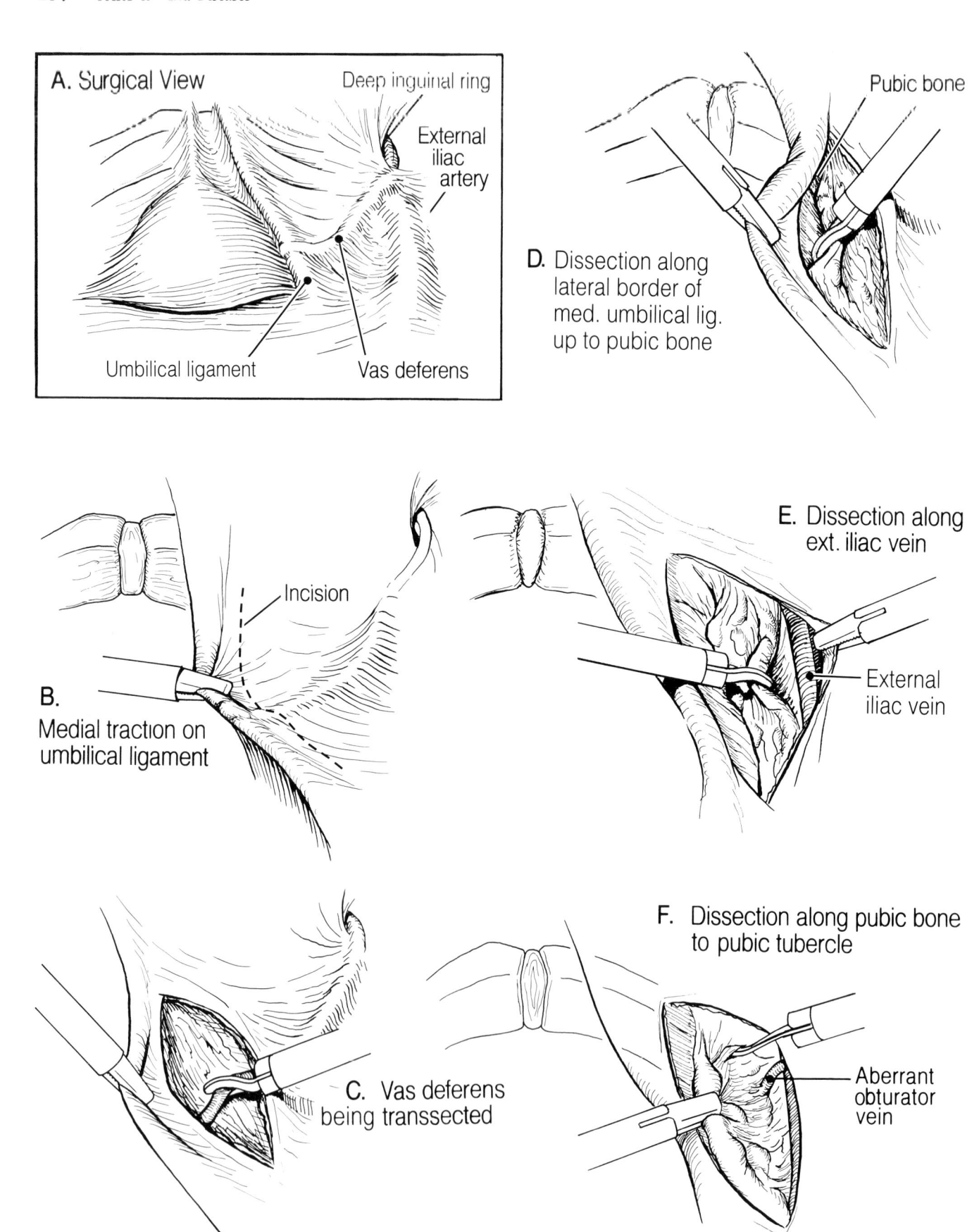

A. Surgical View
- Deep inguinal ring
- External iliac artery
- Umbilical ligament
- Vas deferens

B. Medial traction on umbilical ligament
- Incision

C. Vas deferens being transsected

D. Dissection along lateral border of med. umbilical lig. up to pubic bone
- Pubic bone

E. Dissection along ext. iliac vein
- External iliac vein

F. Dissection along pubic bone to pubic tubercle
- Aberrant obturator vein

G. Nodes released from around obturator vein and nerve

H. Node packet divided at apex

I. Completed dissection

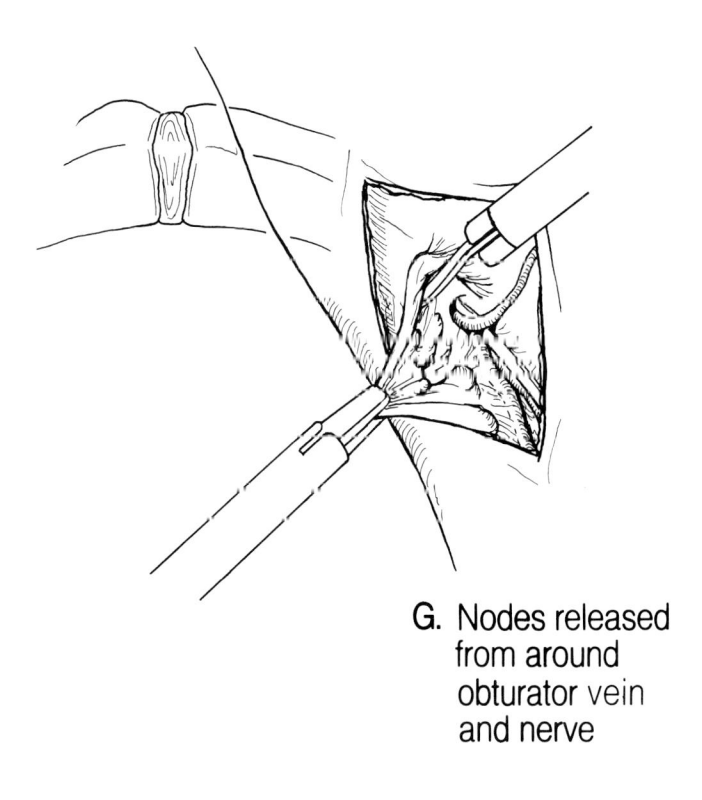

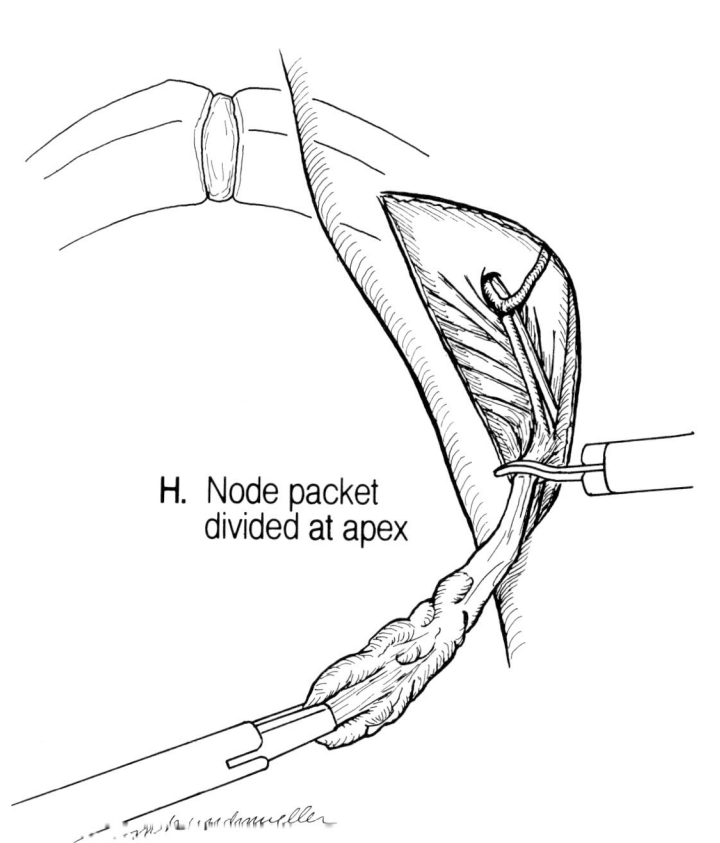

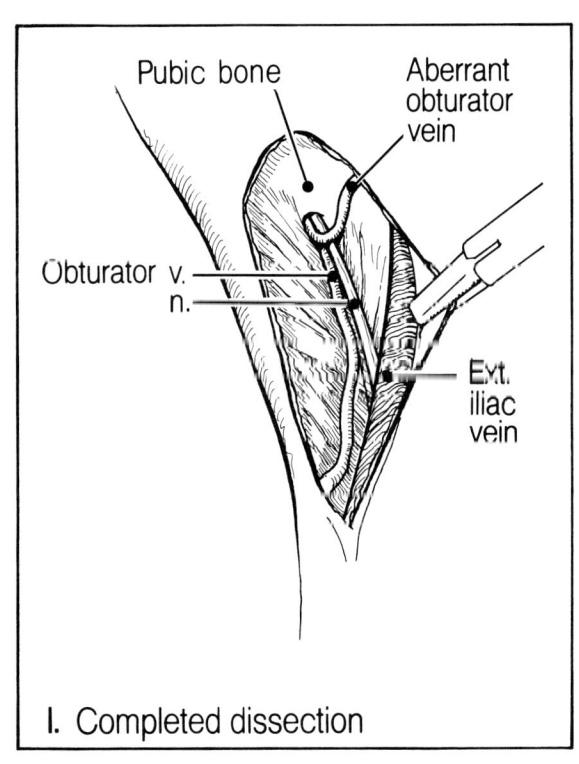

FIGURE 27-3 A. With a laparoscope pointed toward the right groin, the bladder, umbilical ligament, vas deferens, deep inguinal ring, and iliac vessels can usually be seen through the peritoneum. B. The umbilical ligament is grasped and retracted to the patient's left. C. The peritoneum lateral to the umbilical ligament is divided to expose the vas deferens, which is then incised with electrosurgery scissors. D. With the vas deferens divided, the medial extent of the obturator node packet can be visualized and gently teased away from the bladder with closed scissors. E. When the medial aspect of the node packet has been adequately delineated, the lateral margin of the node packet is dissected from beneath the external iliac vein. Blunt retraction of the medial side wall of the external iliac vein aids in this portion of the dissection. F. The node packet is released from the pubic bone. An aberrant obturator vein may be found coursing over the pubic bone at this point. G. The nodes are released from around the obturator vein and nerve. H. The specimen is divided at its apex. I. A completed dissection clearly shows the anatomy of the obturator fossa and external iliac vessels.

is made medial to the medial umbilical ligament, a bladder or ureteral injury may result.

Next, the vas deferens is identified. It traverses the surgical field horizontally on its way to the internal ring. The vas deferens lies directly beneath the peritoneal reflection and is surrounded by a very thin layer of fat. The vas deferens is grasped, held taut, cauterized, and cut. This maneuver opens up the pelvic retroperitoneum and greatly facilitates further dissection of the pelvic lymph nodes.

The retroperitoneal fatty tissue can be gently dissected from the lateral border of the medial umbilical ligament and pushed further laterally. This maneuver helps to define the medial aspect of the nodal packet. The tissue in this area should sweep away easily. If this tissue is unduly vascular or requires sharp dissection to develop the plane, then the operator may be working too close to the bladder. (Tip: Macroscopic hematuria at any time during the dissection, likely indicates a bladder injury. If hematuria is noted, the bladder should be filled with saline stained with indigo carmine. If a bladder perforation is present, it can be repaired immediately, either laparoscopically or by an open surgical approach.) The dissection continues caudal until the pubic bone just lateral to the symphisis pubis can be palpated with either the grasping or dissecting instrument. The overlying tissue is cleared from the pubic bone until the white periosteum can be clearly visualized.

Attention is now turned to the lateral stump of the vas deferens. Pulsations from the external iliac artery can often be noted just posterior to this stump. The tissue just deep to the pulsations is grasped and gently teased away. The underlying external iliac vein should come into view. The vein itself will appear as a blue ribbon; it is usually collapsed as a result of the patient's head-down position and the 15-mmHg pneumoperitoneum. With a gentle spreading action, tissue is swept medially off of the anterior surface of the external iliac vein. The dissection is continued along the anterior surface of the vein in a caudal direction. There should be no branches from the external iliac vein along its anterior surface. This defines the lateral margin of the nodal packet.

Next, the grasper through the ipsilateral 5-mm port is used to roll the anterior surface of the external iliac vein laterally. The grasper via the lower 11-mm port is now used to tease or hold taut the tissue along the medial surface of the external iliac vein so it can be dissected from the underlying obturator internus muscle.

The next step is to complete the dissection of the external iliac vein in the area of the pubic bone. By continuing caudal, along the medial surface of the external iliac vein, the upper edge of an aberrant obturator vein can be identified. This is the only medial, albeit inconstant, side branch from the external iliac vein. The tissue surrounding this vein can be carefully teased away and the vein preserved. Alternatively, if the surgeon desires, the vein can be dissected and secured with metal clips passed via the lower 11-mm port. If this is done, two clips should be placed on either side of the vein. If preserved, the vein can be followed inferiorly as it curves toward the pubic bone to enter the obturator foramen. This can be helpful in leading the surgeon to the obturator vessels and obturator nerve.

If there is no aberrant obturator vein, then as the surgeon dissects along the medial border of the external iliac vein, the pubic bone laterally will be encountered. The pubic bone is cleared of all overlying tissue until the periosteum is clearly visible between the external iliac vein and the area of Cooper's ligament. This tissue may be fatty, and it needs to be carefully dissected, cauterized, and cut. Also lymphatic vessels in this tissue can be identified and cauterized or clipped. The pubic bone defines the inferior border of the nodal packet.

The inferior margin of the packet of tissue along the pubic bone is now grasped and gently pulled cephalad with the ipsilateral 5-mm grasping forceps. The other 5-mm grasping forceps and the electrosurgery scissors are now moved in a sweeping vertical stroking motion along the medial border of the dissection to identify the obturator nerve. This results in the rapid displacement of much of the loose fatty tissue and uncovers the obturator nerve, which appears as a shining white band of tissue. No cutting should be done in this area until the obturator nerve is clearly identified. The obturator vessels can also be identified and dissected. Under most circumstances, these vessels do not need to be incised. Indeed, securing these vessels merely adds time to the procedure and increases the risk of bothersome bleeding without enhancing the yield from the node dissection.

The obturator nerve is followed cephalad until it disappears beneath the internal iliac vein. It is rare to identify the inferior margin of the internal iliac vein. Rather, the dissection is concluded because the surgeon can no longer safely visualize tissue along the upper extent of the obturator nerve. Even if the 0° laparoscope is placed in the lower 11-mm port, the surgical field usually does not change sufficiently to allow for safe dissection of the inferior margin of the internal iliac vein. Via this approach, the entire packet is freed from the obturator nerve, thereby defining the posterior border of the dissection.

The nodal packet is now connected only superiorly to the retroperitoneum by a few strands of tissue running toward the obturator nerve. These are carefully coagulated and incised. During this part of the dissection, it is again important to stay lateral to the medial umbilical ligament to avoid any inadvertent injury to the bladder or ureter. Indeed, at this point in the procedure, the ureter may be seen passing just medial to the medial umbilical ligament (see Fig. 27-3).

The freed nodal packet is now moved to the peritoneal reflection over the rectum and deposited in the cul-de-sac in this area. Retrieval of the packet is done via the lower midline 11-mm port. If the packet is particularly small, a

5-mm grasper with traumatic jaws can be used. However, if the packet is large, then a 10-mm spoon-type grasping forceps or 10-mm rat toothed gallbladder-type grasping forceps can be used to secure the packet and retract it through the 11-mm port.

Careful observation of the retrieval maneuver is important. Specifically, the packet should be watched as it is retracted into the 11-mm port to see if any portion of the packet breaks away and falls onto the underlying bowel. Similarly, when the grasping forceps is reintroduced into the 11-mm port after retrieving some of the nodal packet, the end of the port should be viewed to see if the advancing forceps pushes any residual nodal tissue out of the port. These bits of tissue can be retrieved through either 5-mm port.

As the tissue is pulled into the 11-mm port, a circular twisting motion is helpful to prevent part of the packet from being severed by the opening of the port itself. As the packet is withdrawn further up the shaft of the port, the assistant should remove the 10.5-mm reducer with one hand and, with the other hand, should open the valve on the trocar (desufflate) so that the tissue can be smoothly delivered through the port. If this is not done, then the tissue will become entangled in the valve mechanism of the trocar, thereby decreasing the amount of specimen retrieved and jamming the valve mechanism. This results in a rapid loss of the pneumoperitoneum. If this problem is not immediately resolved, a new 11-mm port will have to be placed.

When the packet is too large to be retrieved in one piece, it may be necessary to use a scissors to divide the packet into several smaller specimens, which can be separately removed. Alternatively, a surgical entrapment sack (Lapsac) has been designed by Cook Urological, Inc., Spencer, IN. This sack has a drawstring along its neck. The sack is introduced via the 11-mm lower midline port. Using the 11-mm port and the ipsilateral 5-mm port, the mouth of the sack is opened. The nodal packet is grasped via the contralateral 5-mm port and deposited in the opened sack. Via the 11-mm lower midline port, a 5-mm grasper is used to secure the drawstrings and pull them taut. The drawstrings and neck of the sack are delivered into the 11-mm port. The port is removed; the drawstrings should lie on the abdominal wall. By pulling on the drawstrings, the neck and entire bag (containing the intact nodal packet) can usually be delivered. If the entrapped packet is too large, a Kelly clamp needs to be introduced into the sack, the nodal packet is fragmented, and the pieces are pulled from the sack, after which the sack is pulled from the abdomen. The 11-mm port is replaced.

After retrieval of the nodal packet, the nodes are sent for frozen section. While waiting for the pathologist's report, the dissection is begun on the contralateral side. The procedure is the same in every aspect as on the initial side. If the frozen-section confirms the presence of metastatic disease, the procedure is immediately terminated because removal of the nodes from the second side is of no value to the patient; continuing the procedure at this point may result in unnecessary and unjustifiable patient morbidity. Despite a recognized false-negative rate of as high as 19 percent on the frozen section, the reduction in patient morbidity by avoiding an unneeded surgical exercise is, in our opinion, sufficient justification to obtain a frozen section diagnosis.[12]

PHASE IV: EXITING THE ABDOMEN

The final step is to exit the abdomen safely. Each of the three non-umbilical port sites needs to be inspected to see if there is any bleeding from the point of abdominal entry. Then, a 5-mm endoscope can be introduced into one of the lateral ports to check the 11-mm umbilical port site. The site of each node dissection is irrigated with approximately 250 mL of irrigant, and the fluid is then aspirated as a final check for bleeding. The bowel is again examined for any injury. The intraabdominal pressure is decreased to 5 mmHg. Both areas of the node dissection are again checked for hemostasis. Next, the umbilical 11-mm port is removed under endoscopic control; as the port is withdrawn, the flapper valve is opened so that a loop of bowel is not inadvertently pulled into the trocar wound. Then, a 2–0 absorbable fascial suture on a 5/6 curved needle is carefully placed to close the 11-mm umbilical incision. For this maneuver, it is helpful to grasp either edge of the fascia firmly with forceps; an eyelid retractor or skin rake can be used to retract the skin. The suture is placed as a figure of eight in the fascia. The same is then done for the lower midline 11-mm port. During the placement of the suture, the pneumoperitoneum is maintained, and the suture placement is monitored endoscopically to preclude any bowel injury. Next, the opposite 5-mm port is withdrawn under endoscopic control. Lastly, the 5-mm endoscope is withdrawn to the end of the 5-mm sheath, and then the entire assembly is removed. The two 11-mm skin incisions are closed with a 4–0 absorbable subcuticular suture. After all the CO_2 is evacuated from the abdomen through the 5-mm port sites, the two 5-mm ports are then closed with a single strip of adhesive (Steri-strip). The nasogastric tube and the Foley urethral catheter can also be removed.

Postoperative Care

Postoperatively, the patient is given another dose of a parental antibiotic (i.e., cefazolin) followed by a broad-spectrum oral antibiotic (i.e., cephalexin) to cover the initial 48 h after the procedure. A clear liquid diet is begun as soon as the patient is awake and alert. Upon resumption of oral intake, the intravenous line is removed. The patient's diet is advanced to a regular meal, usually by the first postoperative morning.

The need for pain medications should be minimal; usually no more than one or two doses of a parenteral narcotic. Within 12 h of the procedure, it is rare for a patient to require analgesics stronger than acetaminophen. The patient is usually discharged after breakfast on the first or second postoperative day.

EARLY WARNING SIGNS

In the immediate postoperative period, the patient may complain of shoulder pain as a result of diaphragmatic irritation from the CO_2 used during the case. Usually this problem resolves spontaneously during the first few hours after laparoscopy. As such, any delayed complaints of severe abdominal pain, especially if the patient was initially pain-free, are worrisome. This may be the first sign of an unrecognized bowel injury.

The presence of macroscopic hematuria postoperatively suggests that an intraperitoneal bladder injury occurred during the procedure. A cystogram should be performed. If a bladder tear is confirmed, then either an immediate repair can be done or a Foley urethral catheter can be placed. If after 1 week of drainage, a repeat cystogram reveals persistent leakage, then a laparoscopic or open surgical repair of the tear will be necessary.

The laparoscopic port skin sites usually heal rapidly. If a superficial wound infection develops, it is treated with drainage and oral antibiotics. However, if this infection is associated with more than localized abdominal signs or if the wound culture produces a mixed aerobic–anaerobic bacterial flora, the possibility of an underlying bowel injury should be entertained, and appropriate diagnostic studies (i.e., flat and upright abdominal radiographs or CT scans with oral contrast medium) should be obtained. Discovery of a bowel injury at this time mandates open surgical exploration and repair.

Also, two other minor problems may arise in about 20 percent of patients: urinary retention and/or abdominal ecchymoses. The problem of urinary retention is managed with a urethral catheter. The patient is discharged with the catheter in place. Usually, 3 to 5 days later, the catheter can be removed either at home or in the office. The second problem, abdominal wall ecchymoses, may not become apparent for several days. However, visually it can be quite impressive and disconcerting to the patient. It resolves spontaneously over a 2-week period. Currently this development has not been a harbinger of a significant vascular injury.

LATE COMPLICATIONS

Late complications of laparoscopic pelvic lymphadenectomy are rare. Herniation through one of the 11-mm trocar sites can occur but it distinctly unusual. Likewise, adhesions with an associated bowel obstruction are rare.

SUBSEQUENT THERAPY

For the urologist, the most vexing problem after a laparoscopic lymphadenectomy, is when to proceed with definitive cancer therapy should the lymph nodes be negative for metastatic disease. If a retropubic prostatectomy is planned, it is prudent to proceed under the same anesthetic, realizing that the frozen-section diagnosis of negative nodes may be incorrect in as many as 19 percent of patients.[12] If the prostatectomy is delayed for 1 week, the periprostatic tissues will still be edematous, and the bowel will often be adherent to the sites of the node dissection. After 3 to 4 weeks, the edema will have resolved, but a loop of bowel may be adherent to the area of the lymphadenectomy. In contrast, if a perineal prostatectomy is planned, this procedure can be safely delayed because the surgical field will not have been at all disturbed during the laparoscopic lymph node dissection. If implant radiation therapy is to be given, this can be done at the same time as the laparoscopic dissection or at a later date depending on the surgeon's wishes. When external beam radiation therapy is planned, the radiation therapist must be informed of the laparoscopic nature of the node dissection. In these patients, radiation to the area of the obturator fossa should be avoided because the bowel may be adherent to this area.

RESULTS

Schuessler, Vancaillie, and associates have had the largest experience with laparoscopic pelvic lymphadenectomy. As of April 1991, they had completed 101 node dissections. Among these patients, 13 percent had positive nodes, and 90 percent were discharged from the hospital within 23 h of the procedure. Their major complication rate has been 1 percent (a single bowel injury necessitating open surgical repair). Recently, Schuessler and coworkers have extended the borders of their pelvic node dissection beyond the external iliac vein and obturator fossa in an effort to stage prostatic cancer more accurately. Currently, their dissection encompasses the distal portion of the common iliac vessels and the internal iliac vein. Results from this more extensive dissection are pending (Schuessler WW, Vancaillie TG. Personal communication, May 1992).

Winfield, See, and colleagues have recently reported their series of laparoscopic node dissection combined with immediate open surgical inspection of the right and left obturator fossae and surgical removal of any remaining obturator nodal tissue. Among 30 patients, the dissection was successfully completed in 73 percent; 23 percent of the patients had positive nodes. On average, 10 nodes were removed laparoscopically from each obturator fossa. Subsequent surgical exploration resulted in retrieval of an additional three nodes per patient. Among these patients, surgical exploration resulted in upstaging to Stage D1 disease in two patients (9 percent) (Winfield NH. Personal communication, May 1992).

CONCLUSION

Overall, laparoscopic pelvic lymphadenectomy offers the patient a less morbid alternative to surgical lymphadenectomy. Although the initial procedure is more lengthy, the hospital stay and, presumably, the convalescence are greatly reduced by a laparoscopic approach. However, there is a steep learning curve, and the procedure itself is not innocuous. Although laparoscopic lymphadenectomy is being routinely offered to patients who are candidates for external beam radiation therapy, radiation implantation therapy, or perineal prostatectomy, its application to patients scheduled to undergo a retropubic prostatectomy should be limited to those patients who are at high risk for nodal metastases.

Finally, on a broader plane, laparoscopic pelvic lymphadenectomy is an invitation to the urologist to become proficient in laparoscopic surgery. Although currently, laparoscopic lymph node dissection and varicocelectomy are the only large-volume urologic procedures to which this methodology is being applied, there is little doubt that, with further experience and technologic advances, many other urologic procedures will be accomplished laparoscopically. Already, there are reports of successful laparoscopic drainage of a pelvic lymphocele, laparoscopic ureterolysis, and laparoscopic nephrectomy. These are but the earliest signs of a new age in surgery in which the disability, discomfort, and disfigurement of incisional surgery will slowly but surely be supplanted by less invasive, yet equally effective, minimally invasive surgical techniques.

REFERENCES

1. Cortesi N, Ferrari P, Zambarda E, et al: Diagnosis of bilateral abdominal cryptorchidism by laparoscopy. *Endoscopy* 1976; 8:33.
2. Winfield HN, Ryan KJ. Experimental laparoscopic surgery. Potential clinical applications in urology. *J Endourol* 1990; 4:1.
3. Schuessler WW, Vancaillie TG, Reich H, et al: Transperitoneal endosurgical lymphadenectomy in patients with localized prostate cancer. *J Urol* 1991; 145:988.
4. Prout GR Jr, Heaney JA, Griffin PP, et al: Nodal involvement as a prognostic indicator in patients with prostatic carcinoma. *J Urol* 1980; 124:226.
5. Oesterling JE, Brendler CB, Epstein JI, et al: Correlation of clinical stage, serum prostatic acid phosphatase and preoperative Gleason grade with final pathological stage in 275 patients with clinically localized adenocarcinoma of the prostate. *J Urol* 1987; 138:92.
6. Kramer SA, Spahn J, Brendler CB, et al: Experience with Gleason's histopathologic grading in prostatic cancer. *J Urol* 1980; 124:223.
7. Catalona WJ: Pelvic lymphadenectomy is essential to staging accuracy in most patients with stages A-2 and B prostate cancer before radical prostatectomy. *Semin Urol* 1983; 1:212.
8. Guinan P, Bhatti R, Ray P: An evaluation of prostate specific antigen in prostatic cancer. *J Urol* 1987; 137:686.
9. Andriole GL, McCarthy JF, Coplen DE, et al: Selection of patients with prostate cancer (CaP) for laparoscopic lymph node dissection: Use of serum PSA and PSA index (PSAI). Presented at the American Urological Association Annual Meeting, 1992.
10. Petros JA, Catalona SJ: Lower incidence of unsuspected lymph node metastases in 521 consecutive patients with clinically localized prostate cancer. *J Urol* 1992; 147:1574.
11. Brendler CB, Cleeve LK, Anderson EE, et al: Staging pelvic lymphadenectomy for carcinoma of the prostate: Risk versus benefit. *J Urol* 1980; 124:849.
12. Catalona WJ, Stein AJ: Accuracy of frozen section detection of lymph node metastases in prostatic carcinoma. *J Urol* 1982; 127:460.

Chapter 28

Emergent and Urgent Laparoscopy

George Berci

Laparoscopy has been employed since the turn of the century,[1] and convincing results were reported from Europe and the United States.[2-4] However, in the past, general surgeons preferred open exploration rather than diagnosis performed through a "keyhole" inspection. Gynecologists recognized the usefulness of laparoscopy in pelvic surgery two decades ago and utilized the technique first in tubal sterilization, followed by diagnostic and staging procedures, oophorectomy, myomectomy, and recently, laparoscopic-assisted hysterectomy.[5] Initially, gastroenterologists were also enthusiastic about laparoscopy as an aid in evaluating liver disease and in performing a more precise biopsy.[6]

The introduction of CT imaging provided a convenient diagnostic tool that largely replaced laparoscopy. It became commonplace, after noting an abnormality on CT scan, to repeat the examination and combine it with guided biopsy. However, a large percentage of aspiration samples obtained in this manner were not informative. Even if cancer cells were identified, the surgeon gained no information regarding staging or operability.

The introduction of laparoscopic cholecystectomy has significantly advanced the acceptance of laparoscopy among general surgeons. At the time of writing this chapter, most surgeons have been trained and are performing laparoscopic cholecystectomy. This has led to a wider employment of laparoscopy in emergency conditions, such as in the assessment of the patient with blunt abdominal trauma or with an abdominal diagnostic dilemma in selected cases.

Accordingly, we initiated emergency minilaparoscopy in 1980,[7] building on the recommendations of Gazzaniga and Carnevale[8,9] for laparoscopy made in 1976 and 1977. We developed the smaller laparoscopic miniset because it was easier to use in the emergency setting.

BLUNT ABDOMINAL TRAUMA

Root and his associates[10] introduced diagnostic peritoneal lavage (DPL) to evaluate the presence of blood or intestinal contents within the abdominal cavity. Experience has shown that patients with blunt abdominal trauma who suffer a minor hemorrhage do not necessarily need a formal exploration. The incidence of unnecessary laparotomies in cases of blunt abdominal trauma is in the range of 10 to 20 percent.[11] These are generally instances in which no active bleeding site is discovered or a coagulum is found at the site of a small injury, even though sufficient blood was spilled to give a positive DPL result. These operations require an investment of time by the medical team, incur needless costs for patient and hospital alike, and result in a small but definite morbidity and mortality. In addition, use of the CT scanner in these cases may reveal fluid (blood) in the peritoneal cavity but does not eliminate the problems of unnecessary exploration.[12]

The advantage of laparoscopy in this setting is that it allows the surgeon to determine whether hemorrhage is ongoing, and in certain cases, minor bleeding sources may be coagulated under laparoscopic control. Additionally, the use of the laparoscope frees the surgeon from having to rely on others for diagnostic information.

Instrumentation

The laparoscopic miniset includes a minitrocar with an outer diameter of 5 mm, through which a 4.2-mm telescope can be introduced. A second similar-sized trocar is employed, through which one may pass a suction–coagulation device that is also used as a palpation probe. A minimal number of instruments are required. One is concerned, not with minute details, but with inspection of the paracolic gutters for blood or intestinal fluid or, when an injury is located, with evaluating the findings and deciding on the appropriate treatment. One may also find it useful to include bowel graspers, with which to "run" the intestines gently.

Modern emergent laparoscopy is performed with an attached television camera, which produces an enlarged image and simultaneously records the procedure on tape. This is useful as a teaching tool and in forming part of the patient's chart. The entire team can follow the procedure on the television screen and coordinate their movements. Furthermore, the complete unit can be transported to the emergency room or the intensive care unit (Figs. 28-1 and 28-2). Additionally, it is necessary to provide a system for irrigation, either a roller pump on the cart or a simple pressure bag. Wall suction should, likewise, be attached to the coagulation probe.

Indications

These are the same as for peritoneal lavage as follows.

1. Obscure clinical picture with questionable physical signs, such as in the patient with an impaired level of consciousness (e.g., head injury, alcoholism, or drug ingestion), in which cases it is often difficult to exclude intraabdominal injuries based on purely clinical grounds).
2. Evidence of blunt or penetrating abdominal trauma.
3. Unexplained hypotension.
4. Equivocal signs during the abdominal examination in a conscious patient.

In many circumstances of multiple trauma, laparoscopy allows treatment to be prioritized and provides the surgeon with a tool that offers a good view of the abdominal cavity. More importantly, it extends the latitude of assessment between exploration and observation.

Contraindications

These depend to a large degree on the surgeon's experience, but include pregnancy, ileus, general peritonitis, and morbid obesity. The previously operated abdomen presents a challenge even to skilled surgical endoscopists, and judgment must be used.

Technique

Laparoscopy may be performed in the emergency room on a stretcher, utilizing local anesthesia with intravenous sedation. Those patients who require intubation for other reasons, of course, would be treated under general anesthesia. The intoxicated or agitated patient requires intravenous sedation, for example, meperidine or diazepam, according to need. An emergency room nurse or house staff officer should monitor vital signs, including pulse, blood pressure, and pulse oximetry. The patient should be sedated to the point of somnolence but remain responsive.

Local anesthetic (1% lidocaine without epinephrine) is injected at the site of the first trocar, which is usually below the umbilicus (for further details, see chap. 21). The telescope with attached television camera is introduced here. The second trocar is inserted under the right costal margin, beside the rectus muscle, under visual control. After local anesthetics are injected, a stab incision is made in the skin below the umbilicus, and the pneumoneedle is inserted. A syringe with saline is attached, and aspiration and slow injection is performed twice to ensure that the needle is not in a blood vessel. If pure blood is aspirated, the position of the needle should be changed and this maneuver repeated. If problems are encountered inserting the needle or if the patient has numerous abdominal scars, the open technique of trocar insertion may be preferred.

When the pneumoneedle is in position, the abdomen is

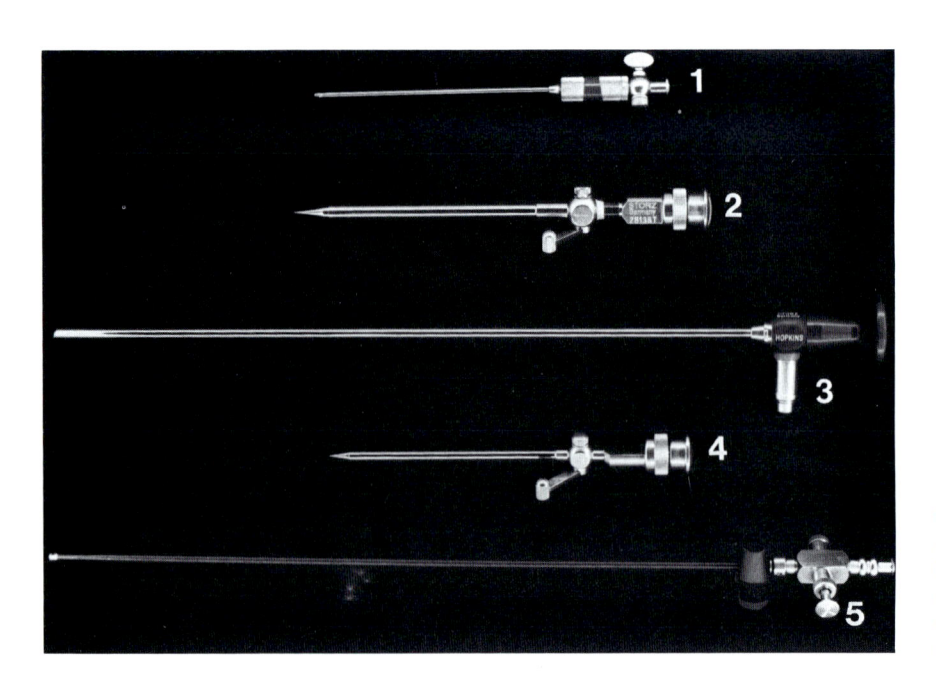

FIGURE 28-1. Basic set. 1. Pneumoneedle. 2. Small (5-mm) trocar. 3. 30° Hopkins II telescope. 4. Second small trocar. 5. Suction–coagulation–palpation cannula. (K. Storz Endoscopy of America, Inc.).

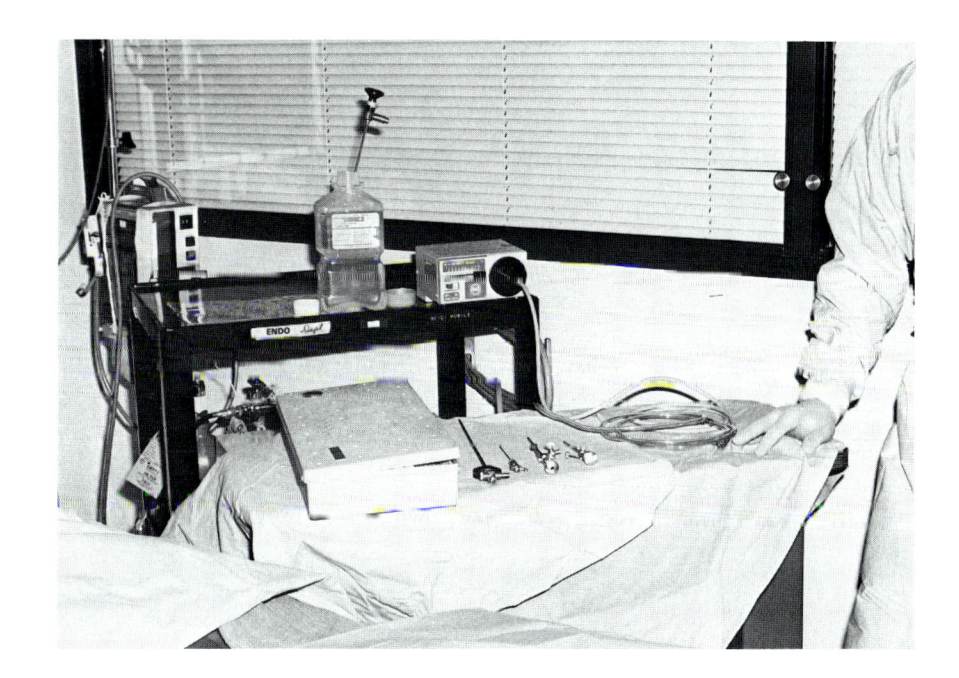

FIGURE 28-2. The entire sterile set is kept in a mobile cart that has an insufflator, light source, and television attached. A sterile camera may be attached. The set can be prepared and ready to go in minutes, enabling performance of laparoscopy in the emergency room or intensive care unit.

insufflated with carbon dioxide or, less commonly, nitrous oxide. The latter gas is slightly less irritating to the peritoneum and is, therefore, better tolerated. The rate of insufflation should not exceed 1 to 1.5 L/min because it is dangerous and uncomfortable. After an appropriate pneumoperitoneum has been achieved (14 to 15 mmHg pressure), the needle is withdrawn, the stab incision is slightly enlarged to ensure a tight fit of the trocar, and the trocar is advanced by penetrating the abdominal cavity with a drilling–pressing motion. If reusable trocars are preferred, it is beneficial to choose one with a stylet that has a central hole, creating a hissing noise as soon as it enters a high-pressure cavity, informing the surgeon that the peritoneum has been pierced.

The telescope is prewarmed to avoid fogging by heating a 1-L plastic bottle of saline in a microwave oven and using a commercially available scope warmer or to apply an antifogging solution. The scope is then dried and inserted, and the sterile television camera is attached after white balancing and focusing is completed.

It is imperative to work fast; the entire procedure should not exceed 15 min, including creation of the pneumoperitoneum. The second trocar is advanced under visual control at the site described, and the workhorse, the suction–coagulation and palpation probe, is introduced. The probe is long enough to reach the left lobe of the liver or the left paracolic gutter. Attention should first be directed to the gutters, which in 50 percent of our cases were free of blood or fluid, in which case the examination can be completed.[11] A view of the pelvic area is recommended before the abdomen is desufflated.

Findings

BLOOD IN THE ABDOMEN

The first step is an overall view for orientation. The falciform ligament should be in the middle of the picture if the telescope with the attached television camera has been introduced in the midline. If blood is found in the paracolic gutters, the volume should be approximately assessed.

MINIMAL HEMOPERITONEUM

If there are streaks of blood among the intestinal loops or a very thin line of blood in the gutters, a systematic search should be initiated. In the case of a motor vehicle accident, deceleration injury is very common, and a laceration is often found on the anterior surface of the liver. The second accessory trocar should be introduced in every case because the palpation probe is the extension of the surgeon's finger. One may use it, not only to convey tactile sensation, but also as a suction and coagulation probe. The left lobe can be completely lifted up and the undersurface of the liver inspected. The right lobe can be only partially elevated. Palpation must be performed in a gentle manner to avoid iatrogenic lacerations. If no liver lesion is discovered, the falciform ligament should be inspected. If this observation proves negative, then attention is drawn to the intestine to expose possible injuries to the mesentery.

In the case of a pelvic fracture, blood may be found in the pelvic area. After a search of 5 to 10 min, if a bleeding site has not been found and the appearance of this minimal hemoperitoneum has not changed, this patient should be observed, with consideration of angiography. The puncture site is closed with clips.

MODERATE HEMOPERITONEUM

Moderate hemoperitoneum denotes that a 5- to 10-mm blood level is found in the gutter. This should be evacuated through the suction–coagulation probe, and an intensive search should commence to locate the bleeding site. If found, a few minutes of observation should be spent to assess the following. Is the bleeding active? Would it be feasible to coagulate a minor ooze? Is it already covered with a coagulum? A decision must then be reached after examination of the area in question as to whether this laceration merits exploration or should merely be observed. After evacuation of accumulated blood and failure to discover a bleeding site, if the blood reaccumulates within 5 to 10 min, this means that the bleeding site is not amenable to laparoscopic evaluation, and the patient should be taken directly to the operating room.

SEVERE HEMOPERITONEUM

If pneumoneedle aspiration results in pure blood, despite repositioning, the patient should be taken immediately to the operating room because this implies free intraperitoneal blood. After creation of the pneumoperitoneum and upon introduction of the telescope, if the intestinal loops are floating on a pool of blood, no further time should be wasted, and the patient should be explored.

SPLENIC INJURIES

In cases of splenic injury, blood will be recovered from the left paracolic gutter. The omentum covering the spleen will appear blue and may be tented as a result of blood or a blood clot underneath. If the vital signs are stable and, after evacuation of the blood and observation of the area for a few minutes, the blood does not reaccumulate, the patient should undergo a CT scan and be observed in the intensive care unit. The normal spleen generally cannot be seen because it is covered by omentum. To inspect the spleen, a steep reverse Trendelenburg position with the left side tilted up is required. This position is obviously difficult to obtain on an emergency room stretcher. In addition, the emergency situation is not an ideal scenario in which to attempt laparoscopic splenectomy.

ORGAN PERFORATION

If yellow or green fluid is observed in the paracolic gutters, the fluid should be aspirated. It may be sent for amylase content but generally, it is an indication for surgery. If several hours have transpired between the actual trauma and laparoscopic examination, findings such as an omental mass covering a particular area or intestinal loops appearing hyperemic provide a clue as to the site of injury. The palpation probe is very useful in moving such loops or adherent omentum to examine the area. Perforation of the retroperitoneal segment of the duodenum or pancreatic injuries cannot be readily visualized, and a high index of suspicion is required to make the diagnosis.

PENETRATING INJURIES

In cases of stab wounds to the abdomen, the entrance wound is temporarily closed with a few stitches to prevent leakage of the pneumoperitoneum. The telescope is introduced, the examiner places one finger on the stab wound, and the abdominal wall is indented. This maneuver is observed from inside through the telescope. If the parietal peritoneum is intact, this indicates that the stab wound has not penetrated. If penetration through the parietal peritoneum is discovered, the area under the stab wound is carefully observed using the palpation probe, and the organs and intestinal loops are lifted up to see whether perforation is present. Obviously, the choice of therapy, be it laparoscopic or open, will depend on the severity of the injury and the skill of the surgeon.

In the majority of gunshot wound cases, laparoscopic evaluation has no role to play. However, in the obese patient with a tangential anterior or lateral small-caliber injury, it may prove useful.[12]

Results

At Cedars-Sinai Medical Center, 150 patients who had sustained blunt abdominal trauma were evaluated by minilaparoscopy in the emergency room with local anesthesia.[13] The criteria for laparoscopic evaluation were those questions that generally prompt the surgeon to perform diagnostic peritoneal lavage, such as uncertain mechanism of injury, unexplained hypotension, or signs of abdominal trauma.

In this series, despite having met these parameters, 56 percent of patients (n = 84) showed no hemoperitoneum on laparoscopy, with none requiring subsequent exploration. A positive laparoscopy was found in 25 percent of cases (38 patients), and only 1 of these needed laparotomy, with the others having minor lacerations that necessitated only close observation. The patient requiring surgery had a missed sigmoid perforation; only a small volume of blood had been seen in the left paracolic gutter at the time of laparoscopy. In 19 percent of patients (28 cases), laparoscopy revealed a severe hemoperitoneum, indicating the need for immediate surgery. In all but one of these cases, the decision to operate was deemed appropriate, the exception being a patient with 700 mL of free blood from no obvious source. There was one complication in the series: a patient with minimal hemoperitoneum resulting from bleeding from the trocar insertion.

These results compared favorably with other techniques of patient triage, but a prospective randomized trial will be needed to define the role of laparoscopy fully in complex situations. There are certain areas of the abdomen that defy visualization, such as the diaphragm, where injuries are notoriously difficult to diagnose using any modality. The use of the laparoscope may be valuable in reducing the number of such missed injuries in cases in which the surgeon has a high level of clinical suspicion.[14]

ABDOMINAL DIAGNOSTIC DILEMMA

In many cases, the diagnosis of an intraabdominal catastrophe can be made on the basis of the clinical assessment, routine laboratory tests, and radiologic examinations. However, there are some patients in whom there is a dilemma regarding the diagnosis or the need for exploration. In these instances, minilaparoscopy can establish a diagnosis and have an impact on patient management.

Young Female Patients

Familiar to every practicing surgeon is the scenario of an acute onset of right lower quadrant pain with a differential diagnosis between acute appendix, ectopic pregnancy, torsion of an ovarian cyst, or pelvic inflammatory disease. A mistaken diagnosis can result in the removal of a normal appendix at laparotomy. Minilaparoscopy can alleviate this risk rapidly and efficiently (see Chap. 16).

Elderly Patients

Elderly patients, especially those with severe atherosclerosis (senility), are often unable to give a precise history and, therefore, present a special challenge. Examination of the abdomen may be noninformative, and the laboratory results are sometimes of little value. However, the intuition and experience of the surgeon may lead to a suspicion of a severe problem. In these cases, laparoscopy facilitates the diagnosis, for example, diverticulitis or organ perforation, and valuable time may be saved before critical peritonitis develops. Similarly, segmental mesenteric ischemia without profound clinical signs or symptoms can be a diagnostic dilemma. These patients often have underlying cardiovascular and respiratory disease that classifies them as a poor operative risk. Laparoscopy enables diagnosis of segmental ischemic bowel and verifies the need for operation early in the patient's management. Hemorrhagic fluid in the paracolic gutter is always indicative of this pathologic condition.

CONCLUSION

The usefulness of emergency laparoscopy was clear at its inception, but its acceptance was hampered by a lack of appreciation and knowledge of the use of this modality. Currently, numerous surgeons have been trained and are performing laparoscopic cholecystectomy. The outlook has, therefore, changed dramatically. Laparoscopy today needs no introduction to the general surgeon, and it is evident that emergency laparoscopy, if used with skill in appropriate cases, can solve emergency room dilemmas. Valuable time is saved, and the priority of treatment in the multiply injured patient is established. Many unnecessary, expensive, and time-consuming laboratory examinations and laparotomies can be eliminated. The laparoscopic examination should be a part of the armamentarium of every surgeon who provides service in the emergency room.

REFERENCES

1. Jacobaeus HC: Kurze Ubersicht uber meine Erfahrungen mit der Laparoskopie. *Munch Med Wochenschr* 1911; 58:2017–2019.
2. Kalk H, Bruhl W: *Leitfaden der Laparoskopie.* Stuttgart, Thieme, 1951.
3. Ruddock JC: Peritoneoscopy. *West J Surg Obstet Gynecol* 1934; 42:392–394.
4. Zoeckler SJ: Peritoneoscopy. A re-evaluation. *Gastroenterology* 1958; 34:969–980.
5. Semm K: *Operative Manual for Endoscopic Abdominal Surgery.* Chicago, Year Book, 1987.
6. Dagnini G: *Clinical Laparoscopy.* Padua, Piccini, 1980.
7. Sherwood R, Berci G, Austin E, et al: Minilaparoscopy for blunt abdominal trauma. *Archs Surg* 1980; 115:672–673.
8. Gazzaniga AB, Slanton WW, Bartlett RH: Laparoscopy in the diagnosis of blunt and penetrating injuries to the abdomen. *Am J Surg* 1976; 131:315–318.
9. Carnevale N, Baron N, Delany HM: Peritoneoscopy as an aid in the diagnosis of abdominal trauma: A preliminary report. *J Trauma* 1977; 17:634–641.
10. Root HO, Hauser CW, McKinley CR, et al: Diagnostic peritoneal lavage. *Surgery* 1965; 57:633–637.
11. Berci G, Dunkelman D, Michel SL, et al: Emergency minilaparoscopy in abdominal trauma. An update. *Am J Surg* 1983; 146:261–265.
12. Sosa JL, Sims D, Martin L, et al: Laparoscopic evaluation of tangential abdominal gunshot wounds. *Arch Surg* 1992; 127:109–110.
13. Berci G, Sackier JM, Paz-Partlow M: Emergency laparoscopy. *Am J Surg* 1991; 161:332–335.
14. Falcone RE, Barnes FE, Hoogeboom JE: Blunt diaphragmatic rupture diagnosed by laparoscopy report of a case. *J Laparoendosc Surg* 1991; 1:299–302.

Chapter 29

Laparoscopic Inguinal Hernia Repair

Jeffrey H. Peters / Adrian E. Ortega

If no other field were offered to the surgeon for activity other than herniotomy, it would be worthwhile to become a surgeon and to devote an entire life to this service.

Halsted[1] states:

"Quite as well, certainly this might be said of the operations for radicle cure of hernia. There is perhaps no other operation which has had so much of vital interest to both physician and surgeon as herniotomy, and there is no operation which, by the profession at large, would be more appreciated than a perfectly safe and sure cure for rupture."

Inguinal hernia repair is a common operation in the United States currently with approximately 500,000 repairs being performed annually.[2] Until recently most of these repairs were performed using the method of Bassini,[3] as originally proposed in 1884, or its modification proposed by McVay[4] in 1948. Bassini is credited with revolutionizing the repair of inguinal hernia by introducing a reconstruction of the inguinal floor. His results, presented before the turn of the century, indicated a recurrence rate of approximately 10 percent. The results of inguinal hernia repair have improved little since that time. Although many surgeons, and a few specialized hernia centers, have reported results showing a 0 to 2 percent recurrence rate, large regional studies have repeatedly found recurrence to be near 10 percent when considering a heterogenous study population.

It has also been stated:

"The main reason for the repair of inguinal hernia remaining a problem is the wide discrepancy between the monotonous excellence achieved in personal series and the uniformly depressing results obtained by impersonal statistical reviews. . . . yet impersonal reviews indicate that the recurrence rate remains excessively high and fairly constant, whatever the method and material is employed."[5]

HISTORIC CONCEPTS

Accompanying the evolution in the treatment of groin hernias has been progress over the centuries in our understanding of hernia development, inguinal anatomy, and social factors mitigating treatment. These events serve as the foundation for the future course of hernia surgery, which is at a very important crossroad, that is, the advent of the laparoscopic inguinal hernia repair. A brief review of where we have been is important to the understanding of where we are going in the era of laparoscopic hernia repair.

The Ancients

The earliest written account of treatment for inguinal hernias dates back to 1500 B.C., when the practice of trussing was described in the Ebers papyrus.[6] Celsus, a Greek immigrant to Rome, is credited with the first operation in 25 A.D. to repair groin herniation. He approached the hernia by means of a scrotal incision, through which the sac was removed, often accompanied by the testis. One hundred years later, a Roman physician named Heliodorus described a twisting of the neck of the sac before transsection and sparing of the testis in his repair. The practices of Celsus and Heliodorus established a Greek versus Roman polemic, centering on the necessity of orchiectomy as a component of hernia repair, which was to rage well into the Middle Ages.

The Middle Ages

The fall of Rome was associated with a decline in science and the arts.[6] Medicine was no exception. Both the Islamic and Christian churches hampered the development of surgical practices. In the Roman Catholic Church, a policy termed *ecclesia abhouret a sanguine* (the Church hates blood) was adopted. The healing arts fell into the realm of priests and monks. Surgery lived on in the modest hands of barbers, hangmen, and itinerant incisors. These practitioners generally could not read or write Greek or Latin and were, thus, systematically prevented from forming a profession or imparting surgical knowledge to either colleagues or successors. Practices were largely empiric—gained from personal experience and handed down within families.

The Medici and Borgia popes of the Middle Ages wished to promote better work by painters and sculptors by authorizing cadaveric dissection.[6] An understanding of the pathologic anatomy of groin hernias began to develop. Ultimately, these activities led to the emergence of such classic anatomic treatises as those written by Scarpa and Cooper.

The Middle Ages also witnessed intense concern about the provision of male sons for the armies of Europe and about the practice of castration during hernia repairs. Monarchs endorsed the "royal operation" attributed to Gerald of Metz, circa 1412 A.D.,[7] in which a gold thread was used to encircle the hernia sac and cord loosely without compromise to testicular blood flow.

The Anatomic Era

The 18th century marked the beginning of the anatomic era of herniology. Maximillian Littre,[8] who was primarily a medical historian, described a hernia of Meckel's diverticulum, hence called Littre's hernia. Heister reported the first successful resection of a gangrenous segment of bowel strangulated within a hernia.[7] In 1756, John Hunter and Percival Pott[9] recognized the congenital nature of some indirect hernias, observing the continuity of the processus vaginalis with the tunica vaginalis. In addition, DeGimbernat[10] described the ligament that bears his name, also referred to as the *lacunar ligament*, and, in 1763, recommended its division in cases of strangulated femoral hernias.

The 19th century can be considered the height of the anatomic era. Antonio Scarpa[11] wrote his classic treatise in 1814 in which he described *hernia en glissade* or the *sliding hernia*. Franz Caspar Hesselbach,[12] a German surgeon and anatomist, reported the triangle bearing his name. It is familiar to most surgeons as the geometric space bounded by the rectus medially, the epigastric vessels laterally, and the inguinal ligament inferiorly, thereby defining direct inguinal hernias. He also described the iliopubic tract. Morton[13] is credited for his documentation of the conjoint tendon. Finally, one of the giants of this period was Sir Astley Paston Cooper, who described the superior pubic ligament, generally referred to as *Cooper's ligament* and the transversalis fascia, which he recognized as being the principle layer of the abdominal wall preventing herniation. Cooper[13a] reported the *shutter mechanism* by which the internal oblique and transversus abdominis muscles contract and reduce the gap between their lower borders and the inguinal ligament and suggested that an inadequate shutter mechanism was implicated in herniagenesis. Although it is unlikely that he ever actually used the superior pubic ligament in a hernia repair, Cooper did suggest its utility for this purpose.

Lister and Antisepsis

One of the most profound influences on hernia surgery occurred in Glasgow, Scotland, where an orthopedic surgeon, Joseph Lister, developed carbolic acid antiseptic spray.[7] In addition to a variety of orthopedic procedures, Lister performed the first antiseptic hernia repair. His technique was spread throughout the world by a number of illustrious pupils, including Marcy, Czerny, Lucas-Championerre, and Kocker. Henry O. Marcy of Massachusetts was Lister's first American protégé, who in 1871 performed the first reported antiseptic herniorrhaphy in this country.[14] His repair entailed opening the hernia sac above the external ring, which was then deeply sutured. Lister's discovery, most importantly, enabled the surgeon to open the fascial planes above the external inguinal ring without fear of deadly infection. Lucas-Championerre was the first to open the inguinal canal and imbricate the roof in its closure.[7]

Edoardo Bassini,[3] born in 1844, is considered to be the father of herniology, not because of any primary discovery, but because his repair revolutionized the treatment of inguinal hernias. For purposes of comparison, two 1890s reviews from Billroth and Bull summarized the European and American experiences with herniorrhaphies.[7] Hernia repairs were associated with a two to seven percent mortality, a 30 to 40 percent 1-year recurrence rate, and a 100 percent recurrence rate by 4 years. Bassini's[3] report in 1889 noted a 10 percent recurrence rate and only 1 death in 262 herniorrhaphy patients. It is interesting to note that the recurrence rate of Bassini's operation has not changed dramatically since his initial report.

William Stewart Halsted[1] described his original hernia operation in 1887. It bore a remarkable resemblance to the Bassini repair except that the cord was transplanted anteriorly to the external oblique aponeurosis. Halsted was also the first to use a relaxing incision in America. In 1898, Lothiessen[15] promulgated a repair utilizing Cooper's ligament, which was subsequently popularized by McVay. The Bassini and McVay repairs became the mainstay of the American surgeon's armamentarium in the 20th century, although the iliopubic tract (Condon) and Shouldice repairs also have their proponents.

The Preperitoneal Repairs

Although the ancient Greeks and Romans approached hernias through a scrotal incision, Hindu practitioners used an abdominal approach. However, Western medicine credits the first noninguinal approach to groin hernias to LaRoque,[16] who performed, in 1919, a superior transperitoneal gridiron incision combined with a Bassini repair. One year later, Cheatle[17] introduced a preperitoneal repair, originally performed through a lower midline incision with cephalad traction of the peritoneum. He amputated the peritoneal protrusions, leaving them in situ. In 1921, he changed his incision to a Pfannenstiel. Despite the obvious utility of the approach, the practices of Cheatle went largely unheeded. A. K. Henry[18] rediscovered the preperitoneal approach in 1936. He sutured the conjoint tendon to the pectineus fascia, and henceforth, the preperitoneal repair became known as the Cheatle-Henry repair.

Mikkelsen and Berne,[19] from Los Angeles County–USC Medical Center, published, in 1954, a series of 113 patients with femoral hernia treated by the Cheatle-Henry repair. There were no recurrences. More importantly this report may have served as the impetus for Nyhus, Condon, and Harkins,[20] who, in 1955, developed a preperitoneal repair utilizing the iliopubic tract. Unfortunately, the repair was associated with a relatively high recurrence rate when applied to inguinal hernias. In 1960, Nyhus introduced the prosthetic patch as an adjunct to the preperitoneal repair. He espoused this approach as being ideal for large bilateral and multiply recurrent hernias. In 1975, he added Marlex mesh to the repair, which was now performed via a lower transverse incision. In 1988, Nyhus and associates[21] reported on 203 recurrent groin hernia repairs in 195 patients. The overall recurrence rate in this series was 1.7 percent. This was a remarkable achievement in light of the fact that herniorrhaphy for recurrent hernias is generally associated with a 20 percent recurrence rate.

Rives and Stoppa and coworkers[22,23] have popularized the "giant prosthetic reinforcement of the visceral sac," known more commonly as a *Stoppa repair*, in which a large chevron-shaped sheet of Marlex is placed preperitoneally after lateralization of the spermatic cords. Stoppa also reported excellent results in a series of predominantly recurrent hernias, with an overall recurrence rate of 1.4 percent.

The Age of Prosthetic Repairs

Since 1968, Lichtenstein has developed two repairs that employ prosthetic materials. His original report described a Marlex plug placed in a recurrent hernia. Among 1276 patients, the recurrence rate was 1.6 percent.[24] Subsequently, Lichtenstein and associates[25] described a tension-free hernioplasty in 1000 patients, followed for 1 to 5 years without recurrences.

The Laparoscopic Era

In 1992, surgeons have a wide variety of hernia operations at their disposal, including the Marcy, Bassini, McVay, Shouldice, anterior iliopubic tract (Condon), preperitoneal iliopubic tract (Nyhus), Stoppa repairs, and most recently, the laparoscopic inguinal herniorrhaphy. No single hernia repair is ideal for all situations. The laparoscopic technique has evolved rapidly since 1989, when the earliest reports described closure of the internal ring, prosthetic plugs, and placement of screens over the inguinal floor from within the abdomen. Overall, there has been a convergence of laparoscopic techniques toward a preperitoneal dissection followed by the placement of Prolene mesh over the inguinal floor. It is well suited for most types of groin hernias and bilateral and recurrent hernias. However, its precise role within the surgeon's armamentarium remains to be determined.

Lichtenstein and colleagues,[25] in 1989, emphasized the fact that traditional methods defy the standard surgical principle of avoiding tension on a suture line; thus, he advocated the "tension-free" hernioplasty. The hallmark of this repair is the placement of an extraperitoneal mesh prosthesis as a means to bridge the hernia defect, avoiding tension in the repair. Many surgeons have adopted this technique, having applied it to large populations of patients with good results. This conceptual "bridge," currently adopted by many, has smoothed the transition from the classic hernia repair toward the application of laparoscopic techniques.

WHY LAPAROSCOPIC HERNIA REPAIR?

Laparoscopic hernia repair is among the most controversial procedures currently in use. The technique of traditional hernia repairs is a proven technique, done without violation of the abdominal cavity and often performed on an outpatient basis under local anesthesia. The potential advantages of laparoscopic hernia repair are, thus, not readily obvious.

The fact is that traditional inguinal hernia repair has associated with it a significant incidence of both complications and recurrence, which were mentioned already. Complications include: (1) painful neuromas of the ilioinguinal nerve, (2) spermatic cord injury, (3) epididymitis and orchitis, (4) prolonged incisional pain, and (5) significant time away from work, especially when the occupation of the herniorrhaphy patient involves heavy lifting. A recurrence rate of 5 to 10 percent for primary hernia repair and 10 to 30 percent for recurrent hernias is apparent when studying large populations.

Standard inguinal hernia repair, therefore, is not a perfect operation. Certainly, attempts at improvement are warranted. It is hoped that carefully controlled trials of laparoscopic hernia techniques will reveal a superior method. Laparoscopic hernia repair falls within this realm and should be investigated. We are early in the evolution of this technique, however, and several concerns stand out. Chief among these is the establishment of an appropriate technique for laparoscopic hernia repair and those questions centered around the use of prosthetic material.

IS THE USE OF PROSTHETIC MESH A CONCERN?

Two significant concerns arise when considering the use of a mesh prosthesis. Will there be a significant incidence of infection? If placed intraabdominally, will adhesion formation, bowel obstruction, and/or fistula formation occur?

Nonabsorbable prosthetic mesh materials, such as polypropylene (Prolene), Marlex, and expanded polytetrafluorethylene (Gortex), have been developed and used extensively for abdominal wall reconstruction. They are safe and effective materials, with a lifetime durability and a low rate of deterioration and fragmentation. Several authors, including the groups led by Lichtenstein,[25] Stoppa,[22] and Nyhus,[21] have reported extensive series of extraperitoneal hernia repairs using these materials, with a very low rate of infection. It seems, therefore, that their use in laparoscopic hernia repair can prognosticate a low incidence of infectious complications. The issues of adhesion formation, bowel obstruction, and fistulization are far from settled and will require further study.

INGUINAL ANATOMY FROM THE LAPAROSCOPIC PERSPECTIVE

The most difficult aspect of laparoscopic hernia repair is understanding the anatomy. Laparoscopy affords a radically different perspective on the inguinal anatomy. With experience, however, the anatomic landmarks and the bounds of laparoscopic dissection become clear. This situation is not dissimilar to the learning process that took place with laparoscopic cholecystectomy, albeit with an increased level of anatomic sophistication. Conceptually, it should be possible for the careful surgeon to achieve reliable lasting results when performing laparoscopic prosthetic repairs.

The anatomic landmarks first seen topographically by the laparoscopic surgeon include the median and lateral umbilical ligaments along the anterior abdominal wall and the external iliac artery and vein coursing through the retroperitoneum (Fig. 29-1). The inferior epigastric artery and vein arise from the external iliac vessels, bridging these structures with the anterior abdominal wall. They are generally visible through the peritoneum. In men, the gonadal vessels arise laterally to join the vas deferens, emerging medially from the pelvic hollow to form the spermatic cord just lateral to the inferior epigastric vessels.

Direct and indirect hernias are generally easily diagnosed as defects in the peritoneum arising medially or laterally to the epigastric vessels. Entering the preperitoneal space, the epigastric vessels are the most anterior structures, often encased in significant amounts of fibrofatty tissue. In such instances, their division opens the pelvic floor and dramatically facilitates identification of the myofascial structures of the pelvic floor.

In 1956, Fruchaud[26] proposed the best anatomic and pathophysiologic model of inguinal anatomy based on the preperitoneal space. He termed structures of the inguinal floor *the myopectineal orifice*. It is a space bound superiorly

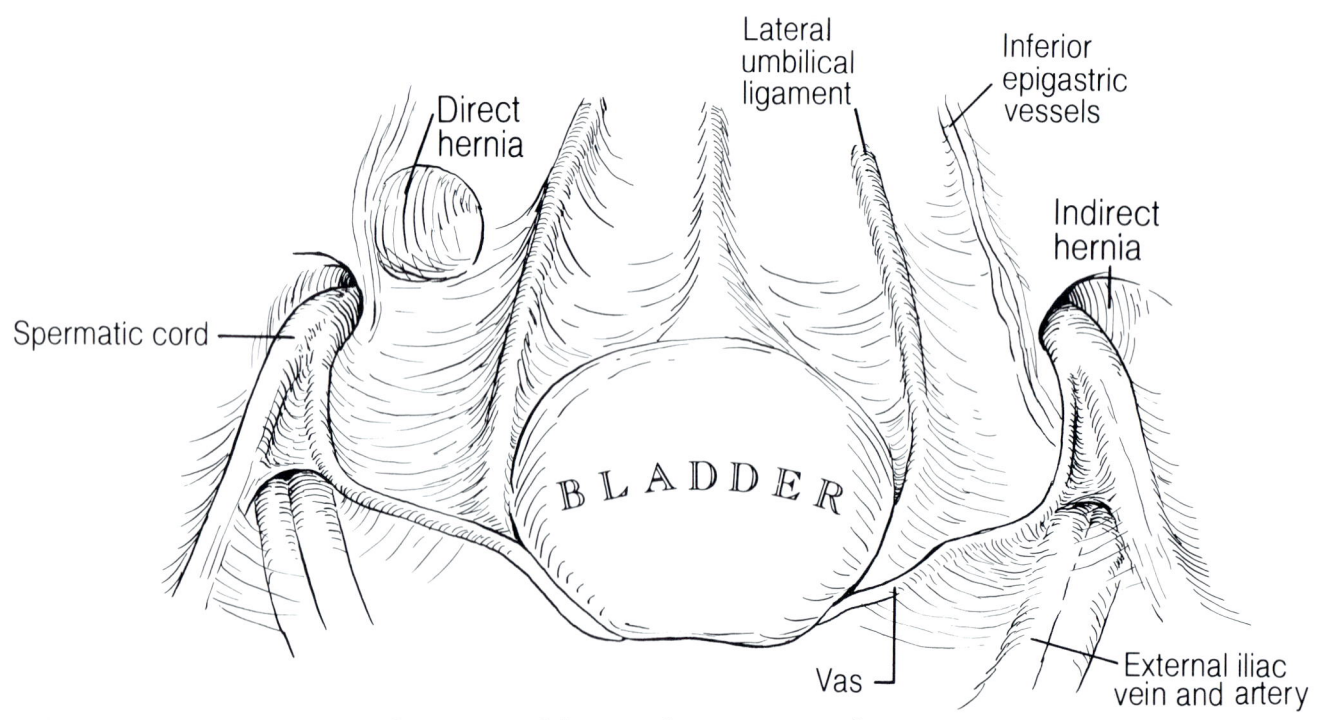

FIGURE 29-1 Laparoscopic topographic anatomy of the inguinal region. In men, the spermatic vessels join the vas deferens to form the spermatic cord. The presence of a fascial defect lateral or medial to the inferior epigastric vessels defines an indirect or a direct hernia, respectively.

by the transversus abdominis and internal oblique muscles, medially by the rectus muscle, inferiorly by the pectin of the pubis, and laterally by the iliopsoas muscle. The myopectineal orifice is spanned in a drum-like or diaphragmatic fashion by the transversalis fascia. From the laparoscopic vantage point, the iliopubic tract is an analogue of the transversalis fascia, which courses anterior to the inguinal ligament—the latter structure is not visible in this plane. The combination of the iliopubic tract and the inguinal ligament just deep to it divides the myopectineal orifice into a vascular compartment through which the external iliac vessels pierce the transversalis fascia posterior or below the iliopubic tract and a cord compartment anterior or superior to this structure. From the laparoscopic perspective, the inguinal ligament is not visible, but is "palpable" as a rigid structure immediately deep to or posterior to the iliopubic tract. Defects within the transversalis fascia define inguinal and femoral hernias. These defects are surgically correctable by either suture repair or replacement of the attenuated transversalis fascia by a prosthetic mesh.

LAPAROSCOPIC HERNIA TECHNIQUES

The technique of laparoscopic hernia repair is to some degree still in evolution. There is, however, a growing consensus for pursuing a transabdominal preperitoneal repair by placement of a mesh prosthesis. Although a variety of other options exist, ranging from simply laying a piece of prosthetic mesh over the hernia defect intraperitoneally and stapling it in place to more complex attempts at suture reconstruction of the inguinal floor, most surgeons have settled upon some variation of the preperitoneal mesh prosthesis. Little to no data exist as to which technique is more effective. Many procedures are being performed outside of classic clinical trials.

Preperitoneal Placement of a Mesh Prosthesis

The transabdominal placement of a preperitoneal prosthetic mesh is the most common repair currently being performed. This approach may be the best and is rapidly becoming the most widely employed technique for both direct and indirect hernias. The technique (described subsequently) involves a peritoneal incision cephalad to the internal inguinal ring, carried from near the midline medially to 2 to 3 cm lateral to the lateral border of the internal inguinal ring. The preperitoneal space is dissected, exposing the superficial epigastric vessels (which can be divided if necessary), the vas deferens, and the spermatic cord structures. Both the direct (medial to the epigastric vessels) and the indirect (lateral to the epigastric vessels) spaces can be covered with a suitably sized mesh prosthesis. The mesh is then tacked in place with laparoscopic hernia stapling devices, and the peritoneum closed over the repair.

Preperitoneal Repair

A number of authors are currently investigating a technique virtually identical to transabdominal placement of a preperitoneal mesh prosthetic, with the exception that the abdominal cavity is not violated and the entire dissection is performed in the preperitoneal space. The repair is begun via a preperitoneal insufflation, with insertion of the laparoscope into the preperitoneal space, and subsequent dissection as described for a transabdominal approach. A major advantage to this technique is that it may lessen, or even negate, any incidence of complications associated with the creation of a pneumoperitoneum. The dissection is considerably more difficult, and the learning curve may be longer than with a transabdominal approach. Given that, aside from these considerations, the method of repair is identical to a transabdominal preperitoneal repair, the results will likely be similar.

Simple Onlay Prosthetic Patch

A relatively easy, and perhaps effective, means of repairing an indirect hernia involves the simple intraperitoneal onlay of a patch of prosthetic mesh, followed by securing it in place.[27] This technique has the advantage of simplicity and speed. There is concern regarding the difficulty of fixing the prosthetic patch in the most inferior aspect where the femoral vessels and vas deferens lie. A second concern is adhesion formation to intraabdominal contents and subsequent complications (e.g., obstruction and fistulization) as a result. Nevertheless, a large multicenter prospective randomized trial is underway utilizing this technique for repair of indirect hernias. Time will provide us with the answer about the usefulness of this procedure.

Suture Techniques

Several investigators have attempted laparoscopic intraperitoneal suture (and mechanical staple closure) repair of both indirect and direct hernias. These techniques have ranged from closure of the internal ring with or without hernia sac reduction to attempts at laparoscopic sewing of the transversalis fascia and the iliopubic tract.[28,29] Simple closure of the internal ring is applicable in a minority of patients with small indirect hernias. More complete suturing techniques are difficult, given the current state of the art, and the results are largely unknown.

Plug Technique

Early in the experience of laparoscopic herniorrhaphy, many practitioners advocated the simple placement of a prosthetic plug into the direct and/or indirect space. Both preperitoneal (after reduction of the sac and a peritoneal incision) and simple intraperitoneal plug techniques were described. Corbitt[30] advocated reduction of the sac, incision of the base of the sac, and then placement of several plugs of preperitoneal Marlex into the inguinal canal, followed by staple transection of the reduced peritoneal sac. Schultz,[31-34] early in his experience, utilized this technique, but has abandoned the simple plug technique after several recurrences. Most surgeons currently believe that a simple plug, whether placed inside or outside of the peritoneum, is not adequate. The technique has been abandoned.

TRANSABDOMINAL PREPERITONEAL PLACEMENT OF A MESH PROSTHESIS

The majority of surgeons performing laparoscopic herniorrhaphy have moved toward performing a repair based upon the preperitoneal placement of a large rectangle of polypropylene mesh covering the inguinal floor. Details of the technique follow.

Positioning and Initiation of the Pneumoperitoneum

The patient is placed in the supine position, in a slight Trendelenburg, with the arms tucked to the side. The anesthesia apparatus is placed just oblique to the operating table on the side opposite the hernia. Such an orientation allows the bowels to fall out of the pelvis and allows the assistant to stand cephalad facing the patient's feet (ipsilateral to the hernia) so as to work unencumbered, high on the side of the hernia. The authors favor an open laparoscopic technique for initiation of the pneumoperitoneum in ALL cases. After placement of a Hasson laparoscopic trocar under direct vision, the abdomen is insufflated to a pressure of 15 mmHg. An angled laparoscope (30 to 45°) greatly facilitates laparoscopic hernia repair because of the tangential orientation of the abdominal wall. The video laparoscope is placed into the abdomen, and the pelvis is inspected. Indirect inguinal hernias are easily recognized as an enlargement of the internal inguinal ring. An unsuspected indirect hernia on the asymptomatic side is commonly seen (the incidence of which is unknown currently). As mentioned, direct defects appear as a concave weakening of the abdominal wall medial to the inferior epigastric vessels (see Fig. 29-1). They are considerably more difficult to recognize than indirect hernias and can be missed if not carefully sought. Both sides should be inspected.

Trocar Placement

Two or three additional operating trocars are then placed (Fig. 29-2). The surgeon's port (10 to 12 mm) is placed

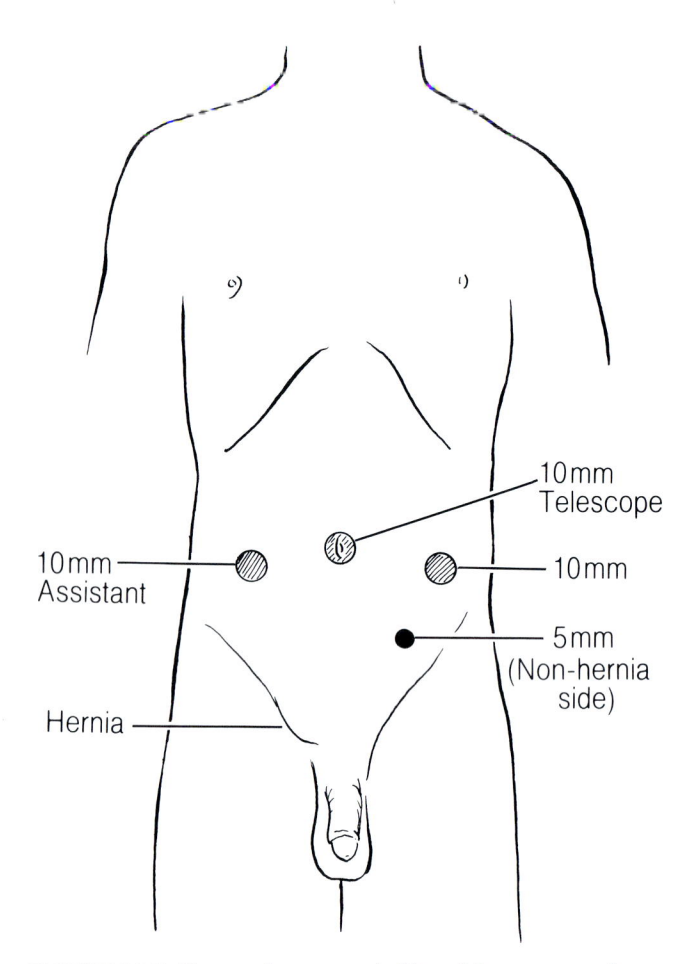

FIGURE 29-2 Trocar placement. A 10 to 11-mm trocar is placed infraumbilically. Two similar trocars are placed at the same level lateral to the rectus sheaths bilaterally. The surgeon stands opposite the hernia. An aditional 5-mm trocar may be placed opposite the hernia, allowing the surgeon to operate with two hands.

opposite the side of the hernia at or slightly below the level of the umbilicus, 1 to 2 cm medial to the iliac crest. The assistant's trocar is placed in an analogous position on the side of the hernia (5 to 12 mm). A larger trocar also can be placed on this side, allowing placement of the hernia stapling device from either side (facilitating fixation of the mesh and closure of the peritoneal incision). The authors commonly place a fourth trocar opposite the side of the hernia to be repaired. We have found the optimal placement of a fourth trocar to be below and medial to the surgeon's trocar, placed one half the distance from the umbilicus to the symphysis pubis (see Fig. 29-2).

Initial Dissection

The procedure begins with an incision in the peritoneum 1 cm cephalad to the internal ring, extending from 2 to 3 cm lateral to the lateral border of the internal ring, and carried through the lateral umbilical ligament nearly to the midline (Fig. 29-3A). An incision of this length is important and allows a complete dissection of the inguinal floor on the affected side. Hemostasis is critical because small amounts of blood obscure the anatomy and absorb light, making further recognition of the structures that are necessary for repair difficult. Curved endosurgical scissors connected to an electrocautery source are an ideal tool for dissection. It should be noted that the lateral umbilical ligament often contains patent umbilical vessels, requiring clipping for control.

The peritoneal flap is developed by extending the peritoneal incision inferiorly toward the patient's dorsum, further exposing the inguinal floor. Early in the dissection, a bundle of fatty tissue containing the inferior epigastric vessels comes into view at approximately the midpoint of the incision. Caution is advised to avoid premature injury to the vascular bundle. The anatomy of the inferior epigastric vascular bundle is variable, depending on the level at which they arise from the external iliac vessels. When arising proximally, they span a V-shaped space, bounded by the peritoneal flap inferiorly and the anterior abdominal wall superiorly, as they course from the external iliac artery and vein to the abdominal wall. When such a configuration exists, the vessels impede the placement of a mesh prosthesis, and we have not hesitated to divide them (Fig. 29-3B). The artery is most commonly single and the vein double, although two arteries and a single vein may be encountered. If doubled, they are carefully dissected, and each is separately doubly clipped proximally and distally and divided. When arising more distally from the external iliac vessels, the inferior epigastric vessels tend to conform to the curve of the abdominal wall (rather than spanning the space developed) and can be preserved by placing the mesh overlying the vessels.

Identification of the inferior epigastric vessels serves as a key to the remainder of the inguinal anatomy. The spermatic cord will be found immediately lateral to the origin of these vessels and Copper's ligament in the depths of the wound medial to the vessels. We prefer to dissect the cord free from its surrounding fibroareolar tissue and encircle it with a vessel loop (brought out adjacent to the trocar opposite the hernia). This allows manipulation of the spermatic cord during placement of the mesh. Caution should be exercised, however, in dissection of the cord because the external iliac vessels course just inferiorly.

Dissection of the Sac

Pseudohernia sacs or protrusions of the peritoneum in the region of Hesselbach's triangle pose no difficulty in dissection. These peritoneal diverticula become part of the inferior peritoneal flap of the preperitoneal dissection. Small indirect hernia sacs (< 2 cm) can also be similarly dissected off the spermatic cord as part of the inferior peritoneal flap. Indirect hernias with sacs extending into the scrotum can pose a formidable challenge for their dissection off the cord. Moreover, the dissection can be associated with increased morbidity secondary to swelling of the cord and possible testicular ischemia.

Perhaps the most prudent approach to the large indirect hernia sac is its circumferential incision at the level of the internal ring, leaving the distal sac in situ along the spermatic cord. Any fluid collections remaining in the retained sac postoperatively are generally innocuous and self-limited.

It cannot be understated that the potential communication pathway between the abdominal cavity and the inguinal canal must be interrupted either by complete dissection of the hernia sac off the spermatic cord or by its transsection to prevent recurrence. After the sac is free of the cord, it can be left invaginated into the abdominal cavity. Incomplete evagination of the hernia sac produces a dimple in the peritoneum along the course of the spermatic cord that acts as a scaffold for rehemiation.

Identification of the Inguinal Anatomy

At this juncture, the inferior epigastric vessels have been identified (and possibly divided) and the spermatic cord encircled (Fig. 29-3C). Cooper's ligament (found deep and medial to the inferior epigastric vessels), the iliopubic tract (and inguinal ligament anteriorly), and the arch of the transversus abdominis aponeurosis are dissected sufficiently for identification and placement of staples for fixation of the polypropylene mesh. The anatomy necessary for repair is now apparent.

Placement of the Mesh Prosthesis

Prolene mesh is preferred because its looser weave aids in placement of staples and visualization of the structures through the mesh. The size of the mesh that is required can be estimated by measuring the dissected space with the span of an endosurgical instrument. Generally, a rectangle of mesh measuring 7 to 8 cm by 11 to 12 cm is required. It is preferable to err with a piece of mesh too large rather than too small to cover the inguinal floor completely. The mesh is notched to allow placement around the spermatic cord in a fashion analogous to that in open hernia repair (Fig. 29-3D). The best orientation of the notch is unknown currently, although we prefer to place it laterally for direct hernias and inferiorly or superiorly for indirect repairs. The mesh is then rolled and placed retrograde into a 10-mm metal reducer sleeve for placement into the abdomen.

Fixation of the Mesh

After it is placed into the abdomen, the mesh is unfolded and placed to cover the entire inguinal floor with the

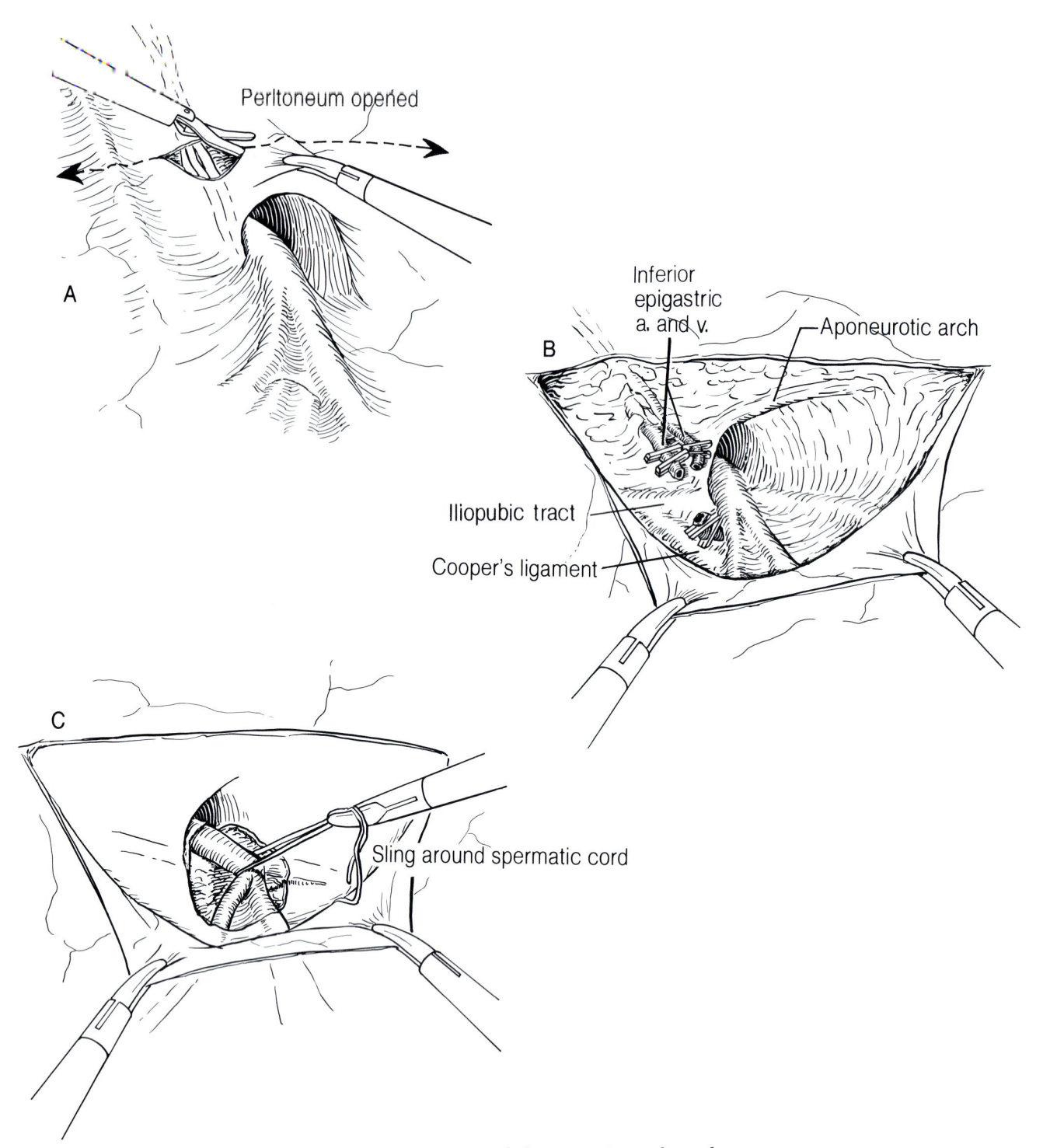

FIGURE 29-3 A. The peritoneum is incised in a transverse fashion 1 to 2 cm above the hernia defect, extending from near the midline to 1 to 2 cm lateral to the hernia defect. B. Individual dissection and division of the inferior epigastric vessels opens the inguinal floor, allowing precise identification of anatomic structures, including Cooper's ligament, the iliopubic tract, and the transverse aponeurotic arch. C. The spermatic cord is encircled with a vesel loop. This maneuver permits atraumatic retraction of the cord and subsequent placement of the mesh prosthesis.

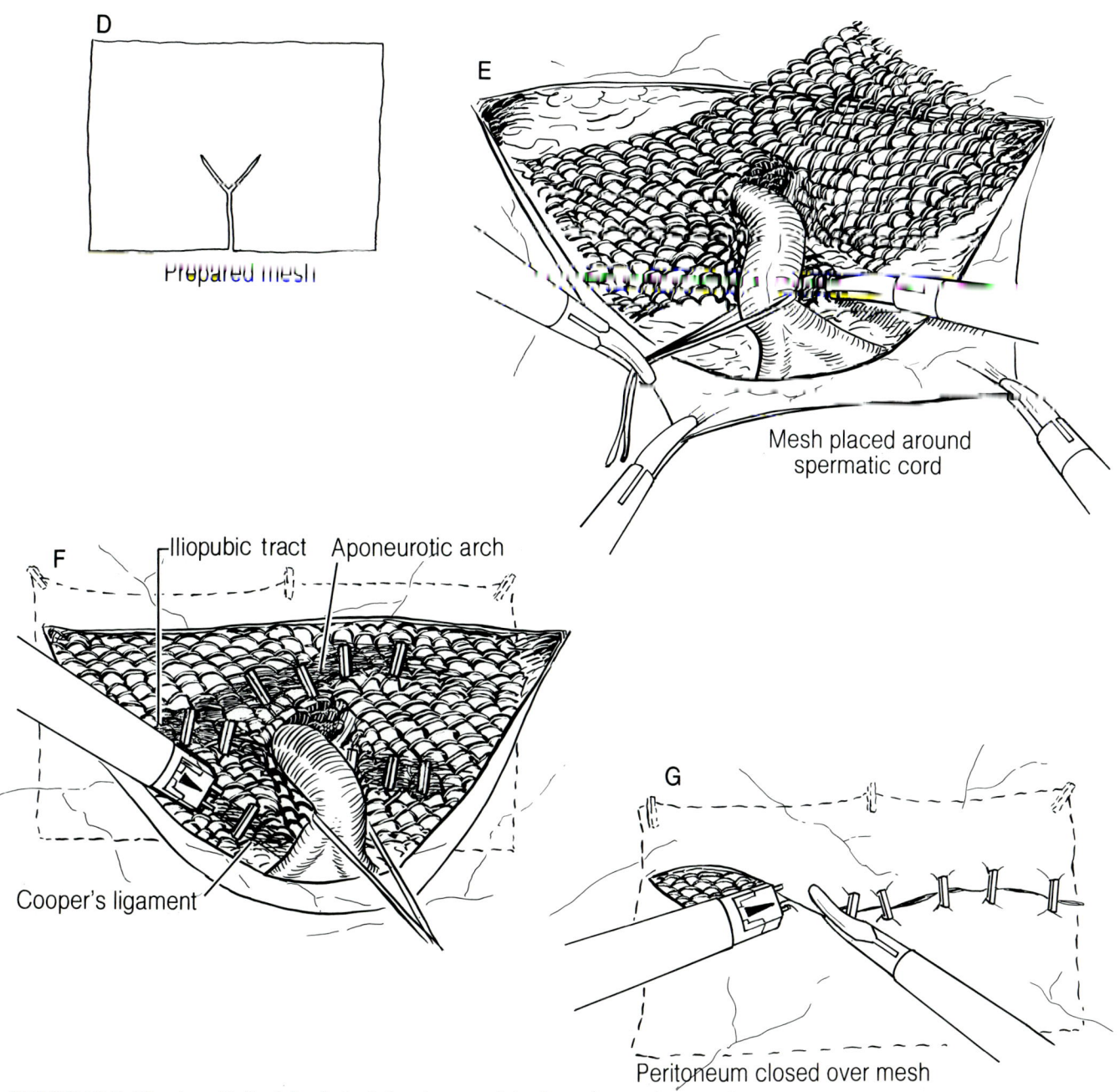

FIGURE 29-3 (Continued) D. A keyhole defect is created in the polypropylene mesh prosthesis to accommodate the spermatic cord. The size of the mesh is estimated to cover the entire inguinal floor. A 3- by 5-in rectangular piece is generally sufficient. E. The polypropylene mesh is placed around the spermatic cord aided by the traction handle created by the vessel loop about the spermatic cord. F. Once in place, the polypropylene prosthetic mesh is secured with endoscopic staples onto known anatomic structures, including Cooper's ligament, the iliopubic tract, and the transverse arch. A few additional staples are placed on the transversus abdominis muscle to eliminate any redundancy of the prosthesis. With the exception of staples placed directly into Cooper's ligament, no staples are placed below the line of the iliopubic tract to avoid injury to the iliac vessels. G. Closure of the peritoneum. The prosthetic mesh is covered by reapproximation of the peritoneal flaps with endoscopic staples to prevent adhesions directly onto the polypropylene mesh.

spermatic cord traversing it (Fig. 29-3E). The mesh is then fixed, utilizing endosurgical hernia staplers. Staples are placed into Cooper's ligament, the iliopubic tract, the arch of the transverse abdominis, and around the periphery of the mesh. The most difficult aspects of mesh fixation occur along the medial superior border (the area of direct inguinal defects) and along the anterior abdominal wall. This latter structure is tangential to the plane of dissection, and the force along the stapling device is toward the patient's feet. Thus, care must be taken not to displace the mesh too far distally on the anterior abdominal wall and to cover the direct space completely. Counterpressure with a hand on the external abdominal wall aids the placement of these staples (Fig. 29-3F).

Closure of the Peritoneum

The peritoneum is then closed. Insufflation pressure is reduced to 7 to 10 mmHg, allowing approximation of the peritoneal leaves (Fig. 29-3G). The peritoneum may be closed via stapling with an endosurgical hernia stapler or, alternatively, may be reapproximated with a running suture. The repair is inspected, the CO_2 evacuated from the abdomen, and the trocar wounds closed with a subcuticular suture of 4–0 polyglycan. Before hernia defects have occurred through large trocar sites, those 10 mm or larger also should be closed with a fascial suture.

REVIEW OF PUBLISHED REPORTS

The success of the laparoscopic cholecystectomy served as the impetus for the laparoscopic approach to repair of inguinal hernias. In 1990, Ger and associates[32] published the first description of laparoscopic hernia repairs, in which he closed the necks of hernia sacs in 15 dogs using a herniastat, or specially designed stapling device. One year later, he reported 24 repairs in human subjects, in which there were two recurrences over a 1- to 14-month follow-up period.[28]

Popp,[33] in 1990, documented a patch repair of an inguinal hernia in a female patient. Most subsequent reports and techniques have focused on either plugs of polypropylene mesh and/or screens placed over the attenuated transversalis fascia. Schultz and associates[34] were the first proponents of the plug technique, with a series of 20 patients published in 1990. The technique entailed incision of the peritoneum over the defect, with placement of two to three rolled pieces of mesh placed within it. Two to three additional 1 by 2-in sheets of mesh were then placed over the defect freely. Of the 20 patients operated on in this manner, 19 were cured after a 3- to 11-month follow-up. Schultz and colleagues reported an average requirement among these patients of 3.3 days to return to normal activities and 3.9 days to return to work. It should be noted that concern has been raised about plug migration, re-creating the patient's sensation of a hernia bulge.

Corbitt[30] developed his own technique, in which the hernia sac was everted and transsected with an Endo-GIA stapling device. He then placed a Mersilene plug and patch graft to repair the hernia defect. Twenty patients were treated using this technique, with one recurrence noted over a maximum of an 8-month follow-up. There were, however, no other complications.

In 1991, Fitzgibbons (Unpublished data, 1991) and Toy and Smoot[27] independently developed very similar techniques consisting of a laparoscopically placed intraabdominal prosthetic patch. The Toy-Smoot laparoscopic hernioplasty entails opening indirect sacs with the placement of an Endoloop, followed by placement of a 5 by 10-cm Gortex patch, which is tailored to cover the hernia defect intraabdominally. The patch is held in place by nylon sutures at each corner and also secured with additional staples. Ten patients were included in this report. There were no complications, and all patients returned to normal activities by the second postoperative day. Fitzgibbons' technique employs the simple placement of large sheet of polypropylene mesh over the peritoneum, which is then stapled in place. Results from a multiinstitutional study utilizing this technique should be forthcoming. Spaw and colleagues[35] published a description of the anatomic basis for the laparoscopic hernia repair based on cadaver dissections.

In 1992, Gazayerli[29] described an anatomic repair for direct and indirect inguinal hernias using the transversalis fascia and the iliopubic tract. The preperitoneal space is entered, where the sac is excised and trimmed. The inferior epigastric vessels are then divided, followed by approximation of the transversus abdominis and transversalis fascia to the iliopubic tract using sutures. A Marlex plug is placed in the space formerly occupied by the hernia sac. A polypropylene mesh is then sutured in place, and the peritoneum is closed with a running or purse-string suture. Fourteen patients were included in this report. Two patients required conversion to an open repair. Twelve patients were available for follow-up. All were discharged within 23 h, and average operating time was 211 min. No patient required narcotic analgesia. Four patients were able to return to work within 72 h.

Arregui and associates[36] performed 61 laparoscopic hernia repairs in 52 patients between October 1990 and December 1991. A preperitoneal dissection was performed in which the inguinal floor defect was tightened with sutures after excision of the hernia sac. A 2.5 by 4.5-in sheet of polypropylene mesh was sutured in place to the transversus abdominis arch, the iliopubic tract or Cooper's ligament, and the transversus abdominis muscle. There were no recurrences, with an average follow-up period of 2.3 months. Of note is that this report included 12 patients with recurrent hernias reoperated upon laparoscopically. These patients reported less postoperative pain and a diminished convalescence period compared to their previous open hernia repairs.

Seid and colleagues[37] published a series of 27 patients who underwent a technique in which the sac of indirect hernias is dissected off the cord and a rolled sheet of polypropylene mesh is sutured onto a screen to prevent migration of the plug. Two additional 4 by 6-cm screens are placed over the plug–screen complex. There were no early recurrences in this series (1 to 7 months follow-up). Patients were able, on average, to return to work within 5 days.

Nolen and associates[38] modified the plug technique by folding the mesh into a fan and then placing it into the space occupied previously by direct and indirect hernias after dissection of these sacs. Sixty-seven repairs in 57 patients were reported in 1992, with one recurrence seen over a 10-month follow-up period. In addition, Hawalsi and associates[39] modified the Schultz technique by placing one to two rolled pieces of mesh into a hernia defect, followed by a mushroom-shaped mesh plug and a 5 by 8-cm mesh screen. This report encompassed 82 repairs in 76 patients, all performed on an outpatient basis. His patients reported pain for 1 to 3 days, a return to full activities within 3 to 7 days, and a return to work by the end of 1 to 2 weeks.

Most recently, McKernan and Laws,[40] in 1992, described a true preperitoneal repair. The preperitoneal space is insufflated with CO_2. Small indirect hernia sacs are dissected off the cord, while large ones are excised, leaving the distal sac in situ on the cord. A 3 by 5-in sheet of mesh is keyholed around the cord and stapled into place. This repair represents a true laparoscopic modification of the Nyhus and Stoppa procedures. Thirty-four repairs were performed. All patients were discharged within 1 day after surgery. No other follow-up was included in the report.

THE PROBLEM OF DATA COLLECTION

Appropriate clinical trials must be carried out and useful data collected. Minimally invasive surgery is clearly on the horizon, and hernia repair will take its place among the procedures performed endoscopically.

Two problems exist with regard to the collection of useful data. First, the technique is in evolution. Many enthusiasts of laparoscopic hernia repair have already modified their technique to the extent that early patient data are not comparable with those from patients operated on more recently. Thus, most series are biased by the lack of a standardized method of repair. Secondly, a long follow-up period is essential. More than 50 percent of recurrences will occur 5 or more years after the original operation,[41] and Ravitch[42] has indicated that up to 20 percent will occur 15 to 20 years postoperatively. It is apparent, therefore, that we will not know the true utility of laparoscopic hernia repair for some years to come. Early reports may be encouraging, but it must be kept in mind that a long-term perspective is needed.

REFERENCES

1. Halsted WS: The radical cure of inguinal hernia in the male, in *Surgical Paper by William Stewart Halsted: The Classics of Surgery Library.* Birmingham, AL, Gryphon Editions, 1984, pp 261–308.
2. Vayda E, Mindell WR, Rutkow IM: A decade of surgery in Canada, England, and the United States. *Arch Surg* 1982; 117:846.
3. Bassini E: *Nuovo Metodo per la Cura Radicale Dell' Ernia Inguinale.* Padua, R. Stabilimento Prosperin, 1889.
4. McVay CB: Inguinal and femoral hernioplasty, an anatomic repair. *Arch Surg* 1948; 57:524.
5. Brandon WJM: Inguinal hernia: The unpredictable result. *Br J Surg* 1946; 34:13.
6. Read RC: The development of inguinal herniorrhaphy. *Surg Clin North Am* 1984; 64:185.
7. Read RC: Historical survey of the treatment of hernia, in Nyhus LM, Condon RE (eds): *Hernia,* ed 3. Philadelphia, JB Lippincott 1989, pp. 3–17.
8. Davis CE Jr: Littre's hernia. *Ann Surg* 1954; 139:370.
9. Pott P: *A Treatise on Ruptures.* London, Hitch & Hawes, 1756.
10. deGimbernat A: *Nuevo Metodo de Operar en la Hernia Crural.* Madrid, Ibrarra, 1793.
11. Scarpa A: *A Treatise on Hernia.* Edinburgh, Thomas Bryce, 1814.
12. Hesselbach FC: *Neueste anatomisch-patholische Untersuchungen uber den Ursprung und das Fortschreiten der Leisten und Schenkelbruche.* Wurzburg, Baumgartner, 1814.
13. Morton T: *The Surgical Anatomy of Inguinal Herniae, the Testis and its Coverings.* London, Taylor & Walton, 1841.
13a. Cooper AP: *The Anatomy and Surgical Treatment of Abdominal Hernia,* 2 vols. London, Longcas, 1864, p 1807.
14. Read RC: Marcy's priority in the development of inguinal herniorrhaphy. *Surgery* 1980; 88:682.
15. Lotheissen G: Zur radicaloperation des schenklhernien. *Zentralbl Chir* 1898; 25:548.
16. La Roque GP: The permanent cure of inguinal and femoral hernias. A modification of the standard operative procedures. *Surg Gynecol Obstet* 1919; 29:507.
17. Cheatle GL: An operation for radical cure of inguinal and femoral hernias. *BMJ* 1920; 2:168.
18. Henry AK: Operation for femoral hernia by a midline extraperitoneal approach with preliminary note on the use of this route for reducible inguinal hernia. *Lancet* 1936; 1230:531.
19. Mikkelsen WP, Berne CJ: Femoral hernioplasty: Suprapubic extraperitoneal (Cheatle-Henry) approach. *Surgery* 1954; 55:743.
20. Nyhus LM, Condon RE, Harkins HN: Clinical experience with preperitoneal hernial repair for all types of hernia of the groin, with particular reference to the importance of transversalis fascia analogues. *Am J Surg* 1960; 100:234.
21. Nyhus LM, Pollak R, Bombeck CT, et al: The preperitoneal approach and prosthetic buttress repair for recurrent hernia, the evolution of a technique. *Ann Surg* 1988; 208:733.
22. Stoppa RE, Rives JL, Warlaumont CR, et al: The use of Dacron in the repair of hernias of the groin. *Surg Clin North Am* 1984; 64:269.
23. Stoppa RE, Warlaumont CR: The preperitoneal approach and prosthetic repair of groin hernia, in Nyhus LM, Condon RE (eds): *Hernia.* Philadelphia, JB Lippincott, 1989, pp 199–225.
24. Shulman AG, Amid PK, Lichtenstein IL: The "plug" repair of 1402 recurrent inguinal hernias: 20-Year experience. *Arch Surg* 1990; 125:265.

25. Lichtenstein IL, Shulman AG, Amid PK, et al: The tension free hernioplasty. *Am J Surg* 1989; 157:188.
26. Fruchaud H: *Anatomie Chirugicale des Hernies de l'Aine*. Paris, G. Doin, 1956.
27. Toy FK, Smoot RT: Toy-Smoot laparoscopic hernioplasty. *Surg Laparosc Endosc* 1991; 1:51.
28. Ger R: The laparoscopic management of groin hernias. *Contemp Surg* 1991; 39:15.
29. Gazayerli MM: Anatomical laparoscopic hernia repair of direct or indirect inguinal hernias using the transversalis fascia and iliopubic tract. *Surg Laparosc Endosc* 1992; 1:49.
30. Corbitt JD: Laparoscopic herniorrhaphy. *Surg Laparosc Endosc* 1991; 1:23.
31. Schultz LS: Laparoscopic inguinal hernia repair. *Laparosc News* 1991; 12:4.
32. Ger R, Monroe K, Duvivier R, et al. Management of indirect inguinal hernias by laparoscopic closure of the neck of the sac. *Am J Surg* 1990; 159:370.
33. Popp LW: Pre-peritoneal prosthetic inguinal herniorraphy in a female patient. *Surg Endosc* 1990; 4:1.
34. Schultz LS, Graber J, Pietrafitta J, et al. Laser laparoscopic herniorrhaphy: A clinical trial—Preliminary results. *J Laparoendosc Surg* 1990; 1:41.
35. Spaw AT, Ennis BW, Spaw LP. Laparoscopic hernia repair. The anatomic basis. *J Laparoendosc Surg* 1991, 1:269.
36. Arregui ME, Davis CJ, Yucel O, et al: Laparoscopic mesh repair of inguinal hernia using a preperitoneal approach: A preliminary report. *Surg Laparosc Endosc* 1992; 2:53.
37. Seid AS, Deutsh H, Jacobson A: Laparoscopic herniorrhaphy. *Surg Laparoscop Endosc* 1992; 2:59.
38. Nolen M, Melichar R, Jennings WC, et al. Use of a Marlex fan in the repair of direct and indirect hernias by laparoscopy. *J Laparoendosc Surg* 1992; 2:61.
39. Hawalsi A: Laparoscopic inguinal herniorrhaphy: The mushroom plug repair. *Surg Laparosc Endosc* 1992; 2:111.
40. McKernan JB, Laws HL: Laparoscopic preperitoneal prosthetic repair of inguinal hernias. *Surg Rounds* 1992; 7:597.
41. Lichtenstein IL, Shore JM: Exploding the myths of hernia repair. *Am J Surg* 1979; 132:307.
42. Ravitch MM: *Repair of Hernia*. Chicago, Year Book Medical, 1969.

Chapter 30

Laparoscopic Splenectomy

Edward H. Phillips

The importance of the spleen has been debated since ancient times. In recent years, its immunologic role has been established, and surgical extirpation for the slightest reason has been replaced by efforts to save all or some of the splenic mass.[1] Nevertheless, occasionally, the entire spleen must be removed because of hypersplenism, intrinsic disease, or for diagnostic reasons. The operative technique for total splenectomy is well known and has not significantly changed in more than 100 years. Splenectomy performed through a generous subcostal or vertical incision has been accomplished with excellent results. However, critically ill patients are often considered for splenectomy, and the risks attendant upon surgical intervention must balance the possible advantages. Some patients are too sick to survive splenectomy. Laparoscopic techniques have been applied to splenectomy in an effort to decrease the morbidity and mortality in these patients and to decrease postoperative discomfort and hospital stay in all patients undergoing splenectomy.

At first consideration, the complex vasculature and the many peritoneal attachments of the spleen seem to defy the laparoscopic approach.[2] In fact, just over 15 years ago, it was commonplace to remove the spleen for even minor tears of the splenic capsule, but surgical experience with splenic salvage and partial splenectomy has increased familiarity with the vascular supply to the spleen.[3] Application of this knowledge and the basic principles of surgery (exposure, tension, countertension, precise dissection, and vessel ligation) under the magnification of the laparoscope has led to the successful removal of the spleen using endoscopic techniques.

At its current stage of development, laparoscopic splenectomy is limited to the elective removal of normal-sized spleens.[4] Slightly enlarged spleens can be removed if the patient is thin and the body habitus permits. Consequently, selected cases have been performed for idiopathic thrombocytopenic purpura and in patients undergoing staging for Hodgkin's disease.[5] Some patients with acquired hemolytic anemia who do not have significant splenomegaly are also candidates for laparoscopic splenectomy when it is indicated to decrease transfusion requirements. The expectation is that more fragile patients (often receiving corticosteroids) may benefit from the lower morbidity and mortality resulting from the lack of an upper abdominal incision and the concomitant early ambulation that the laparoscopic procedure affords.

EQUIPMENT

When undertaking laparoscopic splenectomy, special instrumentation is required. It is not possible to use the laparoscopic cholecystectomy instruments and aim them at the left upper quadrant. The following is a list of essential equipment.

1. A complete tray of open instruments for splenectomy.
2. A 30° forward-oblique viewing laparoscope.
3. A high-intensity xenon light source.
4. A charge coupled device "chip" camera.
5. Two-high definition video monitors.
6. An electric operating room table.
7. An electrocautery unit.
8. An argon beam coagulator (optional).
9. 5-, 10-, and 12-mm trocars (six total).
10. Laparoscopic equipment, including ring forceps (10 mm), right-angled dissector (5 or 10 mm), needle driver, blunt dissector, Babcock grasper (two), fan retractor (two), knot pusher, scissors, and suction–irrigation device (with electrocautery).
11. Pretied Roeder knot loops.
12. A multiple-clip applier.
13. A single-clip applier.
14. A linear endocutter (optional).
15. A specimen bag.

Preoperative Care

Preoperative evaluation and care is particularly critical to the successful outcome of splenectomy. If the splenectomy is being performed for the cure or alleviation of hematologic disease, the workup is usually dictated by the hematologist. Nevertheless, the surgeon should be familiar with the studies performed and the bone marrow results. Sometimes, scans performed during the diagnostic period can point out accessory spleens and alert the surgeon to their location.

Except in emergency situations when time does not permit, pneumococcal vaccine should be given to the patient preoperatively and autologous blood set aside. If this is not possible, two units of banked blood should be typed and crossed. At least six units of platelets should be available if the patient is thrombocytopenic (from a single donor using platelet phoresis, if possible). Preoperative splenic artery embolization should be considered, especially early in a surgeon's experience, and is very helpful in obese patients. It is optional in thin and average weight patients, whose splenic arteries are more easily accessible to the laparoscopic approach through the lesser sac.

TECHNIQUE

It is a matter of routine to give preoperative prophylactic antibiotics, usually a cephalosporin. The patient is then submitted to general anesthesia and intubated. It is preferable not to have the patient's left arm extended, and the left side is elevated 20° degrees with a roll. A nasogastric tube and a Foley catheter are inserted.

A closed Veress needle or open Hasson technique is used to create the pneumoperitoneum. In patients of normal or large body habitus, this is performed at the umbilicus. However, in pediatric or small adult patients, a right paramedian position is preferred as the site for the laparoscope to permit more room and latitude for instrumentation in the left upper quadrant.

Initially, a general intraabdominal exploration with the laparoscope is performed, looking for accessory spleens and other pathologic conditions. Then, a 10- to 11-mm trocar is placed in the subxiphoid position, and a 12-mm (if the linear cutter is going to be used, otherwise a 10- to 11-mm) trocar is placed halfway between the subxiphoid and umbilical trocars. A 10- to 11-mm trocar is placed in the left lower quadrant as laterally as possible (Fig. 30-1). This will be used for the ring forceps, which will grasp, elevate, and inferiorly displace the spleen. A 5- or 10-mm trocar can be placed between the umbilicus and the left lower quadrant trocar to permit the assistant surgeon to use both hands for a grasper or suction.

The operation is commenced by inserting a Babcock grasper, through the subxiphoid trocar, which is used to elevate the stomach. An atraumatic grasper is placed through the left lower quadrant trocar and is used to grasp the transverse colon, providing countertraction. Scissors or an electrocautery hook are then used to make an opening in the gastrocolic omentum. The vessels are secured with clips, a linear cutter, or pretied Roeder loops to make a large enough opening to insert a fan retractor from the left lower quadrant and another fan retractor or a Babcock grasper to elevate the posterior wall of the stomach. Using scissors, an angled dissector, or a right-angled dissector at the superior edge of the pancreas, the splenic artery is identified and clipped (Fig. 30-2). The spleen is then inspected. If there is a line of demarcation, it is usually the lower half of the spleen that has been compromised. In this situation, the artery is dissected more proximally, and the superior branch of the splenic artery is identified and clipped.

After the splenic artery is occluded, or if the artery was embolized preoperatively, platelets are administered, if needed. Attention is then directed to the splenic flexure of the colon. The patient is placed in the Trendelenburg position with the left side up. The surgeon, who is standing on the patient's right side, grasps the greater omentum at the splenic flexure with the left hand, and the assistant surgeon, who is standing on the patient's left side, grasps the

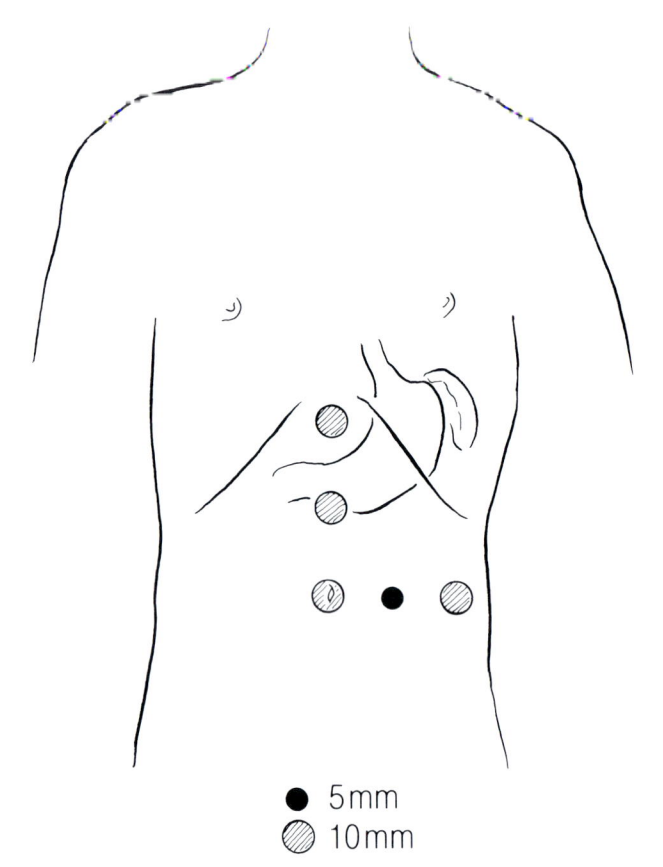

FIGURE 30-1 Trocar site placement.

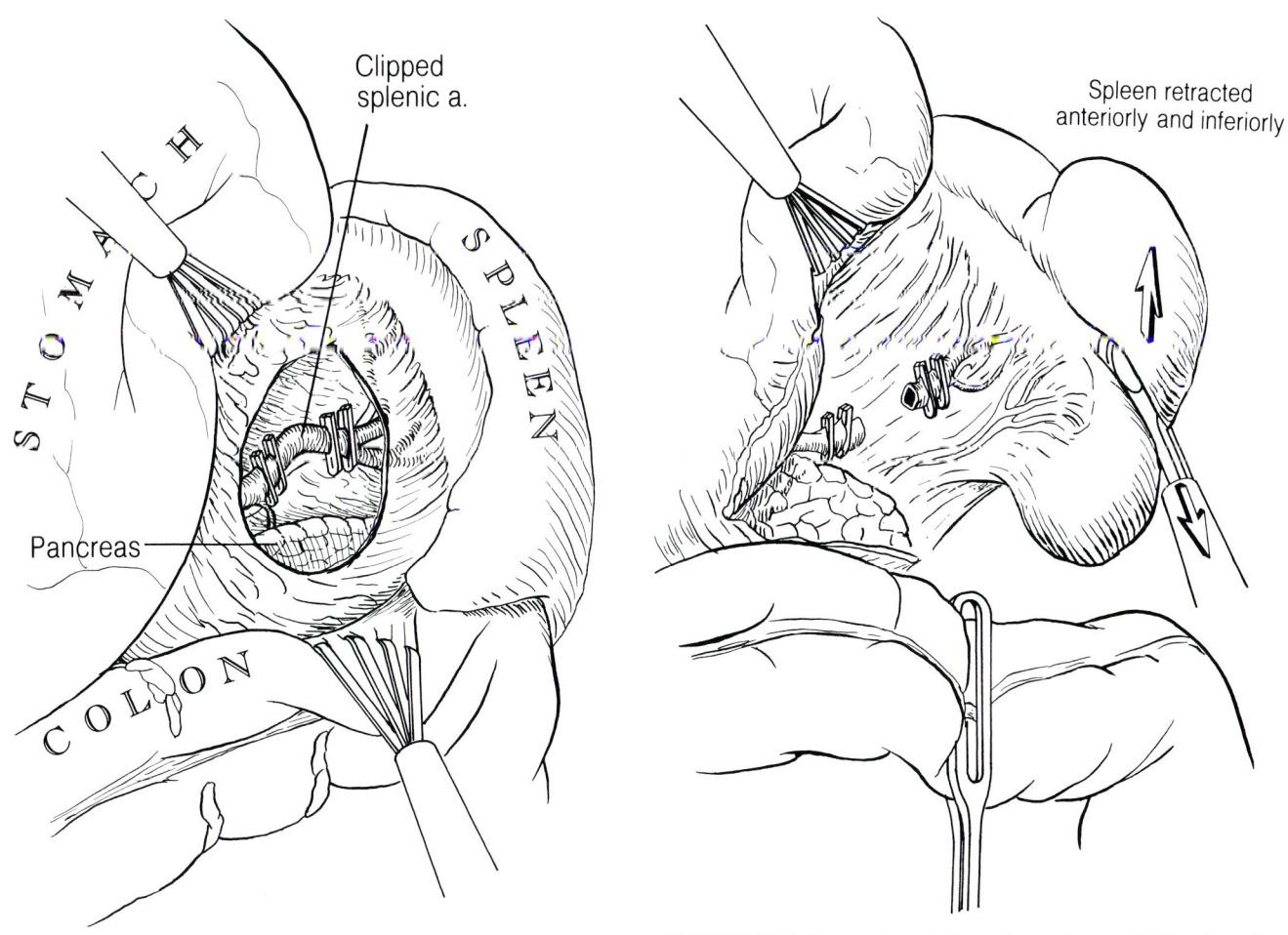

FIGURE 30-2 Clipping splenic artery in lesser sac.

FIGURE 30-3 Retraction of the spleen after mobilization of the splenic flexure of the colon.

descending colon and reflects it medially. We may then use the electrocautery hook or scissors through the mid-abdominal trocar to take down the splenic flexure. In so doing, the omental attachments to the spleen are cauterized.

At this point, the spleen is grasped and elevated by the ring forceps or the linear cutter sizing instrument, thus permitting visualization of the inferior pole vessels (Fig. 30-3). With a fine grasper in the surgeon's left hand and a right-angled dissector in the right hand, the vessels are gently and precisely dissected. When the right-angled dissector is passed around a vessel, it is done so with visualization provided by rotating the laparoscope. The most common problem, leading to hemorrhage, occurs when a posterior branch of the vein being encircled is punctured. It is vital, therefore, to dissect gently within the adventitia on both sides of a vessel to ensure visualization of a posterior branch. After a vessel has been encircled, there are several ligation choices. The easiest is to employ the multiple-clip applier. This is safe only if there is enough length of vessel to allow two clips to be positioned on either side of the site of division. The disadvantage of this technique is that the clips may be knocked off by the passage of multiple instruments, most commonly the fan retractors.

Suture ligature should be performed in the earlier stages of dissection because there are many opportunities to displace clips accidentally during the subsequent dissection. Suture ligation can be accomplished by passing a suture around the vessel and tying an extracorporeal knot with the aid of a knot pusher. After two sutures have been placed, they can be reinforced with clips and the vessel divided. Another alternative is to place a 5-mm trocar, insert a pretied Roeder loop around a grasper, clip the "going" side, grasp the vessel, and secure the loop after dividing the vessel.

After division of the lower pole vessels, the spleen can be retracted medially, and the splenorenal peritoneal attachments are divided (Fig. 30-4). Blunt dissection in that plane helps mobilize the tail of the pancreas, allowing for greater elevation of the spleen. With the spleen lifted toward the

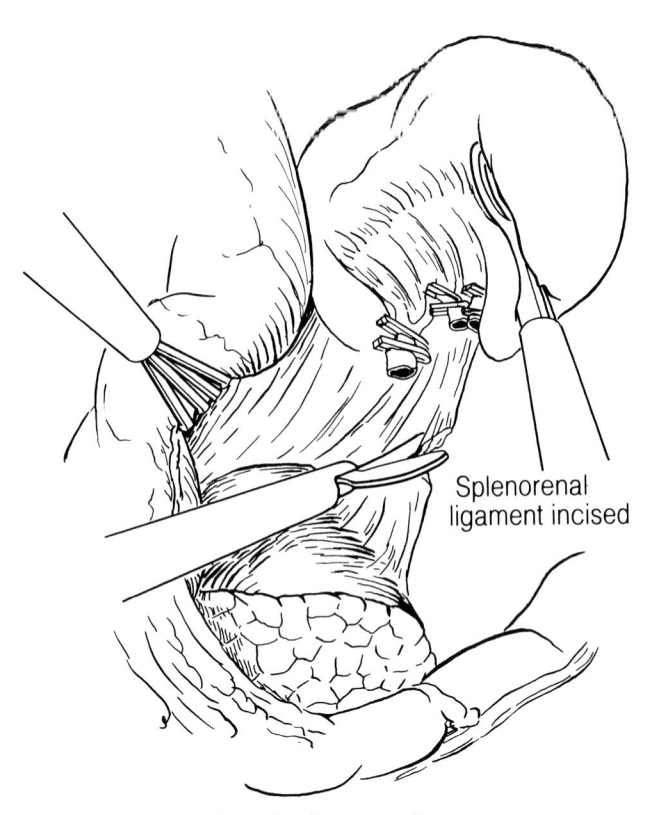

FIGURE 30-4 Incision of splenorenal ligament.

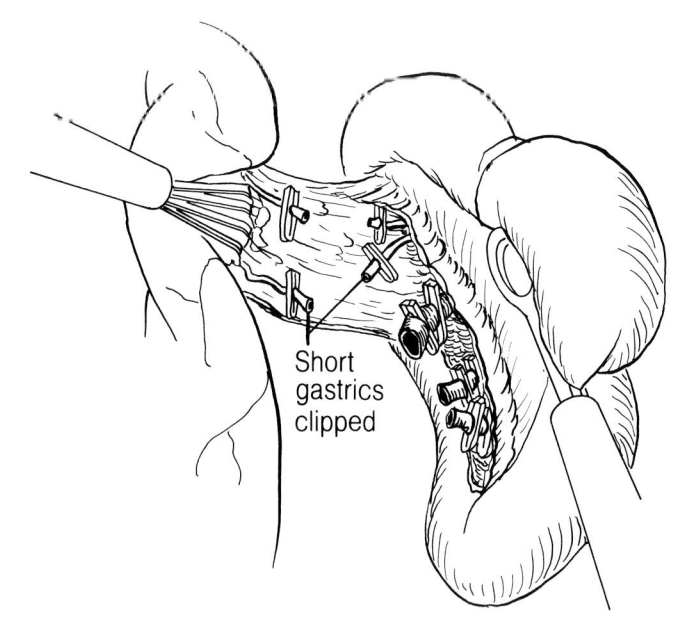

FIGURE 30-5 Clipping of short gastric vessels.

anterior abdominal wall and pulled inferiorly, the hilar vessels are dissected. This maneuver, however, cannot be performed satisfactorily in patients with splenomegaly. The hilar vessels are ligated and divided sequentially until the short gastric vessels are encountered. The splenophrenic attachments are then divided with scissors, and the short gastric vessels can be divided between clips, taking care not include the stomach in the clips (Fig. 30-5).

After the spleen is freed, it is placed in a bag. Currently, the large nylon renal specimen bag (Cook Urologic) is best suited for this purpose. The splenic bed is then carefully inspected because hemostasis must be perfect. Minor bleeding and oozing may be controlled with electrocautery or the laparoscopic argon beam coagulator. More serious bleeding is best managed with suture ligature. Blind clipping will usually result in more bleeding.

Specimen retrieval is the next task. If an intact specimen is not required (e.g., in cases of idiopathic thrombocytopenic purpura), the bag is pulled up into the umbilical trocar site, where a ring forceps can be repeatedly inserted and withdrawn, manually morcellating the specimen (Fig. 30-6). There are automated morcellators available that may also be used. If an intact spleen is required for pathologic examination, a lower midline or Pfannenstiel incision can be performed (e.g., for Hodgkin's disease).

Drainage of the left subphrenic space after splenectomy is controversial. If it is to be done, closed suction drainage should be employed, and this has been performed in some cases of oozing. Since we have employed the argon beam coagulator, fewer cases have required drainage, although this might reflect increased clinical facility.

RESULTS

Scattered isolated reports of successful laparoscopic splenectomy have surfaced in recent months, but no large series has been documented. Our group first attempted laparoscopic splenectomy in January 1992 in a patient with Hodgkin's disease. Currently, we have performed successful laparoscopic splenectomy in two patients with Hodgkin's disease and in six patients with idiopathic thrombocytopenic purpura.

Early in our experience, an obese patient without prior splenic artery ligation in the lesser sac required urgent conversion to open splenectomy as a result of bleeding from a hilar vessel that could not be controlled laparoscopically. Another patient with splenomegaly had to be converted because the enlarged spleen prevented adequate visualization and exposure. Two patients underwent successful preoperative splenic artery embolization and laparoscopic splenectomy. All others had successful splenic artery clipping in the lesser sac.

Patient blood loss averaged 350 mL (range, 75 to 800 mL), and no patient required transfusion. The average duration of surgery was 140 min (range, 120 to 225 min), and the average postoperative hospitalization was 4 days.

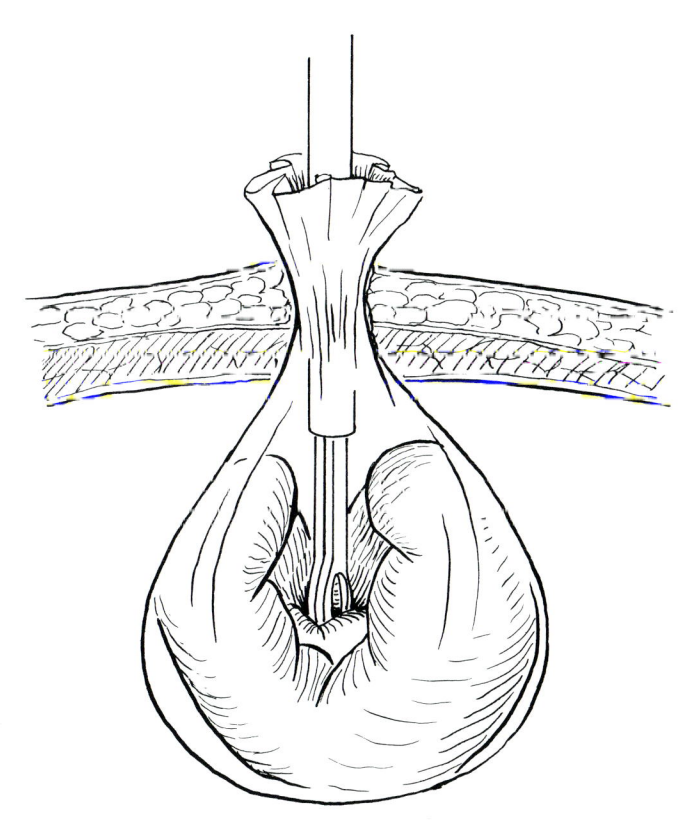

FIGURE 30-6 Morcellating the spleen.

The hospital stay for elective laparoscopic splenectomy in patients with idiopathic thrombocytopenic purpura (without comorbid illness) was 2 days. There were no complications or deaths.

DISCUSSION

As surgeons gain greater familiarity with endoscopic dissection and ligation techniques, more procedures will be performed using laparoscopic surgery. Some advanced laparoscopic procedures will be of questionable safety or advantage to the patient; however, laparoscopic splenectomy clearly has a place in the surgical armamentarium. It is accompanied by less postoperative pain and a shorter postsurgical stay than traditional splenectomy. Although few cases have been performed thus far, the results are as dramatic as the early results of laparoscopic cholecystectomy. Earlier ambulation, recovery of bowel function, and hospital discharge are evident after successful laparoscopic splenectomy. As in the early days of laparoscopic cholecystectomy, select patients were chosen for the first procedures. Currently, more challenging cases of laparoscopic splenectomy continue to be performed.

In the future, the technical problems associated with splenomegaly may be resolved, facilitating laparoscopic splenectomy in these patients. Laparoscopic splenic salvage in trauma cases may be feasible in experienced hands, but it presents considerable challenges of exposure and retraction. Generally, patients selected for laparoscopic splenectomy should have normal-sized spleens. Obese patients should be deferred until experience is gained, and these patients should undergo preoperative splenic artery embolization. As in any surgery, open or laparoscopic, proper training and an appreciation of our skills and limitations make the difference between dangerous and safe surgery. Although the laparoscopic approach benefits our patients, it does so only if is performed safely.

REFERENCES

1. Leonard AS, Giebink GS, Baesl TS, et al: The overwhelming post splenectomy sepsis problem. *World J Surg* 1980; 4:423–432.
2. Kornblith P, Boley S, Whitehouse B: Anatomy of the splanchnic circulation. *Surg Clin North Am* 1992; 72:1.
3. Morgenstern L, Phillips E, Fermelia D, et al: Near-total splenectomy due to Gaucher disease: A new surgical approach. *Mt Sinai J Med* 1986; 53:501–505.
4. Carroll B, Phillips E, Semel C, et al: Laparoscopic splenectomy. *Surg Endoscopy* 1992; 6:183–185.
5. Oza A, Lister T: Diagnosis and staging of Hodgkin's disease. *Curr Opin Oncol* 1990; 2:832–837.

Chapter 31

Endovascular Surgery

Peter F. Lawrence / Samuel S. Ahn

Endovascular surgery is a new field that applies the recently developed techniques of angioscopy, endovascular ultrasound, balloon angioplasty, mechanical atherectomy, and stents. This field uses catheter-based systems delivered through a vascular site remote from the lesion to treat lesions from within the vascular system. It integrates the expertise of vascular surgery, radiology, and cardiology for the treatment of peripheral arterial occlusive disease, using less invasive techniques to enhance and occasionally replace conventional vascular reconstructive procedures.

The field of endovascular surgery is still experimental because most of its devices and techniques have recently been developed and are still unproved. However, the tremendous interest in this field has stemmed from promising early results of procedures that either are less invasive than standard techniques or extend our ability to treat common vascular problems.

ANGIOSCOPY

Angioscopy is a method of visualizing a vessel from within, using a flexible fiberoptic scope, light source, irrigation system, camera, video recorder, and monitor (Fig. 31-1). The angioscope itself consists of quartz fibers for illumination, a light bundle for viewing, and an operating channel for irrigation and/or manipulating instruments.

Indications

The two common indications for angioscopy are: (1) to determine the completeness of thromboembolectomy and endarterectomy[1] and (2) to assist with valve lysis during in situ bypass.[2] Angioscopy has been shown to be superior to angiography for detecting residual intimal flaps after endarterectomy of the iliac artery and carotid endarterectomy.[3] The angioscope can be used to direct a balloon catheter down branching arteries (such as the posterior and anterior tibial) during thrombectomy; it can also be used to determine the completeness of the thrombectomy and facili-

tate removal of residual thrombus, if identified, with a balloon catheter.

Several investigators have also used angioscopy to determine the completeness of valvulotomy during in situ saphenous vein bypass grafting because valvulotomy without direct visualization often leaves retained valves.[4] Chin and associate[5] developed a single-unit angioscopy–valvulotomy system that allows valvulotomy under direct vision.

Other indications for angioscopy include intraluminal inspection of vascular anastomoses, laser-assisted balloon angioplasty, and mechanical atherectomy. Angioscopes can also be used to retrieve foreign bodies by transporting flexible grabbers through the working channel of the angioscope.

Technique

Angioscopy is performed intraoperatively through an open arteriotomy. Control of the proximal vessel is obtained with a vascular clamp; distal back bleeding through collateral vessels is controlled with irrigation fluid infused through the working channel of the angioscope. An irrigation pump controls the volume of fluid infused and enhances the image. The endoscope may be placed directly into the artery or inserted through an introducer sheath with a hemostatic valve and side-arm irrigation channel. Images can be visualized directly on the monitor and recorded for later viewing.

Results

White[6] reported using angioscopy in 160 patients after thrombectomy and found that virtually all patients had residual thrombus. Additional attempts at thrombectomy were performed in 80 percent of patients, although more recently, this group has opted not to remove minor thrombus, reducing the rethrombectomy rate to 40 to 50 percent.

Several other authors utilized angioscopy to identify retained valves in patients undergoing in situ saphenous

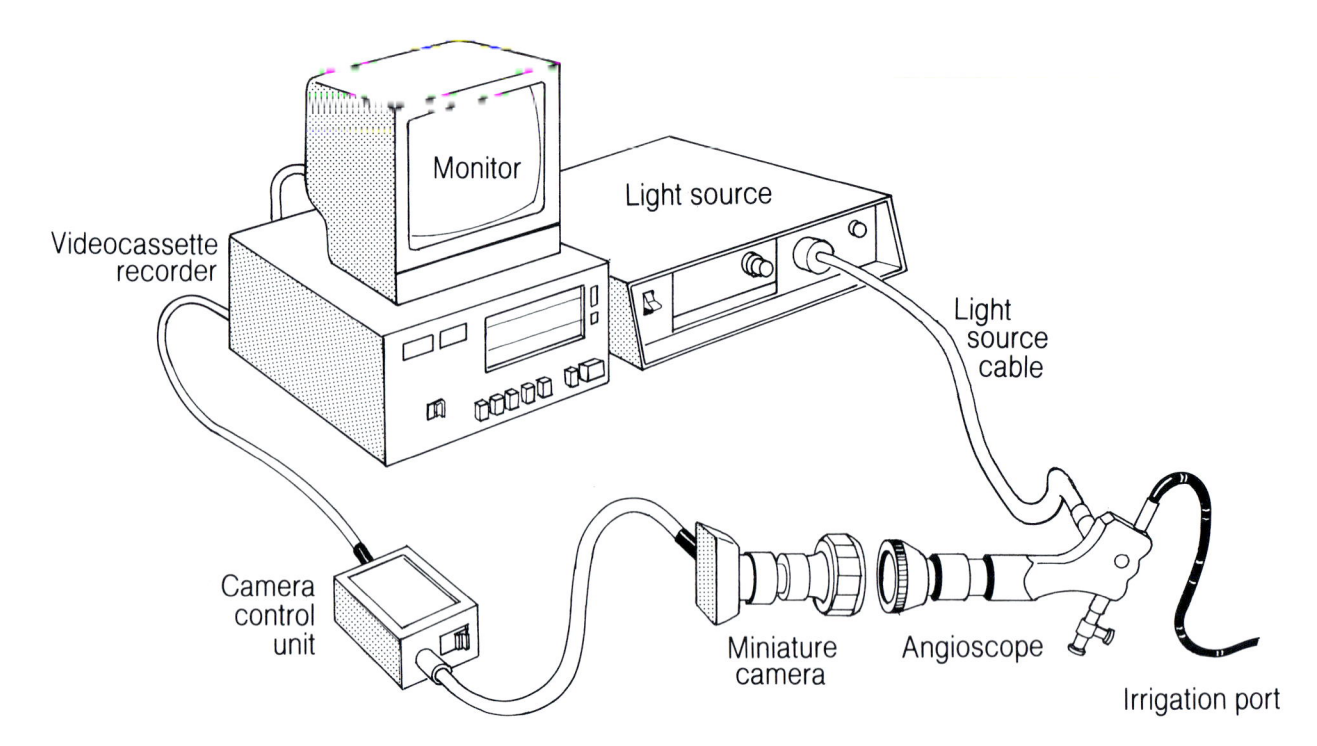

FIGURE 31-1 Angioscopic system.

vein bypass. Miller and colleagues,[7] in a series of 355 lower extremity revascularization procedures, routinely performed angioscopy. There was a 17 percent incidence of incompletely cut valve leaflets, a 33 percent incidence of nonligated tributaries, and a variety of other problems requiring correction. These included recanalized (previously thrombosed) vein, vein stenosis, technically inadequate anastomoses, intimal flaps, and intraluminal thrombus. In all, 155 of 355 patients (44 percent) required significant revision of an anastomosis. In another series, anastomotic problems were identified in 23 percent of patients undergoing surgical bypass, although Olcott[8] noted few intimal flaps or misplaced sutures in anastomotic inspections that required repair. These variations in results may be related to differences in the initial technique and the surgeon's threshold for repairing identified abnormalities.

Limitations and Complications

Angioscopy provides a direct two-dimensional color image of the intima and endovascular disease, without nephrotoxic dye or radiation. However, angioscopy cannot visualize large proximal vessels unless inflow of blood is occluded and does not provide a simultaneous overall picture of the vascular tree. In addition, it may be time consuming to perform, and repeated passes of the angioscope may damage the vessel wall. Furthermore, it is difficult to determine the degree of a stenosis, visualized from the lumen, unless we know the focal length of the angioscope and the distance from the lesion to the lens. Pathologic conditions within the lumen visualized from a distance may look small; those visualized close up may look large.

The greatest limitation of angioscopy is the requirement for irrigation to clear the lumen of blood, because even small amounts of blood can blur or opacify the image. However, excessive irrigation may lead to fluid overload. In addition, the significance of abnormalities identified by angioscopy is difficult to ascertain and may lead to more procedures than are actually necessary.

ENDOVASCULAR ULTRASOUND

Endovascular ultrasound is a promising new technology for imaging in real time all layers of an artery or vein (Fig. 31-2). It was initially developed to visualize intracardiac chambers and valves, but it has recently been used to visualize coronary and peripheral arteries, often performed in conjunction with endovascular procedures, such as balloon angioplasty, laser angioplasty, and atherectomy.

Catheter Design and Principles

Ultrasound transducers are placed on the tip of a catheter, which, for peripheral vessels, is 5- to 8-French and can be lower-frequency (10 to 20 MHz) transducers allow visualization of all three layers of the vessel wall; coronary vessels are visualized using higher-frequency (30 to 40 MHz) transducers, which offer less penetration but higher resolution. The mechanical transducers often are mounted with forward viewing of 30°, so that the vessel can be visualized in front of, and adjacent to, the ultrasonic catheter.

Imaging Capabilities

Endovascular ultrasound offers several theoretical advantages and some disadvantages over more conventional methods of imaging vessels, such as angiography, percutaneous duplex scanning, or angioscopy. It allows visualization of all three layers of the vessel wall, rather than simply the lumen. Consequently, luminal irregularity, such as intimal dissection, can be evaluated with abnormalities of the media. Atherosclerotic plaque can be identified in all layers of the vessel wall and characterized as calcified, fibrous, or fatty. Plaque characterization may have implications in determining optimal methods of treatment (i.e., laser angioplasty versus balloon angioplasty versus atherectomy). In addition, an accurate assessment of luminal stenosis can be obtained using endovascular ultrasound, as shown by a comparison study with angiography.[9] A major advantage of ultrasound is its ability to gain precise information without clearing the vessel of all blood.

Potential Clinical Applications

Although endovascular ultrasound currently is not routinely employed, clinical trials are being conducted to determine its role in a variety of situations. In addition, endovascular technology is rapidly being refined, so that many new clinical applications may be on the horizon.

Endovascular ultrasound may play a role as an independent device to characterize arterial and venous pathologic conditions, similar to angiography or duplex scanning. It can give accurate information on the presence, thickness, and composition of atherosclerotic plaque.[10] It can do this rapidly, with a high degree of resolution, and in real time. In addition, unlike angioscopy, endovascular ultrasound does not require elimination of blood for imaging; in fact, rapidly flowing blood creates less *backscatter* and a clearer image than a slow flowing or static column of blood.

The most promising application of endovascular ultrasound will probably be as an adjunct to endovascular interventions. Balloon angioplasty has been combined with endovascular ultrasound to determine dilatability, control the extent of dilatation, and examine the postdilatation vessel for thrombus, dissection, and flaps.[11] Laser angioplasty ultrasound devices have been developed that more precisely control the laser resection while it is being performed and reduce the risk of perforation. Atherectomy ultrasound systems can more precisely resect the entire

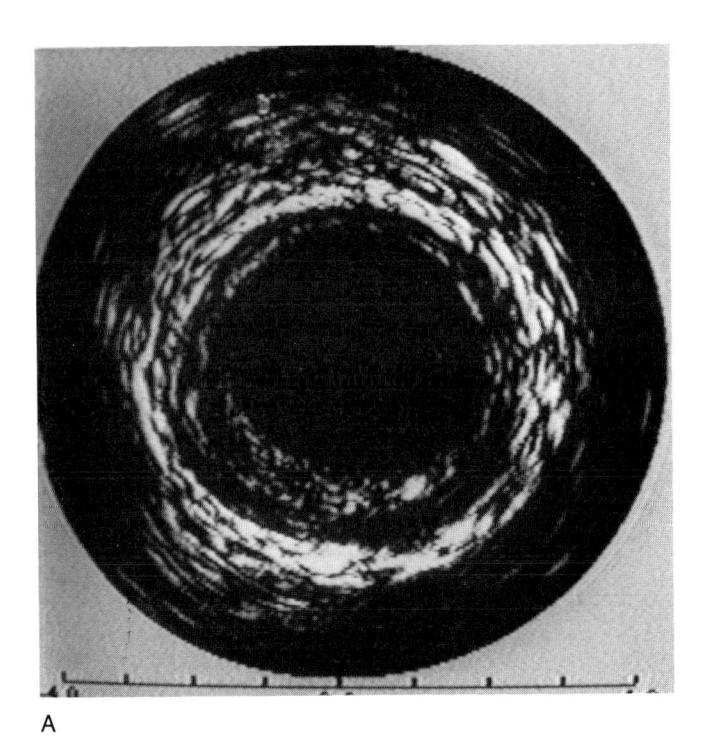

FIGURE 31-2 An endovascular ultrasound image demonstrating (A) normal anatomy, and (B) myointimal thickening in coronary transplant patients.

passed over guide wires from 0.014 to 0.025 in in diameter. The transducer can either be single and mechanically rotated at 1800 rpm or be composed of a multiple-phased array of elements placed circumferentially around the catheter tip, which does not rotate. For peripheral vessels, plaque, leaving normal arterial wall components, such as media and adventitia, behind. One of the few clinical studies using intravascular ultrasound has shown that the Simpson directional atherectomy catheter left an average residual stenosis of 43 percent,[12] although angiography showed the same residual stenosis to be only 14 percent. Stents can also be visualized using ultrasound during and after placement to ascertain that they are fully imbedded in the arterial wall and that they leave no intraluminal irregularities that might stimulate myointimal hyperplasia. Lastly, endovascular ultrasound may help characterize the causes of graft failure by noninvasive examination of all layers of the arterial and graft walls at the sites of anastomosis.

Endovascular ultrasound will have to compete with other evolving technologies in the diagnosis and treatment of vascular disease; however, we can anticipate an increasing role of these devices in the management of peripheral vascular disease.

INTRAOPERATIVE BALLOON ANGIOPLASTY

Most balloon angioplasty procedures should be formed percutaneously before standard surgical revascularization; however, in certain situations, intraoperative balloon angioplasty may be an adjunct to a reconstructive procedure. Percutaneous balloon angioplasty is usually performed in patients with single-level disease who have a good femoral or brachial access vessel. Intraoperative balloon angioplasty is reserved for patients with multilevel disease, which is often treated simultaneously in the operating room with a conventional bypass or endarterectomy procedure combined with balloon angioplasty. Intraoperative balloon angioplasty requires special skills and equipment (Fig. 31-3), which many surgeons may not have. In this case, they should either train in the procedure and gain the experience or invite an interventional radiologist into the operating room to help with the balloon dilatation portion of the procedure.

Indications

The most common indication for intraoperative balloon angioplasty is to establish good inflow for a more distal bypass. An iliac artery stenosis in the presence of an occluded superficial femoral artery is a situation in which the iliac inflow lesion may be treated with intraoperative balloon angioplasty to improve the patency of a femoropopliteal bypass procedure. Similarly, balloon angioplasty of an iliac artery stenosis may be used to provide better inflow for a femorofemoral bypass graft.

Intraoperative balloon angioplasty can also improve outflow after an aortobifemoral bypass graft, femorofemoral bypass graft, or femoral endarterectomy in the presence of a superficial femoral artery stenosis. Similarly, improved outflow for a femoropopliteal bypass is occasionally gained by dilating a distal popliteal or tibial artery stenosis. Adjunc-

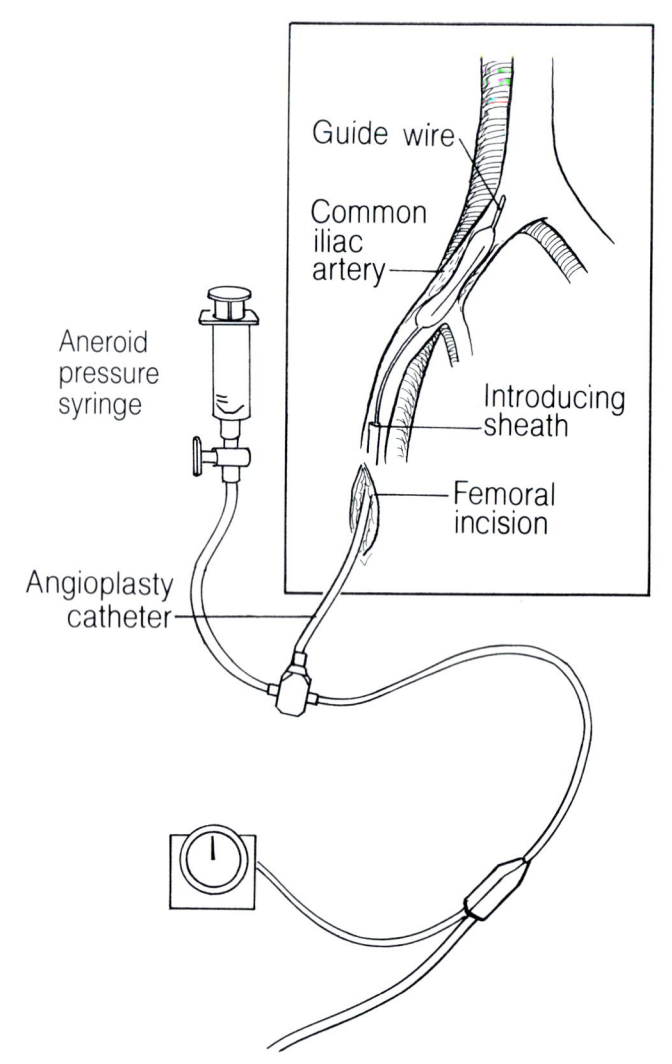

FIGURE 31-3 Illustration of an iliac artery balloon angioplasty.

tive balloon angioplasty of an obstructive popliteal or tibial artery may occasionally allow an above-the-knee, as opposed to a below-the-knee or tibial bypass.

Fogarty and colleagues[13] recently emphasized the importance of treating the underlying atherosclerotic occlusive lesion to maintain vessel patency after a thrombectomy for acute arterial occlusion. For optimal patency, a residual stenosis should be dilated using balloon angioplasty at the time of thrombectomy.

Techniques

The common femoral artery is the most frequent entry site for the balloon catheter; the vessel can be entered either by direct visualization and needle puncture or by arteriotomy. An introducer sheath is directed proximally or distally toward the stenotic lesion; a guide wire is then passed through the introducer sheath and the stenotic lesion. An appropriately sized balloon catheter is passed over the guide wire to the site of the stenotic lesion, and balloon dilatation is performed. After successful balloon angioplasty, angiography with pressure measurements or endovascular ultrasound is used to document the success of the procedure before the surgical bypass.

Results

The contributions of intraoperative balloon angioplasty are difficult to assess because it is combined with vascular reconstruction or thrombectomy. Furthermore, most series have a very short follow-up. However, the increased use of this procedure in selected situations indicates that it should be a part of every vascular surgeon's armamentarium. Lowman and associates[14] reported a series of 16 patients who underwent intraoperative balloon angioplasty in conjunction with a reconstructive procedure, eight iliac angioplasties to improve inflow and eight femoral or popliteal angioplasties to improve outflow. There were no complications, and all procedures were successful. Pfeiffer and colleagues[15] reported 80 patients who underwent iliac, femoral, and carotid artery balloon angioplasty and dilatation of arteriovenous fistulas and vein grafts. One intraoperative embolus occurred, and four late restenoses were identified. Andros and coworkers[16] described in detail the indications and technique of intraoperative balloon angioplasty.

Limitations and Complications

It is important to limit balloon angioplasty procedures to situations in which it is clearly necessary and not meddlesome. Thrombosis of a mildly stenotic iliac balloon angioplasty site can lead to thrombosis of what might have been a satisfactory femoropopliteal bypass. A newly dilated artery has a tendency to be acutely thrombogenic as a result of intimal injury and dissection. Consequently, most vascular surgeons have a preference for preoperative rather than intraoperative balloon dilatation unless the artery is percutaneously inaccessible.

Other complications of intraoperative balloon angioplasty are similar to percutaneous balloon angioplasty: distal emboli, arterial rupture, and groin hematomas. However, surgical exposure of the artery may decrease the frequency of some of these complications because an open technique allows complete control of the artery and suturing of the access site. The balloon angioplasty procedure may add considerable time to the surgical procedure, leading to an increased infection rate, although this complication has not been reported.

LASER ANGIOPLASTY

Laser angioplasty is more properly termed *laser-assisted balloon angioplasty* because a laser is used to recanalize an occluded artery by creating a small channel through which a guide wire and balloon angioplasty system can be delivered. Balloon dilatation creates the final recanalization. Laser angioplasty is a procedure that gained great popularity among patients and some vascular surgeons in the late 1980s as a result of excellent early patency data. However, late results have been so disappointing that this procedure is currently reserved for a very small percentage of patients with arterial occlusive disease; in many hospitals, the procedure has been abandoned.

The destruction of tissue during laser recanalization can be accomplished by several mechanisms. The first, vaporization, is thermal and occurs through rapid heating of water, with rupture of individual cells. The second mechanism occurs through a nonthermal process (*cold laser*) and involves directly breaking intramolecular bonds with precise cutting of the vascular tissue (in this process, large particles may be produced as a result of acoustic shock). The third mechanism occurs when the laser probe is pushed through the plaque, causing mechanical compression, fracture of the plaque, and dilatation.

There are now several systems clinically available for laser-assisted balloon angioplasty. These include the hot thermal metal tip, sapphire thermal tip, direct laser fiber, multifiber coaxial system, angioscopically directed laser system, computer-guided dye laser, and *nonthermal* laser. Many of these laser angioplasty devices are not approved by the Food and Drug Administration and, consequently, are used only in research centers.

Equipment

The metal thermal probe consists of an olive-shaped metal tip that is heated by argon laser energy transmitted through a quartz fiber (Fig. 31-4). The metal tip typically reaches 1000°C in air and 300 to 600°C in tissue and is advanced through the plaque by controlled thermal destruction of the tissue. There is also a hybrid probe that has an aperture at its tip that allows 20 percent of the laser energy to escape directly as light. This combines direct laser recanalization with a thermal hot tip to dilate the arterial stenosis.

Optical thermal probes use sapphire tips and quartz balls to recanalize vessels. Sapphire is a neutral crystal that acts as a lens, focusing the laser energy on the plaque, resulting in recanalization by a combination of direct laser energy and heating.

An excimer laser utilizes a halogen and noble gas to generate laser energy. These gases produce a short wavelength of ultraviolet laser light that is pulsed, allowing bursts of high energy which precisely cut through tissue. The most studied system for arterial disease is the 308-nm pulsed xenon chloride laser, which delivers the laser energy through a flexible quartz fiber.

The computer-guided system incorporates spectroscopic plaque recognition with pulsed-dye laser tissue ablation.

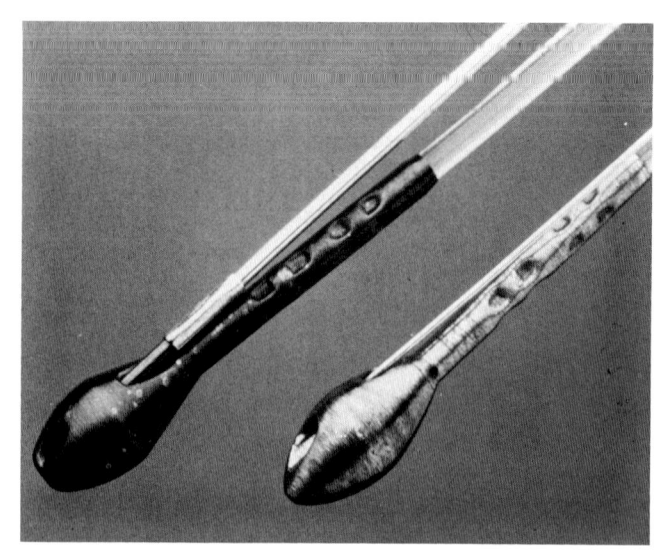

FIGURE 31-4 Two metal thermal probes with an olive-shaped metal cap heated by an argon laser beam.

TABLE 31-1 Likelihood of recanalization of atherosclerotic lesions with laser angioplasty

	Hot tipped	Hybrid	Bare fiber
Short-segment stenosis	Excellent	Excellent	Excellent
Short-segment occlusion	Good	Good	Good
Long-segment stenosis	Fair	Fair	Fair
Long-segment occlusion	Poor	Poor	Poor
Calcified stenosis	Poor	Poor	Poor
Calcified occlusion	Poor	Poor	Poor

The diagnostic portion of the system provides spectral analysis of the fluorescent pattern of the plaque. If the spectral pattern fits parameters consistent with a plaque, the computer instructs a second laser to fire; if it does not, the laser will not fire. A flashlamp-excited dye laser capable of generating high energy during short pulses cuts through the plaque, leaving normal artery behind.

The angioscopically guided laser has an argon laser fiber that runs within the angioscopic catheter sheath. The plaque is visualized, and the laser is then activated under direct vision. The laser fiber is eccentrically placed so that rotation of the tip allows the laser to treat the entire circumference. A balloon–irrigation system is used to clear blood from the lumen, allowing both visualization of the plaque and a clear medium through which to transmit the laser energy.

Indications

Limb-threatening ischemia and severely disabling claudication are the accepted indications for laser-assisted balloon angioplasty, although laser angioplasty was initially advocated for minimal disease. Stenotic lesions can be more easily and rapidly treated with balloon angioplasty alone; consequently, lasers should be reserved for totally occlusive lesions. Even with totally obstructed lesions, a guide wire can often cross the occlusions, so that the laser is unnecessary. In addition, patients with long segment total occlusions are poor candidates for laser angioplasty, based on disappointing long-term patency results, and are better treated with surgical bypass. The likelihood of recanalization is determined by the extent of disease and the type of laser used (Table 31-1). The location of disease also has a major impact on clinical success (Table 31-2). Thus, the current indications for laser angioplasty use are limited and will remain so until second- and third-generation devices are developed that either lessen the damage to the vessel wall or are more effective in recanalizing long segment occlusions.

Technique

Access to the common femoral artery is obtained either percutaneously or through a cut-down procedure. Through a 7- to 9-French introducer sheath, the laser probe or fiber is advanced to the obstructed lesion under fluoroscopic guidance, positioned as closely to the center of the occlusion as possible, and activated. Very gentle pressure is used to advance the catheter, with care taken not to push the catheter too vigorously to avoid perforation. To check the progress, serial angiograms are performed during the laser procedure through the introducer sheath. Although the exact relationship between the laser catheter and arterial wall cannot precisely be identified, alignment of the distal runoff artery and proximal segment of the artery will allow a fairly accurate determination of the catheter position in relationship to the artery. After the occlusive lesion has been crossed, standard balloon angioplasty techniques are used to enlarge the channel to its full diameter. After the procedure is completed, heparinization for 24 h, followed by antiplatelet therapy, is helpful to prevent early thrombosis.

TABLE 31-2 Success of laser angioplasty based on location of disease

Site of arterial disease	Anticipated result
Common femoral	Poor
Proximal superficial	Fair
Profunda femoris	Unknown
Distal superficial femoral	Excellent
Popliteal	Good
Anterior tibial/posterior tibial	Fair–poor
Peroneal	Fair–poor

Results

Cumberland and associates,[17] in 1986, reported an 89 percent initial success rate in clinical trials using thermal hot-tip laser angioplasty; however, these initial results have been duplicated by other investigators only in short (< 3 cm) stenotic lesions. In 1988, the authors updated their results,[17a] having determined that the long-term patency in their patients was similar to that of balloon angioplasty: 90 percent 1-year patency for stenotic and short lesions < 3 cm, 75 percent 1-year patency for lesions 4 to 7 cm, and < 60 percent 1-year patency for lesions > 7 cm.

More recent experience with the thermal metal probe has been even more disappointing. Harrington and colleagues[18] reported their results using the thermal hot tip in 72 limbs with occluded arteries. Although their initial success rate was 82 percent at the time of discharge, only 43 of 72 (60 percent) of the limbs showed clinical improvement. Wright and associates,[19] from the same group of investigators, reported the results of thermal hot tip angioplasty in patients requiring limb salvage. It was initially successful in 10 of 15 cases; within 6 months, 9 of the 10 successfully treated cases had failed. Thus, 14 of 15 patients had unsuccessful results by the 6-month follow-up. Perler and coworkers[20] reported an overall success rate of only 21 of 47 patients (45 percent) and found that those with lesions > 7 cm had the worst results. The overall long-term follow-up revealed a 30 percent clinical success rate at 1 year.

Results using the hybrid argon laser hot tip have been similarly poor. Seeger and associates[21] reported on 46 patients and found a 77 percent initial recanalization rate but only a 48 percent immediate clinical success rate. A 20 percent perforation rate was also noted.

Lammer[22] reported on the Austrian Multi-Center trial using the Surgical Laser Technologies Nd:YAG sapphire contract probe. In 184 patients, the primary success rate was 81 percent, with a 1-year patency of 79 percent, 2-year patency of 73 percent, and 3-year patency of 75 percent. There was a 12 percent dissection or perforation rate in this trial.

The results using excimer laser-assisted balloon angioplasty have been similar. Grundfest and associates[23] reported an initial success rate in 7 of 9 patients with stenotic lesions and 17 of 22 patients with total occlusions. Subintimal dissection or perforation by the excimer laser fiber occurred in five cases. Fortunately, these complications caused no direct adverse results. Long-term follow-up revealed restenosis in 7 of 30 (approximately 25 percent) patients at 9 months.

Nordstom[24] recently reported 1-year follow-up results using the direct argon angioscopically guided laser. The overall initial success rate was 59 of 68 cases (87 percent). In iliac arteries, it was 10 of 14 (71 percent), and in the superficial femoral artery, it was 49 of 54 (91 percent). Three perforations occurred. Life-table analysis revealed an overall 1-year cumulative patency rate of 75 percent. The rate was 75 percent for iliac lesions, 91 percent for femoropopliteal stenosis, and 71 percent for femoropopliteal occlusion.

Leon and colleagues,[25] using the computer-guided laser, reported preliminary results in 129 patients, with an initial success rate of 72 percent (101 of 140). Of these patients, 93 percent underwent subsequent successful balloon angioplasty, for an overall initial success rate of 95 of 140 (72 percent). Mechanical complications caused nine percent of failures. Long-term results are not available, but a comparison of several series of laser angioplasty (Table 31-3) shows a substantial variation in early and late results.

TABLE 31-3 Laser angioplasty—clinical results

Author	Laser	No.	Indications Claudication	Limb salvage	Lesions Stenosis	Occlusions	Initial success Stenosis	Occlusions	Complications	Long-term success
Sanborn	Hot-tipped + balloon	129	66%	34%	16%	84%	100%	85%	9.5%	NR
Wright	Hot-tipped + balloon	15	0%	100%	0%	100%		67%	67%	10%, 6 mo
Diethrich (presented but not published)	Hot-tipped + balloon	770	100%	51%	54%	46%	28–100% (depending on site)		29%	NR
Nordstrom (collected series)	Argon bare fiber + balloon	378	82%	18%	12%	88%	100%	82%	23%	64%, 1yr

NR = not reported

Limitations and Complications

The overall results using laser-assisted balloon angioplasty are no better than balloon angioplasty alone, probably because of the fact that laser is merely a drilling device to provide access for the balloon and still requires dilatation using balloon angioplasty techniques. Laser-assisted balloon angioplasty also carries an additional potential risk of arterial wall perforation and/or dissection, occurring in approximately 10 percent of cases. Furthermore, the usual complications of groin hematoma and/or wound infection, which occur in standard balloon angioplasty, persist and may be more frequent as a result of the large introducer sheaths that are required. Embolic complications occur in one to three percent of cases. In addition, hard calcified plaque is difficult for lasers to penetrate. Calcified plaque contains hydroxyapatite, which has a melting point of 1800°C, and is, thus, resistant to laser thermal ablation. The excimer laser, which uses photodecomposition mechanisms, has had better success in cutting through calcified plaques, although the process is slow. Finally, as in balloon angioplasty, longer lesions have poorer immediate and long-term results. The lesions best treated by laser angioplasty appear to be those < 7 cm in length.

It is clear that current laser-assisted balloon angioplasty techniques will undergo major changes in the next 5 to 10 years. In fact, many technical advances will be necessary before laser angioplasty becomes a routine vascular procedure. We can anticipate the development of lasers that do not require balloon assistance, photodynamic therapy of a plaque to make it more susceptible to a specific laser wavelength, and simpler devices to heat thermal probes. Until a laser is developed that removes plaque from long segments of arteries, with minimal damage to the vessel wall, laser angioplasty will play a limited role in the management of arterial occlusive disease.

PERIPHERAL ATHERECTOMY

Atherectomy is an endovascular procedure that uses a cutting or shaving device to remove atherosclerotic plaque from diseased arteries. The procedure can be performed percutaneously or through a small surgically created arteriotomy remote from the site of disease. Atherectomy offers several theoretic advantages over balloon angioplasty, including: (1) application to elastic plaques that cannot be balloon dilated, (2) more complete debulking of the atheromatous mass, and (3) higher immediate patency caused by a greater reduction in the stenosis and, consequently, higher flow rates. Many different atherectomy devices have been developed, and each offers its own unique features. Four have undergone extensive clinical testing and can, therefore, be compared for efficacy and complications. They are the Simpson Atherocath, Trac-Wright Catheter, Auth Rotoblator, and Transluminal Extraction Catheter.

Indications

Patients with symptomatic atherosclerotic arterial disease of the lower extremities, including claudication, rest pain, or nonhealing ulcers, are candidates for atherectomy. Some investigators who participated in the original clinical trials believe that patients with less severe symptoms and mild claudication should be candidates for atherectomy. Despite an initial low complication rate, however, the long-term restenosis rate approaches or exceeds that of bypass procedures or balloon angioplasty. Therefore, the only compelling argument to liberalize the indications for an atherectomy procedure is the minimally invasive nature of the percutaneous approach and the short hospital stay associated with the procedure. A comparison of the anticipated results for atherectomy is based, to a large extent, on the extent of disease within the vessel (Table 31-4).

Simpson Atherectomy Device

The Simpson atherectomy device consists of a flexible catheter with a distal housing unit that contains a cutter, retrieval chamber, and balloon (Fig. 31-5). The catheter is advanced over a quide wire through a stenotic region of the artery. After the cutting portion of the catheter has been positioned across from the lesion, the balloon is inflated to push the cutter against the plaque. The mobile cutter is then used to resect the protruding plaque by spinning at 2000 rpm. Atheromatous debris is removed and stored in a collection chamber. For long-segment stenoses, the device must be repositioned, and the resection is often slow, with concentric lesions frequently more difficult to resect than eccentric ones. Occlusions cannot be treated using this device.

Simpson and colleagues[26] reported initial experience with 136 lesions in 61 patients. This atherectomy device was used in the iliac, superficial femoral, and popliteal arteries, with initial success in 87 percent of patients. In the unsuccessful cases, the technical inability to remove

TABLE 31-4 Likelihood of recanalization of atherosclerotic lesions with atherectomy

	Simpson	TEC	TRAC-Wright
Short-segment stenosis	Excellent	Good	Good
Short-segment occlusion	Poor	Poor	Fair
Long-segment stenosis	Fair	Fair	Fair
Long-segment occlusion	Poor	Poor	Poor
Calcified stenosis	Fair	Fair	Fair
Calcified occlusion	Poor	Poor	Poor

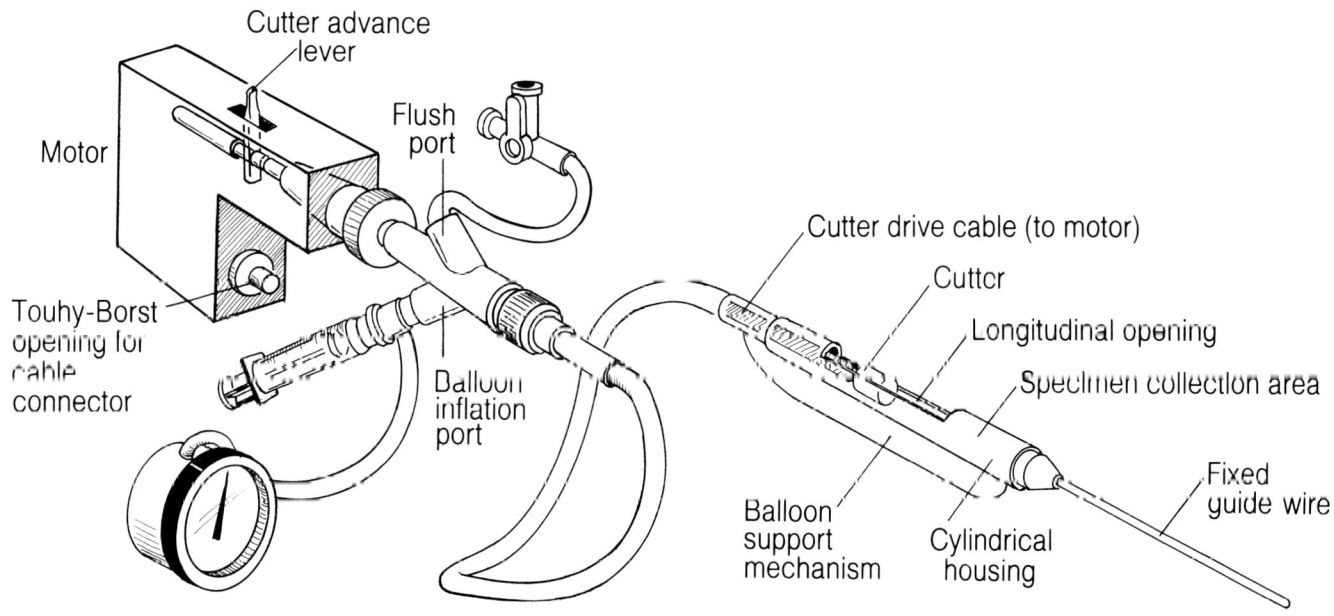

FIGURE 31-5 The Simpson atherectomy device.

atheroma adequately was the primary cause of failure. Among the successfully treated patients, only 69 percent had sustained improvement at the 6-month follow-up. Angiographic studies available in 30 of these patients revealed a restenosis rate of at least 36 percent. The restenosis rate was greater in patients with residual stenosis of > 30 percent at the completion of the atherectomy procedure.

Polnitz and associates[27] reported using Simpson atherectomy procedures in 60 patients with 94 lesions in 77 superficial femoral arteries, 8 popliteal arteries, 8 iliac arteries, and 1 anterior tibial artery. Immediate clinical success occurred in 49 (82 percent) of the 60 patients. Twenty-five patients achieved a 72 percent 1-year clinical patency rate; 16 percent required repeat atherectomy; and 8 percent required surgery for restenosis or occlusion. Six-month angiographic evaluations disclosed restenosis in 13 (24 percent) of 55 lesions: 3 of 13 (23 percent) concentric lesions, 3 of 27 (11 percent) eccentric lesions, and 7 of 15 (47 percent) total occlusions studied. These authors concluded that Simpson atherectomy was best suited for eccentric short-segment stenosis and poorly suited for occlusions or lengthy lesions that diffusely involved the vessel.

The results of Simpson's atherectomy study demonstrated a low initial complication rate. In 136 procedures on 61 patients, two complications occurred, one embolus and one vessel thrombosis. Dissection was a complication in 3 of 61 patients but was related to the guide wire or introducer rather than the atherectomy procedure itself. No perforation was reported, and no patient required emergency surgery for distal emboli.

Trac-Wright (Kensey) Atherectomy Catheter

The Trac-Wright catheter is a 5- or 8-French, high-speed (80,000 to 200,000 rpm) flexible catheter with a distal cam tip designed to chip away at the plaque and develop a lumen that allows balloon angioplasty. In addition, the Trac-Wright catheter infuses saline under high pressure through its distal tip, resulting in secondary arterial dilatation. The device is designed to maintain alignment in the center of the artery without a guide wire; therefore, it can theoretically be used for arterial occlusion and stenosis.

Whittemore[28] reported initial results using the Trac-Wright atherectomy catheter in 10 patients. The procedure benefited one patient; two arterial wall perforations were reported. No peripheral embolization occurred. Snyder and colleagues[29] reported 23 procedures to recanalize superficial femoral artery occlusions; atherectomy was initially successful in only 14 of 23 cases. Eleven of those 14 extremities underwent subsequent percutaneous balloon angioplasty to enlarge the initial channel further. There have been few long-term reports of patency following Trac-Wright atherectomy. Snyder and colleagues[29] reported a 37-month life-table patency after Trac-Wright atherectomy. At 12 months, the patency was 37.5 percent; this poor patency is caused primarily by the initial failure rate of 40 percent.

Unsuccessful use of the Trac-Wright device is frequently related to vessel wall perforation; in fact, one third of all procedures had associated perforation, which usually sealed spontaneously and rarely required operative intervention. Whittemore[28] reported 2 perforations in 10 procedures, with Snyder and colleagues[29] reporting 8 of 23.

The catheter follows the path of least resistance, which is often away from the hard calcified plaque. Although fibrous lesions are amenable to atherectomy, the hard calcified lesions, particularly at the adductor canal, have been resistant to atherectomy. Thromboembolic complications have not yet been reported. Because of the risk of perforation, the Trac-Wright catheter should be used with caution in the iliac arteries. Recent studies of the pulverized debris that passes downstream in the arterial lumen have suggested that this material is large enough to obstruct arterioles and capillaries and may have a detrimental effect on distal tissue. On the basis of this clinical experience, the Trac-Wright device would seem to be most useful in patients who have short-segment noncalcified occlusions of the superficial femoral artery because other procedures and devices are preferable for use in patients with stenosis.

Auth Rotoblator

The Auth Rotoblator is a flexible catheter with a variable-sized football-shaped metal burr on the distal tip. The burr is studded with multiple diamond chips (22 to 45 μm in size) that function as microcutters. The burr comes in various sizes, ranging from 1.25 to 6.0 mm in diameter. The properly sized burr is selected for a given artery and is rotated at 100,000 to 200,000 rpm over a central guide wire. The guide wire must first traverse the lesion before rotational atherectomy can proceed. The high-speed rotation allows the diamond microchips to attack hard calcified atheroma preferentially, while leaving intact the surrounding elastic soft tissue of normal arterial wall. It leaves a smooth polished intraluminal surface and no intimal flaps, but the Rotoblator removes intima from both the normal and diseased portions of the artery as it is passed to and fro. This can result in accelerated atherosclerosis in the treated artery, although the pulverized particles are generally smaller than red blood cells.

Atherectomy is performed through an open arteriotomy that allows the largest-sized burr to be used. An introducer sheath is inserted into the artery through the arteriotomy. Angioscopy or conventional fluoroscopy is used to document the lesion and help with proper placement of the guide wire. A guide wire is passed through the lesion, and the burr is placed over a stiff guide wire and passed to the obstructive lesion. Initially, a 2.0-mm-sized burr is advanced slowly in a to-and-fro manner over the guide wire, recanalizing the artery. After this initial atherectomy, the next-sized burr is inserted, and atherectomy is repeated until an adequately sized lumen is obtained. The patient receives anticoagulation therapy for the first 24 postoperatively to prevent early thrombosis. Aspirin is given for long-term antiaggregate therapy.

The Auth Rotoblator is ideally suited for removal of hard calcified plaque. Recanalization is possible in long and short lesions of the popliteal, superficial femoral, and iliac arteries. Stenotic lesions are best treated because a central guide wire must first traverse the lesion, although occlusions can be treated if the guide wire can be passed through the plaque. Eccentric plaques can be treated because the atherectomy device preferentially attacks hard plaque.

Forty superficial femoral, popliteal, and tibial arteries have been treated at the University of California at Los Angeles.[30] The initial success rate was 38 of 40 arteries (95 percent). Mechanical problems caused two early technical failures; four arteries thrombosed in the early postoperative period. Follow-up revealed that there were seven late failures (29 percent) at 9 months. Overall, only 11 of the original 24 cases (46 percent) had continued vessel patency and clinical benefit. A further analysis revealed that the longer lesions had higher early and late failure rates. Lesions < 7 cm had a 64 percent patency rate; the lesions > 10 cm had only a 20 percent patency rate. The best results occurred in the tibial artery. The worst results were in long superficial femoral artery occlusive lesions.

The Stanford series reviewed 42 patients undergoing Auth Rotoblator procedures (21 open and 21 percutaneous) for superficial femoral artery and popliteal stenosis.[30] The angiographic success rate was 81 percent (34 of 42). The in-hospital clinical success rate was 52 percent (22 of 42); the 6-month patency rate was 43 percent.

Misplacement of the guide wire in a subintimal plane is the most frequent complication and may lead to an intimal flap as the burr tracks over the guide wire. Thromboembolic complications have also occurred; these are mostly microscopic and clinically insignificant. One patient developed diffuse microemboli, and microscopic hemoglobinuria has occurred in several patients, particularly when the larger-sized burrs (4 mm or greater) are used. In the Stanford series, 17 of 42 patients (41 percent) developed complications: six hematomas, two wound infections, four microemboli, three hemoglobinuria, two perforations, and two lost limbs.

INTRAVASCULAR STENTS

Restenosis after transluminal angioplasty and atherectomy has been the greatest limitation of these procedures and has led to the development of intravascular stents that are used to maintain the diameter of an artery after a procedure and limit long-term restenosis. Several types of stents have been described in the literature and have been used experimentally and clinically (Fig. 31-6). These include flexible, rigid, balloon expandable, and self-expanding stents. The Palmaz stent is a balloon expandable, rigid, stainless-steel stent. The Gianturco-Wallace stents are metallic, rigid stents that have properties that allow for self-expansion. The Strecker stent is balloon expandable and flexible; the Wall stent is a stainless-steel, flexible, self-expanding stent. Recently, there have been animal studies testing biodegradable stents.

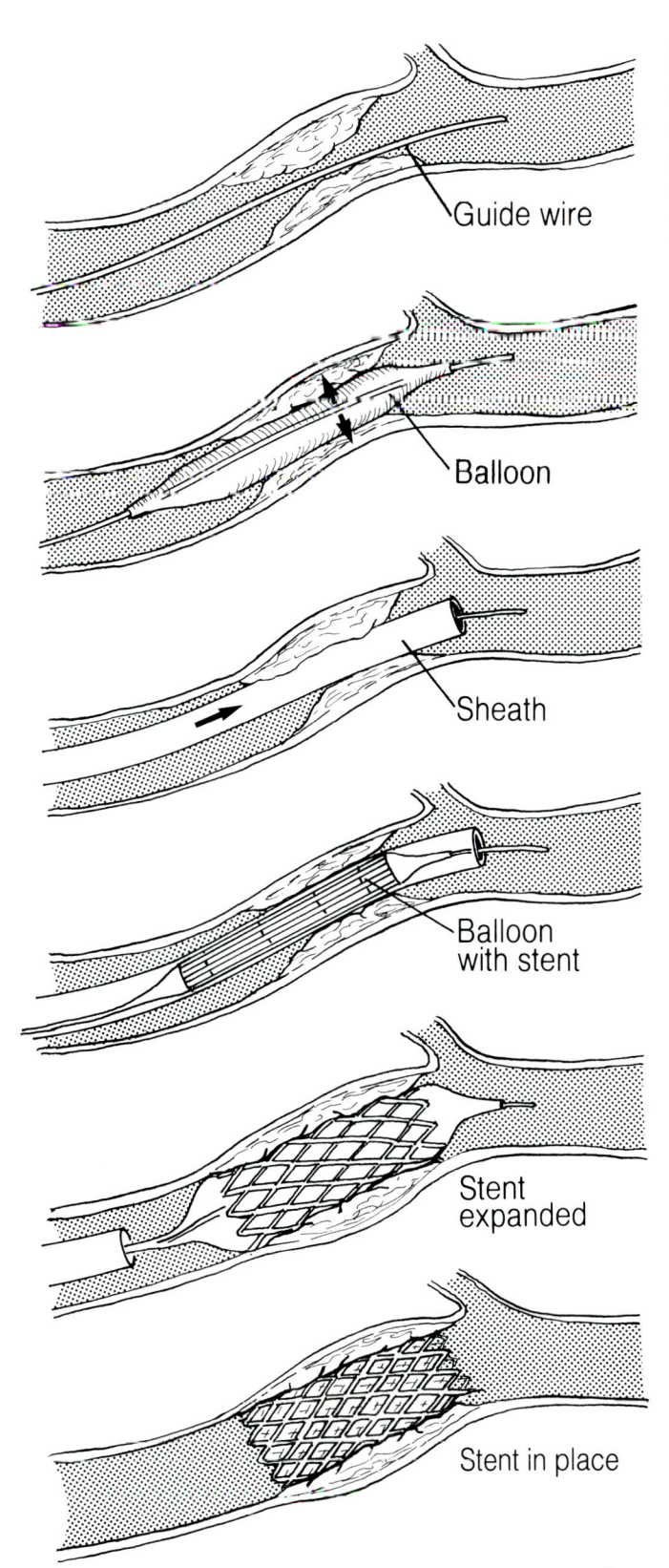

FIGURE 31-6 Illustrations of an intravascular stent expanding the intraluminal surface of a lesion.

Indications

The function of all stents is to provide a scaffold to maintain intraluminal structure and patency of the artery. Stents have been used primarily in occlusive and stenotic lesions in which balloon angioplasty has given an inadequate immediate result as a result of elastic plaque. Stents have also been used to tack dissections that occur after balloon angioplasty. Arteries that show persistent narrowing, despite several balloon dilatation attempts, may benefit from stent placement. Another indication is to prevent restenosis after balloon angioplasty. Stenotic lesions of the distal anastomoses of bypass grafts (intimal hyperplasia), which are notoriously difficult to balloon dilate and maintain in position, have also been successfully stented. The most rapidly expanding clinical application of stents is for maintenance of a fistula between the portal vein and vena cava, a percutaneous portal caval shunt or "TIPS" procedure. Because TIPS is an entirely percutaneous procedure, the technique and results will not be discussed in this chapter.

Technique

Stent placement has primarily been performed percutaneously as an adjunct to percutaneous balloon angioplasty, although intraoperative stent placement after balloon angioplasty has also been reported. The original diameter of the vessel is estimated, and bony landmarks are used to help position the stent before deployment. Superficial femoral arteries are usually stented with 6-mm stents; iliac arteries are usually treated with 8- to 10-mm stents. Multiple stents are occasionally used in a single artery if long segments are stenotic.

With balloon-expanded stents, an introducer sheath is advanced across the stenosis, delivering the stent to the stenotic lesion. With this protective sheath in place, the stent balloon assembly is then advanced within the sheath to the level of the lesion. The sheath is withdrawn, uncovering the mounted stent. The balloon is inflated to expand the stent and lesion simultaneously, leaving the stent mesh flush within the inner lumen. Residual irregularity within, proximal, or distal to the stent is corrected by further dilating the vessel. A second stent may be inserted to dilate residual stenoses proximal or distal to the stent. After stent expansion, the balloon is deflated and withdrawn, and a completion angiogram and pressure measurements are taken.

Self-expanding stents are delivered through an introducer catheter with a rolling membrane or sheath covering the stent. Gradual retraction of the outer membrane or sheath releases the stent, which shortens during release, rendering placement somewhat imprecise. If the catheter is only partially disengaged, the stent can usually be pulled back, but not advanced forward. Repeated stenting is occasionally necessary to obtain optimal results.

Routine anticoagulation and postprocedural antiplatelet

therapy are recommended. There is some preliminary data suggesting that long-term warfarin should be used to prevent early and late thrombosis.

Results

Initial clinical results of intravascular stenting in peripheral arteries have been reported, although long-term results are still accumulating. Most studies involve European testing of the Wall stent. Sigwart and associates[31] reported placing 10 stents during seven procedures in six patients (four femoral and three iliac arteries). Two patients had occluded arteries, and four patients had stenotic arteries that did not respond satisfactorily to balloon angioplasty. In a 6-month follow-up, there were no restenoses, but long follow-up is not available.

Gunther and colleagues[32] treated 45 patients using the Wall self-expanding, flexible stent. Thirty-one patients had lesions of the iliac arteries, and 14 had lesions of the superficial femoral artery. At the 2- to 12-month follow-ups, 40 of 45 patients had patent stents. Two patients had early thrombotic occlusion, and three patients had late intimal hyperplasia restenosis. A sixth patient subsequently developed occlusion at 6 months. Only one of the iliac lesions restenosed; however, 3 of 14 patients with superficial femoral artery stents had restenosis (21 percent).

Rousseau and colleagues,[33] also using the Wall stent, reported 40 femoropopliteal implantations in 36 patients, with a 6-month follow-up in all patients. Seventy-five percent of the lesions were 3 to 7 cm in length; 25 percent of the lesions exceeded 7 cm. Seventy percent were located in the superficial femoral artery, 16 percent in the popliteal artery, and 14 percent in a combination of the arteries. Seven patients had early thrombotic occlusions; restenosis occurred in 10 percent of the remaining patients. The cumulative patency rate was 76 percent at 1 year; however, all nine patients who had received postoperative warfarin did not develop early thrombosis or late restenosis.

Palmaz and associates,[34] in the United States, coordinated a large multicenter trial using the rigid, metallic Palmaz stents. Initial results showed 100 percent patency in the iliac arteries during a follow-up of 6 to 12 months. A further update of this study revealed a 97 percent initial success of stent placement in 165 limbs of 146 patients. Seventy-nine percent of these patients have continued clinical success at the 6-month follow-up. Strecker and coworkers,[35] using the metallic, tantalum filament, flexible stent, reported similar patency rates in the iliac arteries, but they found several restenoses in the superficial femoral artery position.

Limitations and Complications

Most complications of stent placement have been related to percutaneous balloon angioplasty. There have been occasional stent-related complications, such as inability to place the stent in an adequate position and premature dislodgment from the catheter delivery system. In addition, there have been a few reported instances of stent migration and embolization, vessel perforation requiring urgent surgery, and groin hematoma requiring blood transfusion. Other complications have included side-branch occlusion, late thrombosis, and distal emboli. Accelerated intimal hyperplasia has also been noted, particularly in the superficial femoral artery regions. The long-term arterial response to stent placement has not been evaluated for the entire range of patients with arterial disease; therefore, precise recommendations regarding selection of patients and lesions cannot be made at this time. However, the presence of a permanent stent may make reconstructive surgery on the vessel more difficult.

The preliminary results show an excellent patency of stents in the iliac artery position. However, we should note that long-term patency of balloon angioplasty without stents in the iliac arteries is also good, approaching 90 percent patency at 1 year and 80 percent patency at 3 years. So far, the results in the superficial femoral and popliteal positions have been promising. However, there is no substantial evidence that stents reduce restenosis in the superficial femoral or popliteal artery positions. Preliminary testing using biodegradable stents is currently in progress.

Stents have clearly shown their usefulness in certain situations, particularly in improving the early results after failed or inadequate balloon angioplasty that is complicated by intimal dissection or flaps. Stents also play a potential role in proximal renal artery balloon angioplasty and in treatment of stenosis in the distal anastomosis of a bypass graft. There has been preliminary work using endovascular grafts or stents to treat aneurysmal disease. Stents may also play a role in treating recurrent stenosis of arteriovenous hemodialysis access grafts and aortic dissection. Until better long-term information is available regarding the response to these endovascular devices, the indications should be limited, in arterial occlusive disease, to failure of balloon angioplasty.

CONCLUSION

Endovascular surgery is currently in its infancy, and much work is necessary before its full potential can be realized. Because early results of some procedures have been disappointing, enthusiasm regarding all endovascular procedures has become more cautious and realistic. The main challenge for endovascular procedures is in controlling restenosis. The solution may lie with pharmacologic manipulation of myointimal hyperplasia and better understanding of restenosis. It seems likely that the basic research currently underway will lead to a significant reduction in restenosis. If the restenosis problem is solved, then the applications of endovascular surgery will be broader and become a major treatment option in peripheral vascular surgery. It is imperative that vascular surgeons, in particular, continue to maintain an interest in the field, making significant contributions and shaping the future course of endovascular surgery.

REFERENCES

1. White GH, White RA, Kopchock EG, et al: Endoscopic intravascular surgery removed intraluminal flaps, dissections and thrombus. *J Vasc Surg* 1990; 11:280–286.
2. Fleisher HL III, Thompson BW, McCowan TC, et al: Angioscopically monitored saphenous vein valvulotomy *J Vasc Surg* 1986; 4:360–364.
3. Mehigan JT, Olcott C: Video angioscopy as an alternative to intraoperative arteriography. *Am J Surg* 1986; 152:139–154.
4. Grundfest WS, Litvack F, Sherman T, et al: Delineation of peripheral and coronary detail by intraoperative angioscopy. *Ann Surg* 1985; 202:394–400.
5. Chin AK, Fogarty TJ: Angioscopic preparation for saphenous vein in situ bypass grafting, in Moore WS, Ahn SS (eds): *Endovascular Surgery*. Philadelphia, Saunders, 1989, pp 74–81.
6. White GF: Angioscopy to monitor arterial thromboembolectomy, in Moore WS, Ahn SS (eds): *Endovascular Surgery*. Philadelphia, Saunders, 1989, pp 74–82.
7. Miller A, Stonebridge P, Jepsen S, et al: Continued experience with intraoperative angioscopy for monitoring infrainguinal bypass grafting. *Surgery* 1991; 109:286–293.
8. Olcott C: Angioscopic inspection of an anastomosis: Indications and techniques, in Moore WS, Ahn SS (eds): *Endovascular Surgery*. Philadelphia, Saunders, 1989, pp 514–517.
9. Nissen SE, Gurley JC, Grimes CL, et al: Comparison of intravascular ultrasound and angiography in quantitation of coronary dimensions and stenosis in man: Impact of lumen eccentricity, abstracted. *Circulation* 1990; 82(Suppl III):III-440.
10. Barzilai B, Saffitz JE, Miller JG, et al: Quantitative ultrasonic characterization of the nature of atherosclerotic plaque. *Circ Res* 1987; 60:459–463.
11. Isner JM, Rosenfield K, Mosseri M, et al: How reliable are images obtained by intravascular ultrasound for making decisions during percutaneous interventions? Experience with intravascular ultrasound employed in lieu of contrast angiography to guide peripheral balloon angioplasty in 16 patients, abstracted. *Circulation* 1990; 82(Suppl III):III-440.
12. White NW, Webb JG, Rowe MH, et al: Atherectomy guidance using intravascular ultrasound: Quantitation of plaque burden. *Circulation* 1989; 80(Suppl II):II-374.
13. Fogarty TJ, Chin AK, Olcott C, et al: Combined thrombectomy and dilatation for treatment of acute lower extremity arterial thrombosis. *J Vasc Surg* 1989; 10:530–534.
14. Lowman BG, Queral LA, Holbrook WA, et al: Transluminal angioplasty during vascular reconstructive procedures. *Arch Surg* 1981; 116:829–832.
15. Pfeiffer RB Jr, String ST: Adjunctive use of the balloon dilatation catheter during vascular reconstructive procedures. *J Vasc Surg* 1986; 3:841–845.
16. Andros G, Harris RW, Salles-Cunha SX: Technique of intraoperative balloon angioplasty, in Moore WB, Ahn SS (eds): *Endovascular Surgery*. Philadelphia, Saunders, 1992, pp 212–223.
17. Cumberland DC, Sanborn TA, Taylor DA, et al: Percutaneous laser thermal angioplasty: Initial clinical results with a laser probe in total peripheral artery occlusions. *Lancet* 1986; 1:1457–1459.
17a. Sanborn TA, Cumberland DC, Greenfield AJ, et al: Percutaneous laser thermal angioplasty: Initial results and one-year follow-up in 129 femoro popliteal lesions. *Radiology* 1988; 168:121–125.
18. Harrington ME, Schwartz ME, Sanborn TA, et al: Expanded indications for laser-assisted balloon angioplasty in peripheral arterial disease. *J Vasc Surg* 1990; 11:146–155.
19. Wright JG, Belkin M, Greenfield AJ, et al: Laser angioplasty for limb salvage: Observations on early results. *J Vasc Surg* 1989; 10:29–37.
20. Perler BA, Osterman FA, White RI, et al: Percutaneous laser probe femoropopliteal angioplasty: A preliminary experience. *J Vasc Surg* 1989; 10:351–357.
21. Seeger JM, Abela GS, Silverman SH, et al: Initial results of laser recanalization in lower extremity laser arterial reconstruction. *J Vasc Surg* 1989; 9:10–17.
22. Lammer J: Presented at the Seventeenth International Congress of Radiology, Paris, July 1989.
23. Grundfest W, Litvack F, Papaioannou T: Excimer laser angioplasty: From basic science to clinical trials, in Moore WS, Ahn SS (eds): *Endovascular Surgery*. Philadelphia, Saunders, 1989, pp 432–441.
24. Nordstrom LA: Argon laser assisted angioplasty: One-year followup results in peripheral arteries and initial coronary experience abstracted. *Biotronics* 1989; March.
25. Leon MB, Deuek PC, Geschwind HJ, et al: Fluorescence-guided laser assisted balloon angioplasty in peripheral vascular disease, in Moore WB, Ahn SS (eds): *Endovascular Surgery*. 2d edn. Philadelphia, Saunders, 1992, pp 396–405.
26. Simpson JB, Selman MR, Robertson GC, et al: Transluminal atherectomy for occlusive peripheral vascular disease. *J Am Coll Cardiol* 1988; 61:96–101.
27. Polnitz A, Nerlich A, Berger H, et al: Percutaneous peripheral atherectomy: Angiographic and clinical followup of 60 patients. *J Am Coll Cardiol* 1990; 682–688.
28. Whittemore AD: The Kensey catheter: Indications, technique, results and complications, in Moore WB, Ahn SS (eds): *Endovascular Surgery*. Philadelphia, Saunders, 1989, pp 323–326.
29. Snyder SO, Wheeler JR, Gregory RT, et al: Kensey catheter: Early results with a transluminal endarterectomy tool. *J Vasc Surg* 1988; 8:541–543.
30. Ahn S, Eton D: The rotoblator–high-speed rotary atherectomy: Indications, technique, results, and complications, in Moore WS, Ahn SS (eds): *Endovascular Surgery*. Philadelphia, Saunders, 1992, pp 295–307.
31. Sigwart U, Puel J, Mirkowitch V, et al: Intravascular stents to prevent occlusion and restenosis after transluminal angioplasty. *N Engl J Med* 1987; 316:701–706.
32. Gunther RE, Vorwerk D, Bohndorf K: Iliac and femoral artery stenosis and occlusions. Treatment with intravascular stents. *Radiology* 1989; 173:725–730.
33. Rousseau H, Puel J, Joffre F, et al: Self-expanding endovascular prosthesis and experimental study. *Radiology* 1987; 164:709–714.
34. Palmaz JC, Richter GM, Noeldge G, et al: Intraluminal stents in atherosclerotic iliac artery stenosis: Preliminary report of a multicenter study. *Radiology* 1988; 168:727–731.
35. Strecker EP, Lierman D, Barth KH, et al: Expandable, tubular, tantalum stents for treatment of atherosclerotic iliac and femoropopliteal occlusive disease, abstracted. *Biotronics* 1989; March: 33.

Chapter 32

Modern Diagnostic and Therapeutic Thoracoscopy

Randolph M. Kessler

Since the early years of modern thoracic surgery, thoracoscopy has played a role in the diagnosis and treatment of diseases of the chest.[1] Widespread use of endoscopy, in general, followed application of the Edison light bulb to the cystoscope in 1883. Jacobaeus[2] proposed use of the cystoscope for investigation of "serous cavities" in 1910. Although he first used the technique primarily for diagnostic purposes, in 1922, he reported 40 cases of lysis of pleural adhesions to promote artificial pneumothorax in patients with pulmonary tuberculosis. For the next 30 years, the thoracoscope was widely used for pneumonolysis in tuberculosis patients. After effective antibiotics for tuberculosis were developed, use of the thoracoscope waned considerably. In the 1960s, there were only scattered reports of thoracoscopy for evaluation of pleural diseases.[3] However, in 1973, DeCamp and associates,[4] from the Ochsner Clinic, reviewed 126 patients with pleural effusions who had undergone thoracoscopy for diagnostic purposes.

From the time of Jacobeus, who used the thoracoscope primarily as a therapeutic tool for patients with tuberculosis, until very recently, thoracoscopy was employed almost entirely as a diagnostic instrument.[5] During the past few years, there have been increasing numbers of reports about the use of thoracoscopy as a therapeutic modality.[6–9] Included among these are descriptions of thoracoscopy for ablation of pleural blebs, pleurodesis, sympathectomy for hyperhidrosis, drainage and debridement of empyema, hemostasis for traumatic hemorrhage, resection of pulmonary masses, and transthoracic vagotomy, to name a few.

Recent advances in instrumentation have markedly expanded the diagnostic and therapeutic potentials of thoracoscopy. In particular, improvements in optical qualities of video endoscopy, introduction of endoscopic stapling and suturing devices, and the development of other endoscopic instruments, such as needle holders, dissectors, forceps, and irrigation–suction devices, have significantly improved the capability of performing a wide variety of thoracoscopic surgical procedures.

EQUIPMENT

Rigid direct-viewing thoracoscopes have been available for many years and are still useful in simple procedures, such as pleural biopsies and evaluation of pleural effusions.[10,11] The most convenient of these have an offset eyepiece, which allows introduction of instruments through the scope without obscuring vision.[12] Radigan and Glover[13] advocated using a standard rigid sigmoidoscope for thoracoscopic procedures. For very simple procedures, however, a mediastinoscope or rigid laryngoscope passed through an intercostal stab wound will suffice.[14] Exploration can be enhanced by passing a flexible bronchoscope through a rigid endoscope.[15–16]

Renewed interest in thoracoscopy is largely a result of the development of video endoscopic equipment; visualization has been markedly improved, thereby rendering procedures both easier and safer. For most procedures, an end-viewing (0°) 10-mm rigid endoscope, to which can be attached a high-resolution video camera and light source, provides excellent visualization. Occasionally, an angled (30° or 45°) endoscope is useful in procedures requiring visualization around corners or into the various recesses of the chest cavity. Five-millimeter endoscopes are available and are used primarily in pediatric patients. Endoscopic equipment used in the chest is identical to that used for laparoscopic procedures. Dual video monitors positioned on both sides of the patient and toward the head of the bed allow easy visualization by the operator and assistant (Fig. 32-1). Optional console equipment includes a carbon dioxide insufflation device and a video cassette recorder machine (VCR). For most procedures, adequate collapse of the lung is provided by bronchial intubation with a double-lumen endotracheal tube, and additional collapse of the lung by CO_2 insufflation is not necessary. Use of the VCR allows us to review the course of a procedure and to document gross anatomic findings, both of which are particularly advantageous in teaching settings.

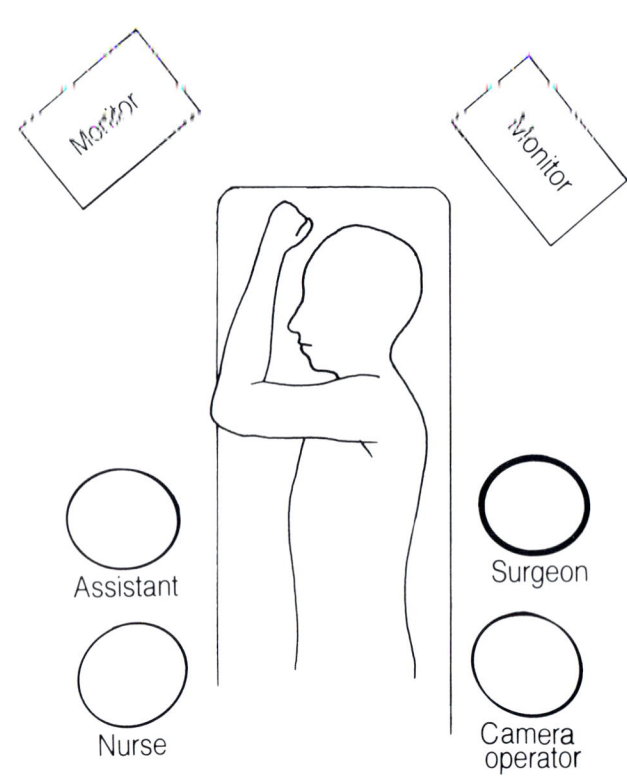

FIGURE 32-1 For most procedures, the patient is placed in a full lateral decubitus position, with surgeon, assistants, and monitors positioned as shown.

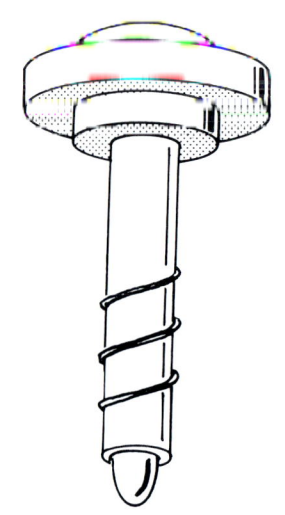

FIGURE 32-2 Disposable ports designed specifically for thoracoscopy (Auto Suture, Norwalk, CT).

The endoscope and instruments are usually introduced through disposable ports. These differ from laparoscopic trocars in that they are shorter, contain no valves, and come with a blunt stylet (Fig. 32-2). Most hand instruments, such as scissors, forceps, and dissectors, fit through 5-mm ports. The 10-mm scope will pass through a 10-mm port, as will most clip appliers. Currently, available stapler devices require a 12-mm port or greater. Adapters are available to convert large-diameter ports to smaller diameters, thus avoiding the need for frequent port changes. However, in most procedures, a tight seal around the instrument is unnecessary. Successful performance of the procedure is not dependent upon positive intrathoracic pressure if lung collapse has been attained by bronchial intubation.

Currently, the range of available endoscopic instruments is expanding at an extremely rapid rate. Most hand instruments are available in disposable (one-time use) or reusable form. Included are a wide variety of forceps, scissors, dissectors, retractors, and needle holders. A particularly useful device is a handle that attaches to an irrigation line, a suction tube, and an electrocautery unit. To this may be attached a variety of tips, with which the operator may dissect, irrigate, suction, or cauterize without removing the instrument from the chest to change modes. The use of disposable instruments is recommended until surgeons gain a realistic perspective on the devices best suited for their practices and operating styles.

Endoscopic clip appliers and stapling devices are invaluable for many thoracoscopic procedures, particularly because suturing and suture ligating are both cumbersome and time consuming. The design and variety of these will undergo significant change in the near future. Currently, single- and multi-fire endoscopic clip appliers are available. Staplers vary from single-staple devices, originally designed for endoscopic hernia repair, to devices that will cut between two double or triple rows of staples 30 or 60 mm in length (Endo-GIA, Auto Suture, Norwalk, CT). Staples have been designed for both vascular and nonvascular use.

Special sutures have been developed to facilitate sewing and knot tying in endoscopic procedures. These include loops, which can be used as ligatures, and sutures with needles of various shapes and sizes. These are designed to allow extracorporeal knot tying and cinching of knots using a knot-sliding device. Although they may be of use in selected thoracic procedures, with the availability of well-designed, effective clip appliers and stapling devices, most thoracoscopic procedures can be performed without resorting to cumbersome and time-consuming suture techniques.

TECHNIQUE OF THORACOSCOPY

Video endoscopy has markedly improved visualization within the chest cavity to the point that, in most circumstances, visualization is better than that obtained with thoracotomy. Video endoscopy has the advantages of magnification, excellent lighting, and the ability to access the entire chest cavity, including recesses difficult to expose by open thoracotomy. Because an assistant, who has the same visualization as the surgeon, can easily manipulate the endoscope, the surgeon's hands are free to operate, which is a distinct advantage over direct-viewing thoracoscopes that require the surgeon also to manipulate the scope.

Currently, the ideal technique for thoracoscopy includes general anesthesia with double-lumen endobronchial intubation and the use of modern video endoscopic equipment. Positioning of the endobronchial tube should be confirmed by careful auscultation and bronchoscopy because control of lung volume is paramount to a successful procedure. We believe that continuous blood pressure monitoring through an arterial catheter should be used in cases in which lung collapse is achieved primarily by insufflation.

For most procedures, a full lateral decubitus position is desirable because it allows the greatest area for port site placement and the best access to the entire hemithorax (see Fig. 32-1). This may be modified, as necessary, depending on the location of a particular lesion or the procedure to be performed. For example, excision of a nodule at the anteromedial surface of the lung may be best performed with the patient rotated 45° backward from the full decubitus position. The uppermost arm should be positioned well cephalad to allow access to the axilla, especially for procedures in the apical region of the chest cavity.

Insufflation may be necessary when endobronchial intubation is impossible, unsuccessful, or unsafe. It may also be useful at the beginning of the procedure to promote and expedite lung collapse and, thereby, avoid lung injury with initial introduction of ports and instruments. The most common situations in which insufflation is of value, if not essential, are: (1) in pediatric cases in which endobronchial intubation is not feasible or safe and (2) in the patient with respiratory failure in need of a lung biopsy who is already receiving mechanical ventilation and too ill to undergo single lung ventilation.

Special insufflating needles exist that have a retractable spring-loaded guard to protect against visceral puncture on entry (Veress needle), but these are not mandatory. An 18-gauge venipuncture catheter will suffice. Insufflation is accomplished using CO_2 instilled at high flow initially through a needle inserted carefully into the chest cavity. A maximum pressure of 10 mmHg must not be exceeded to avoid hemodynamic compromise from a *tension pneumothorax*. Because of this danger, continuous blood pressure monitoring is used in cases in which insufflation is the primary means of lung collapse. After instrument ports are introduced, the CO_2 insufflation line is attached to the side-arm stopcock of the port and insufflation continued. If insufflation is relied on for lung collapse, it is important to maintain a diligent port seal, guarding the chest cavity from atmospheric pressure during the procedure, to maintain satisfactory exposure.

Trocars or thoracoscopy ports are placed according to the procedure to be performed (Fig. 32-3). For most procedures, the endoscope port is placed near the midaxillary line for initial exploration and at approximately the fifth or sixth intercostal space. Most procedures require at least two additional instrument ports, which are typically placed one or two interspaces cephalad or caudal to the endoscopic port and near the anterior and posterior axillary lines. Most trocars are equipped with a removable stylet and a retractable spring-loaded sleeve guard to protect against visceral puncture.

The entry site is prepared by placing a 1-cm skin stab wound, dissecting the subcutaneous and muscular tissues, and entering the intrapleural space over the superior border of a rib with a blunt-nosed clamp. The intercostal muscles are spread with the clamp to accommodate the diameter of the port to be inserted. The port is then introduced through the already created intercostal defect, and the stylet is removed. If a thoracic wall screw anchor is used, the trocar is placed through it before insertion into the chest. The anchor is twisted into place across the chest wall and tightened to the port to prevent movement of the port in or out of the chest. Port lumens are guarded with a membrane or "trapdoor" seal to maintain constant intrathoracic pressure, an essential feature if insufflation is used. If insufflation is

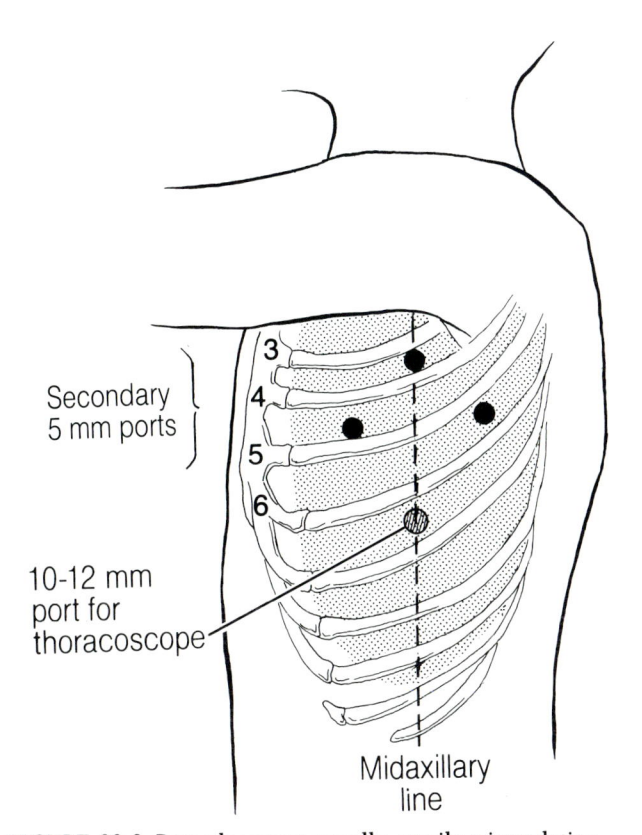

FIGURE 32-3 Port placement usually entails triangulating the instrument ports with respect to the thoracoscopic port. Secondary ports range from 5 mm to small incisions for introduction of standard surgical instruments.

not necessary, a system as simple as the screw anchor by itself allows repeated friction-free access to the chest.

The endoscope port is inserted after collapse of the ipsilateral lung is accomplished. The endoscope is connected to the light source and camera and then introduced through the port. Additional instrument stab wounds are made and ports introduced under direct vision. Adhesions are taken down, and the chest cavity is explored, as indicated. Fogging of the endoscope can be minimized by gently wiping it with a warm moist sponge.

At the end of the procedure, a chest tube should be placed in cases in which lung tissue has been frequently manipulated, retracted, or resected. The chest tube is inserted through one of the port sites and can be accurately placed under direct vision. Other port sites can be sutured closed, preferably in two layers, if a chest tube is not used. A chest tube can be omitted if the operator believes that there is no reason to suspect an air leak. If that is the case, the final stab wound is sutured and sealed with the lung fully expanded, and a chest radiograph is obtained in the early postoperative period.

DIAGNOSTIC PROCEDURES

Evaluation of Pleural Effusions and Masses

When routine thoracentesis has failed to identify the cause of a pleural effusion, thoracoscopy has proven to be diagnostic in more than 80 percent of cases.[17-24] Fluid can be aspirated under direct vision. The entire thoracic cavity is then examined, and suspicious pleural lesions are sampled. Most pleural masses can be easily identified and removed by excision or using bronchoscopic biopsy forceps.[25] Frozen sections are obtained so that, in the case of a malignant pleural effusion, chemical pleurodesis can be performed by instilling (under direct vision) 1 g of doxycycline mixed in 100 mL of normal saline.[26] Alternatively, talc insufflation can be used. However, sterile talc is not readily available and must be prepared by dry heat sterilization of commercial United States Pharmacopeia grade talc (125° for 12 h).

Lung Biopsy

Thoracic surgeons are frequently called on to obtain tissue for diagnosis in cases of respiratory failure as a result of infections or other diffuse parenchymal processes.[27-29] Thoracoscopic biopsy offers a distinct advantage over traditional open lung biopsy because these patients are frequently very ill, immunocompromised, or dependent on mechanical ventilation.[29,30] Usually, an expeditious thoracoscopic lung biopsy can be performed with minimal morbidity and with the added advantage of better visualization than that obtained by thoracotomy. If the intubated patient is too ill to undergo reintubation with an endobronchial tube and one lung ventilation, CO_2 insufflation should be used to promote just enough lung collapse for adequate visualization. A small segment of lung tissue is easily obtained with one or two firings of a stapling–cutting device. Hitomi and associates[31] of Kyoto University, Japan, have developed an ingenious *deep ligator* device specifically for thoracoscopic lung biopsy. Boutin and colleagues[28] advocate excising a small piece of lung with the cautery.

Biopsy of Pulmonary Nodules

Most pulmonary nodules, even when situated deep to the surface of the lung, can currently be easily excised using video endoscopy and endoscopic stapling devices (Fig. 32-4). Successful excision of nodules has also been obtained using precision electrocautery, the argon beam electrocoagulator, and the YAG laser.[32-34] These modalities can be effectively used under video endoscopic monitoring but are more time consuming and may provide less secure aerostasis than stapled excision.

The nodule situated deep to the visceral pleura may be difficult to localize. There are several techniques the surgeon may employ in this situation, including direct palpation with a finger inserted through a stab wound to be used as an instrument port. Through another port, a lung forceps may be inserted to bring the lung up to the palpating finger. Similarly, the lung can often be "palpated" between two lung forceps. For more deeply situated nodules, the radiologist's help may be enlisted for fine-needle localization, very similar to that used for breast masses.[35]

Considering the noninvasive nature, safety, ease, and effectiveness of endoscopic-assisted biopsy of lung nodules, this technique should largely replace attempts at fine-needle aspiration, except in the easily accessible nodule which is strongly suspected of being malignant.

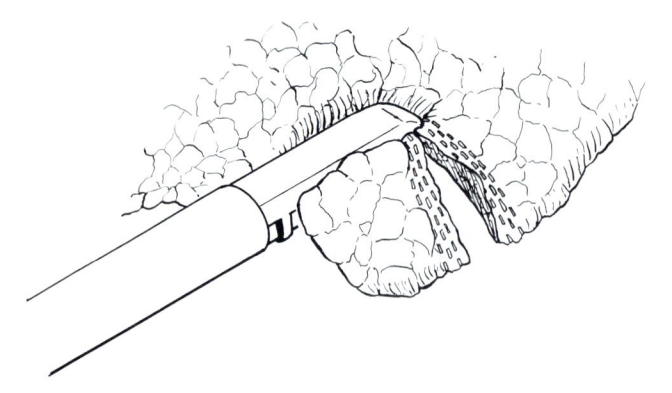

FIGURE 32-4 Lung biopsies and wedge resections are currently easily performed using endoscopic stapling devices that cut between three rows of staples.

Biopsy of Lymph Nodes and Other Mediastinal Masses

Essentially all lymph node stations accessible by thoracotomy can be evaluated by endoscopic-assisted biopsy. After incision of the overlying pleura, nodes can be removed using a combination of blunt, electrocautery, and sharp dissection. This is best performed using the versatile irrigation–suction–cautery–dissection device described earlier.

This technique is especially applicable to stations such as the aortopulmonary window and subcarina, which are not easily reached by mediastinoscopy. Many patients with lung cancer who previously required thoracotomy or anterior mediastinotomy to prove unresectability can be spared unnecessary pain and morbidity using thoracoscopic biopsy of suspicious mediastinal lymph nodes. In the poor-risk patient with lung cancer and limited pulmonary reserve, endoscopic lymph node dissection can be combined with minimal resection for complete staging.

Most mediastinal masses, regardless of location, can also be excised or sampled using video-assisted techniques. This is especially applicable when a malignancy, such as lymphoma, is suspected, which might be best managed by chemotherapy or irradiation.

Evaluation of Chest Trauma

Persistent moderate bleeding from chest tubes placed in an otherwise stable patient after chest trauma may be evaluated, and often treated, thoracoscopically.[36–37] The source is usually a disrupted intercostal vessel in the chest wall.

Thoracoscopy may also be employed when there is uncertainty about a diagnosis of traumatic diaphragmatic hernia. This technique is best performed within 24 h of the injury, before the development of major adhesions.[38]

THERAPEUTIC PROCEDURES

Ablation of Blebs and Pleurodesis for Pneumothorax

Video endoscopy allows full visualization of the entire surface of the lung and, therefore, easy identification of blebs, and often air leaks, associated with spontaneous pneumothorax.[39–41] After initial lung deflation for entry, the lung should be evaluated during ventilation to identify blebs or air leaks which may not be obvious with the lung deflated. This is accomplished by having the anesthesiologist institute controlled ventilation by *hand bagging* to the maximum tidal volumes that still allow adequate visualization. Identification of air leaks can be facilitated by irrigating saline over the surface of the lung.

Small blebs (less than 1 cm) can be easily ablated using a spatula tip to apply electrocautery with a coagulating current at moderate power output. The bleb will turn pale, shrink, and contract. Others have advocated ligation of blebs using an Endoloop ligature (Ethicon, Somerville, NJ).[39] Larger blebs, clusters of blebs, or air leak sites are best excised with an endoscopic stapling device. Alternatively, blebs can be ablated or excised using CO_2 or YAG lasers or the argon beam coagulator,[42–46] although it may be difficult to justify the added equipment, time, and expense, considering the effectiveness of electrocautery and stapled ablation.

Pleurodesis is promoted by stimulating an intense pleural inflammatory process. There are a number of techniques available for this, and we usually employ a combination. The electrocautery can be used over both parietal and visceral pleurae, especially in the apical regions. We routinely perform an apical pleurectomy of the parietal pleura and cauterize the apical surface of the visceral pleura.

At the conclusion of the procedure, chemical pleurodesis can be produced under direct vision to ensure distribution of the agent over the entire surface of the lung. In the past, the intravenous form of tetracycline (currently no longer produced) was used. Because some individuals had adverse reactions to the procaine in the intramuscular form of tetracycline, it should be avoided. Doxycycline has approximately the same acidic pH (2.0) as tetracycline, and this is believed to be responsible for the pleurodesis effect.[26] Clinically, doxycycline has been shown to be equally efficacious as tetracycline. We usually instill 1 g of doxycycline mixed in 100 mL of saline.

The argon beam electrocoagulator device has also been used over the pleural surfaces as an alternative to standard electrocautery to stimulate pleurodesis. It has the advantage of a more uniform distribution of injury, with perhaps less tissue destruction than the standard electrocautery.

Although endoscopic management of pneumothorax and blebs has yet to be fully evaluated, there is no reason to believe it would be less effective than when performed by thoracotomy, assuming adequate ablation of blebs and effective stimulation of pleurodesis. Because of the significant reduction in time, pain, and morbidity with thoracoscopic versus thoracotomy management of spontaneous pneumothorax, consideration should be given to expanding the indications for thoracoscopic intervention. In this regard, we routinely recommend it for all second occurrences and offer it as an option for all first occurrences.

Similar techniques can be applied to management of persistent pneumothoraces of other causes. Included among these would be postsurgical, traumatic, infectious (e.g., from *Pneumocystis carinii*), and emphysematous pneumothoraces.

Resection of Lung Nodules and Mediastinal Masses

Lung nodules and mediastinal masses can be resected as described earlier. When performed for benign neoplasms, the procedure also may be considered therapeutic. Lung cancers should be managed by formal resection and lymph node dissection whenever possible; that is, the approach and degree of resection should not be altered by thoracoscopic capabilities. Techniques and instrumentation are currently available for thoracoscopic segmentectomy, lobectomy, or pneumonectomy; we are restricted primarily by our ability to remove the specimen. Some surgeons are now performing video-assisted resections through limited thoracotomies. As major hemorrhage cannot be easily controlled, such procedures should be undertaken only by a very experienced thoracoscopist and after adequate laboratory trials. For the patient with limited pulmonary reserve and a small peripheral lung cancer, who otherwise would undergo thoracotomy for wedge resection, thoracoscopic wedge resection and lymph node dissection should be considered.

Pericardial Window and Pericardiocentesis

Thoracoscopy provides an excellent approach for diagnosis and drainage of pericardial effusions. For diagnosis, it may provide a safer option over subxiphoid blind pericardiocentesis because it can be performed under direct vision. If there is any concern about recurrence, a segment of pericardium can easily be excised from the left side, taking care to avoid phrenic nerve injury, thus allowing drainage into the left pleural space where fluid can be absorbed. Similarly, it offers a good alternative to a subxiphoid pericardial window for therapeutic drainage of benign or malignant pericardial effusions. Infected effusions are better drained by a subxiphoid approach to avoid contamination of the pleural space.

Transthoracic Vagotomy

The individual who has undergone a peptic ulcer operation or gastrojejunostomy and has ulceration because of incomplete vagotomy may be a good candidate for thoracoscopic vagotomy. Both vagus trunks can be exposed after release of the left inferior pulmonary ligament and mobilization of the distal esophagus from a left-sided approach (Fig. 32-5). Segments of both nerves are excised between hemoclips.

Sympathectomy

When sympathectomy is indicated for refractory cases of reflex sympathetic dystrophy, hyperhidrosis, or Raynaud's phenomenon, the procedure can easily be performed endoscopically.[47,48] Before performing endoscopic sympathectomy, satisfactory response to stellate ganglion block should first be demonstrated.

The approach is through the second or third interspace at approximately the anterior axillary line. The sympathetic

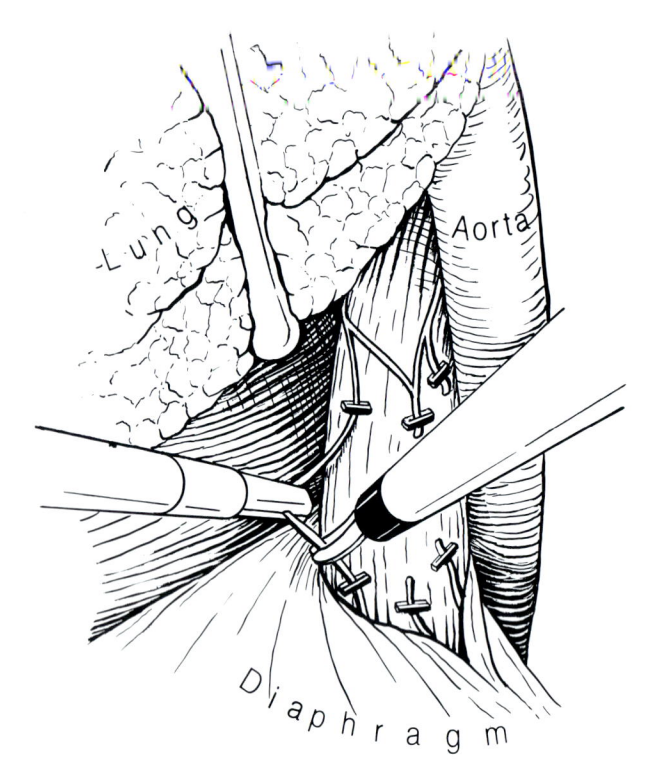

FIGURE 32-5 Thoracoscopic vagotomy. Note that there may be several communicating branches between anterior and posterior trunks above the hiatus.

chain is located and mobilized high in the paravertebral region (Fig. 32-6). There may be one or two stellate ganglia overlying the neck of the first rib, often behind the takeoff of the subclavian artery. The sympathetic trunk is divided sharply, no higher than the inferior border of the inferior stellate ganglion. A 2-cm segment is excised, the caudal limit being approximately the T4 ganglion. The complication of Horner's syndrome can be avoided by minimizing dissection, avoiding use of the electrocautery, and dividing below the inferior stellate ganglion.

Esophageal Myotomy

A modified Heller esophageal myotomy can be performed through the left chest in cases of achalasia in which balloon dilatation has failed, or as an alternative to dilatation. The lung is retracted in a cephalad direction, and the inferior pulmonary ligament is incised up to the inferior pulmonary vein. The pleura overlying the distal esophagus is incised and retracted. A longitudinal esophageal myotomy is then performed from approximately 2 mm beyond the gastroesophageal junction to approximately 5 or 7 cm cephalad. Further dissection onto the gastric wall is avoided to prevent postoperative gastroesophageal reflux. This is done by carefully lifting the muscle and sharply incising until the mucosa is seen to bulge out. The muscle is then dissected laterally in both directions to allow full bulging of the

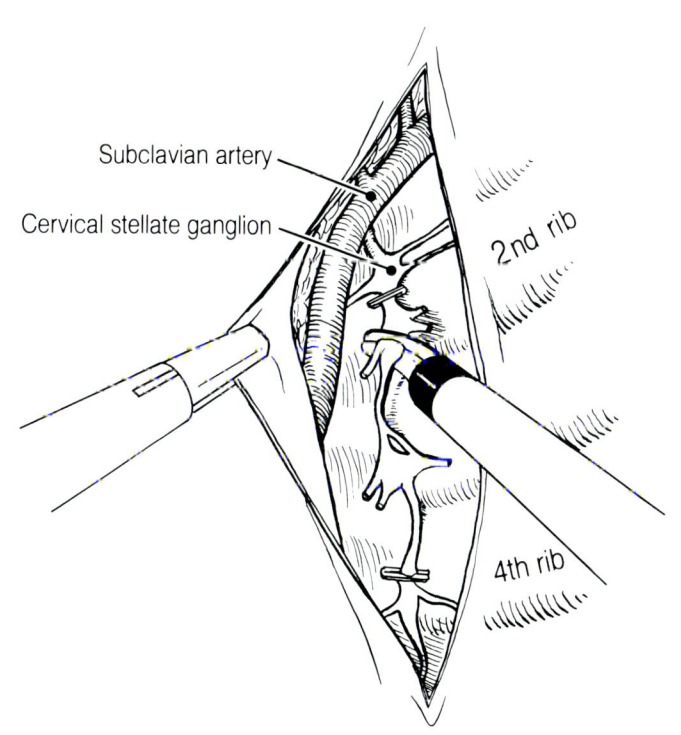

FIGURE 32-6 Thoracoscopic sympathectomy. Note that the upper level of the division must be below the level of the cervical portion of the stellate ganglion to avoid the complication of Horner's syndrome.

mucosa (Fig. 32-7). Care is taken to avoid injury to the vagus nerves.

Again, there are no reports about the effectiveness of this procedure performed endoscopically, but there is every reason to expect good results similar to those obtained with standard thoracotomy.

Decortication and Drainage of Empyema

Ridley and associates[49] and Hutter and colleagues[50] have reported a combined experience of 30 patients with thoracic empyema treated with thoracoscopic debridement and drainage followed by continuous irrigation of the pleural space. Sixty percent of their patients achieved complete resolution, considerably less than we would expect with open thoracotomy and decortication. However, in the case of an early loculated empyema, in which an organized peel has not developed, thoracoscopy for breaking down loculations and guided drainage of entrapped fluid should be considered. If a thick infected peel is encountered, the surgeon should proceed with formal decortication using thoracotomy.

FUTURE APPLICATIONS

With continued refinements in instrumentation and increased operator experience and ingenuity, it is conceivable that virtually any thoracic procedure will have the potential of being performed thoracoscopically.[51] Included among these will be formal pulmonary resections with or without complete mediastinal lymph node dissection, antireflux procedures, repair of diaphragmatic hernias, and resection of esophageal tumors. Thoracoscopy should enhance the safety and exposure for nonthoracotomy blunt esophagectomies.[52] There have been isolated reports or mention of using endoscopic procedures for spinal diskectomies and drainage of disk space abscesses.[53] Patients with pericardial adhesions from previous operations who are in need of automatic internal cardiodefibrillator devices may have the patches placed thoracoscopically along with transvenous sensing lead placement. Epicardial pacemaker leads could similarly be easily and safely positioned.[54] Shirai and associates[55] have recently reported a case of post-pneumonectomy chylothorax treated with thoracoscopic application of fibrin glue. In addition, Hutter and colleagues[56] presented a case of esophageal perforation treated successfully with thoracoscopic irrigation and drainage in a 51-year-old man. Ligation of a patent ductus arteriosus could be performed thoracoscopically by careful dissection and application of clips or ligatures. With the use of percutaneous cardiopulmonary bypass, an internal thoracic artery anastomosis to a left anterior descending artery is conceivable!

CONCLUSION

The advent of new endoscopic equipment, originally developed for abdominal procedures, promises to generate renewed interest in thoracoscopy for both diagnostic and therapeutic applications. Video endoscopy has literally freed the hand and eye of the surgeon, allowing visualization and manipulation of tissues beyond that previously imaginable with older direct-vision endoscopes. Simultaneously, instruments have been developed to allow bimanual dissection and suturing under video endoscopic monitoring. Very recently, stapling devices, clip appliers, and combined suction–irrigation–cautery–dissection devices have been introduced, further expanding the potential of endoscopic surgery. Several groups have reported extensive use of thoracoscopy in pediatric patients.[57–60]

The obvious advantage of endoscopic surgery in the chest is avoiding a painful thoracotomy incision with its attendant morbidity. Acute and chronic pain, loss of pulmonary function, upper extremity weakness, and occasional paraplegia are well-known complications of thoracotomy incisions. In addition, blood loss, wound infections, and unsatisfactory cosmetic results might be expected to increase in patients undergoing thoracotomy rather than thoracoscopy, although this remains to be proved. Another less obvious advantage of thoracoscopy over thoracotomy is its well-illuminated magnified visualization over virtually

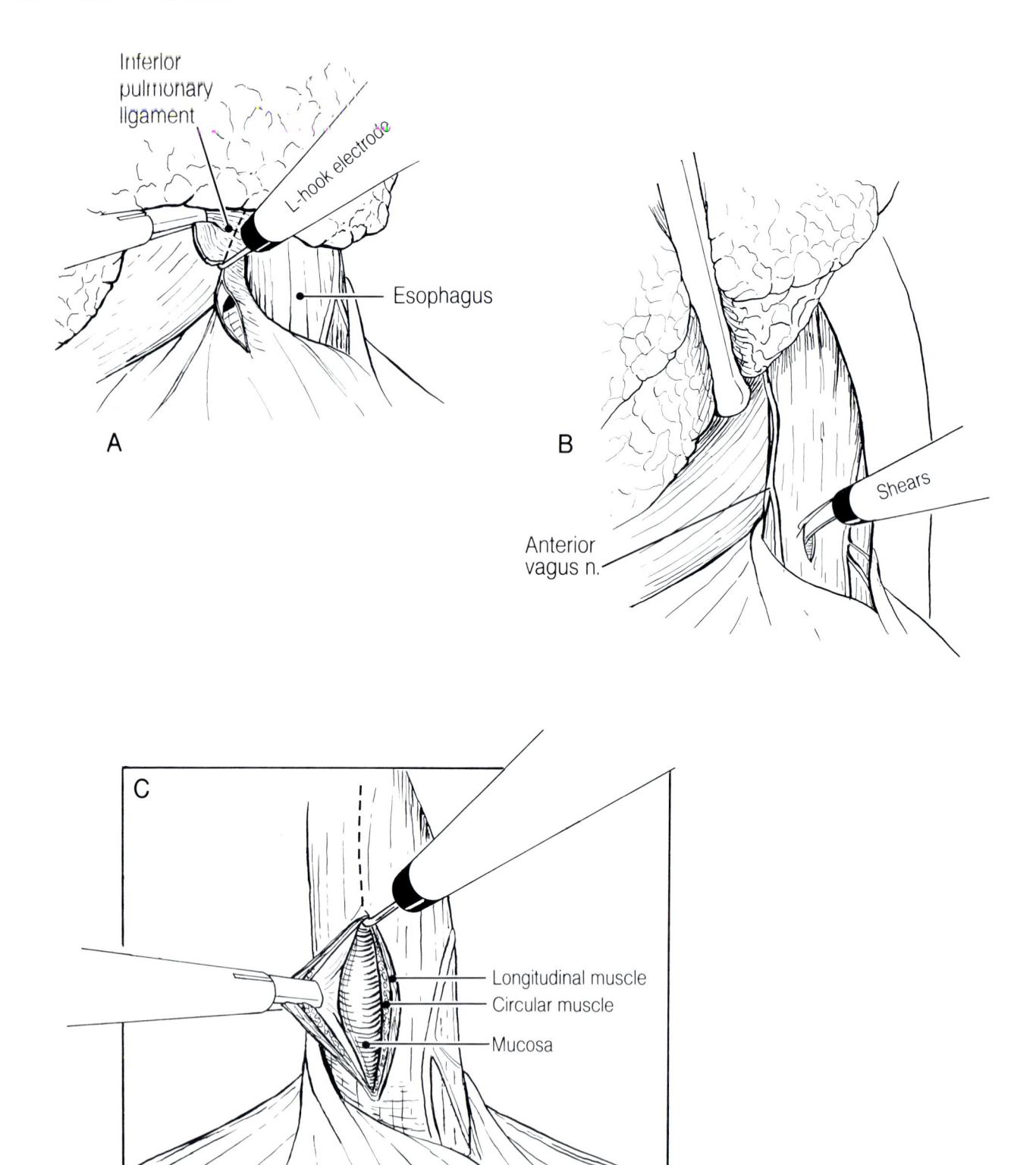

FIGURE 32-7 Thoracoscopic esophageal myotomy. A. The inferior pulmonary ligament is taken down to the level of the inferior pulmonary vein. B. The lung is retracted cephalad with a blunt rod or lung retractor, and the myotomy is initiated with blunt-nosed scissors. C. The longitudinal and circular smooth muscle is retracted away from the mucosa and divided with monopolar or bipolar electrocautery.

the entire chest cavity, especially when performed with full collapse of the lung.

There are, however, distinct disadvantages of thoracoscopy, which must be weighed in the enthusiasm over this technique. Perhaps foremost among these is the inability to palpate the lung and other tissues manually, a source of potential error and frustration for the surgeon accustomed to relying on tactile information for decision making. This is especially problematic in evaluating potential pulmonary metastases in patients with malignancies, in which case excision of all metastatic lesions holds some promise for improved survival. It has been our experience that small and more deeply situated lung masses can be easily missed with thoracoscopic exploration. In adddition, thoracoscopic procedures involving a considerable degree of dissection or suturing are often more time consuming than the same procedure performed by thoracotomy. This may change as the learning curve is traversed. Another potential problem with thoracoscopic procedures involving manipulation or dissection around major vascular structures is the lack of immediate control in the event of sudden severe hemorrhage.

Based on our experience, modern thoracoscopy has proved to be a safe, effective procedure for diagnosis and treatment of a variety of thoracic conditions. It is predicted that, as experience with the procedure grows and as instrumentation is perfected and standardized, many thoracic procedures previously requiring thoracotomy will routinely be done by a thoracoscopic approach.

REFERENCES

1. Bloomberg AE: Thoracoscopy in perspective. *Surg Gynecol Obstet* 1978; 147:434–443.
2. Jacobaeus HC: The practical importance of thoracoscopy in surgery of the chest. *Surg Gynecol Obstet* 1922; 34:289–296.
3. Hatch HB Jr, DeCamp PT: Diagnostic thoracoscopy. *Surg Clin North Am* 1966; 46:1405–1410.
4. De Camp PT, Moseley PW, Scott ML, et al: Diagnostic thoracoscopy. *Ann Thorac Surg* 1973; 16:79–84.
5. Poulos C, Ponn R, Tranquilli M, et al: Thoracoscopy for diagnosis of chest disease. *Conn Med* 1988; 52:201–202.
6. Page RD, Jeffrey RR, Donelly RJ: Thoracoscopy: A review of 121 consecutive surgical procedures. *Ann Thorac Surg* 1989; 48:66–68.
7. Weisberg D, Kaufman M: Diagnostic and therapeutic pleuroscopy: Experience with 127 patients. *Chest* 1980; 78:732–735.
8. Kaiser LR: Diagnostic and therapeutic uses of pleuroscopy (thoracoscopy) in lung cancer. *Surg Clin North Am* 1987; 67:1081–1086.
9. Oakes DD, Sherck JP, Brodsky JB, et al: Therapeutic thoracoscopy. *J Thorac Cardiovasc Surg* 1984; 87:269–273.
10. Oldenburg FA Jr, Newhouse MT: Thoracoscopy: A safe, accurate, diagnostic procedure using the rigid thoracoscope and local anesthesia. *Chest* 1979; 75:45–50.
11. Ash SR, Manfredi F: Directed biopsy using a small endoscope: Thoracoscopy and peritoneoscopy simplified. *N Engl J Med* 1974; 291:1398–1399.
12. Sang CT, Braimbridge MV: Thoracoscopy simplified using the laparoscope. *Thorac Cardiovasc Surg* 1981; 29:129–130.
13. Radigan LR, Glover JL: Thoracoscopy. *Surgery* 1977; 82:425–428.
14. Lewis RJ, Kunderman PJ, Sisler GE, et al: Direct diagnostic thoracoscopy. *Ann Thorac Surg* 1976; 21:536–539.
15. Ben-Isaac FE, Simmons DH: Flexible fiberoptic pleuroscopy: Pleural and lung biopsy. *Chest* 1975; 67:573–576.
16. Senno A, Moallem S, Quijano ER, et al: Thoracoscopy with the fiberoptic bronchoscope: A simple method in diagnosing pleuropulmonary diseases. *J Thorac Cardiovasc Surg* 1974; 67:606–611.
17. Hucker J, Bhatnagar NK, Al-Jilaihawi AN, et al: Thoracoscopy in the diagnosis and management of recurrent pleural effusions. *Ann Thorac Surg* 1991; 52:1145–1147.
18. Weisberg D, Kaufman M, Yurkowski Z: Pleuroscopy in patients with pleural effusion and pleural masses. *Ann Thorac Surg* 1980; 29:205–207.
19. Boutin C, Astoul P, Seitz B: The role of thoracoscopy in the evaluation and management of pleural effusions. *Lung* 1990; 168(suppl):1113–1121.
20. Menzies R, Charbonneau M: Thoracoscopy for the diagnosis of pleural disease. *Ann Intern Med* 1991; 114:271–276.
21. Canto A, Ferrer G, Romagosa V, et al: Lung cancer and pleural effusion: Clinical significance and study of pleural metastatic locations. *Chest* 1985; 87:649–652.
22. Rusch VW, Mountain C: Thoracoscopy under regional anesthesia for the diagnosis and management of pleural disease. *Am J Surg* 1987; 154:274–278.
23. Baumgartner WA, Jark JB: The use of thoracoscopy in the diagnosis of pleural disease. *Arch Surg* 1980; 115:420–421.
24. Canto A, Blasco E, Casillas M, et al: Thoracoscopy in the diagnosis of pleural effusion. *Thorax* 1977; 32:550–554.
25. Krasna M, Flowers JL: Diagnostic thoracoscopy in a patient with a pleural mass. *Surg Laparosc Endosc* 1991; 1:947.
26. Mansson T: Treatment of malignant pleural effusion with doxycycline. *Scand J Infect Dis Suppl* 1988; 53:29–34.
27. Dijkman JH, van der Meer JW, Bakker W, et al: Transpleural lung biopsy by the thoracoscopic route in patients with diffuse interstitial pulmonary disease. *Chest* 1982; 82:76–83.
28. Boutin C, Viallat JR, Cargnino P: Thoracoscopic lung biopsy: Experimental and clinical preliminary study. *Chest* 1982; 82:44–48.
29. Thomas PA Jr: Diagnostic lung biopsy in the immunocompromised patient. *J Thorac Cardiovasc Surg* 1980; 79:471–472.
30. Rodgers BM, Moazam F, Talbert JL: Thoracoscopy: Early diagnosis of interstitial pneumonitis in the immunologically suppressed child. *Chest* 1979; 75:126–130.
31. Hitomi S, Tamada J, Ikeda S, et al: Thoracoscopic lung biopsy using tissue adhesive material and/or deep ligator. *Chest* 1984; 86:155.
32. Rusch VW, Schmidt R, Shoji Y, et al: Use of the argon beam electrocoagulator for pulmonary wedge resections. *Ann Thorac Surg* 1990; 43:287–291.
33. Cooper JD, Pearlman M, Todd TJ Jr, et al: Precision cautery excision of pulmonary lesions. *Ann Thorac Surg* 1986; 41:51–63.
34. Landreneau RJ, Herlan DB, Johnson JA, et al: Thoracoscopic neodymium: yttrium-aluminum garnet laser-assisted pulmonary resection. *Ann Thorac Surg* 1991; 52:1176–1178.
35. Kopans DB, Meyer JE: Versatile spring hookwire breast lesion localizer. *AJR Am J Roentgenol* 1982; 138:586–587.
36. Jones JW, Kitahama A, Webb WR, et al: Emergency thoracoscopy: A logical approach to chest trauma management. *J Trauma* 1981; 21:280–284.
37. Jackson AM, Ferreira AA: Thoracoscopy as an aid to the diagnosis of diaphragmatic injury in penetrating wounds of the left lower chest: A preliminary report. *Injury* 1979; 7:213–217.

38. Adamthwaite DN: Traumatic diaphragmatic hernia. Surg Annu 1983; 15:73–97
39. Nathanson LK, Shimi SM, Wood RAB, et al: Videothoracoscopic ligation of bulla and pleurectomy for spontaneous pneumothorax. Ann Thorac Surg 1991; 52:316–319.
40. Vanderschueren RG: The role of thoracoscopy in the evaluation and management of pneumothorax. Lung 1990; 168(suppl): 1122–1125.
41. Verschool AC, Ten Velde GP, Greve LH, et al: Thoracoscopic pleurodesis in the management of spontaneous pneumothorax. Respiration 1988; 53:197–200.
42. Locicero J, Frederiksen JW, Hartz RS, et al: Experimental air leaks in lung sealed by low energy carbon dioxide laser irradiation. Chest 1985; 87:820–822.
43. Locicero J, Hartz RS, Frederikson JW, et al: New applications of the laser in pulmonary surgery: Hemostasis and sealing of air leaks. Ann Thorac Surg 1985; 40:546–550.
44. Wakabayashi A: Thoracoscopic ablation of blebs in the treatment of recurrent or persistent spontaneous pneumothorax. Ann Thorac Surg 1989; 48:651–653.
45. Torre M, Belloni P: YAG laser pleurodesis through thoracoscopy: New curative therapy in spontaneous pneumothorax. Ann Thorac Surg 1989; 47:887–889.
46. Wakabayashi A, Brenner M, Wilson AF, et al: Thoracoscopic treatment of spontaneous pneumothorax using carbon dioxide laser. Ann Thorac Surg 1990; 50:786–790.
47. Milewski PJ, Hodgson SP, Higham A: Transthoracic endoscopic sympathectomy. J R Coll Surg Edinb 1985; 30:221–223.
48. Kux M: Thoracic endoscopic sympathectomy in palmar and axillary hyperhidrosis. Arch Surg 1978; 13:264–266.
49. Ridley PD, Brambridge MV: Thoracoscopic debridement and pleural irrigation in the management of empyema thoracis. Ann Thorac Surg 1991; 51:161–161.
50. Hutter JA, Harari D, Braimbridge MV. The management of empyema thoracis by thoracoscopy and irrigation. Ann Thorac Surg 1985; 39:517–520.
51. Miller J: Therapeutic thoracoscopy: New horizons for an established procedure. Ann Thorac Surg 1991; 52:1036–1037.
52. Leahy PF, Pennino RP, Hinshow JR, et al: Minimally invasive esophagogastrectomy: An approach to esophagogastrectomy through the left thorax. J Laparoendosc Surg 1990; 1:53–62.
53. Obenchain TG: Laparoscopic lumber discectomy: Case report. J Laparosc Surg 1991; 1:145–149.
54. Beaulieu M, Despres JP, Benichou J, et al: Xiphoid mediastinoscopy for permanent myocardial implantation of a modified electrode: Preliminary report. J Thorac Cardiovasc Surg 1971; 61:968–974.
55. Shirai T, Amano J, Takabe K: Thoracoscopic diagnosis and treatment of chylothorax after pneumonectomy. Ann Thorac Surg 1991; 52:306–307.
56. Hutter JA, Fenn A, Braimbridge MV: The management of spontaneous esophageal perforation by thoracoscopy and irrigation. Ann Thorac Surg 1985; 39:517–520.
57. Janik JS, Nagaraj HS, Groff DB: Thoracoscopic evaluation of intrathoracic lesions in children. J Thorac Cardiovasc Surg 1982; 83:408–413.
58. Ryckman FC, Rodgers BM: Thoracoscopy for intrathoracic neoplasia in children. J Pediatr Surg 1982; 17:521–524.
59. Rodgers BM, Ryckman FC, Moazam F, et al: Thoracoscopy for intrathoracic tumors. Ann Thorac Surg 1981; 31:414–420.
60. Rodgers BM, Moazam F, Talbert JL: Thoracoscopy in children. Ann Surg 1979; 89:176–180.

Chapter 33

High Tech Surgery: Speculation on Future Directions*

Richard M. Satava

Predicting the future trends in any profession jeopardizes the credibility of the author. Few persons would have given credence to laparoscopic cholecystectomy as little as 3 years ago; yet this book is a testimonial to the way laparoscopic procedures have revolutionized the practice of surgery. Interestingly, all of the technologies involved in laparoscopic surgery are at least 10 to 20 years old. Gynecologists have been routinely performing laparoscopy for decades, video cameras were available in the late 1970s, and video endoscopy was introduced by Sivak and associates[1] in 1984. Many of the laparoscopic instruments are traditional or modified urologic and gynecologic instruments. It is evident that the current revolution has been under our noses for years. The critical factor was not inventing a new technology, but recognizing those relevant advanced technologies and combining them for a specific surgical application. Few, if any, medical advances have come from pure medical research; most have been derived from academia, business (computers), industry (aerospace), and government.

There are two categories of technology to investigate: parallel and convergent. Parallel technologies solve similar problems with the same technology, such as when cardiologists and plumbers both use *roto-rooters*. Convergent technologies use different solutions for a common problem, such as urologists who use lithotripsy or physicists who use lasers to disintegrate stones.

As an example of parallel technology, flexible fiberoptic endoscopy is derived from the aerospace industry where, in the early 1950s, the flexible fiberoptic boroscope was introduced to inspect the interior components of jet turbine engines for stress fractures and defects. Rather than having a maintenance technician spend hours tearing down, inspecting, and reassembling an engine, the fiberoptic boroscope was used to inspect the interior of engines for flaws. The instrument was subsequently converted to a video boroscope (then came the video endoscope), and now advanced research is focused on utilizing microrobots for the same purpose. In a letter to the editors of the *New England Journal of Medicine* in 1990, Fleischer[2] has expressed an incredibly perceptive concept (while applying it to *cloggology*) as follows: many of the medical and surgical disciplines are working on the same problem and share a common goal ". . . to establish flow in an occluded biologic cylinder." We must also recognize that many medical problems share a common denominator with nonmedical fields; the Alaskan oil pipe line has been inspected, unclogged, and repaired by robots for years. Not only do clogged coronary arteries, bronchus, colon, and ureter present a similar challenge, but this common problem (a clogged cylinder or pipe) is currently under aggressive research by oil companies, miners, plumbers, and space shuttle engineers.

Convergent technologies are best typified by the approach to common bile duct stones. Lasers developed in physics laboratories, chenodeoxycholic acid from the chemists, directed energy weapons (lithotripsy) from military research, and miniature instruments from mechanical engineers have all been adapted for removing biliary tract stones. For laparoscopic surgery, it was the convegence of video imaging, lasers, high-flow insufflation, and laparoscopy that provided the breakthrough. From these examples, it is apparent that there is an inherent critical principle. In this era where complex problems are conquered with high-technology solutions, it is essential to cultivate a broad perspective and become familiar with advanced technology in many disparate fields.

As with any innovation, after the initial blush of excitement, there is a careful analysis of the technology, which reveals many limitations and areas for improvement. For example, laparoscopic surgery begs for solutions; some of the more obvious areas are acquiring three-dimensional

---

*The opinions or assertions contained herein are the private views of the author and are not to be construed as official, or as reflecting the views of the Department of the Army or the Department of Defense.

vision, providing sensory feedback from the instruments to the surgeon, and improving the dexterity of the instruments. Surveying academia, government, and industry reveals that the answers to these limitations are already under vigorous pursuit. Among the vast number of directions of research, there are a few that appear to have particular potential for application to general surgical practice. Three of these (out of a multitide) are robotics and microrobotics, virtual reality and telepresence surgery and newer application of lasers.

ROBOTICS AND MICROROBOTICS

Robots have always held the imagination to replace human manual tasks by a machine that can more accurately, efficiently, and rapidly perform a task. The first of these robotic surgical machines to come on the clinical horizon is applied to artificial hip replacement (Fig. 33-1). Dr. R. H. Taylor of the International Business Machine Corp. T. J. Watson Research Center and Dr. H. A. Paul of the University of California at Davis[3] have developed a robotic device that is capable of extreme accuracy in coring the femoral shaft to accept a femoral prosthesis precisely, thereby dramatically increasing the precision of the femur–prosthesis interface and decreasing the play which results in the need for future replacement. Using CT scanning, the femur is precisely mapped to the prosthesis on the computer. This data is then fed to a robotic arm with an orthopedic drill, which actually performs the procedure by coring out the femur to match the size of the prosthesis precisely. Currently, this is being performed in routine veterinary practice for dogs while further research and certification is obtained.

The next-generation robots may come from the laboratory of Dr. Stephen Jacobsen of the University of Utah where the Utah/MIT dexterous hand (Fig. 33-2) brings dexterity, tactile sensation, and force feedback to the operator's hand.[4] Delicate tasks, such as replacing a light bulb without breaking it, demonstrates the level of dexterity and sensory input that has been achieved. In a parallel project at Dr. Jacobsen's laboratory, the dexterous telerobotic arm (Fig. 33-3) has pioneered multisensory input remote robotic manipulation. By inserting your arm and hand into the master exoskeleton, manipulation of a distant robotic arm

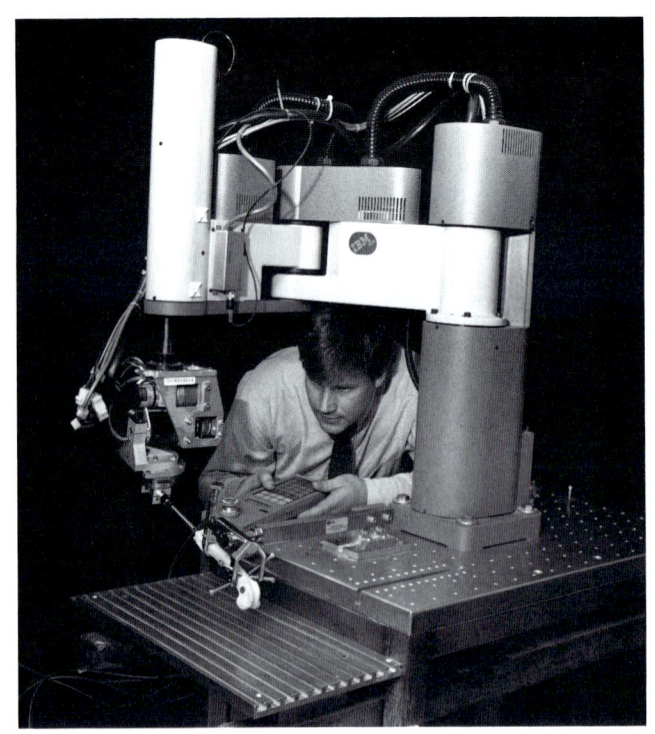

FIGURE 33-1 Robotic hip replacement. University of California at Davis graduate student Brent Mittelstadt tests "Robodoc" on a model thigh bone in the laboratory. (Courtesy of University of California, Davis School of Medicine.)

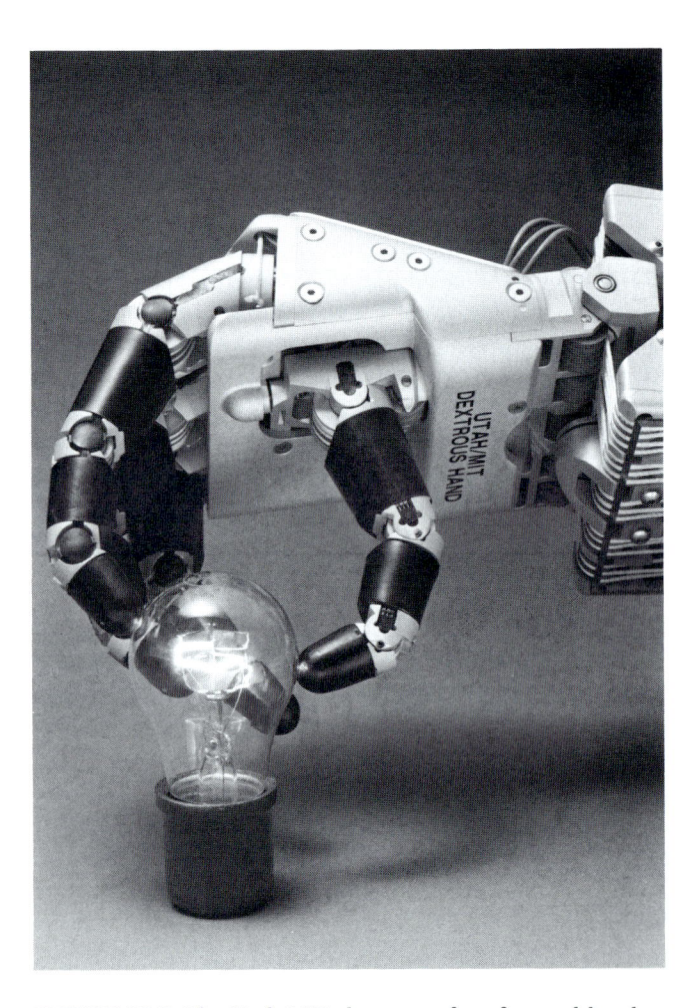

FIGURE 33-2 The Utah-MIT dexterous four-fingered hand. (Courtesy of S.C. Jacobsen, University of Utah, Salt Lake City, UT.)

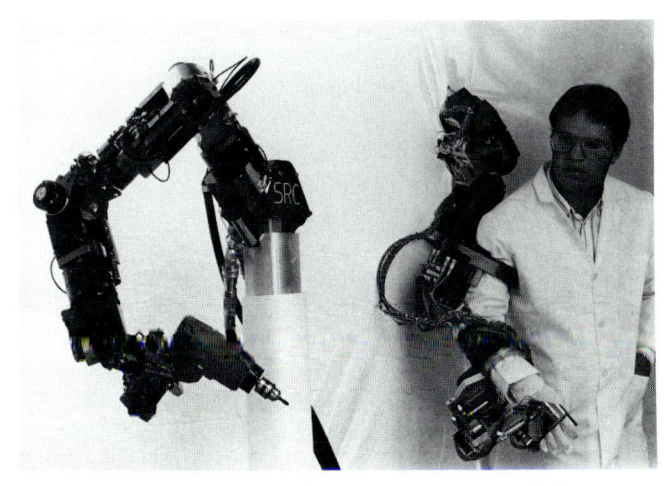

FIGURE 33-3 Dexterous teleoperation system with force-reflecting exoskeleton master and slave. (Courtesy of S. C. Jacobsen, University of Utah, Salt Lake City, UT.)

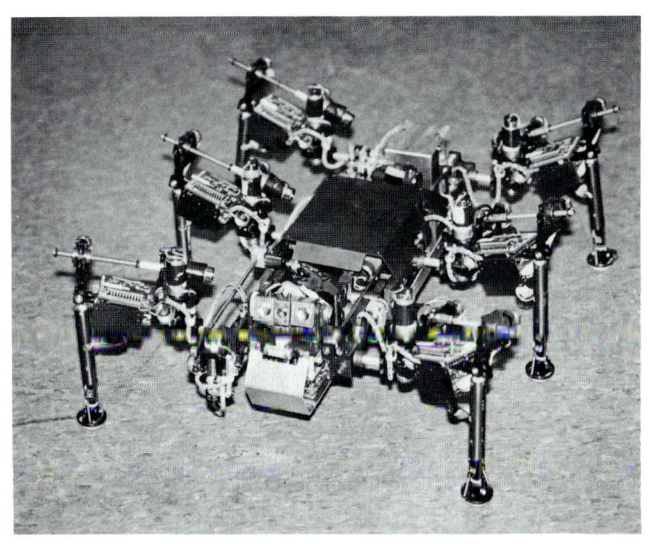

FIGURE 33-5 Atilla. Second-generation intelligent robot. (Courtesy of Anita Flynn, MIT Artificial Intelligence and Mobile Robotic Laboratory, Boston, MA.)

can permit precision performance of tasks. These sophisticated machines point to a future where the ability of a surgeon performing a difficult surgical procedure may be enhanced by robotic control, or where a surgical procedure can be remotely performed in a place too dangerous or distant for the surgeon actually to be present (see section on telepresence surgery).

Another form of robots under intense investigation are miniature and microrobots. Pioneered at the Massachusetts Institute of Technology Artificial Intelligence and Robotics Laboratory under the direction of Dr. Rodney Brooks and associate Anita Flynn, intelligent miniature robots have been developed.[5,6] Two of the newer generation robots, Genghis Kahn (Fig. 33-4) and Attila (Fig. 33-5) have a limited artificial intelligence and autonomy. Rather than being programed for a specific task, they have been programed for a behavior, such as walking while avoiding or crawling over objects. They use sensory input feelers and microchip vision to navigate the world. Their size of 6 to 12 in appears to be too large for specific surgical application; however, Squirt (Fig. 33-6) is a robot about twice the size of a quarter with mobility and vision. The latest generation gnat robot (Fig. 33-7) is a prototype that is approaching the size which could, in the distant future, be employed much in the same fashion as an endoscope.

With further miniaturization and integration, it might be possible to develop a robot that is small enough to be placed in the gastrointestinal tract (by the rectum or swallowed) and navigated through the tortuous curvatures much more effectively than current-generation endoscopes. Admittedly, much research will be required to produce a truly working model; however, the initial concept appears valid. But the problem of size has already been addressed by the rapidly developing field of micromachines and microsensors. These microscopic devices, which are some of the essential component parts of robots, are as small as 10 to 100 μm in size. The rotary motor pictured in Figure 33-8 is capable of producing torque; other motors can provide translational motion. Microsensors can relate information concerning strain, pressure, sheering force, and temperature. The Advanced Intelligent Mechanical Sensors of the University of Utah are microscopic devices that are designed to be incorporated into a silicon chip or at distal working sites ". . . to implement local intelligence necessary for functions such as self-calibration, correction for subsystem failure, and interaction with adjacent sensors."[7] As

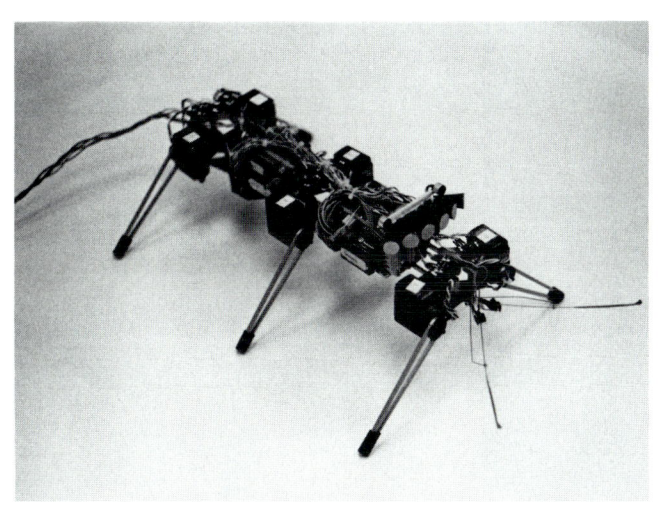

FIGURE 33-4 Genghis Khan. First-generation intelligent robot. (Courtesy of Anita Flynn, MIT Artificial Intelligence and Mobile Robotic Laboratory, Boston, MA.)

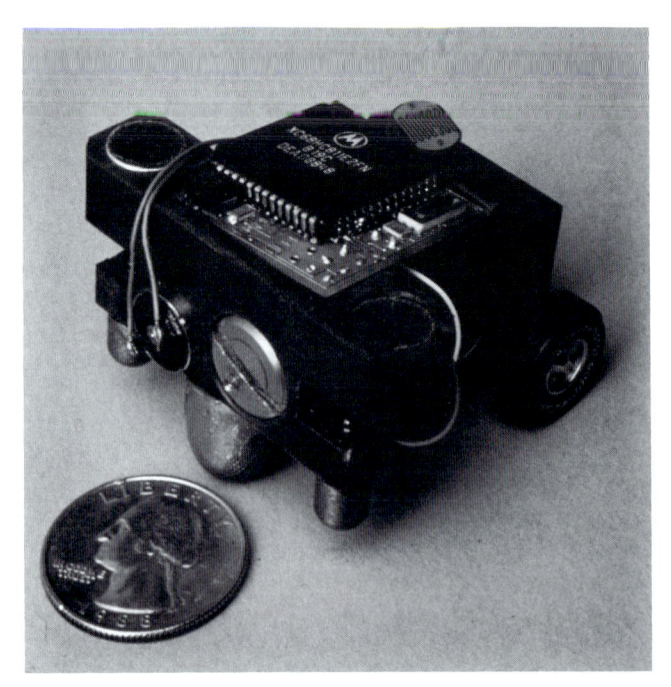

FIGURE 33-6 Squirt, the microrobot, compared with a quarter. (Copyright 1990, Bruce H. Frisch.)

these microscopic engineering parts become more readily available, the construction of an even smaller more complex level of miniature intelligent robotics will be possible.

VIRTUAL REALITY AND TELEPRESENCE SURGERY

A revolutionary field of computer science may change the very fabric of our society: virtual reality. Until now, computer drawings and graphs have been displayed in two or three dimensions and then simply viewed or animated to understand interactions. Virtual reality takes this a giant step forward; the viewer can actually enter into a three-dimensional drawing (called a *world*) and move around and minipulate objects as if the computer-generated world existed. It is an imaginary or virtual world, not a real world, yet the experience approaches reality even though it is entirely contained within the computer. To achieve this level of credibility, a head-mounted display and DataGlove are used (Fig. 33-9). The first is a helmet with two miniature televisions mounted directly in front of the eyes to provide stereoscopic vision, and binaural speakers to provide stereophonic sound. The DataGlove is a *gesture input device* with fiberoptic sensors along the fingers. As viewers move their hands or point fingers, they appear to move or fly forward or backward in the world; making a fist allows objects to be grasped and manipulated. The result is that as the world is entered, the viewer is totally surrounded by the computer-generated image (immersion) and cut off from the real world. By turning the head, the viewer "sees" what is behind. By pointing the glove, the viewer can "fly" from one point to another or even inside an object (such as a

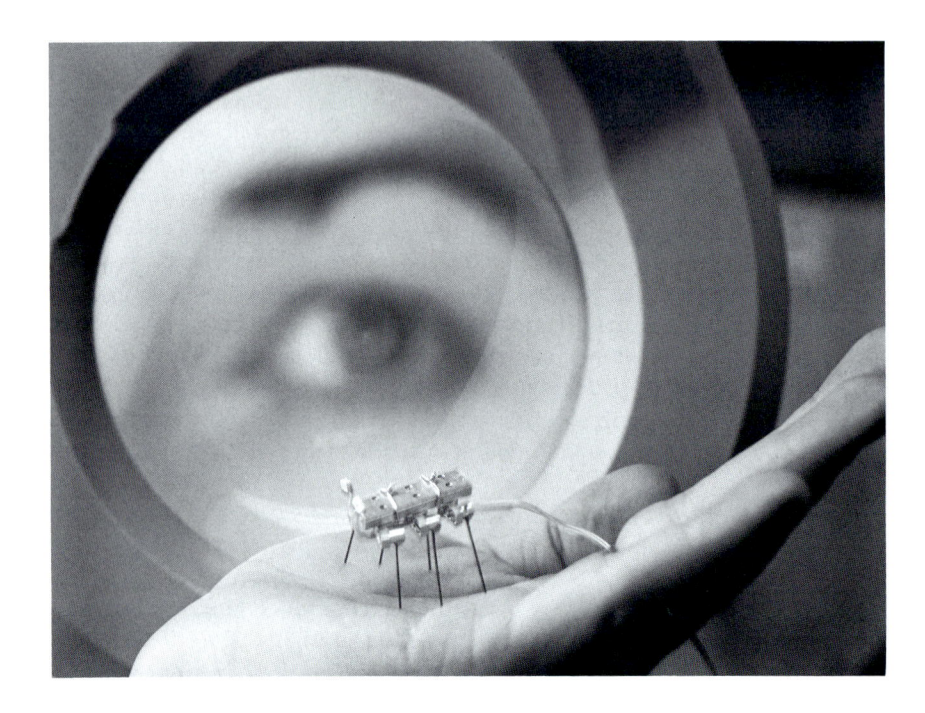

FIGURE 33-7 Gnat robot on the hand of researcher Anita Flynn. (Copyright 1991, Peter Menzel.)

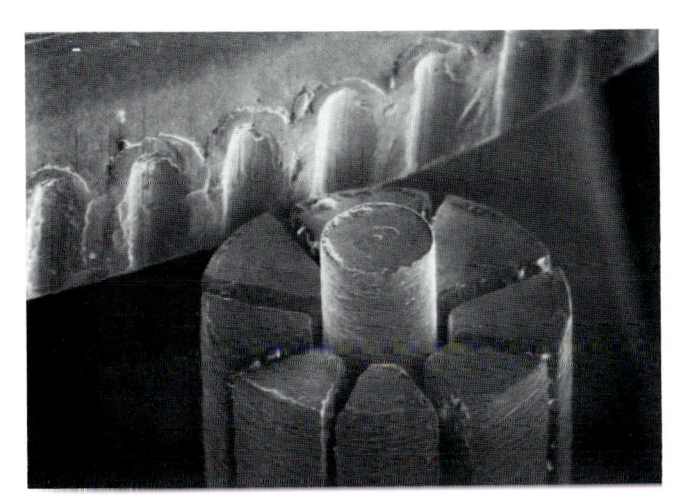

FIGURE 33-8 Microscopic-size rotary motor compared with the edge of a dime. (Courtesy of S. C. Jacobsen, University of Utah, Salt Lake City, UT.)

refrigerator or blood vessel) or can pick up and manipulate various objects (such as balls, pizzas, or scalpels) in the world. For example, architects are creating an entire virtual-reality building; "walking" through it with their clients to visualize problems with spaces, lighting, and other design flaws; and then making necessary design corrections without every hammering a single nail or laying a single brick.

In addition, more than one person can enter the world at the same time. Herein lies the power of virtual reality; people can interact in this imaginary space (also referred to as *cyberspace*, from a novel written in 1984 by William Gibson called *Neuromancer*) as if they were actually together face to face having a discussion or performing the task. Because the virtual world is a digital creation, it can be networked worldwide. The military uses SIMNET, a specialized computer network with re-creations of various battlefields (complete with terrain, tanks, and helicopters) to bring together aviators, infantry, and tank commanders located in various areas of the United States to participate in a simulated battle simultaneously. A helicopter being "flown" by an aviator in one part of the United States can destroy a tank being "driven" by someone from another state.

A virtual world can also become a powerful research tool. An interesting concept at the computer research laboratory of Dr. Frederick Brooks of the University of North Carolina is the creation of a chemical molecule's world, which resembles a universe of atoms. The various elements, carbon, hydrogen, and nitrogen, are represented by colored spheres; the user "grabs" the elements, and changes them to form new chemicals. Being able to fly around, above, behind, and inside the molecules and feel the strength of the chemical bonds provides an entirely new dimension to chemical engineering. Research in DNA modeling, genetic engineering, and antigen–antibody interaction are benefiting from this new research tool, called molecular engineering.

As indicated in the introduction, it was the convergence of many technologies that made laparoscopic surgery possible; these technologies are currently pointing to another

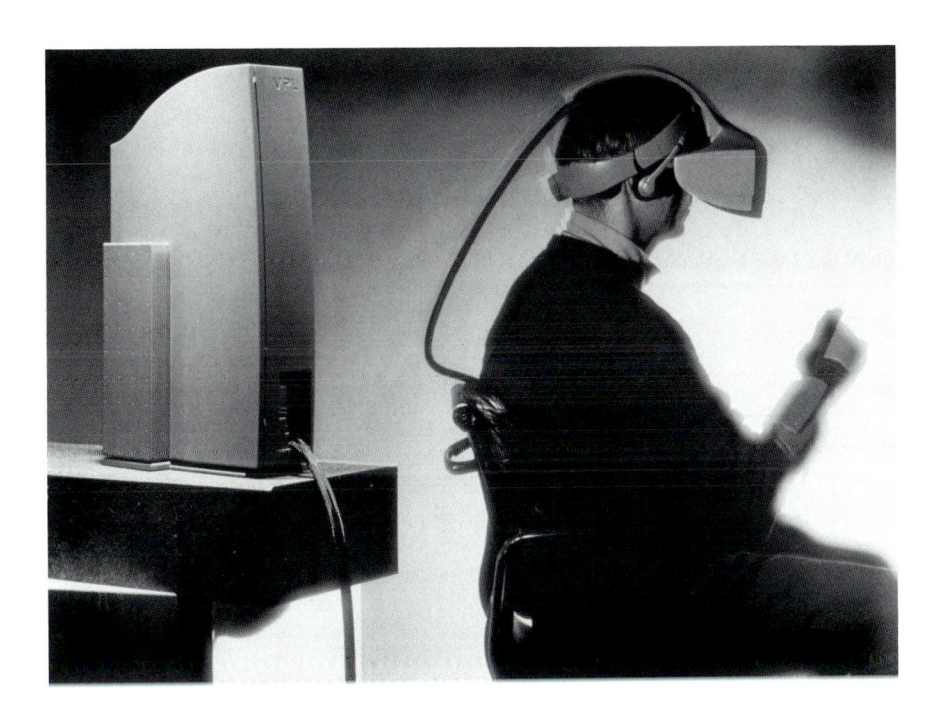

FIGURE 33-9 The head-mounted display and DataGlove used to view a virtual reality world. (Courtesy of VPL Research, Inc., Redwood City, CA.)

advance: telepresence surgery. Remote manipulation or robotics can have increasing levels of complexity, and telepresence is near the top. In a review of robotics by Professor Tom Sheridan[8] there is a hierarchy which can be viewed as follows (Table 33-1): teleoperation, a master arm simply moves a slave arm by moving up and down, or right and left; telerobotics, input from the master causes the robotic arm to perform a preprogrammed task, such as pick up; supervisory control, a robotic system performs an entire complex task under the remote supervision of a master control, such assemble a widget; and telepresence, the master controls the slave at a remote site, but with full sensory (three-dimensional vision, tactile and force feedback, and stereophonic sound) input so that the master teleoperators feel as if they were at the remote site. Above this, the next level is virtual reality, with complete individual immersion to a point of not being able to distinguish the virtual world from a real world. Artificial virtual reality is a completely synthetic world, such as inside a chemical molecule, which a person could never physically occupy. Natural virtual reality is a situation that could physically exist, for example, a surgical procedure on a realistic re-creation of a human body. Obviously, the fine line between telepresence and natural virtual reality becomes more arbitrary as the level of realism increases.

There is currently a prototype telepresence system for surgical procedures, the Green Telepresence Surgery System, designed by Dr. Philip Green, Director of the Biomedical Engineering Research Laboratory at Stanford Research Institute (SRI, International, Stanford, CA). The system consists of two components: the operative site and the surgical work station. At the operative site, there is a pair of charged coupled device video cameras mounted at the proper distance and angle to permit transmission of stereoscopic vision, a stereophonic microphone pickup, and a remote manipulator with four degrees of freedom, force feedback, and tactile feedback. The work station consists of a high-resolution monitor with the three-dimensional video image and a joystick shaped like a surgical instrument with full sensory force feedback. Preliminary experiments demonstrated dexterity to a degree that the remotely manipulated scalpel could slice a grape into 1-mm sections, precisely touch the head of a pin 25 consecutive times, and perform simple dissection on an isolated porcine kidney. From these modest beginnings, there will be development of a complete telepresence system as described by Green and associates.[9] This system is conceived as the next logical step for laparoscopic surgery. Compared with laparoscopic cholecystectomy (Fig. 33-10), telepresence is begun in an identical fashion; however, a stereoscopic video camera will be inserted though the umbilical port and the instruments will be dexterous, six degree-of-freedom, force-feedback instruments. The camera and instruments will be attached to the remote controlling device (Fig. 33-11). The surgeon will then go over to the surgical work station (Fig. 33-12) and complete the operation remotely. This system is a combination of teleoperation, sensory feedback, three-dimensional imaging, and micromachines (instrumentation) to name a few. Combining this system over a network, similar to the military SIMNET, would permit surgical procedures to be performed remotely at a dangerous distant site, such as a space station or Antarctica. Alternatively, two surgeons in different cities could both operate on the same patient because both will be operating on a virtual patient. After remote surgery is perfected, then a telepresence system with miniature tools and a microscope can be developed, theoretically leading to the eventual capability to perform microsurgery on a single cell.

An obvious extension is to create a virtual world of the abdomen of a patient and connect it to the Green Telepresence Surgery System; the system could be used for either a real patient or a simulation, with the flick of a switch. This could be the ultimate surgical "flight simulator," which could be used to train a resident or used by a surgeon to practice a difficult procedure before actual execution. As the virtual world becomes more realistic, the day may come when it would not be possible to determine if an operation were being performed on a real or computer-generated patient. Such a virtual reality surgical simulator is under development by Satava and associates in conjunction with VPL Research, Inc. (Redwood City, CA). The abdominal organs have been created in a three-dimensional world and the surgeon is able to fly in and around the organs. The next step is to develop virtual surgical instruments to practice on these organs. Major barriers need to be overcome to make a more realistic simulation, such as representing tissue deformation when an organ is grasped or incised, inclusion of tissue resistance, and the addition of blood vessels that actually bleed. But the threshold has been crossed, and a new world is forming that is half real and half imaginary.

As speculative as applications may appear, it is important to emphasize that these technologic advances are being generated by a need to overcome the limitations of current

TABLE 33-1 Levels of complexity in robotics/reality

Teleoperation	One-to-one master–slave remote manipulation
Telerobotics	Master selects robotic preprogrammed task
Supervisory control	Programmed independent task is supervised by master
Telepresence	Master has multisensory input and dexterity with illusion of being at a remote site
Virtual reality (cyberspace)	Total sensory immersion in artificial world with illusion of being inside the world and can manipulate imaginary objects

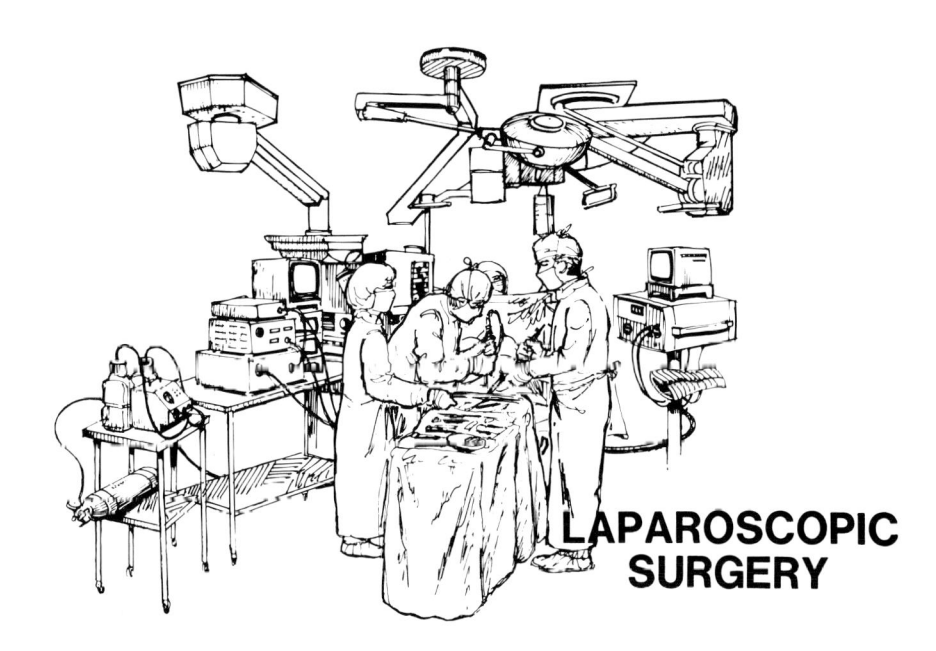

FIGURE 33-10 Laparoscopic surgery, as currently performed.

LAPAROSCOPIC SURGERY

surgical procedures (such as laparoscopic surgery) and an ever-present desire to introduce new educational modalities. Whether the hypothetic virtual world of cyberspace ever reaches the dimension where multiple surgeons can interact and communicate is yet to be seen. Extrinsic factors, such as unfamiliarity of the potential, inconvenience, impracticality, or cost may determine the future direction.

LASERS

Lasers have been on the leading edge of technology for decades and continue to reveal new applications. Their use in tissue destruction and ablation, for cutting and coagulation, and for blasting apart various renal or biliary stones has become commonplace. A powerful new application is just being introduced: laser tissue welding. At the laboratory of Dr. Michael Treat of Columbia University in New York City, preliminary studies demonstrate that tissues can be welded together using a laser and a tissue solder, which consists of fibrinogen and indocyanine green dye.[10] The advantages of a laser weld is that there is no foreign body to produce an inflammatory reaction, the weld is water or fluid tight, and a welded anastomosis has the ability to grow compared with sutured anastomoses. Dr. Jude Sauer and colleagues[11] originated an automated laser tissue welding

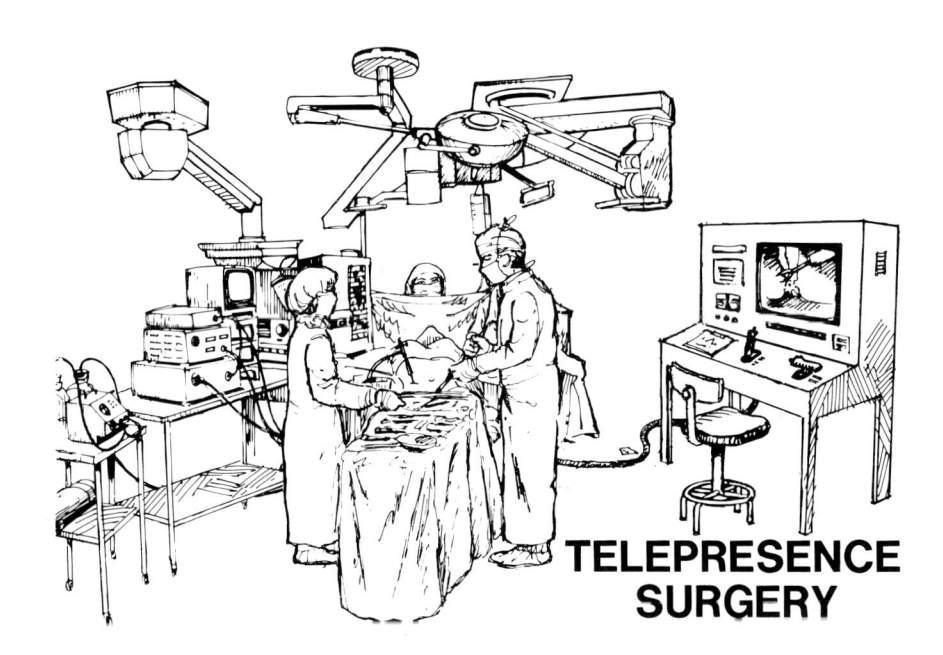

FIGURE 33-11 Telepresence surgery. Setting up the system identical to laparoscopic surgery but attaching the instruments and camera to robotic controls.

TELEPRESENCE SURGERY

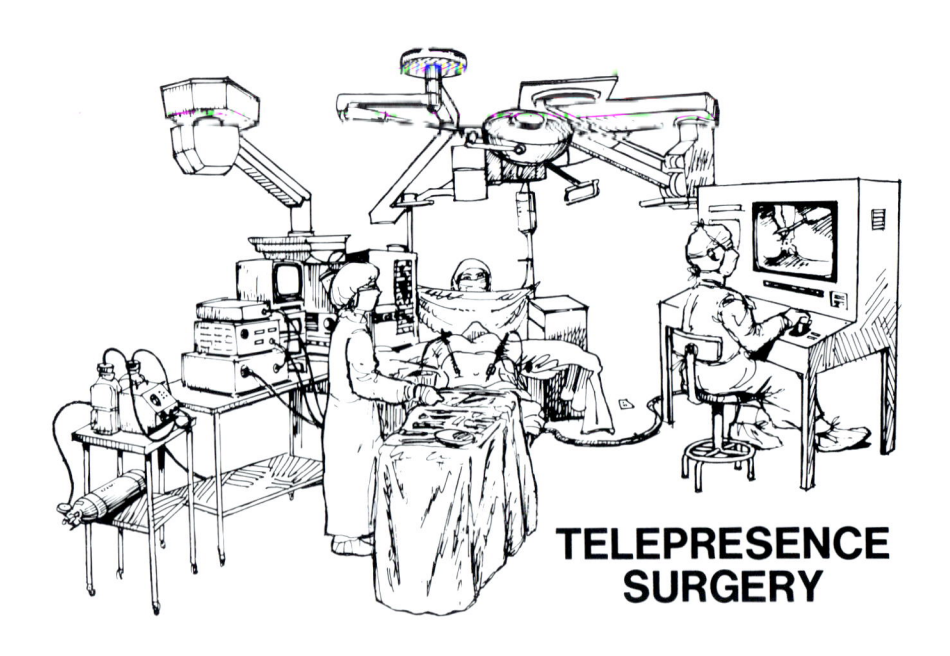

FIGURE 33-12 Telepresence surgery. Performing surgery remotely from the surgical work station.

device called the ExoScope, which utilizes an absorbable stent and circumferential clamping mechanism with embedded laser fibers. The stent sets the edges of an end-to-end anastomosis, and a strong serosal weld is accomplished by a computer-controlled laser. Douglas Dew[12] is performing laser welding to accomplish skin closure on a pig model. Other areas of investigation include vascular anastomoses, including arteriovenous fistula and vasovasotomy.

The mechanism of tissue welding is unknown; there are two major competing hypotheses. The first is that welding is achieved with high temperature, inducing covalent bonding of the structural proteins, such as collagen. The second hypothesis is that laser-treated protein is denatured and hydrogen or disulfide bonds are responsible for the welding bond. Regardless of the controversy over the mechanism, Dr. Rodney White and associates[13] have demonstrated clinical application in a series of laser-welded arteriovenous fistulae. After 4.5 years of follow-up, the patency rate is at least 70 percent.

Once again, there is the recurring theme of making parallel advances on Fleischer's biologic cylinder. Regardless of the speciality, attempts are being made to connect together two ends of a cylindric structure more accurately and quickly with a water-tight stronger bond. Cross pollination of ideas is driving the research forward.

OTHER ENABLING TECHNOLOGIES

It is impossible to mention many of the other technologies that are crossing paths with surgery and may have a major impact on future directions. When looking for a common denominator, it is extraordinary that nearly all of the innovations are dependent on computers to perform their task. Lasers require computers to drive the system, robotics are regulated by computers, and virtual worlds are composed entirely in the computer. The current generation of computers appear to be reaching a plateau in their growth of speed, programming, data storage, and processing ability because only so much can be physically etched onto a silicon chip. There are two areas that are emerging that may once again provide quantum leaps forward: organic computers and neural networks. Rather than using silicon for the computer, biophysicist Dr. Robert Birge of the Syracuse University's Center for Molecular Electronics[14] is cultivating a microbiologic chemical bacteriorhodopsin as a substrate for an organic computer. By scanning this compound with a laser, the molecule can be flipped from one energy state to another in the same manner as an electron might flow through the etched switches on a silicon wafer. By functioning on a molecular level rather than a microscopic level (like silicon-based computers), organic computers and data storage disks can provide the tremendous requirement for speed and data storage that will be required as more technologies depend on computational power.

Complementary to this development is neural networks, a configuration of a computer that could lead to a primitive artificial intelligence. Neural networks are a manner of processing information, especially applicable to highly complex information such as images. Many identical processing elements (each chip is actually an entire microcomputer) are connected to others in a web-like arrangement, each connection having a variable influence on other connections, analogous to the networking of the human brain. Although conventional computer architecture requires a program to run the computer, one with the neural network has no program but learns like a baby. As each new piece of information is fed into the network, it uses the data to distinguish among the numerous possible outcomes. This is particularly valuable in image processing to either recognize a specific item or to compare different images.

These two innovations have been highlighted because they appear to provide potential solutions to some critical rate-limiting steps in computer technology. However, there are a vast number of other fields of development that could just as easily be a major turning point for the future.

SUMMARY

As we approach the 21st century, where the trend will be toward more and more specialization, we must keep our intellectual horizons broad. Parallel and convergent technologies, both within the medical disciplines and outside in academia, government, business, and industry, must be aggressively pursued. We must heed the advice of Fleischer to focus our quest on broad, unifying principles, such as the biologic cylinder, no matter what seemingly unlikely bridge must be crossed, even into the domain of plumbers, physicists, and astronauts. We must be prepared to embrace cross fertilization of specialties to gain new insight into old problems. The gallstone is no longer the private domain of surgeons but must be shared with radiologists, endoscopists, and gastroenterologists. Robots, microrobots, telepresence, virtual reality, lasers, welding, organic computers, and neural networks are just a few of the emergent technologies, any one of which could be a pivotal seed for a new direction for surgery. Pundits will always pontificate to secure their own familiar views and positions, but it is the innovator who braves the unknown territory that shall force the tides of change.

REFERENCES

1. Sivak MV, Fleischer DE: Colonoscopy with a videoendoscope: Preliminary experience. *Gastrointest Endosc* 1984; 30:1.
2. Fleischer DE: Unclogging the obstructed biologic cylinder (letter to the editor). *N Engl J Med* 1990; 322:477.
3. Preising B, Hsai TC, Mittelstadt B: A literature review. Robots in medicine. *IEEE Engi Med Biol* 1991; 10:13–22.
4. Jacobsen SC, Knutti DF, Johnson RT, et al: Design of the Utah/MIT dextrous hand. Presented at the IEEE International Conference of Robotics and Automation, San Francisco, CA, April 1986.
5. Brooks RA. Robust layered control system for a mobile robot. *IEEE Robotics Automation* 1991; RA-2:14–23.
6. Yeaple JA: Robot insects. *Popular Science* 1991; 3:52–56.
7. Jacobsen SC, Knutti DF, Johnson RT, et al: Advanced Intelligent Mechanical Sensors (AIMS). Presented at the IEEE Transducers, 6th International Conference on Solid State Sensors, San Francisco, CA, June 1991.
8. Sheridan TB: Telerobotics. *Automatica* 1989; 25:487–507.
9. Green PE, Piantanida TA, Hill JW, et al: Telepresence: Dexterous procedures in a virtual operating field, abstracted. *Am Surg* 1991; 57:192.
10. Treat MR, Oz MC, Bass LS: New technologies and future applications of surgical lasers. *Surg Clin North Am,* in press.
11. Sauer JS, Hinshaw, JR, McGuire KP: The first sutureless laser-welded, end-to-end bowel anastomosis. *Lasers Surg Med* 1989; 9:70–73.
12. Dew DK: Review and status report on laser tissue sealing—1990. *Proc SPIE* 1990; 1200:38.
13. White RA, Kopchock GE: Laser vascular tissue fusion: Development, current status and future perspectives. *J Clin Laser Med Surg* 1990; 47–54.
14. Freedman DH: Bytes of life. *Discover* 1991; 12:67–72.

Index

Page numbers in *italic* indicate figures; page numbers followed by "t" indicate tables.

Abdominal team, for perivisceral dissection of esophagus, 84–85
Abdominal trauma
  blunt. *See* Emergent/urgent laparoscopy
  penetrating, 294
Abscess, laparoscopic drainage of, 181–182
Adenocarcinoma, Barrett's change and, 93–94
Adenoma, villous, rectosigmoid. *See* Villous adenoma, rectosigmoid
Adhesion, biomaterials and, 51–54
Alkaline reflux, 92
Ammeter, electrosurgical desiccation and, 37
Anastomoses
  ductal, intracorporeal suturing of, 154
  gastrointestinal. *See* Sutured laparoscopic gastrointestinal anastomosis
Anesthesia. *See under specific procedures*
Angioplasty
  balloon, intraoperative. *See* Intraoperative balloon angioplasty
  laser. *See* Laser angioplasty
Angioscopy, 315–316, *316*
  indications for, 315
  limitations and complications of, 316
  results of, 315–316
  technique for, 315
Antireflection coating, 8
Antireflux surgery, laparoscopic, 97–108
  anatomic considerations in, 99
  contraindications to, 98
  functional considerations in, 98
  hiatal dissection and mobilization of esophagus and esophageal junction in, 99–101, *100, 101*
  insertion of vascular sling around esophagus and, 100–101, *102*
  posterior mobilization of crura and upper stomach and, 101, *103*
  hiatus repair and total fundoplication in, 101, 103–104, *104*
    continuous suturing method and, 104, *105*
    interrupted suturing method and, 103–104, *104*
  indications for, 97–98, 98t
  instrumentation for, 99, 99t
  outcome of, 108
  patient positioning and trocar placement for, 99, *99*
  reduction repair and total fundoplication for large hiatal hernias in, 105, *106*
    anterior partial fundoplication in, 106, *108*
    ligamentum teres cardiopexy in, 106, 108, *108*
    posterior crurally fixed partial fundoplication in, 105–106, *107*
Appendectomy, laparoscopic, 171–176
  current perspective on, 176
  diagnostic problems and, 171–172
  history of, 171–172
    acute and complicated appendicitis and, 172–173
    chronic appendicitis and, 173
    incidental appendectomy and, 172
    unsure diagnosis and, 172
  methods of, 173–175, *173–175*
  results of, 175–176
Appendicitis. *See also* Appendectomy, laparoscopic
  diagnosis of, 171–172
  unsure, 172
Argon beam coagulator (ABC), for telescopic surgery, 60
Argon laser, in rectosigmoid laser therapy, 131–132
Atherectomy
  peripheral, 322–324
    Auth Rotoblator and, 324
    indications for, 322, 322t
    Simpson atherectomy device and, 322–323, *323*
    Trac-Wright atherectomy catheter and, 323–324
Attila, 341, *341*
Auth Rotoblator, 324

Balloon angioplasty, intraoperative. *See* Intraoperative balloon angioplasty
Barium enema, in diagnosis of appendicitis, 171
Barrett's esophagus, gastroesophageal reflux disease and, 93–94
Baskets
  for choledochoscopy, 237
  for fluoroscopically guided common duct stone retrieval, 233, 233–235
BICAP tumor probe, in esophageal cancer. *See* Esophageal cancer, BICAP tumor probe in
Biliary disease. *See also* Common bile duct exploration, laparoscopic
  confirmation of bile duct tumors and, 200–201

349

Biliary disease (Cont.):
  endoluminal treatment of bile duct stones and, 209–211, *210, 211*
  endoluminal treatment of bile duct tumors and, 207–208, *208, 209,* 210–211
  interventional radiologic procedures in, 197–206
    bile duct stones and, 202–203
    gallbladder and cystic duct ablation and, 205–206
    stenting of bile duct strictures and. *See* Stents, bile duct strictures and
    symptomatic gallstones and, 203–205, *204*
Biliary system, ultrasound imaging of, 17
  laparoscopic intracorporeal ultrasonography and, 19–20, *20*
Bioactive surfaces, 53
Biocompatibility, 44–45
  definition of, 44
Biolite carbon, 53
Biomaterials, 43–54
  biocompatibility and, 44–45
  biological and biodegradable, 50–51
  cardiovascular, 49
  criteria for, 46, 48
  definition of, 44
  improving polymers for, *51,* 51–54
    bioactive surfaces and, 53
    biodegradable and bioresorbable polymers and, 54
    biomembrane surfaces and, 51, *52*
    cell encapsulation and, 53
    cell seeding and adhesion and, 51–53
    polyethylene oxide surfaces and, 53
    titanium surfaces and, 53–54
    vapor-deposited carbon coatings and, 53
  natural, 51
  polyurethane, 48
  silicone rubber, 48
  surface interactions as determinants of performance of, 45–46, *47*
  surfaces of, 45, 51, *52,* 53–54
  for surgical mesh, 49–50
  for sutures, 48–49
  for wound dressings, 49
Biopsy
  laparoscopic, of liver, 265–266, *266*
    ascites and, 266
    techniques for, 265
  thoracoscopic
    of lung, 332
    of lymph nodes and mediastinal masses, 333
    of pulmonary nodules, 332, *332*
Bipolar electrosurgery, energy source for, 217
Blebs, thoracoscopic ablation of, 333
Bleeding
  as complication of laparoscopic cholecystectomy, 227
  intraperitoneal, transjugular intrahepatic portosystemic shunt and, 276
Blood, in abdomen, emergent/urgent laparoscopy and, 293
Blunt abdominal trauma. *See* Emergent/urgent laparoscopy
Bowel. *See also specific bowel procedures*
  occlusion of, sutured laparoscopic anastomosis and, instrumentation for, 159–160, *160*
Bowel clamps, atraumatic, 160
Burn risks, with electrosurgery
  laparoscopes and, *38,* 38–39, *39*
  monopolar, 37–38

Cameras
  for choledochoscopy, 236
  for documentation of laparoscopic cholecystectomy, 217–218
  for emergent/urgent laparoscopy, 291–292
  for laparoscopic cholecystectomy, 216
  positioning, for laparoscopic suturing and tissue approximation, 146
  for telescopic surgery, 61
  videoendoscopy and, 13
Cancer. *See also specific types and sites*
  staging of, endoscopic ultrasound and, 18
Capacitive coupling, 38–39, *39,* 40
Cardiopexy, ligamentum teres, in laparoscopic antireflux surgery, 106, 108, *108*
Cardiovascular grafts, 49
  cell seeding and adhesion and, 52–53
Cavitronic ultrasound aspirator (CUSA), energy source for, 217
Cecopexy, laparoscopic, 182–183, *183*
Cell encapsulation, biomaterials and, 53
Cell seeding, biomaterials and, 51–54
Charge-coupled device (CCD), 13
Chest pain, in gastroesophageal reflux disease, 95

Chest trauma, thoracoscopic evaluation of, 333
Childhood, gastroesophageal reflux disease in, 98
Cholangiocarcinoma, strictures in, 198, 200
Cholangiography, 162–163
  laparoscopic cholecystectomy and, 218–219, *219*
Cholecystectomy
  laparoscopic, 213–228, 291
    anesthesia for, 220
    camera for, 216
    cholangiography and, 218–219, *219*
    clip applier for, 218
    complications and results of, 226–228
      acute cholecystitis and, 226, *226*
      bleeding and, 227
      converting to open cholecystectomy and, 227
      postoperative management and, 227–228
      spilled stones and, 227
    contraindications to, 214–215
    documentation of, 217–218
    energy source for, 216–217
      bipolar electrocautery and, 217
      cavitronic ultrasound aspirator and, 217
      contact laser and, 217
      free beam laser and, 217
      harmonic scalpel and, 217
      hydrodissection and, 217
      monopolar electrocautery and, 216–217
    hand instruments for, 219–220
    indications for, 213–214
    insufflator for, 216
    irrigation for, 217
    laparoscope cleaner for, 218
    light source for, 216
    mixing desk for, 218
    needle for, 218
    patient preparation for, 215–216
    pretied catgut loops for, 218
    suction for, 217
    sutures and needle holders for, 218
    technique for, 220–225, *220–226*
    telescope for, 218
    television screens for, 216
    trocars for, 218
  laparoscopic intracorporeal ultrasonography during, 19–20, *20*
  retrograde, 219

Cholecystitis, acute
  as complication of laparoscopic cholecystectomy, 226, 226
  as contraindication to laparoscopic cholecystectomy, 214
Cholecystojejunostomy, sutured laparoscopic anastomosis in. See Sutured laparoscopic gastrointestinal anastomosis, in cholecystojejunostomy
Choledochoscopy, 236–239
  equipment for, 236–238
  procedure for, 238, 238–239, 239
Chromophores, tissue absorption of laser light and, 28
Cimetidine, in gastroesophageal reflux disease, 97
Cirrhosis, as contraindication to laparoscopic cholecystectomy, 214
Clip(s)
  in laparoscopic appendectomy, 173, 174
  in telescopic surgery, 62
Clip appliers
  for laparoscopic cholecystectomy, 218
  for thoracoscopy, 330
Coagulopathy, as contraindication to laparoscopic cholecystectomy, 214
Coherent bundle, 9
Coherent light, 24, 24
Cold laser, angioplasty and, 319
Colectomy, sigmoid, exit site for tissue in, 64
Collagens, biomaterials and, 50
Colocolostomy, sutured laparoscopic anastomosis and. See Sutured laparoscopic gastrointestinal anastomosis, in colocolostomy
Colon and rectal surgery. See also specific procedures
Colon and rectal surgery, laparoscopic, 179, 179–187. See also Colostomy, laparoscopic
  abdominoperineal resection of rectum, 186–187
  total abdominal colectomy and, 187
  colectomy, 185–186
    left hemicolectomy, 185–186, 186–188
    right hemicolectomy, 185, 185
    total abdominal, 187
  equipment for, 180, 181
  patient preparation for, 181
  reversal of Hartmann's procedure, 184, 184–185
  techniques in, 181–182
    for abscess drainage, 181–182
    for ileostomy, 181, 182
    for repair of full-thickness excision of bowel wall, 181
    for repair of injured bowel, 181, 181
  training for, 180
Colorectal ultrasound, 18–19
Colostomy, laparoscopic, 182–184, 183
  cecopexy and, 182–183, 183
  rectopexy and, 183–184, 184
Columnar-epithelium-lined esophagus (CELO), gastroesophageal reflux disease and, 93–94
Common bile duct exploration (CBDE), 231
  laparoscopic, 231–243
    choledochoscopy and, 236–239
      equipment for, 236–238
      procedure for, 238, 238–239, 239
    fluoroscopically directed stone removal and, 232–236
      equipment for, 232–234, 233–235
      procedure for, 234–236
    laparoscopic choledochotomy and, 240–241
      equipment for, 240
      procedure for, 240–241, 241
    results of, 241–243, 242, 243t
Computed tomography (CT), in esophageal cancer, 70, 71
Computers, organic, 346
Contact tips, 26
Containers, for specimens, 63, 63–64, 64
Cryotherapy, hepatic ablation with, 257
Cyberspace, 343
Cystic duct, ablation of, 205–206
Cystotomy, laparoscopic, 267, 267–268

Dacron grafts, 49
  knitted and woven, 52–53
Dacron mesh, 50
DataGlove, 342–343, 343
Desiccation
  electrosurgical, 36, 36–37
    bipolar, 37
  radiofrequency, hepatic ablation with, 260, 261, 261
Dexon mesh, 50
Dexterous hand, 340, 340
Dexterous telerobotic arm, 340–341, 341
Diagnostic peritoneal lavage (DPL), 291
Diet, in gastroesophageal reflux disease, 97
Dilation, in esophageal cancer, 79, 79
Dissecting tools, for telescopic surgery, 59–61
Dissection, in telescopic surgery. See Telescopic surgery, dissection and resection methods in
Documentation, of laparoscopic cholecystectomy, 217–218
Doppler ultrasonography, 16
Drug therapy, in gastroesophageal reflux disease, 97
Ductal anastomoses, intracorporeal suturing of, 154
Duodenogastric reflux, gastroesophageal reflux disease and, 91–92
Dysphagia
  in gastroesophageal reflux disease, 94–95
  hiatal hernia and, 88

Ecchymoses, of abdominal wall, laparoscopic pelvic lymphadenectomy and, 288
Electrocautery, in laparoscopic appendectomy, 174
Electrohydraulic fragmentation devices, for telescopic surgery, 59
Electrohydraulic lithotripsy (EHL), 203, 237–238
Electroshield Monitoring System, 39, 40
Electrosurgery. See also Laparoscopic electrosurgery
  telescopic, 59
Emergent/urgent laparoscopy, 291–295
  contraindications to, 292
  diagnostic dilemmas and, 295
    in elderly patients, 295
    in young female patients, 295
  findings of, 293–294
  indications for, 292
  instrumentation for, 291–292, 292, 293
  results of, 294–295
  technique for, 292–293
Empyema, thoracoscopic decortication and drainage of, 335
Encephalopathy, transjugular intrahepatic portosystemic shunt and, 276
End-to-end anastomosis, intracorporeal suturing of, 154
End-to-side anastomosis, intracorporeal suturing of, 154
Endoluminal ultrasonography (EUS), staging of rectal carcinoma and, 102

Endoscopic ultrasonography (EUS), 17–19, *19*
  in esophageal cancer, 70, *71*
Endoscopy. *See also specific procedures and disorders*
  in gastroesophageal reflux disease, 96, 97t
  optical principles of, 7–9
    fiberoptic endoscope and, 8–9, *9, 10*
    lens endoscope and, 7–8, *8*
    videoendoscopy and, 13
Endovascular surgery, 315–327. *See also specific techniques*
Energy, control of, in telescopic surgery, 60
Energy sources, for laparoscopic cholecystectomy. *See* Cholecystectomy, laparoscopic
Energy sources, for telescopic surgery, 58
Enteral nutrition, 113–119
  laparoscopically guided feeding jejunosotomy and, 117–119
    results with, 119
    technique for, 117, *117, 118,* 119
  laparoscopically guided gastrostomy and, 119, *119, 120*
  percutaneous endoscopic gastrostomy for. *See* Percutaneous endoscopic gastrostomy
  percutaneous endoscopic jejunostomy and, 116–117
Esophageal cancer, 69–80
  BICAP tumor probe in, *75,* 75–76
    follow-up examinations and, 76
    postprocedure for, 76
    results with, 76
    technique for, 75–76
  dilation in, *79,* 79
  esophageal prostheses and, 77–78
    complications with, 78, *78*
    indications for, 77
    postprocedure for, 78
    technique for, 77, 77–78
  injection therapy in, 79–80
  iridium-192 radiotherapy in, 75
    results with, 75
    technique for, 75
  laser ablation of, 69–74, *70*
    indications for, 69–70, 70t
    patient evaluation for, 70–71, *71, 72*
    postprocedure for, 73
    results with, 73–74
    subsequent sessions and, 73
    technique for, 71–73, *73*
  perivisceral dissection of esophagus in, 83–86
    equipment for, *83,* 83–84

operative procedure for, 84–85, *85*
patient, team, and theater setting for, 84, *84*
postoperative management and, 85
preoperative assessment and indications for, 84
preoperative management and anesthesia for, 84
results with, 86
photodynamic therapy in, 74
  results with, 74
  technique for, 74
Esophageal clearance, gastroesophageal reflux disease and, 91
Esophageal motility disorders, gastroesophageal reflux disease associated with, 98
Esophageal mucosal resistance, gastroesophageal reflux disease and, 90–91
Esophageal webs, gastroesophageal reflux disease and, 92
Esophagitis, histopathology of, 92
Esophagogastroduodenoscopy (EGD), 71
Ethyl alcohol
  gallbladder and cystic duct ablation with, 205–206
  hepatic ablation with, 257–259, *258*
Excimer laser, angioplasty and, 319
Exit-pupil, 7
ExoScope, 346
Exposure, in telescopic surgery, 61–62
Extracorporeal knot-tying, *152,* 152–153, *153*
  in laparoscopic appendectomy, 173, *174*
  in laparoscopic choledochotomy, 240
Extracorporeal shock wave lithotripsy (ESWL), 203, 251–252
Eye–hand coordination, for laparoscopic suturing and tissue approximation, 144–145
Eyepiece, 7

Feeding jejunostomy, 113
Feeding jejunostomy, laparoscopically guided
  results with, 117–119
  technique for, 117, *117, 118,* 119
Fiberoptic endoscope, 8–9, *9, 10*
Fiberoptics, 7–13. *See also* Endoscopy
  laser Doppler and, 12–13
  pressure monitoring with, 9–11, *10*
  videoendoscopy and, 13

in vivo oximetry with, 10–12, *11, 12*
Fibrin implants, compression-molded, 50–51
Film dressings, 49
Fluoroscopically guided common duct stone retrieval (FGSR), 232–236
  equipment for, 232–234, *233–235*
  procedure for, 234–236
Flutter-valve theory of lower esophageal competence, gastroesophageal reflux disease and, 89
Foam dressings, 49
Fulguration, electrosurgical, *35,* 35–36, *36*
Fundoplication. *See* Antireflux surgery, laparoscopic

Gallbladder
  ablation of, 205–206
  carcinoma of, as contraindication to laparoscopic cholecystectomy, 215, *215*
  porcelain, as contraindication to laparoscopic cholecystectomy, 215, *215*
Gallstones, rotational contact lithotripsy and, 203–205, *204*
Gastric factors, gastroesophageal reflux disease and, 91
Gastric juice, gastroesophageal reflux disease and, 91–92
Gastric lymphoma, endoscopic ultrasound and, 18
Gastric muscle, oblique, gastroesophageal reflux disease and, 88
Gastric outlet obstruction, 202
Gastroesophageal reflux disease (GERD), 87–108
  clinical features of, 94t, 94–96
  complications of, 92–94, 98
  etiology of, 88–91
    esophageal clearance and, 91
    gastric factors and, 91
    mechanical factors in, 88–89
    mucosal resistance and, 90–91
    sphincteric and motor factors in, 89–90
  investigations in, 96, 97t
  laparoscopic surgical treatment of. *See* Antireflux surgery, laparoscopic
  medical therapy of, 96–97
  pathology and clinical features of hiatal hernia and, 87–88
  pathology of, 91–94
    gastric juice and, 91–92
    histopathology of esophagitis and, 92

patterns of reflux and, 91
Gastroesophageal varices. *See* Transjugular intrahepatic portosystemic shunt
Gastrojejunostomy, sutured laparoscopic anastomosis in. *See* Sutured laparoscopic gastrointestinal anastomosis, in gastrojejunostomy
Gastroscopy, laparoscopic cholecystectomy and, 215, *215*
Gastrostomy. *See also* Percutaneous endoscopic gastrostomy
  laparoscopically guided, 119, *119, 120*
Genghis Kahn, 341, *341*
Gesture input device, 342
Ginaturco-Rösch Z-stent, 272–273, *274*
Globus hystericus, in gastroesophageal reflux disease, 95
Gnat robot, 341, *342*
Grasping forceps, for sutured laparoscopic anastomosis, 157, *158, 159*
Green Telepresence Surgery System, 344
Guide wires, for choledochoscopy, 236–237
Gynecologic surgery, exit site for tissue in, 64

H_2 blockers
  in gastroesophageal reflux disease, 97
  in peptic ulcer disease, 123
Harmonic scalpel, energy source for, 217
Hartmann's procedure, laparoscopic reversal of, *184*, 184–185
Head-mounted display, 342
Heartburn, in gastroesophageal reflux disease, 94
Hematoporphyrin derivative (HpD), in photodynamic therapy, 74
Hemicolectomy
  left, laparoscopic, 185–186, *186–188*
  right, laparoscopic, 185, *185*
Hemoperitoneum, emergent/urgent laparoscopy and, 293–294
Hemorrhage
  as complication of laparoscopic cholecystectomy, 227
  intraperitoneal, transjugular intrahepatic portosystemic shunt and, 276
Hepatic cysts, benign, laparoscopic approach to, 267

Hepatic malignancies, percutaneous interstitial ablation of, 255–262, 262t
  cryotherapy and, 257
  ethanol injection and, 257–259, *258*
  laser hyperthermia and, 259, 261
  materials and protocol for, 255–256
  procedure for, 256–257
  radiofrequency desiccation and, *260, 261, 261*
  radiotherapy and, 259
  results of, 257–261
Hepatic reserve, 256
Hernia
  hiatal. *See also* Gastroesophageal reflux disease
    pathology and clinical features of, 87–88
  inguinal, repair of. *See* Inguinal hernia repair, laparoscopic
High-pressure zone (HPZ), gastroesophageal reflux disease and, 89–90
Hopkins rod–lens system, 7
Hydrocolloid dressings, 49
Hydrogel dressings, 49
Hydrophilic surfaces, 45
Hydrophobic surfaces, 45
Hyperthermia, laser, interstitial, hepatic ablation with, 259, 261

Ileocolostomy, sutured laparoscopic anastomosis and. *See* Sutured laparoscopic gastrointestinal anastomosis, in ileocolosotomy
Ileostomy, laparoscopic, 182, *182*
Iliopubic tract, 301
Implants, polymeric biomaterials for. *See* Biomaterials
In vivo oximetry, 10–12, *11, 12*
Incision, extension of, for tissue removal, 63
Incoherent bundle, 9
Infancy, gastroesophageal reflux disease in, 98
Informed consent, for laparoscopic pelvic lymphadenectomy, 280
Inguinal hernia repair, laparoscopic, 297–307
  data collection and, 307
  history of, 297–299
  inguinal anatomy and, *300*, 300–301
  prosthesis placement and, 302–306, *305*
  closure of peritoneum and, *305, 306*
  dissection of sac and, 303

fixation of mesh and, 303, *305, 306*
  identification of inguinal anatomy and, 303, *304*
  initial dissection and, 302–303, *304*
  positioning and initiation of pneumoperitoneum and, 302
  trocar placement and, 302, *302*
prosthetic mesh and, 299–300
published reports on, 306–307
reasons for, 299
techniques for, 301–302
  peritoneal repair and, 301
  plug placement and, 301–302
  prosthesis placement and, 301
  simple onlay prosthetic patch and, 301
  suturing and, 301
Injection therapy, in esophageal cancer, 79–80
Insufflation, for emergent/urgent laparoscopy, 291
Insufflators
  for laparoscopic cholecystectomy, 216
  for telescopic surgery, 57, 60
Internal reflection, total, 8
Intracorporeal ligation techniques, in telescopic surgery, 62
Intracorporeal suturing, 153–154
  of ductal anastomoses, 154
  knot-tying and, 149–152
    in laparoscopic choledochotomy, 240
    square knot and, 149, *150–151, 152*
  of linear incisions and lacerations, 153–154
    continuous suturing for, 153–154
    interrupted suturing for, 153
Intraoperative balloon angioplasty, *318*, 318–319
  indications for, 318
  limitations and complications of, 319
  results of, 319
  techniques for, 318–319
Intravascular stents. *See* Stents, intravascular
Iridium-192 seed placement, in biliary disease, 201, *201*
Irrigation, for laparoscopic cholecystectomy, 217
Irrigation pump, for telescopic surgery, 60

Jejunostomy, feeding. *See* Feeding jejunostomy

Klatskin tumors, 200
Knot-tying
   extracorporeal, 152, 152–153, 153
      in laparoscopic appendectomy, 173, 174
      in laparoscopic choledochotomy, 240
   intracorporeal, 149–152
      in laparoscopic choledochotomy, 240
      square knot and, 149, 150–151, 152

Laparoscope cleaner, for laparoscopic cholecystectomy, 218
Laparoscopic cecopexy, 182–183, 183
Laparoscopic colostomy, 182–184, 183
   cecopexy and, 182–183, 183
   rectopexy and, 183–184, 184
Laparoscopic cystotomy, 267, 267–268
Laparoscopic electrosurgery, 33–41
   effects of electrical energy on tissue temperature and, 33–34, 34
   effects of temperature on tissue and, 33, 34
   history of, 33
   laparoscopy and, 38–40, 38–40
   misconceptions about, 40
   monopolar, risks of, 37–38, 174
   results with, 37–40
   risks of, 37–40, 38–40
   technique of, 34–37
      desiccation and, 36, 36–37
      fulguration and, 35, 35–36, 36
      vaporization and, 35
Laparoscopic ileostomy, 182, 182
Laparoscopic intracorporeal ultrasound (LICU), 19–20, 20
Laparoscopic liver biopsy, 265–266, 266
   ascites and, 266
   techniques for, 265
Laparoscopic liver resection, 268
Laparoscopic rectopexy, 183–184, 184
Laparoscopic surgery, relevance of microsurgery to, 141
Laparoscopic suturing and tissue approximation, 141–154
   entrance and exit bites for, 148–149
      amount of bite and, 148–149
      exit bite and, 149
      selection of entrance point and, 148
   extracorporeal knot-tying techniques for, 152, 152–153, 153

eye–hand coordination and, 144–145
hand instruments for, 143
intracorporeal knot-tying techniques for, 149–152
   square knot and, 149, 150–151, 152
intracorporeal suturing techniques for, 153–154
   for ductal anastomosis, 154
   for linear incisions and lacerations, 153–154
in laparoscopic appendectomy, 173, 174
needle control for, 146–148
   adjusting needles and, 147
   grasping and loading in needle driver and, 146, 147
   needle deflection and remedy and, 147–148, 147–149
   setup and angles of approach for, 145–146
      instrument locations and, 146, 146
      laparoscope and camera location and, 146
sutures and, 142–143
   handling characteristics of, 142
   material for, 143
   needle profile and diameter and, 142
   tips and, 142
techniques for, 145–149
tissue approximation methods, 141–142
   choices for, 141
   preferences for, 141–142, 142
tissue handling and, 145, 145
trocars for, 142
video magnification for, 144
visual perception and, 143–144
Laparoscopic techniques. See also specific procedures and disorders
   benign hepatic cysts and, 267
   emergent and urgent. See Emergent/urgent laparoscopy
Laparoscopically guided enteral feeding access
   feeding jejunostomy, 117–119
      results with, 119
      technique for, 117, 117, 118, 119
   gastrostomy, 119, 119, 120
Laparotomy, conversion to, cholecystojejunostomy and, 164
Laser(s), 23–31. See also Nd:YAG laser; Rectosigmoid laser therapy; headings beginning with term Laser
   argon, in rectosigmoid laser therapy, 131–132

cold, angioplasty and, 319
contact, energy source for, 217
delivery systems for, 25–26, 26
excimer, angioplasty and, 319
free beam, energy source for, 217
free-electron, 27, 27
future development of, 345–346
nonthermal, angioplasty and, 319
photodynamic therapy using, 29–30, 30
physics of, 23, 23–24, 24
pulsing, 25, 25
for telescopic surgery, 60
tissue interaction and, 27, 27–29
   absorption of laser light and, 28, 28
   laser pulsing and, 29, 29
   scattering of laser light and, 28–29
wavelengths of monochromatic light and, 26, 26–27
welding with, 31
Laser angioplasty, 319–322
   equipment for, 319–320, 320
   indications for, 320, 320t
   limitations and complications of, 322
   results of, 321, 321t
   technique for, 320
Laser Doppler, 12–13
Laser hyperthermia, hepatic ablation with, 259, 261
Laser lithotripsy, 237
Laser therapy, in rectosigmoid tumors. See Rectosigmoid laser therapy
Lens endoscope, 7–8, 8
Light source, for laparoscopic cholecystectomy, 216
Lipid membranes, polymerizable, 51, 52
Lithotripsy
   electrohydraulic, 203, 237–238
   extracorporeal shock wave, 203, 251–252
   intraductal, 237
   laser, 237
   rotational contact, 203–205, 204
      procedure for, 204–205
Liver. See also Hepatic malignancies
   ultrasound imaging of, 17
Liver biopsy, laparoscopic, 265–266, 266
   ascites and, 266
   techniques for, 265
Liver resection, laparoscopic, 268
Lung biopsy, thoracoscopic, 332
Lymph nodes, thoracoscopic biopsy of, 333

Lymphadenectomy, pelvic. *See* Pelvic lymphadenectomy, laparoscopic

Marlex mesh, 49–50
Mechanical factors, gastroesophageal reflux disease and, 88–89
Mediastinal masses
 thoracoscopic biopsy of, 333
 thoracoscopic resection of, 333–334
Mediastinal team, for perivisceral dissection of esophagus, 84–85
Medical therapy, in gastroesophageal reflux disease, 96–97
 failure of, as indication for surgery, 97–98
Mersilene mesh, 50
Mesh
 in laparoscopic inguinal hernia repair. *See* Inguinal hernia repair, laparoscopic
 surgical, 49–50
Microrobotics, *341*, 341–342, *342*
Microsurgery. *See also* Laparoscopic suturing and tissue approximation; Transanal endoscopic microsurgery
 relevance to laparoscopic surgery, 141
Minilaparoscopy, 291
Minimally invasive surgery. *See also specific techniques*
 advantages of, 4–5
 applications of, 4
 definition of, 3–4
 disadvantages of, 5
 impact of, 6
 technology and, 4
 training for, 5–6
Mixing desk, for laparoscopic cholecystectomy, 218
Monopolar electrosurgery (MPES)
 energy source for, 216–217
 risks of, 37–38, 174
Morcellators, for telescopic surgery, 64
Motor factors, gastroesophageal reflux disease and, 89–90
Mucosal resistance, esophageal, gastroesophageal reflux disease and, 90–91
Myopectineal orifice, 300–301
Myotomy, esophageal, thoracoscopic, 334–335, *336*

Nasogastric intubation, disadvantages of, 113
Nasopancreatic decompression, 250, 250t

Nd:YAG laser
 in rectosigmoid laser therapy, 131–132
 scattering of light and, 28–29
 for telescopic surgery, 60
Needle(s)
 for laparoscopic cholecystectomy, 218
 for laparoscopic suturing and tissue approximation. *See* Laparoscopic suturing and tissue approximation
Needle driver, for laparoscopic suturing and tissue approximation, 143
 grasping and loading, 146, *147*
 positioning, 146, *146*
Needle holders
 for laparoscopic cholecystectomy, 218
 for sutured laparoscopic anastomosis, 157–158, *158*, *159*
Neural networks, 346–347
Neutral reflux, 92
Nonthermal laser, angioplasty and, 319

Obesity, as contraindication to laparoscopic cholecystectomy, 214
Objective, of lens endoscope, 7
Odynophagia, in gastroesophageal reflux disease, 94
Omeprazole, in gastroesophageal reflux disease, 97, 98
Operating room setup. *See also under specific procedures*
 for telescopic surgery, 58
Operative ultrasonography, 16–17
Organ perforation, emergent/urgent laparoscopy and, 294
Organic computers, 346
Oximetry, in vivo, 10–12, *11*, *12*

Pacemaker, as contraindication to laparoscopic cholecystectomy, 214
Pain
 in chest, in gastroesophageal reflux disease, 95
 in gastroesophageal reflux disease, 94
Pancreas. *See also specific pancreatic disorders*
 endoscopic ultrasound and, 18, *19*
 ultrasound imaging of, 17
Pancreatic cancer, 201
Pancreatic endoprostheses, 250–252, *251*, *252*

Pancreatitis, acute
 endoscopic intervention after, 246–248
  idiopathic pancreatitis and, 246–247, *247*
  massive pancreatic necrosis and, 248
  preoperative "road map" for, 247–248, *248*
 endoscopic intervention during, 245–246
  gallstone pancreatitis and, 245–246, 246t
  traumatic pancreatitis and, 246
Pancreatitis, chronic, endoscopic intervention in, 248–252
 diagnostic considerations with, 248–249, 249t
 recurrent postoperative symptoms and, 249
 technique for, 249t, 249–252
Papillary adenoma, of common bile duct, endoluminal treatment of, 207, *208*
Pelvic lymphadenectomy, laparoscopic, 279–289
 complications of, 288
 indications for, 279–280
 informed consent for, 280
 instrumentation for, 280–281
 patient preparation for, 280
 postoperative care and, 287–288
 procedure for, *281*, 281–287, *283–285*
  exiting abdomen and, 287
  pneumoperitoneum and, 281
  trocar placement and, 281–282
 results of, 288–289
 subsequent therapy and, 288
 technique for, 280–288
Penetrating injuries, emergent/urgent laparoscopy and, 294
Peptic ulcer disease, laparoscopic treatment of, 123–129
 bilateral truncal vagotomy with forced pyloric endoscopic balloon dilation in, *127*, 127–128
  peritonitis from perforated ulcer and, 128–129
  technique for, *128*, 128–129
  treatment indications for, 129
 posterior truncal vagotomy with anterior seromyotomy in, 124–126
  creation of pneumoperitoneum and trocar positioning for, *124*, 124–125
  equipment for, 124
  operating room setup for, 124
  patient preparation for, 124

Peptic ulcer disease (Cont.):
 procedure for, 125–126, 125–127
 results of, 129
 posterior truncal vagotomy with hyperselective anterior vagotomy in, 128, 128
Percutaneous endoscopic gastrostomy (PEG), 113–116
 complications of, 116
 contraindications to, 113
 indications for, 113
 patient positioning for, 114, 114
 patient preparation for, 113–114
 postoperative care and, 116
 technique for, 114, 115, 116
 alternatives for, 116
Percutaneous endoscopic jejunostomy (PEJ), 116–117
Pericardial window, thoracoscopy and, 334
Pericardiocentesis, thoracoscopic, 334
Photodynamic therapy (PDT), 29–30, 30, 74
 in esophageal cancer, 74
 results with, 74
 technique for, 74
 sensitizers for, 74
Phrenoesophageal membrane, gastroesophageal reflux disease and, 89
Pleural effusions, thoracoscopic evaluation of, 332
Pleural masses, thoracoscopic evaluation of, 332
Pleurodesis, thoracoscopic, 333
Pneumoperitoneum
 for laparoscopic inguinal hernia repair, positioning and initiation of, 302
 for laparoscopic pelvic lymphadenectomy, 281
Pneumothorax, thoracoscopic ablation of blebs and pleurodesis for, 333
Polidocanol, in injection therapy, in esophageal cancer, 80
Polyethylene oxide (PEO) surfaces, 53
Polymeric biomaterials. See Biomaterials
Polyhydroxy alkanoate polymers, 54
Polyhydroxybutyrate polymers, 54
Polysaccharide dressings, 49
Polyurethane biomaterials, 48
Postcholecystectomy syndrome, 215, 215
Posture, in gastroesophageal reflux disease, 97
Pregnancy, as contraindication to laparoscopic cholecystectomy, 214

Pressure monitoring, fiberoptic, 9–11, 10
Pretied catgut loops, for laparoscopic cholecystectomy, 218
Prostatic cancer, laparoscopic pelvic lymphadenectomy in. See Pelvic lymphadenectomy, laparoscopic
Pseudocysts, pancreatic, endoscopic intervention in, 252
Pulmonary nodules
 thoracoscopic biopsy of, 332, 332
 thoracoscopic resection of, 333–334
Pulsing, of laser beams, 25, 25
 tissue effects of, 29, 29
Pyrosis, in gastroesophageal reflux disease, 94

Q-switch, 25

Radiofrequency desiccation, hepatic ablation with, 260, 261, 261
Radiotherapy
 interstitial, hepatic ablation with, 259
 intraluminal, in esophageal cancer, 75
 results with, 75
 technique for, 75
Receptive relaxation, gastroesophageal reflux disease and, 90
Rectal polyposis, rectosigmoid laser therapy in, 138–139
 outcome of, 138–139, 139
 patient cohort and, 138
Rectal surgery. See specific procedures
Rectopexy
 endoscopic, transanal, 195–196, 196
 laparoscopic, 183–184, 184
Rectosigmoid laser therapy, 131–139
 in cancer, 132–134, 135
 outcome of, 133, 133–134
 patient cohort and, 132t, 132–133, 133
 in rectal polyposis, 138–139
 outcome of, 138–139, 139
 patient cohort and, 138
 surgery versus, 139
 technique for, 131–132
 in villous adenoma, 134–138, 137t
 outcome of, 136, 136–137, 137
 patient cohort and, 134–136, 135
Regurgitation, in gastroesophageal reflux disease, 95–96
Resection, in telescopic surgery. See Telescopic surgery, dissection and resection methods in
Retracting tools, for telescopic surgery, 61, 61

Robotics, 340–342, 340–343
 levels of complexity in, 344, 344t
Rotary motor, for robots, 341, 342
Rotational contact lithotripsy, 203–205, 204
 procedure for, 204–205

Scalpels, harmonic, energy source for, 217
Scalpels, ultrasonic, 60
Scissors, for telescopic surgery, 59
Seromyotomy, in peptic ulcer disease. See Peptic ulcer disease, laparoscopic treatment of
Shuttle, for specimens, 64, 64
Side-to-side anastomosis, intracorporeal suturing of, 154
Silicone rubber biomaterials, 48
Simpson atherectomy device, 322–323, 323
Sodium tetradecyl sulfate (STS), gallbladder and cystic duct ablation with, 205–206
Sparking, electrosurgery and, 40
Sphincter of Oddi dysfunction, endoscopic intervention in, 249–250, 250t
Sphincteric factors, gastroesophageal reflux disease and, 89–90
Sphincterotomy, endoscopic
 in acute pancreatitis, 245–246, 246t
 in biliary disease, 207–210, 210, 211
 in chronic pancreatitis, 248
 in sphincter of Oddi dysfunction, 250
Splenectomy, laparoscopic, 309–313
 equipment for, 309–310
 preoperative care and, 310
 results of, 312–313
 technique for, 310–312, 310–313
Splenic injuries, emergent/urgent laparoscopy and, 294
Square knot, intracorporeal knot-tying and, 149, 150–151, 152
Squirt, 341, 342
Stapling
 in laparoscopic appendectomy, 173–174, 174
 stapled and sutured anastomosis and
 in cholecystojejunostomy, 163–164, 165
 in gastrojejunostomy, 167–168
 in ileocolostomy, 168
Stapling devices, 141
 for thoracoscopy, 330

Stents, 77, 77. *See also* Transjugular intrahepatic portosystemic shunt
  bile duct strictures and, 197–202, *198–201*
    benign strictures and, 202, *202, 203*
    malignant strictures and, 198, 200–202, *201*
  in esophageal cancer. *See* Esophageal cancer, esophageal prostheses in
  intravascular, 324–326, *325*
    indications for, 325
    limitations and complications of, 326
    results with, 326
    technique for, 325–326
  metal
    for biliary cancer, 198, *200, 201,* 201, 208
    self-expanding, 78, *78*
  plastic, for biliary cancer, 201, 208, *209*
Stones, bile duct, 202–203. *See also* Choledochoscopy; Fluoroscopically guided common duct stone retrieval
  endoluminal treatment of, 209–211, *210, 211*
  lithotripsy and, 203
  removal of, 210, *211*
  spilled, 227
Strictures
  of bile duct, 239. *See also* Stents, bile duct strictures and
  dilation of, in esophageal cancer, 79, *79*
  in gastroesophageal reflux disease, 92, 95
Suction, for laparoscopic cholecystectomy, 217
Surface free energy, 45
Surface tension, 45
Surgical machines, robotic, 340–342, *340–343*
Surgical mesh, 49–50
Surgical team, for telescopic surgery, 58
  perivisceral dissection of esophagus and, 84–85
Suture(s)
  absorbable, 48–49
  biomaterials for, 48–49
  for laparoscopic cholecystectomy, 218
  for laparoscopic choledochotomy, 240
  for laparoscopic suturing and tissue approximation, 142–143
  nonabsorbable, 49

  in telescopic surgery, 62
Sutured laparoscopic gastrointestinal anastomosis, 157–170
  basic technique for, 157–161
    bowel occlusion and, 159–160, *160*
    grasping forceps and, 157, *158*
    instrument access and port placement and, 160–161, *160–162*
    needle holders and sutures and, 157–159, *158, 159*
  in cholecystojejunostomy, 161–164
    cholangiography and, 162–163
    conversion to laparotomy and, 164
    patient positioning, port placement, and exposure for, 161–162, *163*
    patient selection for, 161
    postoperative recovery and, 164
    stapled and sutured anastomosis and, 163–164, *165*
  in colocolostomy, 169–170
    bowel mobilization for, 169
    localization of luminal pathologic findings and, 169
    patient position and port placement for, 169
    patient selection for, 169
    proximal control of colon, specimen excision, and extraction in, 169–170
    sutured anastomosis and, 170
  in gastrojejunostomy, 164, 166–168
    patient positioning and port placement for, 164, 166
    patient selection for, 164
    stapled and sutured gastrojejunostomy and, 167–168
    sutured anastomosis and, 166, *167*
  in ileocolostomy, 168
    exposure and control of peritoneal contamination and, 168
    patient position and port placement for, 168
    patient selection for, 168
    stapled and sutured anastomosis and, 168
Suturing. *See also under specific procedures*
  continuous
    intracorporeal, for linear incisions and lacerations, 153–154
    in laparoscopic antireflux surgery, 104, *105*

  interrupted
    intracorporeal, for linear incisions and lacerations, 153
    in laparoscopic antireflux surgery, 103–104, *104*
  laparoscopic. *See* Laparoscopic suturing and tissue approximation
  of gastrointestinal anastomoses; Sutured laparoscopic gastrointestinal anastomosis
Sympathectomy, thoracoscopic, 334, 335
Symptom scoring, in gastroesophageal reflux disease, 96, 96t

Technology, 4
  development of, 339–347
Teflon mesh, 49
Telescope
  for laparoscopic cholecystectomy, 218
  for perivisceral dissection of esophagus, 83, *83*
  for transanal endoscopic microsurgery, 191
Telescopic surgery, 57–65. *See also* Esophageal cancer, perivisceral dissection of esophagus in
  dissection and resection methods in, 59–62
    dissecting tools and, 59–61
    portal placement, exposure, cutting, and securing and, 61–62, *63*
    retracting tools and accessories and, 61, *61*
  equipment for, 57–58
  operating room setup for, 58
  removal methods in, 63–64
    containers for, *63,* 63–64, *64*
    incision extension and conversion to larger ports for, 63
    morcellators for, 64
    site choice for, 64
  single-surgeon technique for, 58–59
  surgical team for, 58
  two-handed, 59
  two-surgeon technique for, 58
Television screens, for laparoscopic cholecystectomy, 216
Thoracoscopy, 329–337
  diagnostic procedures and, 332–333
    chest trauma and, 333
    lung biopsy and, 332
    lymph node and mediastinal mass biopsy and, 333
    pleural effusions and masses and, 332

Thoracoscopy (Cont.):
  pulmonary nodule biopsy and, 332, 332
  equipment for, 329–330, 330
  future applications of, 335
  technique of, 330–332, 331
  therapeutic procedures and, 333–335
    ablation of blebs and pleurodesis for pneumothorax, 333
    decortication and drainage of empyema, 335
    esophageal myotomy, 334–335, 336
    pericardial window and pericardiocentesis, 334
    resection of lung nodules and mediastinal masses, 333–334
    sympathectomy, 334, 335
    transthoracic vagotomy, 334, 334
Through-the-scope technique, 17
Tissue
  detachment from parent organ, in telescopic surgery, 62, 63
  effects of temperature on, 33, 34
  polymeric biomaterials and. See also Biomaterials
    biocompatibility of, 44–45
  removal of
    choice of site for, 64
    in colon and rectal surgery, 180
    in laparoscopic splenectomy, 312, 313
    in telescopic surgery, 63–64
  temperature of, effect of electrical energy on, 33–34, 34
Tissue approximation, laparoscopic. See Laparoscopic suturing and tissue approximation
Tissue handling, for laparoscopic suturing and tissue approximation, 145, 145
Tissue interaction, of lasers. See Laser(s), tissue interaction and
Tissue welding, 346
  with lasers, 31
Titanium surfaces, 53–54
Total internal reflection, 8
Trac-Wright atherectomy catheter, 323–324
Training, for minimally invasive surgery, 5–6
Transanal endoscopic microsurgery (TEM), 191–196
  equipment for, 191–195
  indications for, 191–192
  patient, team, and operating room setting for, 193
  postoperative management and, 195
  preoperative assessment for, 192–193, 193
  preoperative management and anesthesia for, 193
  procedure for, 193–195, 194
  rectopexy, 195–196, 196
  results of, 195
Transanal endoscopic rectopexy (TER), 195–196, 196
Transient lower esophageal sphincter relaxation (TLESR), gastroesophageal reflux disease and, 90
Transjugular intrahepatic portosystemic shunt (TIPS), 269–277, 275t
  history of, 269
  indications for, 270
  technique for, 270, 271–274, 272–274
Trocars. See also under specific procedures
  for laparoscopic cholecystectomy, 218
  for laparoscopic suturing and tissue approximation, 142
Tumor probes, in esophageal cancer. See Esophageal cancer, BICAP tumor probe in

Ulcers
  Barrett's, 93
  gastroesophageal reflux disease and, 92–93
  peptic. See Peptic ulcer disease, laparoscopic treatment of
Ultrasonography, 15–20
  in diagnosis of appendicitis, 171
  Doppler, 16
  endoscopic, 17–19, 19
  endovascular, 316–318, 317
    catheter design and principles for, 316–317
    imaging capabilities of, 317
    potential clinical applications of, 317–318
  hepatic malignancies and, 256
  intracorporeal, laparoscopic, 19–20, 20
  laparoscopic cholecystectomy and, 215, 215
  operative, 16–17
  physics and instrumentation for, 15t, 15–16
Ureters, injury to, preventing, 180
Urgent laparoscopy. See Emergent/urgent laparoscopy

Urinary retention, laparoscopic pelvic lymphadenectomy and, 288

Vagal reflex, gastroesophageal reflux disease and, 90
Vagotomy
  parietal cell, in gastroesophageal reflux disease, 90
  in peptic ulcer disease. See Peptic ulcer disease, laparoscopic treatment of
  transthoracic, thoracoscopic, 334, 334
  truncal, in gastroesophageal reflux disease, 90
Vapor-deposited carbon coatings, 53
Vaporization, electrosurgical, 35
Varices
  gastroesophageal. See Transjugular intrahepatic portosystemic shunt
Vascular embolectomy catheters, for fluoroscopically guided common duct stone retrieval, 233
Veress needle, for laparoscopic cholecystectomy, 218
Vicryl mesh, 50
Videoendoscopy, 13, 330–331
Video magnification, for laparoscopic suturing and tissue approximation, 144
Video tape, of laparoscopic cholecystectomy, 217
Villous adenoma, rectosigmoid, laser therapy in, 134–138, 137t
  outcome of, 136, 136–137, 137
  patient cohort and, 134–136, 135
Virtual reality, 342–345, 343, 344t, 345, 346
  levels of complexity in, 344, 344t
Visual perception, for laparoscopic suturing and tissue approximation, 143–144

Wallstent, 198, 272, 272, 273
Wavelength, for medical use, 26, 26–27
Webs, esophageal, in gastroesophageal reflux disease, 92
Wiggler, 27
Wound abscess, following laparoscopic appendectomy, 175
Wound dressings, biomaterials for, 49

Yttrium aluminum garnet (YAG), 23